Cancer Symptom Science

Measurement, Mechanisms, and Management

Cancer Symptom Science

Measurement, Mechanisms, and Management

Edited by

Charles S. Cleeland

Michael J. Fisch

Adrian J. Dunn

CAMBRIDGE
UNIVERSITY PRESS

CAMBRIDGE UNIVERSITY PRESS
Cambridge, New York, Melbourne, Madrid, Cape Town,
Singapore, São Paulo, Delhi, Dubai, Tokyo, Mexico City

Cambridge University Press
The Edinburgh Building, Cambridge CB2 8RU, UK

Published in the United States of America by Cambridge University Press, New York

www.cambridge.org
Information on this title: www.cambridge.org/9780521869010

First published 2011

Printed in the United Kingdom at the University Press, Cambridge

A catalogue record for this publication is available from the British Library

Library of Congress Cataloguing in Publication data

Cancer symptom science : measurement, mechanisms, and management / [edited by] Charles S. Cleeland, Michael J. Fisch, Adrian Dunn.
p. cm.
ISBN 978-0-521-86901-0 (hardback)
1. Cancer–Pathophysiology. 2. Symptoms. I. Cleeland, Charles S. II. Fisch, Michael J., 1964- III. Dunn, Adrian J.

RC269.C366 2011
616.99′4071–dc22 2010034378

ISBN 978-0-521-86901-0 Hardback

Contents

Section 3: Clinical Perspectives In Symptom Management and Research

Section 4: Symptom Measurement

Section 5: Government and Industry Perspectives

Section 6: Conclusion

Contributors

Sonia Ancoli-Israel, PhD
Department of Psychiatry, University of California San Diego, La Jolla, California, USA

Vickie E. Baracos, PhD
Department of Oncology, University of Alberta, Edmonton, Canada

Jessica A. Boyette-Davis, PhD
Department of Pain Medicine, The University of Texas M. D. Anderson Cancer Center, Houston, Texas, USA

Joanna M. Brell, MD
Community Oncology and Prevention Trials Research Group, National Cancer Institute, Rockville, Maryland, USA

Tristin D. Brisbois Clarkson, PhD
Department of Agricultural Food and Nutritional Science, University of Alberta, Edmonton, Canada

Michael A. Burke, MD
Department of Psychiatry and Behavioral Sciences, Winship Cancer Institute, Emory University School of Medicine, Atlanta, Georgia, USA

David Cella, PhD
Department of Medical Social Sciences, Northwestern University Feinberg Medical School and The Robert H. Lurie Comprehensive Cancer Center of Northwestern University, Chicago, Illinois, USA

Victor T. Chang, MD, FACP
Section of Hematology Oncology, VA New Jersey Health Care System, East Orange, New Jersey, USA; Department of Medicine, UMDNJ-NJMS, New Jersey, USA

Charles S. Cleeland, PhD
Department of Symptom Research, The University of Texas M. D. Anderson Cancer Center, Houston, Texas, USA

Robert Dantzer, PhD, DVM
Integrative Immunology and Behavior Program, Departments of Animal Sciences and Medical Pathology, University of Illinois, Urbana, Illinois, USA

Patrick M. Dougherty, PhD
Department of Pain Medicine, The University of Texas M. D. Anderson Cancer Center, Houston, Texas, USA

Adrian J. Dunn, PhD
Department of Psychology and Pacific Biosciences Research Center, University of Hawaii at Manoa, Honolulu, Hawai'i, USA

Diane L. Fairclough, DrPH
Department of Biostatistics and Informatics, University of Colorado, Denver, Aurora, Colorado, USA

Michael J. Fisch, MD, MPH
Department of General Oncology, The University of Texas M. D. Anderson Cancer Center, Houston, Texas, USA

Perry N. Fuchs, PhD
Departments of Psychology and Biology, Center for the Study of Health and Illness, The University of Texas at Arlington, Arlington, Texas, USA

Sergio A. Giralt, MD
Adult Bone Marrow Transplant Service, Memorial Sioan-Kettering Cancer Center, New York, New York, USA

Luca Imeri, MD
Department of Physiology and Giuseppe Moruzzi Centre for Experimental Sleep Research, University of Milan Medical School, Milan, Italy

Edward F. Jackson, PhD
Department of Imaging Physics, The University of Texas M. D. Anderson Cancer Center, Houston, Texas, USA

Aminah Jatoi, MD
Department of Oncology, Mayo Clinic, Rochester, Minnesota, USA

Juan Miguel Jimenez-Andrade, PhD
Department of Pharmacology, Arizona Cancer Center, University of Arizona, Tucson, Arizona, USA

Valen E. Johnson, PhD
Department of Biostatistics, The University of Texas M. D. Anderson Cancer Center, Houston, Texas, USA

Keith W. Kelley, PhD
Integrative Immunology and Behavior Program, Departments of Animal Sciences and Medical Pathology, University of Illinois, Urbana, Illinois, USA

Nisha Lassi, MD
Department of Medicine, Mayo Clinic, Rochester, Minnesota, USA

Bang-Ning Lee, PhD
Department of Hematopathology, The University of Texas M. D. Anderson Cancer Center, Houston, Texas, USA

Richard T. Lee, MD
Department of General Oncology, The University of Texas M. D. Anderson Cancer Center, Houston, Texas, USA

Lianqi Liu, MD
Department of Psychiatry, University of California San Diego, San Diego, California, USA

Patrick W. Mantyh, PhD, JD
Department of Pharmacology, Arizona Cancer Center, University of Arizona, Tucson, Arizona, USA; Research Service, VA Medical Center, Minneapolis, Minnesota, USA

Mary W. Meagher, PhD
Department of Psychology, College of Liberal Arts, Texas A&M University, College Station, Texas, USA

Tito R. Mendoza, PhD
Department of Symptom Research, The University of Texas M. D. Anderson Cancer Center, Houston, Texas, USA

Christina A. Meyers, PhD
Department of Neuro-Oncology, The University of Texas M. D. Anderson Cancer Center, Houston, Texas, USA

Andrew H. Miller, MD
Department of Psychiatry and Behavioral Sciences, Winship Cancer Institute, Emory University School of Medicine, Atlanta, Georgia, USA

Lesley-Ann Miller, PhD, MS
Department of Drug Use Policy and Pharmacoeconomics, The University of Texas M. D. Anderson Cancer Center, Houston, Texas, USA

Lori M. Minasian, MD
Community Oncology and Prevention Trials Research Group, National Cancer Institute, Rockville, Maryland, USA

Ruchika Mohla, MS
Department of Psychiatry, University of Medicine & Dentistry of New Jersey – New Jersey Medical School, Newark, New Jersey, USA

Ann O'Mara, PhD, RN, FAAN
Community Oncology and Prevention Trials Research Group, National Cancer Institute, Rockville, Maryland, USA

Mark R. Opp, PhD
Department of Anesthesiology and Pain Medicine, University of Washington, Seattle, Washington, USA

T. Dorina Papageorgiou, PhD, MHSc
Department of Neuroscience, Baylor College of Medicine, Houston, Texas, USA

Russell K. Portenoy, MD
Department of Pain Medicine and Palliative Care, Beth Israel Medical Center, New York, New York, USA

Charles L. Raison, MD
Department of Psychiatry and Behavioral Sciences, Winship Cancer Institute, Emory University School of Medicine, Atlanta, Georgia, USA

James M. Reuben, PhD
Department of Hematopathology, The University of Texas M. D. Anderson Cancer Center, Houston, Texas, USA

Jane A. Scott, PhD
Mapi Values, PLC, Macclesfield, Cheshire, UK

Maria Sgambati, MD
Biomedical Consultant, Washington DC, USA

Qiuling Shi, MD, PhD
Department of Symptom Research, The University of Texas M. D. Anderson Cancer Center, Houston, Texas, USA

Allan Siegel, PhD
Department of Neuroscience & Neurology, University of Medicine & Dentistry of New Jersey – New Jersey Medical School, Newark, New Jersey, USA

Ellen Stovall
National Coalition for Cancer Survivorship, Silver Spring, Maryland, USA

Javier O. Valenzuela, PhD, MS
Department of Symptom Research, The University of Texas M. D. Anderson Cancer Center, Houston, Texas, USA

Lynne I. Wagner, PhD
Department of Medical Social Sciences, Northwestern University Feinberg Medical School and The Robert H. Lurie Comprehensive Cancer Center of Northwestern University, Chicago, Illinois, USA

Xin Shelley Wang, MD, MPH
Department of Symptom Research, The University of Texas M. D. Anderson Cancer Center, Houston, Texas, USA

Jane C. Weeks, MD, MSc
Dana Farber Cancer Institute, Harvard Medical School, Boston, Massachusetts, USA

Jeffrey S. Wefel, PhD
Department of Neuro-Oncology, The University of Texas M. D. Anderson Cancer Center, Houston, Texas, USA

Loretta A. Williams, PhD, RN, MSN, BSN
Department of Symptom Research, The University of Texas M. D. Anderson Cancer Center, Houston, Texas, USA

Wendy V. Wismer, PhD
Department of Agricultural Food and Nutritional Science, University of Alberta, Edmonton, Canada

Randall T. Woodruff, BS
Department of Psychiatry, University of Medicine & Dentistry of New Jersey – New Jersey Medical School, Newark, New Jersey, USA

Steven S. Zalcman, PhD
Department of Psychiatry, University of Medicine & Dentistry of New Jersey – New Jersey Medical School, Newark, New Jersey, USA

Haijun Zhang, MD
Department of Pain Medicine, The University of Texas M. D. Anderson Cancer Center, Houston, Texas, USA

Foreword

> ...For the secret of the care of the patient is in caring for the patient.
>
> Francis W. Peabody

Cancer...Symptom...Science. Simply reading the three words grouped together in the title of this book signals that we have indeed entered a new age in the way we will consider how to treat a person diagnosed with cancer. To those of us who have long advocated for integrative, evidence-based cancer care that recognizes, assesses, and then treats the whole person with cancer, this book is a welcome addition to the body of research that finally puts the biology of cancer in line with the real experiences of patients. And perhaps most importantly, this book now substantiates the case to all of us – health professionals, patients, and those who finance health care – for treating them accordingly. As this book so importantly points out, we now know how to measure the severity of symptoms that wreak havoc with a cancer patient's recovery and to examine what is happening biobehaviorally, even though it was not so long ago that this realm of research was relegated to an area of science considered to be "soft" and not easily quantifiable. Today, quality cancer care is ideally based not only on familiar, quantitative "hard" science, but on a marrying of the quantitative with the qualitative – the subjective experiences of people with cancer – to determine the best intervention for any one person or a population of people.

My own experiences with cancer have motivated my support of cancer-related and disability rights causes for more than 40 years, the last 20 of them at the National Coalition for Cancer Survivorship (NCCS). Nearly six years ago, I was invited to speak to a meeting of researchers interested in symptom management that was hosted by Dr. Charles Cleeland at The University of Texas M.D. Anderson Cancer Center. A long-time admirer of Dr. Cleeland's work, I did not hesitate to accept. As I considered how in 20 minutes or less to discuss my organization's strategy for making the treatment of cancer-related symptoms a health care priority for policymakers in Washington DC, I realized that I would have a friendly audience, and that the real challenge would be to ensure we had the evidence base that would allow us to take that message to our lawmakers and to those who determine what is valued in health care today.

My message 22 years ago, when I became an activist for quality cancer care, and my message six years ago, when I spoke to Dr. Cleeland's colleagues, are no different from what I am writing today. The difference is that we now have a contemporary body of evidence that can support the interventions needed to minimize the many domains of distress that often come with a diagnosis of cancer.

My own cancer survivorship began nearly four decades ago when on December 23, 1971, two events got my attention. One was very personal, and the other quite political. On that day, I began treatment for stage IV Hodgkin's lymphoma, and the news programs on television that night began with the announcement that President Richard Nixon had signed into law the National Cancer Act, officially declaring a "war on cancer." On that day, I began my education about how we, as a nation, have made cancer a political issue, and how one individual with cancer, under the best of privileged circumstances, experiences our health care system when dealing with a life-limiting illness.

The 1970s were an era where a diagnosis of some common cancers in children was no longer an immediate death sentence, yet where pain and suffering for adults diagnosed with cancer was not uncommon, where outcomes for most adult cancers was virtually uncertain, and where most of the research on the psychosocial and behavioral aspects of cancer was concerned with whether or not to tell the diagnosis, how to prepare for death, how to manage bereavement, and generally, how to reduce suffering (that overly simplified snapshot of cancer care looks very different today).

When I was diagnosed in 1971, I wanted to take part in a clinical trial that was testing some new combination of anticancer drugs, but I was considered ineligible because I was four weeks postpartum. Instead, I was treated with radiation alone, which at the time was not considered to be curative for my stage and type of disease. The cobalt 60 total nodal irradiation virtually rendered all who received it infertile – an outcome that was not discussed with me prior to my treatment, out of concern on the part of my doctors that I might defer or refuse the treatment. I lived for 12 years without a recurrence, but with lingering short-term and late effects of the radiation treatment, including early-onset menopause, infertility, radiation-induced pericarditis, costochondritis, and cardiac arrhythmia, precipitous deterioration of my lumbar and cervical spine, recurrent bladder inflammations, and a painful and somewhat debilitating chronic condition called avascular necrosis. In 1984, I had a recurrence and was treated with the very chemotherapy regimen that was tested in the 1971 clinical trial, but which left me with painful neuropathy in my feet and hands that persists to this day. That recurrence also left me with a level of apprehension that was only effectively managed with excellent psychotherapy and a short course of medication. In 2007, I was diagnosed with significant coronary vessel and valve damage, concluded to be consequential to radiation exposure, and then bilateral breast cancer, also most likely to be a late effect of prior treatment.

Today, I am thankfully cancer-free, but never will I be free of cancer or its consequences. My desire to be part of a clinical trial in 1971 and the inability to participate has made me an ardent advocate for quality cancer care, with a special respect for the clinical trials process as a way of advancing new therapies for people diagnosed with cancer. I have carried out my work as an advocate over the last two decades working for the National Coalition for Cancer Survivorship. For nearly 25 years, NCCS has been at the forefront of the cancer survivorship movement – a movement that today includes scores of cancer survivor-led information, support, and advocacy organizations. The survivorship movement did not exist prior to the founding of NCCS. The founders included a public health physician, oncology professionals (including oncology nurses and social workers), experts in disability law, insurance reform, psychosocial research, and biomedical research, and cancer survivors who had led peer-support groups in their communities. Together, they created a new language for cancer, beginning with defining the word "survivor" as anyone with a history of cancer – from the moment of diagnosis and for the remainder of life. The founders of NCCS were expansive in their approach to using this new language, by including in their definition of "survivor" a cancer patient's family, friends, and anyone who supports the person with cancer – recognizing the devastating effect this diagnosis has on everyone involved in the life of an individual undergoing cancer treatment.

Nearly all of us diagnosed with cancer will tell you that it affects us on a physical, emotional, social, economic, and spiritual level. With some exceptions, cancer survivors are eager to tell you their stories and all of the health professionals who work with cancer survivors know that learning from their patients' experiences can provide insights into the true nature of illness and how individuals experience it. At NCCS, we know that being an informed and empowered consumer, as well as finding ways to improve the quality of one's life while being treated for cancer, can make a tremendous difference in how well or how poorly an individual adjusts to a diagnosis of cancer. Communicating with others about our hopes and fears as well as about how our family relationships and functioning have been affected by cancer is very important. For many survivors, reaching out to others – whether seeking psychosocial support from individual professionals or participating in support groups in person, over the Internet, and over the telephone – is key, and many have found hope by listening to and sharing with others their own stories of survivorship.

I am a privileged cancer survivor. Through all of my cancer and related health issues, I experienced them under the best circumstances. I have often considered over the last four decades what would have happened if I had not been living in the Washington metropolitan area where access to quality cancer care was so readily available. What if I had not had adequate health insurance coverage or had been underinsured? What if I had not had a supportive employer? What if I had been raised by a family that viewed my cancer diagnosis as a shameful event that put a curse on our household, as some survivors have told me was their experience? What if my spouse had not been able to cope with my difficulties reentering our family life, as so often is the case with less fortunate survivors?

To answer some of these questions as they apply more generally, we turn to the policies and politics of cancer. Those of us whose work is found in cancer-related advocacy have a rich history of involvement that has informed cancer policy. Starting with the grassroots, from 1992 to 1994 NCCS held a series of talks in Town Halls in cities across America to listen and learn from people living in diverse communities about how they were experiencing cancer, with a special interest in how their quality of care and quality of life were having an impact on their daily living. Taking what we learned from these Town Halls, and wanting to bring together many of the community leaders we met in our travels, NCCS assembled the broader cancer community in 1995 by convening the First National Congress on Cancer Survivorship. This three-day Congress was our effort to bring what we had heard from ordinary people to the attention of a broader audience in Washington DC and to work with them to come up with a set of essential elements for quality cancer care. The consensus findings and recommendations from this assembly were published by NCCS in our *Imperatives for Quality Cancer Care.*[1] These Imperatives for the first time defined quality cancer care in a written document, with recommendations that were informed by the patients' perspectives. The Imperatives call for treating the whole person with cancer, with a multidisciplinary team of care providers across the full continuum of care. The National Cancer Institute responded to the recommendations in the Imperatives by establishing the Office of Cancer Survivorship in 1996 and by making one of the authors of the Imperatives, Dr. Julia Rowland, director of this office. Two of the key principles outlined in the Imperatives:

- People with cancer should be provided with a range of benefits by all health care plans, including primary and secondary prevention, early detection, initial treatment, supportive therapies to manage pain, nausea, fatigue and infections, long-term follow-up, psychosocial services, palliative care, hospice care, and bereavement counseling.
- The provision of psychosocial services must be safeguarded and promoted. Persons diagnosed with cancer should receive psychosocial assessments at critical junctures along the continuum of cancer care to determine availability of needed support and their ability to seek information and to advocate on their own behalf.

These principles are part of the best practices used by many oncology professionals today in treating people with cancer. As further evidence in support of these interventions, in 1999 the Institute of Medicine (IOM) researched and published the first in a decade-long series of reports, beginning with *Ensuring Quality Cancer Care*,[2] that cited these principles as integral to the provision of quality cancer care. What cancer survivors experience – the qualitative, anecdotal, day-to-day living with and dying from this disease – does not always find its way into the research, because the dollars to adequately fund it simply haven't been allocated. Subsequent reports issued by the IOM have given us a robust body of additional evidence for how much this research is needed and that we will, in the not too distant future, be able to proudly point out how much the interventions addressed in *Cancer Symptom Science* will truly help people with cancer live better lives and, when the time comes, have better deaths.

Over the years of my survivorship, I have read many beautifully expressed stories of extraordinary people who live their survivorship and their dying with grace and dignity. One story in particular is vividly etched in my memory. It was written in an essay entitled "Under Toad Days" by physician and cancer survivor Elizabeth McKinley.[3]

> After my very last radiation treatment for cancer, I lay on a cold steel table, hairless, half-dressed, and astonished by the tears streaming down my face. I thought I would feel happy about finally reaching the end of treatment, but instead, I was sobbing. At the time, I wasn't sure what emotions I was feeling. Looking back, I think I cried because this body had so bravely made it through 18 months of surgery, chemotherapy, and radiation. Ironically, I also cried because I would not be coming back to that familiar table where I had been comforted and encouraged. Instead of joyous, I felt lonely, abandoned, and terrified. This was the rocky beginning of cancer survivorship for me.
>
> I'm DONE, according to the medical profession. But I don't really FEEL done. I think we survivors are never truly done. We just move from the quantifiable, treatable disease to the immeasurable uncertainty of survivorship. Being in the midst of active treatment means being seen regularly by a nurse or a physician – being truly CARED for. As I got up off that radiation table for the last time and walked away, I found myself alone with a cancer ghost who would not let me forget where I had been or allow me to freely choose where I might be going.

> We cancer survivors are millions strong, and our ranks will continue to grow as improved cancer treatments extend our lives. But because this struggle with uncertainty after treatment is completed is usually a silent battle waged outside of the physician's office, most physicians don't think or talk about it. In my life as a primary care physician before cancer, I certainly did not. Now I believe that we physicians need to talk with our cancer survivors about the unique struggles of survivorship. Oncologists need to focus on preparing us cancer patients for survivorship. That is, they must address the loss experienced by survivors when active treatment is over and they are sent away from a very intense environment. They must help survivors understand the impact of fear and uncertainty on their lives and what might help to reduce these stresses.

For Dr. McKinley and millions of others, some of the questions we have left to explore include, but are not limited to, the following:

- What are the most common short-term and late effects of cancer treatment and who is at risk for developing them?
- Are there ways to evaluate who might be at highest risk for these effects and can they be prevented or minimized?
- What is the best way to follow cancer survivors for late effects of treatment, and to monitor for recurrence in those at highest risk?
- What are the costs of providing this follow-up care?
- Do behavioral or psychosocial interventions reduce physical or other morbidities in these populations?

The book you hold in your hands begins to address some of these questions, combining the work of basic and clinical scientists, whose research can often be neatly quantified and measured, with the work of behavioral scientists, whose research is often based on subjective patient report – all to create this new discipline called symptom research. Here we can learn about the true science of biobehavioral research that takes a deeper dive into our understanding of how we can better manage many of the consequences of a cancer diagnosis. The important work of this interdisciplinary symptom-research community tells the story of thousands of my fellow survivors who have become part of a documented history of cancer survivorship. This work tells the very human stories of the way people with cancer cope with the distressing symptoms – the physiological and psychosocial consequences that people experience as they live with and, sadly, die from cancer. We survivors know how this work can be measured; we know how valuable it is; and we also know that it needs to be valued by those who pay for health care, and by the health professionals who deliver that care.

When I first began to advocate for quality care for people with cancer, a colleague sent me a paper by Dr. Stanley Reiser, published in *JAMA* and titled "The Era of the Patient," in which he wrote about using the experience of illness in shaping the mission of health care.[4] He referenced an article quoting Vaclev Havel's views of the politics of the world. He cited Havel's critique and its similarities to science and medicine's continual evolution and development. Havel wrote:

> Things must once more be given a chance to present themselves as they are, to be perceived in their individuality. We must see the pluralism of the world and not bind it by seeking common denominators or reducing everything to a single common equation. We must try harder to understand than to explain. The way forward is not in the mere construction of universal systemic solutions, to be applied to reality from the outside; it is also in seeking to get to the heart of reality through personal experience.

Over many decades, cancer survivors have discussed their fears and their hopes, their feelings of anxiety and uncertainty, with many in the health professions. They have reported their symptoms to their oncologists, to their nurses, social workers, and others – only too frequently to be undertreated. Thankfully, with the publishing of this book, we have reason to hope that quality care for people with cancer will truly be integrative and leave no patient without proper symptom management throughout their survivorship – from the moment of diagnosis and for the remainder of life – for after all, it is the quality of living that we seek to preserve.

Cancer survivor and author Arthur Frank, in his book *At the Will of the Body: Reflections on Illness*,[5] put it this way:

I am trying, in this third year after cancer, to be a little less afraid. Some days the world seems immensely fearful…and I realize that the only real difference between people is not health or illness, but the way each holds onto a sense of value in life. When I feel I have no time to walk out and watch the sunlight, my recovery has gone too far. A little fear is all right. It is all right to know that in a month I could be lying in a hospital bed asking myself how I spent today. Holding onto that question – how did you spend today? – reminds me to feel and see and hear. When the ordinary becomes frustrating, I have to remember those times when the ordinary was forbidden to me. Now that I am back in the ordinary, I have to retain a sense of wonder at being here.

Ellen Stovall, April 2010

References

1. Clark EJ. *Imperatives for Quality Cancer Care: Access, Advocacy, Action, and Accountability*. Silver Spring MD: National Coalition for Cancer Survivorship, 1996.
2. Hewitt ME, Simone JV, National Cancer Policy Board (US). *Ensuring Quality Cancer Care*. Washington DC: National Academy Press, 1999.
3. McKinley ED. Under Toad days: surviving the uncertainty of cancer recurrence. *Ann Intern Med* **133**(6):479–480, 2000.
4. Reiser SJ. The era of the patient: Using the experience of illness in shaping the missions of health care. *JAMA* **269**(8):1012–1017, 1993.
5. Frank AW. *At the Will of the Body: Reflections on Illness*. Boston: Houghton Mifflin, 1991.

Credits and acknowledgements

This volume would not have been possible without the editorial talents, patience, and downright doggedness of Jeanie F. Woodruff, ELS, of the Department of Symptom Research at The University of Texas M. D. Anderson Cancer Center. In so many ways, it is her book. In addition to her wordcraft, she has been a master of administering doses of reminders, encouragement, advice, and, where appropriate, tweaks of guilt – all for the purpose of getting this book into your hands.

It has taken an extraordinary amount of time for the book to find its way into print. First, cancer symptom science is a developing area of investigation, and the collective knowledge base for the field is dynamic and rapidly evolving. This has led to course corrections along the way. Second, we have engaged a highly heterogeneous group of very busy clinical and laboratory investigators who often had to do some background preparation by learning about complementary research areas before they could make a contribution to this very multidisciplinary book. We thank them for this extra effort. Certainly the editors have learned much in this process, and we hope that the contributors have gained from it as well.

One consequence of this delay is that it potentially detracts from those who got their contributions in on schedule, as both their own and others' research may have moved on to provide information not included in these chapters. The laggards and procrastinators have benefited by having a more up-to-date look at their topic. This problem is easily remedied: a quick literature search by the authors' names should bring you up to date.

We are indebted to the staff of Cambridge University Press for their expertise, professionalism, patience, and encouragement as we embarked on this adventure and worked to bring it to completion. Although we were privileged to collaborate with many Cambridge staffers, we particularly thank Nisha Doshi, Nick Dunton, Chris Miller, Laura Wood, and Betty Fulford for their invaluable assistance throughout this project.

Finally, we would like to note, in memoriam, those of the editors' families who have died of cancer and have suffered the symptoms that this book addresses – Abby, Linda, Joseph, Gus, and Louis Doctor; John Charles Dunn; E. M. and Martha Helen Flake; and Eclas Houston Patterson. Were we able to include the names of all the family members of the contributors to this book who have suffered, and possibly died, from cancer and its effects, this remembrance would likely fill a page.

It is to them, whether known to us by name or not, that we dedicate this work.

Section 1 Chapter 1

Introduction

Introduction to cancer symptom science

Charles S. Cleeland, Michael J. Fisch, and Adrian J. Dunn

More than 11 million people in the United States have a history of cancer, and more than 1.4 million new cases of the disease are diagnosed every year. Due to progress in the prevention and treatment of cancer, approximately 68% of patients now survive for at least 5 years after diagnosis; nonetheless, 18% will die, often after months of painful, progressive illness.[1]

The symptoms experienced by patients with cancer and even cancer survivors are well known to cause significant distress, affect the ability to function, and impair rehabilitation. Whereas many of these symptoms are the result of disease, it is increasingly recognized that pain, neuropathy, fatigue, sleep disturbance, cognitive dysfunction, and affective symptoms can also be caused by the treatments for the cancer. Treatment-related symptoms may persist for weeks, months, or years and may worsen, even when the cancer improves; they can limit vocational activity and inhibit social recovery.

In many cases, cancer can be managed much like other serious chronic diseases – thus extending for many years the need for continued treatment accompanied by the frequent monitoring and managing of treatment-related symptoms. And, as patients survive cancer for increasingly longer periods, persistent residual treatment-related symptoms are becoming more prevalent and pose an increasing barrier to the resumption of predisease functioning. Treatment-related symptoms can directly affect survival if they become so severe that patients abandon potentially curative therapies. Having the ability to control or even prevent such symptoms would be of potential benefit to thousands of cancer patients and survivors.

Symptoms and symptom burden

A symptom is a sensation or perception of change related to health function. Symptoms, such as fatigue, pain, and nausea, may be classified based on their severity and perceived impact on function. A symptom that leads to a diagnosis is called a cardinal symptom. In a medically correct sense, a symptom is a subjective report.

In contrast, a sign – such as elevated blood pressure or abnormal appearance of the retina – is objective evidence of the presence of a disease or disorder. A symptom can thus more simply be defined as any feature that is noticed by the patient, whereas a sign is noticeable by others; it is not necessarily the nature of the sign or symptom that defines it, but who observes it. The same feature may be noticed by both doctor and patient, and so is at once both a sign and a symptom. Some events, such as pain, can only be symptoms. Other indicators, such as a blood cell count measured by a doctor or a laboratory, can only be signs.

Moderate and severe cancer-related symptoms greatly affect a patient's quality of life and ability to function, collectively creating a "symptom burden" upon the patient that can be thought of as the subjective counterpart of the tumor burden caused by the disease. Anyone who has or has had cancer or who treats patients with cancer knows that multiple symptoms clearly coexist and that symptoms may exacerbate the severity of one another (eg, pain is often linked with affective disturbance, sleep problems, difficulties with concentration, and fatigue), yet only recently has serious attention been paid to this fact. And despite broad appreciation for the distress caused by cancer-related symptoms, relatively little is known about how biobehavioral mechanisms may cause or contribute to the emergence of symptoms or symptom clusters (two or more symptoms that co-vary in onset and severity) from cancer or cancer therapy.

The possibility that many symptoms are induced by a common mechanism finds its expression in the characteristics of animal models of sickness behavior, which resemble the expression of symptoms in patients with cancer.[2–5] "Sickness behavior" refers to a constellation of behavioral and physiological

Cancer Symptom Science: Measurement, Mechanisms, and Management, eds. Charles S. Cleeland, Michael J. Fisch, and Adrian J. Dunn.
Published by Cambridge University Press.

responses observed in animals after administration of inflammatory agents or specific proinflammatory cytokines.[6,7] Findings in animals need to be strongly linked to symptom expression in cancer patients, and the study of symptoms in cancer patients needs to inform the development of animal models. If such associations could be established and specific mechanisms be identified, we could manage multiple symptoms via their underlying mechanisms rather than by the use of empirical treatments for individual symptoms, such as stimulants for fatigue or opioids for pain.

A better understanding of symptom mechanisms may bring a melding of treatments directed at tumor burden with those that reduce symptom burden. Ultimately, the goal in the treatment of cancer is to achieve a clinical response that offers the best quality of remission for the longest period.[8] This is especially important for patients with cancer that is currently incurable – where survival time has increased but quality of life is often diminished by aggressive therapy that causes intolerable symptoms. The development of new, targeted therapies represents an opportunity to reduce the burden of typical chemotherapy-induced side effects at the same time that disease control improves. However, these newer agents also bring novel side effects that will need further exploration and management to reduce the symptom burden and functional disturbance of patients who require therapy for malignancy.

The emerging science of symptom research

The emergence of a field of cancer symptom science – the inspiration for the creation of this book – in some ways parallels the types of collaboration that must be developed to gain a scientific understanding of a disease: the biological and behavioral aspects of the disease have to be understood, ways of measuring the prevalence and severity of the disease must be identified, existing treatments have to be tested to determine whether they are effective against the disease, and new treatments must be developed. When a new disease emerges, methods for its prevention and treatment do not yet exist. The research required to understand its biology, its behavioral ramifications, and the best way to treat it is not in place. Investigators must be attracted to the area, disciplines must talk to each other to develop appropriate methods of research, and investigators must be trained and funded. If hypotheses about the genesis of symptoms can be formulated and tested, those that withstand empirical tests should lead to the proposal of novel treatment methods.

The need for new approaches to symptom management in cancer is well recognized. The Institute of Medicine of the National Academy of Sciences lists the control of pain due to cancer as one of the top 20 health care priorities for improving health care.[9] A report of the National Cancer Advisory Board of the Institute of Medicine[10] called for a significant increase in symptom-directed research, noting that the feasibility of symptom-control research has been demonstrated. That report cited a broad range of recent advances, including the growing acceptance of subjective patient reports about symptoms as reasonable measures in the conduct of clinical and laboratory research. New investigational methods present unique opportunities to understand the biology underlying symptom expression and severity. Emerging methods in longitudinal modeling of symptom patterns, genetic screening (genomics), and longitudinal assays of the relationship between symptoms, cytokines, and neurotransmitters (proteomics) should provide information about patient–environment and treatment–environment factors that facilitate or inhibit symptom expression. Functional and molecular imaging methods should help us understand the cortical representation of symptoms and the specific molecules that are associated with cancer-related fatigue, pain, cognitive impairment, and other nonspecific symptoms.

The purpose of this book

The editors are pleased to offer *Cancer Symptom Science* as a resource for those interested in the goal of preventing or reducing the symptom burden of cancer. The overarching aim of this volume is to collect the developing threads of new approaches to understanding cancer-related symptoms and to illustrate how diverse areas of science can share findings that will stimulate novel approaches to symptom management. We offer contributions from component disciplines that are now poised to make major contributions to understanding the biobehavioral basis of symptoms and to test, in both preclinical models and clinical trials, new agents that may have a broad spectrum of effects on multiple symptoms simultaneously. Our chief aspiration in presenting this book is to promote an interdisciplinary research effort that will provide a framework for:

- merging behavioral and biological disciplines to clarify the mechanisms of symptom evolution;
- developing animal models that parallel the behaviors of people with symptoms from cancer or its treatment;
- incorporating new technologies (eg, genetics, protein measurement, and functional and molecular imaging) that have been applied to other biological problems;
- testing potential novel agents for symptom control in both preclinical studies and clinical trials with cancer patients;
- developing new statistical models to integrate longitudinal symptom reports with multiple biological data points obtained during clinical studies; and
- promoting cross-disciplinary discussions that will create interdisciplinary-minded thinkers and expand the investigator base for sustaining this type of research.

Whatever the potential mechanistic basis of symptoms and their management will be, the interdisciplinary approach to understanding symptoms may look very much like a combination of the specific approaches presented in the following chapters.

We are hopeful that the synergy between the various disciplines described in the next chapters will inspire new ways to prevent the development of symptoms and to develop new or enhanced treatment methods for the symptoms of cancer and cancer treatment. The target of all of these efforts is the ultimate improvement in patient functioning, stress level, satisfaction with and willingness to endure therapy, and quality of life, both during and after cancer treatment.

References

1. National Institutes of Health, National Cancer Institute. Surveillance Epidemiology and End Results (SEER) cancer statistics review 1975–2006. Available from: URL: http://seer.cancer.gov/csr/1975_2006/browse_csr.php. Accessed Aug 14, 2009.
2. Cleeland CS, Bennett GJ, Dantzer R, et al. Are the symptoms of cancer and cancer treatment due to a shared biologic mechanism? *Cancer* **97**(11): 2919–2925, 2003.
3. Dantzer R, O'Connor JC, Freund GG, Johnson RW, Kelley KW. From inflammation to sickness and depression: when the immune system subjugates the brain. *Nat Rev Neurosci* **9**(1):46–56, 2008.
4. Lee BN, Dantzer R, Langley KE, et al. A cytokine-based neuroimmunologic mechanism of cancer-related symptoms. *Neuroimmunomodulation* **11**(5):279–292, 2004.
5. Miller AH, Ancoli-Israel S, Bower JE, Capuron L, Irwin MR. Neuroendocrine-immune mechanisms of behavioral comorbidities in patients with cancer. *J Clin Oncol* **26**(6):971–982, 2008.
6. Hart BL. Biological basis of the behavior of sick animals. *Neurosci Biobehav Rev* **12**(2):123–137, 1988.
7. Kent S, Bluthé RM, Kelley KW, Dantzer R. Sickness behavior as a new target for drug development. *Trends Pharmacol Sci* **13**(1):24–28, 1992.
8. Durie BG. New approaches to treatment for multiple myeloma: durable remission and quality of life as primary goals. *Clin Lymphoma Myeloma* **6**(3):181–190, 2005.
9. Patrick DL, Ferketich SL, Frame PS, et al. National Institutes of Health State-of-the-Science Conference statement: symptom management in cancer: pain, depression, and fatigue, July 15–17, 2002. *J Natl Cancer Inst* **95**(15):1110–1117, 2003.
10. Foley KM, Gelband H. *Improving Palliative Care for Cancer*. Washington DC: National Academy Press, 2001.

Section 1 Chapter 2

Introduction

Researching the mechanisms underlying the symptoms of patients with cancer

Adrian J. Dunn

The overarching goals of the science of symptom research are to prevent the development of symptoms and to establish new or enhanced treatment methods for the symptoms of cancer and cancer treatment, which may in turn lead to improvement in patient function, stress level, satisfaction with and willingness to endure therapy, and quality of life both during and after cancer treatment. To design treatments for the symptoms experienced by patients with cancer, it would be extremely useful to know the underlying mechanisms of those symptoms. In many areas of medicine, animal models have proven useful for suggesting underlying mechanisms of diseases and for testing appropriate therapies.

In this chapter we briefly discuss the theories underlying the use of animal models in cancer symptom research. Chapter 3 builds on this foundation with a review of animal research that may be appropriate for modeling the symptoms associated with cancer and its treatment.

The rationale for animal models

Using animal models in research

In principle, animal models can be used to mimic certain disease states, to identify potential underlying mechanisms and to test potential therapies – pharmacological, surgical, or otherwise. The primary rationale for using animal models is that certain experimental procedures are difficult to perform or would be considered unethical to perform in humans. Most often the justification is that the measurement of some important variable is too intrusive to measure in humans, or that a proposed experimental therapy carries unknown risks. In the most common examples, a drug known to affect a metabolic process may be tested in animals for its efficacy and/or to reveal unforeseen, unacceptable, or toxic side effects.

Animal models can have limited validity. For example, a treatment that works in rats may not work in humans in the same way and may induce unforeseen side effects. In general, animal models work best when the method for inducing the model is related to the underlying cause of the disease. This may not be too difficult when the underlying cause of the disease is known or suspected, but may be particularly difficult in the case of affective symptoms, especially symptoms like depression or psychosis. Do we really know that a rat or a mouse can experience depression as humans do? Assuming a rat can become psychotic, how would we recognize the psychosis?

Developing appropriate animal models

The most successful animal models have been developed on the basis of the disease state of interest. For example, in studies of Parkinson's disease, it was learned that the disease was associated with the death of certain neurons in the brain that use the neurotransmitter dopamine. Accordingly, dopamine depletion was induced in experimental animals using the neurotoxin 6-hydroxydopamine to create a model for Parkinson's disease. This resulted in the use of L-DOPA (levodopa), a precursor for dopamine, to ameliorate the depletion of brain dopamine, first in rats and later in humans.

Another example would be the use of methylphenidate (Ritalin®) to treat attention deficit hyperactivity disorder (ADHD) in children. Experiments showed that when rats were treated with the neurotoxin 6-hydroxydopamine, which depletes dopamine in the brain, the rats became hyperactive. This result was considered paradoxical because activity normally is increased by drugs that *stimulate* dopamine release, such as amphetamines. Also paradoxically, the hyperactivity in rats could be reversed by treatment with amphetamines and related drugs.[1] The changes pursuant to 6-hydroxydopamine treatment most likely

Cancer Symptom Science: Measurement, Mechanisms, and Management, eds. Charles S. Cleeland, Michael J. Fisch, and Adrian J. Dunn.

occurred because the numbers of postsynaptic receptors for dopamine were upregulated (sensitized) by the 6-hydroxydopamine treatment in response to the lack of dopamine – the bodily mechanisms presumably attempting to normalize the system. Subsequently, amphetamine-like drugs, such as methylphenidate, were tested in children diagnosed with ADHD to enhance dopaminergic activity. This treatment has proven to be very successful in many patients, although not all patients respond appropriately. The most likely reason that this model was successful is that the neurotoxin-treated rat exhibited changes that resembled those in the human disease.

With respect to animal models, it is important to distinguish between an animal model and an animal test. A *model* is a procedure used to induce a state in the animal that resembles the disease to be studied. A *test*, however, is a procedure that can be used to detect signs or symptoms of the human disease (preferably quantifying them). For example, in the case of depression, most animal models have relied on chronic stress paradigms, because depression is often preceded by a stressful life event. On the other hand, *tests* for depression would include procedures such as the forced-swim test or the tail-suspension test, which have been used in experimental animals to assess depression-like activity or antidepressant efficacy.

Animal models and the mechanisms of cancer symptoms

It has been argued that the most appropriate model for the symptoms experienced by patients with cancer is so-called sickness behavior, which includes hypomotility (lethargy), hyperthermia, hypophagia (anorexia), decreased curiosity (for example, exploring new things), decreased libido, and increased time spent sleeping. "Sickness behavior" is a term coined by Benjamin Hart in a review in which he argued that the behavior of sick animals (and humans) was not just a nonspecific set of symptoms, but was a defensive strategy.[2] He wrote: "The behavior of a sick individual is not a maladaptive and undesirable effect of illness but rather a highly organized strategy that is at times critical to the survival of the individual if it were living in the wild state."

In fact, Hart was not the first to recognize the existence of sickness behavior. Several decades earlier, Hans Selye, then in medical school in Prague, noted that patients displayed certain symptoms that did not appear to reflect the specific aspects of their particular illness. He subsequently wrote: "Just look around and examine sick people. They are all indisposed, they look tired, have no appetite, gradually lose weight, they do not feel like going to work, they prefer to lie down rather than to stand up. Today, we would say they show non-specific manifestations of disease. They all present a syndrome simply indicative of being ill. That is why I baptized this state that so attracted my attention as 'the syndrome of just being sick.'"[3]

Selye and Hart both noted the similarities between sickness behavior and a variety of illnesses, but Hart's concept that sickness behavior was adaptive clearly indicated that whereas nonspecific symptoms did exist, some of the behaviors were indeed adapted to the specific problems presented by the disease. Thus sickness behavior is adaptive in the sense that at least some of the specific behaviors expressed may be specific for the disease. For example, if increasing body temperature would help to fight the disease, the body may invoke a fever, thus inhibiting the reproduction of certain viruses and enhancing the immune system's ability to kill the virus. A good example of the adaptability of sickness behaviors is found in the realm of sexual behavior, which is inhibited in sick females but not in males.[4] A sick female would not be well served by becoming pregnant, because this would place major demands on her body and very likely impair the growth and development of the fetus. On the other hand, males have little to lose, and sexual activity may enable the transmission of the males' genes.

Sickness behavior and inflammatory cytokines

Most or all of the sickness behaviors are induced when humans or animals are infected with viruses or other pathogens. Recently, there has been much focus on cytokines as mediators of sickness behavior, because infections and tissue damage induce a cytokine cascade involving the production of interleukin (IL)-1, IL-6, and tumor necrosis factor (TNF)-α, among others. In patients acutely ill from viral infections, Vollmer-Conna et al.[5] found that circulating concentrations of IL-1β and IL-6 spontaneously released from peripheral blood mononuclear cell cultures were consistently correlated with reported manifestations of a cluster of symptoms reflecting acute sickness behavior, including fever, malaise, pain, fatigue, mood, and poor concentration.

Administration of cytokines to animals has induced a number of physiological and behavioral responses. These include changes in body temperature[6] and activation of certain endocrine systems, most notably the hypothalamic-pituitary-adrenal axis. Behavioral effects can be profound, including decreases in activity, feeding, exploration, and social behavior; increased sleep; and impairment of cognitive behaviors.[7,8] Neurotransmission in the brain is also affected and may underlie the endocrine and behavioral changes.[9] Administration of endotoxin (lipopolysaccharide, LPS) induces the synthesis of IL-1, IL-6, TNF-α, interferon (IFN)-γ, and perhaps other cytokines.

Particular attention has been focused on IL-1, because administration of this cytokine induces sickness behavior in several animal species, as further discussed in Chapter 3. Peripheral administration of IL-1 in animals has been associated with a variety of classic sickness behaviors, including increased sleep[10] and decreases in general activity,[11] feeding,[11,12] exploration of the environment,[13–15] social interactions,[16] and sexual activity.[17] (For reviews of the effects of IL-1 on behavior, see Dantzer et al.,[16] Kent et al.,[18] and Larson and Dunn.[8]) In addition, IL-1 affects memory[19] and motivation.[20]

Cancer symptoms and inflammatory cytokines

The behavioral activity of cytokines raises the possibility that cytokines secreted in cancer patients undergoing therapy may be responsible for some of the adverse neurobehavioral responses these patients experience.

It is well known that symptoms and increases in specific proinflammatory cytokines, primarily IL-1, IL-6, and TNF-α, are produced by both disease and treatment. Recent studies of rheumatoid arthritis, Crohn's disease, and depression have suggested that inflammation plays a central role in the production of multiple symptoms in diseases other than cancer, and that reduction of inflammation by targeted cytokine therapies produces amelioration of pain and other symptoms.[21–23] What is not known is whether these cytokines actually cause the emergence of symptoms and/or symptom clusters, and accordingly, whether modulation of these cytokines could affect the prevalence and severity of symptoms that cancer patients experience. This knowledge would support the development of symptom management strategies based on underlying symptom mechanisms rather than on the use of empiric treatments. (Bisphosphonates for bone pain and erythropoietin for fatigue and anemia are examples of mechanism-based treatments; the use of stimulants for fatigue and opioids for pain are examples of empiric treatments.)

A popular hypothesis is that excess IL-1 is responsible for inducing depressive illness, because depressed patients typically exhibit many sickness behaviors. However, this theory is controversial because, whereas early reports from Maes' laboratory indicated that stimulation of macrophages obtained from depressed patients stimulated with LPS *in vitro* showed increased secretion of IL-1,[24] subsequent studies have not demonstrated consistent increases in circulating concentrations of IL-1 (see Chapter 9).

Conclusion

The mechanisms underlying the production of symptoms in cancer are likely to be rather complex and may well differ among populations of patients; they would almost certainly depend on the organ(s) affected and the nature of the cancer. Animal models of cancer-related and cancer treatment-related symptoms may suggest a direction for future programmatic research into the mechanisms of symptoms. Careful description of cancer-related symptoms and correlation of these symptoms with clinical laboratory data, coupled with both laboratory and clinical research studies, is an important direction for future research. Clinical research needs to be complemented by animal and *in vitro* studies that directly examine cytokine dysregulation caused by cancer and cancer therapies, and agents that attenuate the inflammatory consequences of cancer therapies should be investigated. Such studies could lead to the control and possibly even the prevention of individual or clusters of cytokine-related symptoms.

The next chapter by Zalcman et al. reviews the research that has been performed using animal models that may be appropriate for modeling the symptoms associated with cancer and its treatment. Chapters 4–15 offer paired discussions of animal and clinical research for each of six symptoms commonly experienced by patients with cancer: pain, cognitive impairment, depression and affective impairment, fatigue, appetite loss and cachexia, and sleep disorders.

References

1. Shaywitz BA, Klopper JH, Yager RD, Gordon JW. Paradoxical response to amphetamine in developing rats treated with 6-hydroxydopamine. *Nature* **261**(5556):153–155, 1976.
2. Hart BL. Biological basis of the behavior of sick animals. *Neurosci Biobehav Rev* **12**(2):123–137, 1988.
3. Selye H. *The Stress of My Life: a Scientist's Memoirs,* with a 32-page section of photographs, 2nd ed. New York: Van Nostrand Reinhold, 1979.
4. Yirmiya R, Avitsur R, Donchin O, Cohen E. Interleukin-1 inhibits sexual behavior in female but not in male rats. *Brain Behav Immun* **9**(3):220–233, 1995.
5. Vollmer-Conna U, Fazou C, Cameron B, et al. Production of pro-inflammatory cytokines correlates with the symptoms of acute sickness behaviour in humans. *Psychol Med* **34**(7):1289–1297, 2004.
6. Blatteis CM, Sehic E. Cytokines and fever. *Ann N Y Acad Sci* **840**:608–618, 1998.
7. Dantzer R, Kelley KW. Twenty years of research on cytokine-induced sickness behavior. *Brain Behav Immun* **21**(2):153–160, 2007.
8. Larson SJ, Dunn AJ. Behavioral effects of cytokines. *Brain Behav Immun* **15**(4):371–387, 2001.
9. Dunn AJ. Effects of cytokines and infections on brain neurochemistry. In: Ader R, Felten DL, Cohen N, eds. *Psychoneuroimmunology.* San Diego, CA: Academic Press, 2001:649–686.
10. Krueger JM, Majde JA. Microbial products and cytokines in sleep and fever regulation. *Crit Rev Immunol* **14**(3–4):355–379, 1994.
11. Otterness IG, Seymour PA, Golden HW, Reynolds JA, Daumy GO. The effects of continuous administration of murine interleukin-1 alpha in the rat. *Physiol Behav* **43**(6):797–804, 1988.
12. McCarthy DO, Kluger MJ, Vander AJ. Suppression of food intake during infection: is interleukin-1 involved? *Am J Clin Nutr* **42**(6):1179–1182, 1985.
13. Dunn AJ, Chapman Y, Antoon M. Endotoxin-induced behavioral changes of mice in the multicompartment chamber are distinct from those of interleukin-1. *Neurosci Res Commun* **10**:63–69, 1992.
14. Lacosta S, Merali Z, Anisman H. Influence of interleukin-1beta on exploratory behaviors, plasma ACTH, corticosterone, and central biogenic amines in mice. *Psychopharmacology (Berl)* **137**(4):351–361, 1998.
15. Spadaro F, Dunn AJ. Intracerebroventricular administration of interleukin-1 to mice alters investigation of stimuli in a novel environment. *Brain Behav Immun* **4**(4):308–322, 1990.
16. Dantzer R, Bluthé RM, Castanon N, et al. Cytokine effects on behavior. In: Ader R, Felten DL, Cohen N, eds. *Psychoneuroimmunology*. San Diego, CA: Academic Press, 2001:703–727.
17. Avitsur R, Donchin O, Barak O, Cohen E, Yirmiya R. Behavioral effects of interleukin-1 beta: modulation by gender, estrus cycle, and progesterone. *Brain Behav Immun* **9**(3):234–241, 1995.
18. Kent S, Bluthé RM, Kelley KW, Dantzer R. Sickness behavior as a new target for drug development. *Trends Pharmacol Sci* **13**(1):24–28, 1992.
19. Pugh CR, Fleshner M, Watkins LR, Maier SF, Rudy JW. The immune system and memory consolidation: a role for the cytokine IL-1 beta. *Neurosci Biobehav Rev* **25**(1):29–41, 2001.
20. Larson SJ, Romanoff RL, Dunn AJ, Glowa JR. Effects of interleukin-1beta on food-maintained behavior in the mouse. *Brain Behav Immun* **16**(4):398–410, 2002.
21. Raison CL, Capuron L, Miller AH. Cytokines sing the blues: inflammation and the pathogenesis of depression. *Trends Immunol* **27**(1):24–31, 2006.
22. Stack WA, Mann SD, Roy AJ, et al. Randomised controlled trial of CDP571 antibody to tumour necrosis factor-alpha in Crohn's disease. *Lancet* **349**(9051):521–524, 1997.
23. Taylor PC. Anti-TNFalpha therapy for rheumatoid arthritis: an update. *Intern Med* **42**(1):15–20, 2003.
24. Maes M. Evidence for an immune response in major depression: a review and hypothesis. *Prog Neuropsychopharmacol Biol Psychiatry* **19**(1):11–38, 1995.

Section 1 Chapter 3

Introduction

Cytokines and sickness behavior: a model for cancer symptoms

Steven S. Zalcman, Randall T. Woodruff, Ruchika Mohla, and Allan Siegel

The term "sickness behavior" refers to a series of behavioral and physiological changes that occur after exposure to an inflammatory or infectious agent, or after administration of recombinant proinflammatory cytokines.[1] Symptoms of sickness behavior include social withdrawal, anhedonia, cognitive impairment, anorexia, fever, and other symptoms. Behavioral changes associated with sickness behavior are transient in nature and serve adaptive purposes that help the individual mount an effective immune response.

Considerable attention has focused on the role of centrally acting cytokines in mediating sickness behavior. As might be expected, abnormal increases in cytokines appear to result in psychopathological outcomes. Indeed, sickness behavior and clinical depression (among other psychiatric disturbances) are evident in patients receiving cytokine therapy.[2] Increased proinflammatory cytokine activity has been implicated in the etiology of depression, schizophrenia, and other psychiatric disorders.[3]

Cancer-related symptoms are strikingly similar to the symptoms associated with cytokine-induced sickness behavior.[4] On the basis of this observation and coupled with evidence that behavioral disturbances in patients with cancer may occur coincident with abnormal increases in proinflammatory cytokines,[5] it has been suggested that common cytokine-related signaling pathways underlie sickness-related and cancer-related symptoms.[4,6] In this chapter, we will discuss similarities between cancer-related symptoms and sickness behavior, and we will examine potential common mediators and mechanisms, including proinflammatory cytokines and subsequent interactions with neurotransmitter and molecular signaling pathways.

Cancer-related symptoms

Cancer-related symptoms refer to physical and psychiatric manifestations produced by the disease process or treatment (including chemotherapy, radiotherapy, immunotherapy, and surgical procedures).[7] Cancer-related symptoms may be categorized as physical, cognitive, or affective. Physical symptoms include fatigue, pain, cachexia, gastrointestinal difficulties, and shortness of breath. Cognitive symptoms include memory deficits and impaired concentration. Affective symptoms include depression, irritability, and anxiety.

Symptoms may be directly or secondarily related to the disease process. For example, the pain induced by cancer or its treatment adversely affects a patient's mood and level of activity.[6] Multiple symptoms are typically present and may occur in clusters, such as the often-seen co-occurrence of pain, fatigue, and depression.[8,9] It has been suggested that analyses of symptom clusters can shed light on the extent to which common biological mechanisms underlie given symptoms.[10] However, there are disparities across studies about the extent to which specific symptoms cluster together. This is likely related to differences in the way in which symptoms are categorized, the diagnostic instruments used, and the heterogeneous nature of patient populations.[8] Despite these differences, investigators have observed that symptoms comprising cancer-related clusters are also characteristic of sickness-related behaviors.[4,11] Thus, insight into sickness behavior and the biological mechanisms underlying it could shed important light on mechanisms underlying cancer-related symptoms.

Sickness behavior

A series of alterations in neural and behavioral activity occurs in response to immunological challenge. Neural alterations serve to regulate the ongoing immune response (Figure 3.1).[12] For example, alterations of hypothalamic monoamine activity[12,13] are induced in sites mediating sympathetic outflow to immune organs,[14,15] which, in turn, modulates the

Cancer Symptom Science: Measurement, Mechanisms, and Management, eds. Charles S. Cleeland, Michael J. Fisch, and Adrian J. Dunn.

ongoing response.[16] The behavioral changes, collectively referred to as sickness behavior, help the individual mount an effective immune response.[17]

Animal models of endotoxin and cytokine challenge

Sickness behavior has been studied extensively in animals by the use of endotoxin (lipopolysaccharide, or LPS) challenge and administration of proinflammatory cytokines. LPS, a component of the cell wall of gram-negative bacteria (eg, *Escherichia coli*, *Salmonella*), is released when bacteria are lyzed. In animal models, LPS is injected in purified form to induce a series of immunological, physiological, and behavioral changes that are characteristic of gram-negative bacterial infections. LPS challenge induces macrophage and endothelial cell production and the release of proinflammatory cytokines, notably interleukin (IL)-1, IL-6, IL-8, tumor necrosis factor (TNF)-α, and interferon (IFN)-γ. LPS also induces an increase in proinflammatory cytokine activity in the brain.[18,19] Cytokines in turn stimulate the production of prostaglandins and leukotrienes. This cascade of events results in inflammation, fever, and behavioral alterations. The peripheral and central actions of cytokines released during the individual's response to an infectious or inflammation-inducing agent, among other factors,[20] likely mediate these behavioral changes. Similarly, administration of exogenous cytokines induces signs of sickness behavior.

Symptoms of sickness behavior

A range of behavioral changes, reminiscent of cancer-related symptoms, is induced by LPS challenge. Behavior changes include fatigue, depressive-like activity (including hypoactivity, social withdrawal, and anhedonia), cognitive difficulties, lack of appetite, altered response to predators, and sleep disturbances.[17] Such sickness-related behaviors are adaptive in nature. For example, depressive-like activity decreases metabolic demands that are otherwise taxed by increased immune activity and limits exposure to pathogens and predators, which could result in additional infection. Reduction in food consumption helps to deprive pathogens of nutrients. It should be emphasized that these behavioral changes are transient; persistent changes would be expected to result in psychopathological outcomes.[17]

Cytokines and sickness behavior

There is a striking overlap between cancer-related symptoms and sickness behavior. For example, classic symptoms of sickness behavior, such as fatigue, cognitive impairment, lack of appetite, depression, and pain, are evident in patients with cancer. It has been well established that proinflammatory cytokines induced in the periphery and in the brain during the host response to infection act as important mediators of sickness behavior. In patients with cancer, there is also evidence that symptoms occur coincident with increases in proinflammatory cytokines.[5] For example,

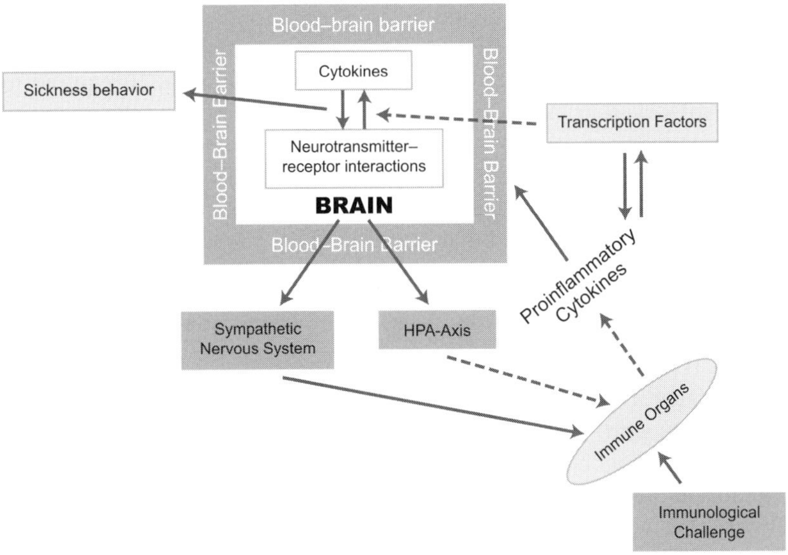

Figure 3.1. A schematic illustration of neuroimmune interactions. Alterations in peripheral and brain cytokine activity occur after immunological challenge. Cytokines may gain entry into the brain via transport across the blood–brain barrier or through circumventricular organs. Cytokines may also activate afferent nerves, which in turn alter brain activity. Immune-to-brain signaling serves to modulate activity in brain regions that mediate sympathetic outflow to immune organs and to stimulate HPA-axis activity. Cytokine–neurotransmitter and molecular interactions also underlie adaptive behavioral changes that are characteristic of sickness behavior.

depressive-like activity and cognitive impairment can be induced by injections of proinflammatory cytokines; similarly, proinflammatory cytokines have been implicated in the etiology of clinical depression (which develops in a subset of cancer patients receiving cytokine therapy), schizophrenia, and other psychiatric disorders.[1,3] In patients with metastatic colorectal cancer, increases in IL-6, TNF-α, and transforming growth factor-α have been shown to be correlated with increased fatigue, loss of appetite, reduced emotional and social functioning, and worsening performance status.[21]

In this section, we discuss representative overlapping behavioral alterations that are characteristic of sickness behavior and cancer-related symptoms, along with suggested underlying cytokine-related mechanisms.

Reduction in food intake

Reduced food consumption is a common consequence of illness, including cancer, and occurs after exposure to a variety of immunological challenges. For example, marked reductions in food consumption are induced in response to LPS challenge.[17,22,23] Administration of proinflammatory cytokines that mediate the host's response to LPS also results in a reduction in food intake.[24–26] Central microinjections of IL-1β into the ventromedial hypothalamus potently reduce food consumption in rats, indicating that this brain region may play a fundamental role in mediating the suppressive effects of IL-1 on feeding.[27] Of further importance, IL-1-induced anorexia activity and reductions in food consumption were prevented by pretreating rats with a serotonin synthesis inhibitor, suggesting that these effects are mediated by alterations in serotonergic mechanisms.[28] However, Swiergiel and Dunn[29] failed to find evidence in ad lib fed mice for the involvement of serotonin in IL-1-induced or LPS-induced reductions in milk intake.

Other cytokines, including IL-6, TNF-α, and IFN, also decrease food consumption, although their effects are less potent and are more dependent upon their route of administration.[1,30–32] Despite the parallels between LPS-induced and IL-1-induced reductions in food intake, combined antagonism of IL-1, IL-6, and TNF-α is required to attenuate the anorectic effects of LPS.[23] It should also be mentioned that treatment with a nonsteroidal anti-inflammatory drug (NSAID), which inhibits cyclooxygenase-2, attenuated body weight loss that was induced in mice treated with concanavalin A and in rats administered carbon tetrachloride.[33] These findings provide support for the use of NSAIDs, which have been employed to treat cachexia in cancer patients.

A significant number of patients with AIDS experience cachexia and reductions in food intake. HIV-related abnormalities are not due to the virus itself because neurons are not infected with the virus. Instead, it is thought that interactions among several factors are involved. These factors include viral elements (notably the HIV-1 viral envelope glycoproteins gp120 and Tat), and the induction of inflammatory cytokines secreted by infiltrating microglia. The latter occurs subsequent to the binding of gp120 to a receptor on glial cells,[34] which in turn stimulates production of various substances, including proinflammatory cytokines (eg, IL-1β). In rats, single intracerebroventricular injections of gp120 result in several neural and behavioral alterations, including reduced intake of standard laboratory chow.[35–39] It has been suggested that IL-1β is the principal mediator of gp120-induced effects, because pretreatment with IL-1 receptor antagonist (IL-1RA) blocks certain gp120-induced reductions in food intake.[35] IL-1RA selectively binds to the IL-1 type I receptor (IL-1RI) with the same affinity as IL-1β; thus, it has been concluded that this effect of gp120 is mediated centrally via IL-1RI. Further, the effects of acute gp120 administration on food intake are not related to alterations of central TNF-α.[36] In contrast with its modulatory effects on food intake, intracerebroventricular microinjections of IL-1RA do not block gp120-induced reductions in open-field activity.

As mentioned above, combined antagonism of proinflammatory cytokines, rather than antagonism of a given proinflammatory cytokine, is required to attenuate LPS-induced anorexia. Thus, the extent to which a given cytokine contributes to reductions in food intake after immune activation varies across different immunological challenges. It may also be concluded that a cytokine may play an important role in mediating the effects of an immunological challenge on food intake without having pronounced effects alone.

Psychiatric abnormalities

Direct evidence linking cytokines with sickness behavior and psychiatric abnormalities derives from studies using immunotherapy to treat various malignancies (and other illnesses).[2] In these studies, patients receive chronic high-dose injections of recombinant IFN-α, IL-2, or both. Sickness behavior is commonly observed during the early stages of therapy. As treatment continues over weeks or months, a subset of patients develop psychiatric disturbances such as depression, anxiety, mania, psychosis, and cognitive impairment. Two overlapping syndromes – depression-specific (disturbances of mood, anxiety, and cognition) and neurovegetative (fatigue, anorexia, psychomotor slowing, and pain) – have been described in patients. Certain patients appear to be at greater risk for developing these symptoms: notably, depression is more likely to develop in patients exhibiting mood and anxiety symptoms before onset of cytokine immunotherapy.[40] Thus, a history of psychiatric abnormalities increases sensitivity to the psychopathological consequences of cytokine administration, suggesting that cytokines modulate activity in brain regions that underlie given psychopathological outcomes.

Depressive-like behavior

Major features of clinical depression that are evident in patients with cancer include feelings of sadness and anhedonia (ie, the inability to experience pleasure). In animal models, food reward (consumption of a palatable substance) has been extensively used to study the effects of events or substances on hedonic behavior. Significant reductions in food reward are evident after LPS challenge[41] and after peripheral or central injections of cytokines involved in the host's response to LPS.[17,25] For example, a single injection of IL-1β reduces consumption of a palatable substance.[42–44] The effects of IL-1β on food reward are independent of its effects on food intake *per se*.[1,45,46] Although consumption of standard laboratory chow and the effort expended for food reward are both reduced by a single injection of IL-1β, the time courses for these effects differ.[25] Moreover, IL-1β-induced decreases in consumption of a palatable substance are maximal in animals that are not food deprived and are most evident as the number of responses per unit of reinforcer (ie, "response cost") increases.[46]

Other inflammatory cytokines (IL-6, TNF-α), which with IL-1β, comprise a "cascade" of cytokines after LPS challenge, also influence hedonic behavior and reward processes. For example, sucrose consumption is significantly reduced in animals infected with an IL-6 adenovector.[31] Moreover, TNF-α modulates the rewarding effects of methamphetamine.[47] Specifically, TNF dose-dependently blocks methamphetamine-induced place preference, indicating that TNF blocks rewarding aspects of drug administration. Additionally, pretreatment with TNF resulted in a decrease in the number of Fos positive cells in the nucleus accumbens core and shell of methamphetamine-treated mice. Because these proinflammatory cytokines induce differential effects on central monoamine activity,[48] including activity in the nucleus accumbens,[49] different cytokine-neurotransmitter interactions may underlie their effects on reward.

Although sickness behavior typically refers to behavioral and physiological changes associated with LPS challenge or proinflammatory cytokine administration, exposure to other immunological challenges also may induce marked alterations in motivational state. For example, it was shown that rates of responding for intracranial self-stimulation elicited from the nucleus accumbens are significantly reduced at the time of the peak antibody response to a T-cell-dependent antigen.[50]

A cytokine involved in this immune response likewise reduces rates of responding in the mesolimbic system. Specifically, IL-2 treatment results in marked decreases in rates of responding for intracranial self-stimulation elicited from the ventral tegmental area.[51,52] Interestingly, IL-2 potently modulates dopamine release and membrane conductance in the mesolimbic system, including the ventral tegmental area and nucleus accumbens.[48,49,53–56] The direction of these effects depends on various factors, including cytokine dose and stressor environment, among others. In addition to modulating dopamine release, IL-2 appears to influence dopamine D_1 and D_2 receptor binding in the frontal cortex and D_2 binding the nucleus accumbens.[57] Moreover, it has been shown that IL-6 and TNF in the nucleus accumbens potently modulate dopamine activity.[47]

Performance deficits in cognitive tasks

Memory loss and distractibility are evident in patients with cancer and patients receiving chronic cytokine (IL-2, IFN) therapy.[40] Animal models have provided further evidence of IL-2-related deficits in attention and performance in cognitive tasks. For example, inappropriate exploration of a novel environment or a novel stimulus is induced after peripheral or central administration of IL-2.[55,58,59] Chronic IL-2 treatment also induces performance deficits in the Morris water maze, suggesting that IL-2 influences spatial memory and neural activity in the hippocampus.[57,60,61] Single injections of IL-2 have no effect on performance; thus, IL-2's effects are related to the chronicity of treatment. This finding is of unique importance because cognitive difficulties observed in patients after cytokine immunotherapy emerge with repeated cytokine injections. That the IL-2 gene is an important factor in development of the hippocampus is evidenced in IL-2 knockout mice, which display hippocampal abnormalities and spatial-memory deficits.[62] Together, these data suggest a parallel between human and animal studies: in humans, IL-2 treatment induces cognitive deficits; in rodent studies, repeated injections of IL-2 induce performance deficits in cognitive tasks.

Alterations in aggressive behavior

Psychological distress has been shown to be associated with hostility in patients with cancer.[63] Increased levels of aggressiveness among patients are associated with cytokines, including IFN-α2b and IL-2, used to treat cancer and other disorders.[40] In a hierarchical cluster analysis of cancer-related symptoms, Cleeland et al.[6] showed that sadness clusters with irritability and distress; McHutchison et al.[64] showed that anger, hostility, and irritability are increased in patients receiving cytokine immunotherapy. However, it is possible that other factors such as infection, drug treatment, and hospitalization may have interacted in generating aggressive reactions.

The linkage between increases in aggressive behavior and increases in cytokine production and immune cell activity has been provided from animal studies. Using the resident-intruder model for the study of aggressive behavior, Stefanski and Ben-Eliyahu[65] found that rats receiving mammary tumor cells one hour into a seven-hour confrontation had increased tumor retention, and that this effect was blocked by a β-adrenergic antagonist. Petitto et al.[66] showed that production of IFN and IL-2 and proliferation of T cells were higher in mice bred for high aggression (based on frequency of attacks after contact) than in mice bred for low aggression. Avitsur et al.,[67] using a paired fighting model to determine the effects of fighting on measures of splenic cell distribution and function, found that six daily sessions resulted in increased levels of monocytes and neutrophils. These investigators also observed a decrease in the percentage of lymphocytes. These effects were likely related to the actions of glucocorticoids because they occurred coincident with a state of glucocorticoid resistance in splenocytes.

Taken together, these studies demonstrate that exposure to an aggressive confrontation can enhance immune cell and cytokine activity; however, the type of confrontation and behavioral response influences the nature of the immunological changes. Thus, it is important to consider that a number of factors affect the cytokine–aggression relationship.

A recent line of research has focused on identifying the modulatory role of cytokines associated with specific neuronal pathways over which aggressive behavior is elicited. Several studies conducted systematic analyses of a particular feline model of aggression called defensive rage behavior, which involves pronounced affective signs such as vocalization, marked pupil dilatation, retraction of the ears, arching of the back, and unsheathing of the claws.[68,69] Moreover, the cat will frequently modify its response by striking at a moving object. This response is ethologically significant in that it occurs under natural conditions when the animal, its territory, or its kittens are threatened by another animal of the same or a different species. Defensive rage behavior is elicited reliably by electrical stimulation of the medial preoptic hypothalamus and by electrical or chemical stimulation of the periaqueductal gray.[68] The primary descending pathway from the medial hypothalamus mediating defensive rage behavior is directed to the periaqueductal gray, which in turn projects back to the medial hypothalamus, completing a reciprocal feedback loop.[68]

In one study, microinjections of IL-1β into the medial hypothalamus potently facilitated defensive rage behavior elicited from the periaqueductal gray.[70] These effects were blocked by pretreatment with either an IL-1 type 1 receptor antagonist (IL-1RA) or with an IL-1 antibody. Pretreatment of the defensive rage site in the hypothalamus with a serotonin receptor (5-HT_2) antagonist blocked the potentiating effects of IL-1. Moreover, immunocytochemical evidence indicated that 5-HT_2 and IL-1 type I receptors in the medial hypothalamus were colocalized, thus providing further support for the linkage of IL-1 and serotonin receptors.[71] IL-1 and serotonin receptors in the periaqueductal gray likewise facilitate defensive rage behavior when elicited from the medial hypothalamus, suggesting that IL-1 receptors in both regions associated with defensive rage behavior mediate similar functions.[72]

Other evidence indicates that IL-2 modulates defensive rage behavior in a somewhat different manner. In contrast with the effects of IL-1 upon defensive rage, microinjections of IL-2 into the medial hypothalamus induced a potent dose-dependent suppression of this form of aggression.[73] This effect was blocked by pretreating the injection site with an antibody against the α-subunit of the IL-2 receptor. Of further importance, a gamma-aminobutyric acid receptor antagonist ($GABA_A$) blocked the suppressive effects of IL-2. The latter effect is consistent with the fact that inhibition of defensive rage is associated with $GABA_A$ receptors in the hypothalamus.[68] In contrast to the findings observed after microinjections of IL-2 into the medial hypothalamus, microinjections of IL-2 into the periaqueductal gray facilitated defensive rage behavior elicited from the medial hypothalamus; the potentiating effects were mediated through a neurokinin-1 receptor mechanism in the periaqueductal gray.[74]

On the basis of these studies, it may be concluded that IL-1 and IL-2 potently modulate a form of aggressive behavior. The facilitation or inhibition of defensive rage behavior is mediated by highly selective cytokine-specific, neurotransmitter-specific, and brain-region-specific mechanisms.[72]

Fatigue

The most common cancer-related symptom is fatigue. Fatigue is a fundamental symptom associated with exposure to infectious agents that stimulate a proinflammatory cytokine cascade. This, along with the fact that fatigue is seen in cancer patients receiving IFN or IL-2 therapy, suggests a mechanistic role for these cytokines. Relatively few animal studies have examined the immune–fatigue relationship; however, inoculation of mice with *Brucella abortus* or *Corynebacterium parvum* has been shown to result in a fairly persistent (approximately two-week) suppression of running.[75,76] In C57Bl/6J mice, this effect is paralleled by elevations in brain IL-1β and TNF-α mRNA. Moreover, IFN has been implicated in the fatigue-inducing effects of polyinosinic polycytidylic acid, a synthetic double-stranded RNA that induces an immune response similar to that associated with viral infection.[76]

Fatigue is also linked with Epstein-Barr virus (EBV). Antibodies to EBV-encoded enzyme antibodies, which are elevated in various disorders linked with EBV, were shown to enhance the ability of human peripheral blood mononuclear cells to produce proinflammatory cytokines and to induce symptoms of sickness behavior *in vivo*.[77]

Molecular mechanisms

Proinflammatory cytokines are capable of inducing various symptoms of sickness behavior. However, certain cancer-related symptoms that are likewise characteristic of sickness behavior are induced by different cytokine-neurotransmitter mechanisms. Lee et al.[4] offered an intriguing unifying hypothesis: that nuclear factor κB (NF-κB), a transcription factor that regulates innate and adaptive immune responses, plays a fundamental role in underlying these behavioral alterations. NF-κB is induced in various types of cancer, immune responses, and stressful events, and it is activated by chemotherapy. Of note, NF-κB is reciprocally linked with cytokines and enzymes involved in inflammation. Thus, Lee et al. hypothesized that NF-κB is a common endpoint that underlies cancer-related and sickness-related symptoms. Support for this hypothesis was provided by Nadjar et al.[78] These investigators showed in rats that brain microinjections of NF-κB essential modulator (NEMO) binding domain peptide, which inhibits NF-κB activation, markedly attenuated IL-1β-induced depressive-like behavior and reductions in food consumption. This treatment also attenuated IL-1-induced variations of c-Fos expression in the hypothalamus and amygdala.

Molecular mechanisms underlying the relationship among cytokines, sickness behavior, and cancer-related symptoms were examined in mice by Wood et al.[41] These investigators examined the behavioral, immunological, and molecular effects of etoposide, a cancer chemotherapy drug that activates p38 MAPK. Etoposide administration resulted in various symptoms of sickness behavior, including decrease in body weight, fever, and reductions in food consumption and running activity. These effects coincided with increases in serum levels of IL-6. The extent to which a given molecular signaling pathway underlies symptoms related to cancer or cancer therapy is yet to be determined. Nonetheless, these studies underscore the need to identify molecular mechanisms and could have important implications in the development of treatments for cancer-related symptoms.

Conclusion

Behavioral changes that are characteristic of sickness behavior are mediated by the individual or combined actions of proinflammatory cytokines via cytokine neurotransmitter receptor and molecular mechanisms. In light of the striking similarity between sickness-related and cancer-related symptoms, it may be suggested that they are mediated by common cytokinergic mechanisms. Support for this suggestion is provided from studies showing that (1) increases in proinflammatory cytokines occur coincident with behavioral disturbances in patients with cancer, and (2) psychopathological outcomes are induced in patients receiving cytokine immunotherapy. To be sure, the precise cytokine, neurochemical, and molecular mechanisms that underlie given symptoms of sickness behavior remain to be fully elucidated. Identification of these mechanisms would provide additional insight into mechanisms underlying given cancer-related symptoms or symptom clusters and would suggest therapeutic interventions.

References

1. Dantzer R, Aubert A, Bluthé RM, et al. Mechanisms of the behavioural effects of cytokines. *Adv Exp Med Biol* **461**:83–105, 1999.
2. Raison CL, Demetrashvili M, Capuron L, Miller AH. Neuropsychiatric adverse effects of interferon-alpha: recognition and management. *CNS Drugs* **19**(2):105–123, 2005.
3. Müller N, Schwarz MJ. Neuroimmune-endocrine crosstalk in schizophrenia and mood disorders. *Expert Rev Neurother* **6**(7):1017–1038, 2006.
4. Lee BN, Dantzer R, Langley KE, et al. A cytokine-based neuroimmunologic mechanism of cancer-related symptoms. *Neuroimmunomodulation* **11**(5):279–292, 2004.
5. Kurzrock R. Cytokine deregulation in cancer. *Biomed Pharmacother* **55**(9–10):543–547, 2001.
6. Cleeland CS, Bennett GJ, Dantzer R, et al. Are the symptoms of cancer and cancer treatment due to a shared biologic mechanism? *Cancer* **97**(11):2919–2925, 2003.
7. Cleeland CS. Cancer-related symptoms. *Semin Radiat Oncol* **10**(3):175–190, 2000.
8. Cleeland CS, Mendoza TR, Wang XS, et al. Assessing symptom distress in cancer patients: the M. D. Anderson Symptom Inventory. *Cancer* **89**(7):1634–1646, 2000.
9. Portenoy RK, Thaler HT, Kornblith AB, et al. Symptom prevalence, characteristics and distress in a cancer population. *Qual Life Res* **3**(3):183–189, 1994.
10. Miaskowski C, Aouizerat BE. Is there a biological basis for the clustering of symptoms? *Semin Oncol Nurs* **23**(2):99–105, 2007.
11. Chen ML, Tseng HC. Symptom clusters in cancer patients. *Support Care Cancer* **14**(8):825–830, 2006.
12. Besedovsky H, del Rey A, Sorkin E, Da Prada M, Burri R, Honegger C. The immune response evokes changes in brain noradrenergic neurons. *Science* **221**(4610):564–566, 1983.
13. Zalcman S, Shanks N, Anisman H. Time-dependent variations of central norepinephrine and dopamine following antigen administration. *Brain Res* **557**(1–2):69–76, 1991.
14. Williams JM, Peterson RG, Shea PA, Schmedtje JF, Bauer DC, Felten DL. Sympathetic innervation of murine thymus and spleen: evidence for a functional link between the nervous and immune systems. *Brain Res Bull* **6**(1):83–94, 1981.
15. Nance DM, Hopkins DA, Bieger D. Re-investigation of the innervation of the thymus gland in mice and rats. *Brain Behav Immun* **1**(2):134–147, 1987.
16. Nance DM, Sanders VM. Autonomic innervation and regulation of the immune system (1987–2007). *Brain Behav Immun* **21**(6):736–745, 2007.
17. Dantzer R. Cytokine-induced sickness behavior: where do we stand? *Brain Behav Immun* **15**(1):7–24, 2001.
18. Layé S, Parnet P, Goujon E, Dantzer R. Peripheral administration of lipopolysaccharide induces the expression of cytokine transcripts in the brain and pituitary of mice. *Brain Res Mol Brain Res* **27**(1):157–162, 1994.
19. Rivest S. Molecular insights on the cerebral innate immune system. *Brain Behav Immun* **17**(1):13–19, 2003.
20. Swiergiel AH, Smagin GN, Johnson LJ, Dunn AJ. The role of cytokines in the behavioral responses to endotoxin and influenza virus infection in mice: effects of acute and chronic administration of the interleukin-1-receptor antagonist (IL-1ra). *Brain Res* **776**(1–2):96–104, 1997.
21. Rich T, Innominato PF, Boerner J, et al. Elevated serum cytokines correlated with altered behavior, serum cortisol rhythm, and dampened 24-hour rest-activity patterns in patients with metastatic colorectal cancer. *Clin Cancer Res* **11**(5):1757–1764, 2005.
22. Dunn AJ. Effects of cytokines and infections on brain neurochemistry. In: Ader R, Felten DL, Cohen N, eds. *Psychoneuroimmunology.* San Diego: Academic Press, 2001:649–686.
23. Yirmiya R. Endotoxin produces a depressive-like episode in rats. *Brain Res* **711**(1–2):163–174, 1996.
24. Asarian L, Langhans W. Current perspectives on behavioural and cellular mechanisms of illness anorexia. *Int Rev Psychiatry* **17**(6):451–459, 2005.

25. Merali Z, Brennan K, Brau P, Anisman H. Dissociating anorexia and anhedonia elicited by interleukin-1beta: antidepressant and gender effects on responding for "free chow" and "earned" sucrose intake. *Psychopharmacology (Berl)* **165**(4):413–418, 2003.

26. Plata-Salamán CR. Cytokines and feeding. *Int J Obes Relat Metab Disord 25(Suppl* **5**):S48–S52, 2001.

27. Kent S, Bret-Dibat JL, Kelley KW, Dantzer R. Mechanisms of sickness-induced decreases in food-motivated behavior. *Neurosci Biobehav Rev* **20**(1):171–175, 1996.

28. Zubareva OE, Krasnova IN, Abdurasulova IN, Bluthé RM, Dantzer R, Klimenko VM. Effects of serotonin synthesis blockade on interleukin-1 beta action in the brain of rats. *Brain Res* **915**(2):244–247, 2001.

29. Swiergiel AH, Dunn AJ. Lack of evidence for a role of serotonin in interleukin-1-induced hypophagia. *Pharmacol Biochem Behav* **65**(3):531–537, 2000.

30. Plata-Salamán CR, Sonti G, Borkoski JP, Wilson CD, French-Mullen JM. Anorexia induced by chronic central administration of cytokines at estimated pathophysiological concentrations. *Physiol Behav* **60**(3):867–875, 1996.

31. Sakić B, Gauldie J, Denburg JA, Szechtman H. Behavioral effects of infection with IL-6 adenovector. *Brain Behav Immun* **15**(1):25–42, 2001.

32. Weingarten HP. Cytokines and food intake: the relevance of the immune system to the student of ingestive behavior. *Neurosci Biobehav Rev* **20**(1): 163–170, 1996.

33. Okamoto T. NSAID zaltoprofen improves the decrease in body weight in rodent sickness behavior models: proposed new applications of NSAIDs (Review). *Int J Mol Med* **9**(4):369–372, 2002.

34. Sharpless NE, O'Brien WA, Verdin E, Kufta CV, Chen IS, Dubois-Dalcq M. Human immunodeficiency virus type 1 tropism for brain microglial cells is determined by a region of the env glycoprotein that also controls macrophage tropism. *J Virol* **66**(4):2588–2593, 1992.

35. Barak O, Weidenfeld J, Goshen I, Ben-Hur T, Taylor AN, Yirmiya R. Intracerebral HIV-1 glycoprotein 120 produces sickness behavior and pituitary-adrenal activation in rats: role of prostaglandins. *Brain Behav Immun* **16**(6):720–735, 2002.

36. Barak O, Goshen I, Ben-Hur T, Weidenfeld J, Taylor AN, Yirmiya R. Involvement of brain cytokines in the neurobehavioral disturbances induced by HIV-1 glycoprotein120. *Brain Res* **933**(2):98–108, 2002.

37. Glowa JR, Panlilio LV, Brenneman DE, Gozes I, Fridkin M, Hill JM. Learning impairment following intracerebral administration of the HIV envelope protein gp120 or a VIP antagonist. *Brain Res* **570** (1–2):49–53, 1992.

38. Opp MR, Rady PL, Hughes TK, Jr., Cadet P, Tyring SK, Smith EM. Human immunodeficiency virus envelope glycoprotein 120 alters sleep and induces cytokine mRNA expression in rats [published errata appear in Am J Physiol 1996 Aug;271(2 Pt 2):section R following table of contents and 1996 Dec;271(6 Pt 3):section R following table of contents]. *Am J Physiol* **270**(5 Pt 2):R963–R970, 1996.

39. Pugh CR, Johnson JD, Martin D, Rudy JW, Maier SF, Watkins LR. Human immunodeficiency virus-1 coat protein gp120 impairs contextual fear conditioning: a potential role in AIDS related learning and memory impairments. *Brain Res* **861**(1):8–15, 2000.

40. Capuron L, Ravaud A, Miller AH, Dantzer R. Baseline mood and psychosocial characteristics of patients developing depressive symptoms during interleukin-2 and/or interferon-alpha cancer therapy. *Brain Behav Immun* **18**(3):205–213, 2004.

41. Wood LJ, Nail LM, Perrin NA, Elsea CR, Fischer A, Druker BJ. The cancer chemotherapy drug etoposide (VP-16) induces proinflammatory cytokine production and sickness behavior-like symptoms in a mouse model of cancer chemotherapy-related symptoms. *Biol Res Nurs* **8**(2):157–169, 2006.

42. Brebner K, Hayley S, Zacharko R, Merali Z, Anisman H. Synergistic effects of interleukin-1beta, interleukin-6, and tumor necrosis factor-alpha: central monoamine, corticosterone, and behavioral variations. *Neuropsychopharmacology* **22**(6):566–580, 2000.

43. Dunn AJ, Swiergiel AH. The reductions in sweetened milk intake induced by interleukin-1 and endotoxin are not prevented by chronic antidepressant treatment. *Neuroimmunomodulation* **9**(3):163–169, 2001.

44. Larson SJ, Romanoff RL, Dunn AJ, Glowa JR. Effects of interleukin-1beta on food-maintained behavior in the mouse. *Brain Behav Immun* **16**(4):398–410, 2002.

45. Kent S, Rodriguez F, Kelley KW, Dantzer R. Reduction in food and water intake induced by microinjection of interleukin-1 beta in the ventromedial hypothalamus of the rat. *Physiol Behav* **56**(5):1031–1036, 1994.

46. Larson SJ, Dunn AJ. Behavioral effects of cytokines. *Brain Behav Immun* **15**(4):371–387, 2001.

47. Nakajima A, Yamada K, Nagai T, et al. Role of tumor necrosis factor-alpha in methamphetamine-induced drug dependence and neurotoxicity. *J Neurosci* **24**(9):2212–2225, 2004.

48. Zalcman S, Green-Johnson JM, Murray L, et al. Cytokine-specific central monoamine alterations induced by interleukin-1, -2 and -6. *Brain Res* **643**(1–2):40–49, 1994.

49. Song C, Merali Z, Anisman H. Variations of nucleus accumbens dopamine and serotonin following

systemic interleukin-1, interleukin-2 or interleukin-6 treatment. *Neuroscience* **88**(3):823–836, 1999.

50. Zacharko RM, Zalcman S, Macneil G, Andrews M, Mendella PD, Anisman H. Differential effects of immunologic challenge on self-stimulation from the nucleus accumbens and the substantia nigra. *Pharmacol Biochem Behav* **58**(4):881–886, 1997.
51. Hebb AL, Zacharko RM, Anisman H. Self-stimulation from the mesencephalon following intraventricular interleukin-2 administration. *Brain Res Bull* **45**(6):549–556, 1998.
52. Miguelez M, Lacasse M, Kentner AC, Rizk I, Fouriezos G, Bielajew C. Short- and long-term effects of interleukin-2 on weight, food intake, and hedonic mechanisms in the rat. *Behav Brain Res* **154**(2): 311–319, 2004.
53. Anisman H, Kokkinidis L, Merali Z. Interleukin-2 decreases accumbal dopamine efflux and responding for rewarding lateral hypothalamic stimulation. *Brain Res* **731**(1–2):1–11, 1996.
54. Lapchak PA. A role for interleukin-2 in the regulation of striatal dopaminergic function. *Neuroreport* **3**(2):165–168, 1992.
55. Petitto JM, McCarthy DB, Rinker CM, Huang Z, Getty T. Modulation of behavioral and neurochemical measures of forebrain dopamine function in mice by species-specific interleukin-2. *J Neuroimmunol* **73**(1–2):183–190, 1997.
56. Ye JH, Tao L, Zalcman SS. Interleukin-2 modulates N-methyl-D-aspartate receptors of native mesolimbic neurons. *Brain Res* **894**(2):241–248, 2001.
57. Hanisch UK, Neuhaus J, Rowe W, et al. Neurotoxic consequences of central long-term administration of interleukin-2 in rats. *Neuroscience* **79**(3):799–818, 1997.
58. Zalcman S, Murray L, Dyck DG, Greenberg AH, Nance DM. Interleukin-2 and -6 induce behavioral-activating effects in mice. *Brain Res* **811**(1–2):111–121, 1998.
59. Nisticò G, De Sarro G. Behavioral and electrocortical spectrum power effects after microinfusion of lymphokines in several areas of the rat brain. *Ann N Y Acad Sci* **621**:119–134, 1991.
60. Araujo DM, Lapchak PA, Collier B, Quirion R. Localization of interleukin-2 immunoreactivity and interleukin-2 receptors in the rat brain: interaction with the cholinergic system. *Brain Res* **498**(2):257–266, 1989.
61. Lacosta S, Merali Z, Anisman H. Influence of acute and repeated interleukin-2 administration on spatial learning, locomotor activity, exploratory behaviors, and anxiety. *Behav Neurosci* **113**(5): 1030–1041, 1999.
62. Petitto JM, McNamara RK, Gendreau PL, Huang Z, Jackson AJ. Impaired learning and memory and altered hippocampal neurodevelopment resulting from interleukin-2 gene deletion. *J Neurosci Res* **56**(4):441–446, 1999.
63. Deimling GT, Kahana B, Bowman KF, Schaefer ML. Cancer survivorship and psychological distress in later life. *Psychooncology* **11**(6):479–494, 2002.
64. McHutchison JG, Gordon SC, Schiff ER, et al. Interferon alfa-2b alone or in combination with ribavirin as initial treatment for chronic hepatitis C. Hepatitis Interventional Therapy Group. *N Engl J Med* **339**(21):1485–1492, 1998.
65. Stefanski V, Ben-Eliyahu S. Social confrontation and tumor metastasis in rats: defeat and beta-adrenergic mechanisms. *Physiol Behav* **60**(1):277–282, 1996.
66. Petitto JM, Lysle DT, Gariepy JL, Lewis MH. Association of genetic differences in social behavior and cellular immune responsiveness: effects of social experience. *Brain Behav Immun* **8**(2):111–122, 1994.
67. Avitsur R, Stark JL, Dhabhar FS, Sheridan JF. Social stress alters splenocyte phenotype and function. *J Neuroimmunol* **132**(1–2):66–71, 2002.
68. Siegel A, Roeling TA, Gregg TR, Kruk MR. Neuropharmacology of brain-stimulation-evoked aggression. *Neurosci Biobehav Rev* **23**(3):359–389, 1999.
69. Siegel A. *The neurobiology of aggression and rage.* Boca Raton: CRC Press, 2005.
70. Hassanain M, Zalcman S, Bhatt S, Siegel A. Interleukin-1 beta in the hypothalamus potentiates feline defensive rage: role of serotonin-2 receptors. *Neuroscience* **120**(1):227–233, 2003.
71. Hassanain M, Bhatt S, Zalcman S, Siegel A. Potentiating role of interleukin-1beta (IL-1beta) and IL-1beta type 1 receptors in the medial hypothalamus in defensive rage behavior in the cat. *Brain Res* **1048**(1–2):1–11, 2005.
72. Zalcman SS, Siegel A. The neurobiology of aggression and rage: role of cytokines. *Brain Behav Immun* **20**(6):507–514, 2006.
73. Bhatt S, Zalcman S, Hassanain M, Siegel A. Cytokine modulation of defensive rage behavior in the cat: role of GABAA and interleukin-2 receptors in the medial hypothalamus. *Neuroscience* **133**(1):17–28, 2005.
74. Bhatt S, Siegel A. Potentiating role of interleukin 2 (IL-2) receptors in the midbrain periaqueductal gray (PAG) upon defensive rage behavior in the cat: role of neurokinin NK(1) receptors. *Behav Brain Res* **167**(2):251–260, 2006.
75. Ottenweller JE, Natelson BH, Gause WC, et al. Mouse running activity is lowered by *Brucella abortus* treatment: a potential model to study chronic fatigue. *Physiol Behav* **63**(5):795–801, 1998.

76. Sheng WS, Hu S, Lamkin A, Peterson PK, Chao CC. Susceptibility to immunologically mediated fatigue in C57BL/6 versus Balb/c mice. *Clin Immunol Immunopathol* **81**(2):161–167, 1996.

77. Glaser R, Padgett DA, Litsky ML, et al. Stress-associated changes in the steady-state expression of latent Epstein-Barr virus: implications for chronic fatigue syndrome and cancer. *Brain Behav Immun* **19**(2):91–103, 2005.

78. Nadjar A, Bluthé RM, May MJ, Dantzer R, Parnet P. Inactivation of the cerebral NFkappaB pathway inhibits interleukin-1beta-induced sickness behavior and c-Fos expression in various brain nuclei. *Neuropsychopharmacology* **30**(8):1492–1499, 2005.

Section 2 Chapter 4

Cancer Symptom Mechanisms and Models: Clinical and Basic Science

The clinical science of cancer pain assessment and management

Victor T. Chang and Russell K. Portenoy

The assessment and management of cancer pain is a complex enterprise. This chapter will describe key elements of assessment and management, critique the emerging supportive evidence base, and discuss the basis for future studies of the underlying science.

Assessing cancer pain

Aspects of clinical practice

The goals of cancer pain assessment include characterization of the pain complaint and integration of information in a manner that leads to inferences about underlying pathophysiology and syndrome recognition. This understanding is the foundation for diverse management strategies that often rely on multiple modalities to relieve pain while minimizing side effects and treatment burden.

Pain measurement

Pain may be evaluated in terms of severity, location, quality, and other aspects. Among the most salient elements is measurement of pain intensity, which may be viewed as the cutting edge of the longstanding effort to develop a scientific foundation to assessment.

The scientific basis of patient ratings of pain intensity began more than half a century ago with the early development of clinical trials methodology for the evaluation of analgesics.[1,2] These studies confirmed that a subjective experience like pain can be validly measured using self-reported rating scales. In the clinical setting, however, the measurement of cancer pain intensity often is beset by practical problems. Some patients are not able to respond with numerical descriptors. Other patients may have an impaired cognitive status or are simply unable to answer questions. This is an area where much work still needs to be done.[3]

Although most patients can provide a pain measurement, the interpretation of these ratings may be a clinical challenge. Although pain measurement yields scores that can be validly manipulated to determine treatment effects, these scores clearly encompass more information. The relevance of pain intensity as a mediator of function and quality of life has been affirmed in large surveys,[4] and the manner in which pain intensity interacts with other symptoms, dimensions of function, and specific quality of life domains are areas of ongoing study.

The complexity of this interpretation of pain intensity scores also is evident in the observed lack of consistency of scoring across patients or times of assessment. Patients with the same disease and similar imaging studies may have markedly different levels of pain. Current trends in research suggest that not only are underlying disease processes important, but psychological mechanisms, genetics, expectations, and the social environment may also affect pain severity.

Severe pain adversely affects all domains of quality of life. The clearest example of the impact it may have is observed in the phenomenon of pain crisis, in which cancer pain crescendos over a number of days into unmanageable pain. An empirical definition of "pain crisis" is a pain severity of eight or greater on a self-reported numerical scale of pain intensity (where 0 = no pain and 10 = worst pain) that is sustained for at least six hours and that escalates over a course of several hours to days.[5] These episodes may precipitate hospital admission and provide a unique opportunity to study severe cancer pain, its management and multiple consequences.[6] Such exacerbations of pain represent an urgent clinical need that underlies the development of cancer pain as a symptom science.

Assessing the mechanisms of cancer pain

A key step to translate the evaluation of cancer pain, including its measurement, into actionable information is the integration of data into inferences about pain mechanisms. An important aspect of this process

Cancer Symptom Science: Measurement, Mechanisms, and Management, eds. Charles S. Cleeland, Michael J. Fisch, and Adrian J. Dunn.

involves interpretation of verbal descriptors about the pain. Patients with pain describe the experience using any of a wide variety of descriptors, such as aching, stabbing, burning, or crampy. These descriptors, once combined with findings on the physical examination and data from imaging studies or other objective tests, can be used by clinicians to make inferences about the underlying mechanisms that are sustaining the pain. Empirically, individual descriptors are not very specific,[7] and the strategy to classify pain by inferred mechanism focuses more on patterns of descriptors.[8]

A mechanism-based approach to cancer pain, and to pain in general, has been a key goal of pain research. Although the complexity of the diverse pathophysiologies that underlie clinical pain makes it likely that simplified systems will continue, the hope is that a diagnosis that contains information about high-probability mechanisms will improve rational diagnosis and treatment. At present, the diagnostic categories are extremely simple and begin with a major distinction between so-called "nociceptive" pain and "neuropathic" pain. Nociceptive pain describes a syndrome in which an inference is made that the pain is predominantly sustained by ongoing activation of a relatively intact nervous system. It usually is divided into "somatic" and "visceral" pain. Neuropathic pain, in contrast, is a label applied to pain syndromes inferred to be sustained by aberrant somatosensory processing in the peripheral or central nervous system. In other words, nociceptive pain is perceived to be directly related to ongoing tissue injury, whereas neuropathic pain is perceived to be related to disease or dysfunction of the nervous system. Although this categorization is simplistic it has become common clinical practice, largely because of the insights it offers into treatment selection.

Somatic nociceptive pain. Somatic pain is related to injury to somatic structures, including skin, bone, joints, or muscle. Cutaneous pain includes pain from masses on the skin, radiation dermatitis, and wounds; stretching pain from edema and ascites; and discomfort from epidermal growth factor receptor (EGFR) inhibitors. Relatively little is known about the specific mechanisms underlying many of these cutaneous pain syndromes.

Bone pain, the most common type of cancer pain, is conventionally considered a form of nociceptive pain. Important examples of bone pain include focal pain from lytic or blastic lesions and pathological fractures. A history of new pain with weight bearing or movement usually initiates an evaluation that includes imaging of bone. An interesting manifestation of bone pain is the flare, an exacerbation of bone pain that can be seen after radiation therapy or after administration of bisphosphonates, hormonal agents in some cancers, or growth factors.[9,10]

In practice, somatic nociceptive pain usually is adequately responsive to nonsteroidal anti-inflammatory drugs (NSAIDs) and opioids.

Visceral nociceptive pain. Patients with visceral pain syndromes include those with obstructed viscera secondary to tumor or injury to mesentery or similar structures. The pain related to some types of obstructed viscera may be poorly localized and crampy; other visceral pains are sharp and well-localized to referral sites. Some visceral syndromes appear to be relatively less responsive to opioids, and treatment often rests on relieving the obstruction or performing a nerve block. Laboratory work in visceral pain is relatively new compared with studies of somatic nociceptive pain, and has been directed primarily at understanding the basis of functional pain syndromes.

Neuropathic pain. Although the best definition of neuropathic pain remains an area of debate,[11] the basic principle is that neuropathic pain is not the result of persistent activation of a physiological system, but rather is the result of aberrant neural processes that generate the perception of pain. Examples exist with lesions at every level of the neuraxis, including painful polyneuropathy (eg, chemotherapy-induced), painful mononeuropathy or plexopathy due to tumor or surgery, painful radiculopathy (eg, from spinal tumor or postherpetic neuralgia), or central pain due to a spinal cord or brain lesion. Descriptors of neuropathic pain often include terms such as shocklike, shooting, stabbing, numb, and tingling. However, the relation of descriptors to underlying mechanisms remains unclear,[12] and descriptors may not be specific for pain etiology in patients with chronic neuropathic pain.[7]

Diagnosing neuropathic pain remains challenging in cancer, both because there are no unique descriptors or physical findings and because syndromes commonly have complex pathology that may lead to multiple pain mechanisms. Neuropathic pain is usually inferred if there is clear injury to a neural structure or if sensory neurological findings are abnormal, irrespective of imaging studies or electrodiagnostic studies (see Chapter 23 on symptom assessment). Screening instruments have been developed and their usefulness for studies in the cancer pain population remains to be see.[13]

Assessing cancer pain syndromes

Another key element in the pain assessment is the identification of a pain syndrome. Syndrome recognition has been a focus of cancer pain research for decades, and numerous syndromes have been defined from a constellation of clinical findings supported by imaging and other data.[14] In practice, recognition of a syndrome may help determine the need for more evaluation, clarify prognosis, and point the way toward preferred treatments.

Cancer pain syndromes comprise those related to the disease itself, those related to oncological treatments, and those unrelated to the tumor or its therapy. As the number of cancer survivors increases, cancer pain syndromes related to treatment of the cancer (for example, chemotherapy-related neuropathic pain syndromes[15] and the aromatase inhibitor musculoskeletal syndrome[16]) are increasing in importance (Table 4.1). As novel molecules are used to target pathways in cancer treatments, the potential for new treatment-related pain syndromes is likely to increase as well.

Table 4.1. Examples of treatment-related pain syndromes

Syndrome	Manifestation
Chemotherapy-related pain syndromes	
Chemotherapy-induced peripheral neuropathy	
Bortezomib	
Epothilones	
Thalidomide	
Oxaliplatin	
Taxanes	
Vinca alkaloids	
Aromatase inhibitor arthralgias	
Procedural pain	
Radiation-related pain syndromes	Plexopathy
	Mucositis
	Dermatitis
Surgery-related pain syndromes	Postthoracotomy pain syndrome
	Postmastectomy pain syndrome
	Postradical neck dissection pain syndrome
	Phantom pain

Evidence base for cancer pain assessment

Reviews suggest that pain assessment instruments are valid and can be used for clinical trials.[17] Many areas for further work have already been mentioned. An NIH review panel recommended more longitudinal studies of cancer pain, pain in special populations (cognitively impaired patients, geriatric and pediatric patients, palliative care patients, cancer survivors, and patients stratified by gender), pain in various cultures, and the relation of pain to other constructs, such as quality of life, symptom clusters, and sleep.[18] These areas would build on the limited existing evidence base, exploring some of the implications of the scientific advances that have been made in cancer pain assessment.

Implications of research

Basic science methodologies

Newly characterized physiological processes include the concepts of peripheral nociceptor activation and sensitization, central sensitization with or without glial activation, and descending inhibition. Work is proceeding rapidly to clarify the neurophysiology and neurochemistry of these mechanisms. Understanding the receptors and channels that subserve nociceptive processing, and the neurochemistry involved at each, will lead to more sophisticated classification of inferred mechanisms for pain. Similarly, understanding the types of perturbations in these systems that may underlie specific types of injury or be associated with specific types of subjective and objective phenomena may allow subclassification of both nociceptive and neuropathic pains. The inflammatory skin and bone pain models (presented in Chapter 5) exemplify this type of modeling. Can the inflammatory model of pain completely describe the genesis of cancer pain? Are there various tumor-specific combinations of chemokines and cytokines that generate pain? New methods for correlating symptoms with laboratory measurements have been described.[19]

Ultimately, it may be possible to proceed from a clinical pain assessment to an inference about a specific process or set of processes underlying the pain. In the future, clinicians may be able to make meaningful guesses that a pain is predominantly related to sodium channel dysfunction, or overexpression of nerve growth factor, or any of many other potential abnormalities that may lower the threshold for persistent pain. If this can be done, the next step would be to determine whether treatments that target a specific mechanism (eg, sodium channel blockers or modulators for pain disorders inferred to be related, at least in part, to sodium channel dysfunction) may be relatively more efficacious than the current approach to treatment selection. This would raise the approach to clinically relevant mechanism-based therapy to the next level of sophistication.

Clinical methodologies

An NIH review panel found that there were more than 100 instruments for assessing pain, and the large number has led to calls for a consensus on what components should be included.[20] A more uniform assessment scheme is needed for comparability across studies.[21]

The problems inherent in capturing subjective assessments from a population that is medically ill are being addressed in various ways. The identification of pain syndromes allows establishment of reasonably homogeneous groups. From the perspective of pain-intensity measurement, work in developing pain ratings from item response theory, described in Chapter 23, has the potential for helping to making pain ratings more consistent and comparable across patients.[22,23] Further, technological approaches to record patient assessment in real time are being developed. This real-time clinical evaluation may be adopted with the concepts of ecological momentary assessment.[24]

Efforts to inform the analysis of subjective clinical information with data that are relatively more objective also have begun. The role of quantitative sensory testing in characterizing neuropathic pain remains to be determined.[25] The development of pain imaging also may help determine which pathways and receptors will be relevant to improved diagnosis or treatment selection. Genomic studies have the potential to help explain individual differences in response to pain stimuli, and susceptibility to pain,[26] an approach that may allow more sophisticated analysis of pain data.

Managing cancer pain

Aspects of clinical practice

Although pain can be well controlled for most patients using opioid-based pharmacotherapy, some patients do not experience significant pain relief and require additional interventions. A variety of approaches should be available, both to improve the results of partially effective systemic drug therapy and to address the needs of the small proportion whose pain is poorly responsive to medication.

Nonpharmacological approaches

Psychological and physical medicine approaches. The importance of psychosocial aspects of cancer pain have long been recognized,[27] and psychological interventions have long been supported in clinical guidelines. These strategies represent an aspect of pain management that until recently had no counterpart in animal models.[28] A wide range of psychological approaches have been developed for management of cancer pain, including supportive-expressive therapy, cognitive behavioral therapy, education, narrative therapy, hypnosis, and other types of psychotherapy.

Physical therapy interventions range from splints to massage, to various modalities such as transcutaneous electrical nerve stimulation, ultrasound, and others. These approaches are reviewed in textbooks of supportive care and palliative medicine. Although these are time-honored approaches, more research is required here.

Disease-modifying approaches

Therapies that are antineoplastic that or otherwise address tumor burden may have analgesic effects. These include radiation therapy, chemotherapy and biological therapies, and surgery.

Radiation therapy. Radiation therapy is a long-accepted means of cancer-pain control. Most of the published research in cancer pain has been devoted to radiation therapy dosing for treatment of bone metastases and epidural spinal cord compression, and for the management of radiation-induced pain syndromes, such as mucositis and dermatitis. For pain specifically, radiation to bone lesions has received the most attention, with evaluation of a wide variety of radiation delivery methods (external beam radiation therapy, brachytherapy, large field radiation, and radioactive nuclides). When pain is addressed with radiation, relief is only partially related to the underlying histology, and onset of pain relief usually occurs before recalcification.[29] The mechanism of pain relief with radiation remains unclear.[30] Improved understanding of the inflammatory mechanisms underlying cancer pain may help generate hypotheses on how radiation therapy leads to pain relief.

The mechanisms underlying radiation-related dermatitis and mucositis are unknown. It is not surprising that successful treatments are few, despite multiple large-scale trials.

Chemotherapy. There is evidence that chemotherapy can improve pain and other aspects of quality of life. The mechanisms by which this occurs are presumably complex. In some cases, pain relief is linked to reduction in tumor burden, but in others, it can occur with only minimal reduction in tumor size as measured by CT scans. With these chemotherapies, mechanisms other than tumor lysis may be important.

Surgery. Examples of surgical interventions for pain relief include neurosurgical interventions for epidural disease, orthopedic interventions for bone metastases, general surgical interventions for relief of obstructed viscera, and amputation. The reporting of postsurgical pain outcomes tends to be limited. Large-scale randomized trials have been uncommon, with a few notable exceptions.[31]

Pain-modifying approaches

Pharmacotherapy. Pharmacological interventions represent the mainstay of cancer pain management. At present, the treatment guidelines that are commonly followed derive from a very large clinical experience gleaned over several decades. With an increasing number of agents and routes, however, the need for a more evidence-based approach has evolved.

A number of problematic areas exist. For example, should a medication be chosen according to pain severity, disease process (syndrome), or inferred pain mechanism(s)? Choosing a medication for a patient with cancer neuropathic pain or breakthrough pain is most problematic, with inferred mechanisms, potential for drug interactions, and comorbidities as leading considerations. It is unknown whether one should start with a combination of an opioid and other analgesics, or with one first and then others added as needed. The role of the NSAIDs continues to evolve with emerging evidence that the toxicity profiles of the cyclooxygenase (COX)-2 inhibitors, including prothrombotic effects and adverse gastrointestinal effects, may increase risk in the medically ill to an extent that has not been appreciated heretofore. Balancing these risks with pain relief in an otherwise refractory pain syndrome in a patient with limited survival is difficult.

One interesting example that illustrates the lack of certainty involving drug selection is the pain from herpetic neuralgia. When this disorder occurs in a patient with metastatic disease, the clinical inclination would be to treat with an opioid first and add one of the adjuvant analgesics used for neuropathic pain, such as gabapentin, next. A recent randomized clinical trial that compared oxycodone to gabapentin found oxycodone superior in providing pain relief[32] and provided a better rationale for this strategy. Nonetheless, it is not the typical approach used when zoster-associated pain occurs in patients who are cured of cancer, or who never had a cancer illness. In these populations, the first-line approach typically is the gabapentanoid. The differences in strategies used for the same condition in related but not identical populations highlight the limitations of the evidence and the clinical reliance on conventional practice patterns.

Opioids remain the mainstay of pharmacology cancer therapy. The cancer pain clinician daily confronts areas of controversy in the use of these drugs. On the basic science level, the discovery of opioid receptors has been followed by the cloning and characterization of the opioid receptor genes and related splice variants. Selection of drug and route and the management of side effects remain important areas of research (Table 4.2).

The use of adjuvant analgesics for neuropathic pain illustrates the rapid growth in the availability and utility of these drugs. Adjuvant analgesics comprise a large number of agents in multiple classes (Table 4.3). The most important drugs are the gabapentinoids and the analgesic antidepressants, of which

Table 4.2. Areas of opioid-related research interest

Opioid equianalgesic dosing
Opioid drug–receptor interactions
Opioid rotation
Opioid toxicity and side effects
Opioid-induced bowel dysfunction
Opioid-induced hyperalgesia
Opioid-induced dysimmune effects
Opioid metabolism and side effects
Pharmacogenomics of opioids
Tolerance
Opioids in special populations (eg, patients with impaired organ function)
Role of methadone, buprenorphine, and new centrally acting dual-mechanism drugs

Table 4.3. Categories of adjuvant analgesics

Purpose	Analgesic
Multiple purposes	Corticosteroids
	Antidepressants
	Alpha-2 adrenergic agents
	Topical drugs
Neuropathic pain	Anticonvulsants
	NMDA receptor antagonists
	Sodium channel blockers
	GABA agonists
	Cannabinoids
Bone pain	Bisphosphonates
	Calcitonin
Pain related to bowel obstruction	Anticholinergic drugs
	Somatostatin analogues

NMDA indicates N-methyl-d-aspartate; GABA, gamma-aminobutyric acid. Readers may wish to examine the list of pain trials at the National Institutes of Health, http://www.clinicaltrials.gov.

the older tricyclic antidepressants and the newer dual reuptake inhibitors such as duloxetine and milnacipran have strong evidence of analgesic efficacy. Many of these drugs are being developed and tested.[33] In addition to the gabapentinoids and the analgesic antidepressants, other classes of adjuvant analgesics that may prove useful in cancer pain management include other anticonvulsants, sodium channel blockers, *N*-methyl-d-aspartate inhibitors, cannabinoids, gamma-aminobutyric acid (GABA) agonists, and alpha-2 adrenergic agonists. Other adjuvant analgesics are used in the context of bone pain (eg, the bisphosphonates) or malignant bowel obstruction (eg, anticholinergic drugs and the somatostatin analogue, octreotide). Although there are very few trials of any of these drugs in cancer pain, extrapolation of their use to medically ill populations provides a variety of strategies that empirically improves outcomes over opioid therapy alone.

Interventional techniques. Interventional approaches include injections, nerve blocks, and implanted devices that may deliver medication or provide neurostimulation. While only 5% to 10% of patients are estimated to require interventional measures for pain control, patients with severe pain are more likely to be seen by palliative care teams or pain specialists and to be evaluated as candidates for these kinds of interventions. Patient selection and the timing of these interventions in the disease course (sooner or later) are important clinical variables. Patients with severe cancer pain that may require invasive approaches are often also terminally ill, and the clinician has to balance the burden of intervention with the necessity of pain relief.[34] Despite their long history of use, the published literature on most interventional approaches is limited.

Intraspinal (so-called neuraxial) infusion may be performed with a variety of techniques, ranging from inserting a percutaneous catheter into the epidural space to implantation of a pump to deliver medication into the cerebrospinal fluid. Multiple medications may be used, including various opioids, local anesthetics, clonindine, ziconotide, and others. The doses that must be delivered are very small given the proximity between the site of delivery and the site of drug action in the spinal cord or adjacent routes, and for this reason it is often possible to provide pain relief with fewer side effects than would be possible with systemically administered drugs.

An extensive literature for neuraxial infusion is mostly related to the post-operative setting. One large randomized study has been done in cancer patients.[35] Study design recommendations for consideration in future trials are presented in Table 4.4.[36] In addition to timing, clinical research questions include when to use combinations of agents, and if so, which ones.

Neurolytic blocks are often considered when conventional pain interventions have been unsuccessful or are causing unacceptable side effects for the patient. The prototype is the neurolytic celiac plexus block for patients with pancreatic cancer, where a recent large randomized controlled trial demonstrated superiority in pain relief compared to sham control.[37]

Evidence base for cancer pain management

Recent reviews of the literature in cancer pain (and other symptom) management have concluded that the quality of studies has been inferior to those done for the treatment of cancer itself. In a 2001 systematic review funded by the Agency for Health Quality Research, a search of Medline, CancerLit and Cochrane Controlled Trials Registry for the period 1966 to December 1998 yielded 19000 titles in English about cancer pain. From this review, 24 epidemiological surveys and 188 randomized clinical trials were identified. The median number of patients enrolled on trials

Table 4.4. Recommendations regarding the cancer pain management evidence base

Recommendations for analgesic trials	Recommendations for spinal epidural trials[a]
Specify presumed underlying pain mechanisms	Clearly define the demographic characteristics of the sample
Include standard error of the pain outcome measures	Use validated scales to measure pain, and describe associated factors
Incorporate double-blind assessment whenever possible to avoid bias in patient-rated outcomes	Specify inferred etiology of the pain
Improve quality of reporting of pain trials	Compare study drug with other analgesics and other routes of administration
Study further the effects of sex, age, genetics, ethnicity, and culture on pain experience, report, and relief	Prospectively assess side effects
Additional features of well-designed analgesic trials include:	Perform power analysis to determine sample size prior to starting a controlled trial
• enrollment of larger numbers of patients for longer observation intervals than have generally been studied	Evaluate neurotoxicity of study drug
• comparisons with active placebo groups, when a placebo arm is ethically appropriate, or a standard treatment if a placebo is unacceptable	List inclusion criteria for patients in terms of prior therapy
• incorporation of washout intervals to avoid drug carryover effects	Describe drug delivery methods
• integration of quality-of-life measurements	Include pharmacokinetic data for trials with prolonged spinal administration
• standardization of methods to assess rest, incident, and breakthrough pain, as well as side effects of treatment	Describe duration of follow-up (several months) to fully define side effects, dropout rates, and technical complications
	Evaluate outcomes

[a]Adapted from Walker et al.[36]

was 70 or less. Heterogeneous reporting of outcomes, pain measurements, and other data precluded all but three meta-analyses. Randomized controlled trials on cancer pain did demonstrate effectiveness for modalities, but constituted only 1% of published trials.[38]

In a follow-up study published in 2004,[39] the same investigators identified 24822 reports and 213 randomized clinical trials. NSAIDs, opioids, selected adjuvant medications, bisphosphonates, radionuclides, external radiation, palliative chemotherapy, and neurolytic celiac plexus block were each deemed efficacious in relieving cancer pain. Patient preferences, the relative efficacy of different routes of drug administration, the side effects of analgesics, and the relation of pain control to quality of life had not been studied comprehensively. The quality of scientific evidence was poor for a variety of reasons. As before, randomized controlled trials of cancer pain control often enrolled few subjects, had low methodological quality, offered little detail about pain characteristics and mechanisms, and involved heterogeneous interventions and outcomes. One particular point was the heterogeneity of outcomes instruments employed: of 218 retrieved trials, there were 125 distinct pain outcomes assessed.

Separate Cochrane database analyses have been reported for radiation for painful bone metastases (CD001793, 2000), radioisotopes for painful bone metastases (CD003347, 2003), bisphosphonates for painful bone metastases (CD002068, 2002), NSAIDs (CD005180, 2005), calcitonin for bone metastasis pain (CD003223, 2006), oral morphine (CD003868, 2007), methadone (CD003971, 2007), prevention of oral mucositis (CD000978, 2007), treatment of oral mucositis (CD001973, 2007), and transcutaneous electrical nerve stimulation (CD006276, 2008). In each case, the reviewers could identify a limited number of studies and could only draw tentative conclusions about the role of bisphosphonates, radioisotopes, calcitonin, and transcutaneous electrical nerve stimulation.

Few other systematic reviews have been reported. In a meta-analysis of radiation trials for bone cancer that compared single and multiple fractions, Chow et al.[40] found a reproducible assessable complete response rate in 30% of patients and an overall response rate of 74%, concluding that single fractions yielded the same amount of pain relief.

For some treatments used in cancer pain, such as neuraxial analgesia,[35] only one or two randomized controlled trials have been conducted and the overall level of evidence is weak. In the case of psychological and complementary treatments, the level of evidence varies with the approach. For example, many case series have been reported for hypnosis,[41] but by modern standards the evidence of effective pain relief from this method is lacking.[42] In contrast, a meta-analysis of randomized clinical trials of cognitive behavioral therapy for patients with breast cancer found cognitive behavioral therapy to be effective for both distress and pain.[43] Ongoing research issues include the relation of depression to pain, the relation of fear to pain and catastrophizing responses, the role of the caregiver and environment in helping patients cope,[44] and the role of narrative medicine.[45] The biological mechanisms that underlie the effectiveness of psychological approaches remain unknown.

Finally, many of the specific treatments used in cancer pain, ranging across disease-modifying therapies, drug therapies, interventional approaches, and other adjunctive techniques, are applied despite a complete lack of evidence or are based on data that cannot simply be extrapolated across the populations studied. A recent evidence-based and expert panel review conducted to develop quality-of-care guidelines for cancer pain found that many randomized clinical trials could not be used because of the difficulty in applying the results to this population of patients. The panel could only recommend that cancer pain should be assessed, and that radiation therapy should be used to manage bone pain and epidural cord compression.[46]

Implications of basic science for cancer pain management

The burgeoning knowledge about pain mechanisms in general (reflected in Chapter 1 and Basbaum and Bushnell[47]) provide a real opportunity for developing new interventions. The increased understanding of nociception and the pathophysiology that may be involved in sustaining painful perceptions promises advances in the development of new classes of analgesics and new ways to sequence and combine analgesics, and the potential for new ways of delivering analgesics and manage clinical phenomena such as tolerance and side effects. However, much of the experimental data comes primarily from laboratory systems and experimental pain paradigms in animal models. The physiology of animals may differ from humans, and animals are unable to rate symptoms and side effects the way patients can. Although the development of animal cancer pain models[48] holds great promise, the applicability of pain findings from animal models requires careful evaluation.[49,50]

The role of analgesics and their metabolites in mediating analgesia and side effects remains an important area, as are interactions between drugs. The emerging field of pharmacogenomics may provide new understanding of analgesic actions and side effects.

Future clinical research directions

A large number of studies have demonstrated that cancer pain is poorly controlled. The reasons for this are many, and may be related to the health care system, the patient, or both. Overcoming the barriers to effective pain management is a subject that is extensively addressed in the literature and that in any event is beyond the scope of this chapter; suffice it to say that patients with cancer will not experience relief from their pain unless they are treated for it. This section describes clinical research approaches that may strengthen the evidence base for improving cancer pain management.

Observational studies

Observational studies do not provide high-quality evidence but are important for a number of reasons. They can evaluate the wide variety of cancer patients and pain syndromes, provide information about treatment safety and tolerability in real-life settings, and assist in generating hypotheses for testing. One approach is to prospectively study large cohorts, an approach employed by an Italian study conducted at 100 different centers using Internet-based methods.[51]

Analytical strategies may increase the information available from nonrandomized patient cohorts.[52] The propensity score is an example of an approach that adjusts for selection bias in observational studies of treatments.[53] A propensity score-based approach was used to assess the potential of nabilone, a cannabinoid analogue, for future analgesic trials.[54] Instrumental variable analysis is an observational method used in econometrics that is finding application in studies of health care delivery where large datasets are available. An instrumental variable can be thought of as an intervening variable in the dataset that acts as a randomizer. The variable has to be related to variations in terms of who gets a particular treatment, but has no effect on the outcome of treatment.[55]

Quality of care approaches in health care services research that examine administration or performance provide a promising approach in motivating and enabling pain interventions.[56] The availability of computerized records containing treatment data, usually for billing purposes, affords an opportunity to examine large datasets as records of health care delivery.

Clinical trials

Clinical trials remain an important source of evidence but have been difficult to do in patients with cancer for a number of reasons. First is the heterogeneity of pain syndromes. For clinical trials to detect effects, the patient population should be as homogeneous as possible. For an adequately powered trial, where the prevalence of any pain syndrome is low, large-scale multicenter studies will be needed. Second, patients with severe cancer pain are likely to be clinically unstable, and the study sample often demonstrates significant attrition over weeks. For US Food and Drug Administration (FDA) registration purposes, this is problematic because longer-term follow-up (three to six months) is required to demonstrate the safety of a proposed medication. Phase III studies may demonstrate efficacy, but their generalizability is unknown.

Nevertheless, an essential and key area in improving the evidence base is more and better clinical trials. A number of new developments in clinical trial methodology do offer the promise of enhancing the feasibility and usefulness of clinical trial data.

Types of clinical trials

Recent interest in comparative effectiveness trials highlights the relative lack of such comparisons for adjuvant analgesics and for combinations. Many trials have compared new analgesic agents against placebo, and these remain the standard for establishing efficacy in selected populations. There is a large gap in the evidence base both for "head to head" comparisons and for establishing effectiveness, ie, the clinical utility of a treatment over time in the population of interest. In this context, there are distinct methodological differences between superiority trials, noninferiority trials, and equivalence trials, as well as the regulatory implications (pertaining to drug approval and labeling) that surround the data collected from these approaches.[57,58] Combinations of modalities, such as psychological and medical approaches, represents another new area in clinical trial design.[59]

Methodological elements

To reduce dropout, run-in periods to identify patients who are more likely to be stable, or other so-called enrichment strategies, may be considered. Another important issue is the severity of the pain at time of treatment. The investigator has to balance the need to control pain with the observation that analgesic effects are more easily detected if the patient has moderate to severe pain at baseline.

The power to detect differences between study groups requires an adequate sample size. Large-scale studies in the treatment of cancer pain have been implemented in the last two decades by the National Cancer Institute cooperative study groups, and by the pharmaceutical industry (see Chapters 20 and 21). A challenge in cancer pain research is the development of large-scale, simple pragmatic trials to answer treatment questions in a generalizable study population. Adaptive trial designs, described in Chapter 25, can add more flexibility and efficiency to trial designs.

Outcomes assessment in cancer clinical trials has been evolving for decades. Assessment of pain intensity and pain relief remains an area for further work.[60] Originally, placebo-controlled studies emphasized patient ratings of pain and pain relief.[61] Attention then turned to clinically significant changes in pain ratings.[39,62] Outcomes have been defined for patients in radiation therapy trials for bone pain.[63] The Initiative on Methods, Measurement, and Pain Assessment in Clinical Trials (IMMPACT) has issued statements developed for patients with chronic pain that may be relevant for studies of patients with cancer pain.[64,65] Of particular relevance are guidelines for evaluation of multiple outcomes.[66] More recent work has come from the field of patient-reported outcomes. Guidelines have been developed for calculating the responsiveness of patient-reported outcomes,[67] and in 2009 the FDA published guidance for the use of patient-reported outcomes in developing labeling claims.[68] New statistical methods have been developed for displaying data from clinical trials.[69]

Clinical trials of analgesic combinations

Analgesic combinations will become more important because of the multiplicity of mechanisms that are likely to be active in cancer pain. Most studies to date have focused on drug combinations in neuraxial infusion[36] and nonmalignant neuropathic pain.[70] One recent study demonstrated that the combination of morphine and gabapentin was superior to morphine alone for patients with noncancer neuropathic pain.[71]

There is great clinical interest in whether lower doses of two drugs can yield greater analgesia with fewer side effects ("synergy"). Even additive analgesia is useful if there are no additional side effects. An isobologram is defined as the combination of two drugs required to yield a given effect, where each drug dose is based on the D50 (or ED50), the dose at which there will be a half-maximal response to the drug. For two drugs with a constant relative potency, interactions can have additive effects, synergistic additive effects, or antagonistic effects.[72] Studies have demonstrated that, when the relative potency between drugs is not constant, or full and partial agonists are combined, nonlinear isoboles occur, which can confuse the assessment of synergistic and antagonistic interactions.[73] Further, prior knowledge of dose–response curves and substantial patient sample sizes are needed and this has led to questions about the practical applicability of the isobologram model to studies of patients with neuropathic pain.[74]

Response surface modeling has been proposed as a way to capture these interactions with smaller numbers of patients. The advantage of a response surface modeling approach is the ability to study higher numbers of agents given concurrently, and to study a wider range of doses. Drugs that are agonists at one dose level may become partial agonists or even antagonists at other doses.[75] The development of rapid optimization schemes that minimize the number of patients needed for these studies should increase the popularity of this research approach.[76] Other important concepts include response free models and the factorial design.

Translational approaches

Translational studies historically have focused on moving compounds that have proved to be antinociceptive in animal models into clinical trials. New approaches may focus on pharmacogenomic correlates, genomic correlates, pain-related gene families, or inflammatory markers as biological correlates of pain or as predictors of therapeutic response. These strategies may enable testing of hypothesized mechanisms underlying cancer pain, or potentially identify variables that can be used clinically to increase the likelihood of a favorable response to a treatment.[77]

Conclusion

A 1956 paper on cancer pain[78] outlined the anatomical causes of pain and therapeutic approaches directed at the disease and its complications. It then summarized modification of pain pathways (neurolytic blocks and neurosurgical interruption of pathways), modification of pain perception through the use of analgesics (opioids, antipyretics, and other agents), and psychotherapeutic approaches. Our understanding of pain mechanisms, modes of treatment effects, and the disease itself has increased dramatically since then, but the fundamental questions have not changed significantly. Even so, we are in an era of refining the evidence that will guide the assessment and management of cancer pain in the future. Readers are referred to the 2009 International Association for the Study of Pain (IASP) conference on cancer pain[79] for new updates in these and other areas.

Dedication

This chapter is dedicated to Dr. Raymond Houde and Dr. Mitchell Max.

References

1. Beecher HK. The measurement of pain; prototype for the quantitative study of subjective responses. *Pharmacol Rev* **9**(1):59–209, 1957.
2. Houde RW. Methods for measuring clinical pain in humans. *Acta Anaesthesiol Scand Suppl* **74**:25–29, 1982.
3. Buffum MD, Hutt E, Chang VT, Craine MH, Snow AL. Cognitive impairment and pain management: review of issues and challenges. *J Rehabil Res Dev* **44**(2):315–330, 2007.
4. Serlin RC, Mendoza TR, Nakamura Y, Edwards KR, Cleeland CS. When is cancer pain mild, moderate or severe? Grading pain severity by its interference with function. *Pain* **61**(2):277–284, 1995.
5. Hagen NA, Elwood T, Ernst S. Cancer pain emergencies: a protocol for management. *J Pain Symptom Manage* **14**(1):45–50, 1997.
6. Moryl N, Coyle N, Foley KM. Managing an acute pain crisis in a patient with advanced cancer: "this is as much of a crisis as a code". *JAMA* **299**(12):1457–1467, 2008.

7. Rasmussen PV, Sindrup SH, Jensen TS, Bach FW. Symptoms and signs in patients with suspected neuropathic pain. *Pain* **110**(1–2):461–469, 2004.
8. Dworkin RH, Jensen MP, Gammaitoni AR, Olaleye DO, Galer BS. Symptom profiles differ in patients with neuropathic versus non-neuropathic pain. *J Pain* **8**(2):118–126, 2007.
9. Ingham J, Seidman A, Yao TJ, Lepore J, Portenoy R. An exploratory study of frequent pain measurement in a cancer clinical trial. *Qual Life Res* **5**(5):503–507, 1996.
10. Loblaw DA, Wu JS, Kirkbride P, et al. Pain flare in patients with bone metastases after palliative radiotherapy: a nested randomized control trial. *Support Care Cancer* **15**(4):451–455, 2007.
11. Treede RD, Jensen TS, Campbell JN, et al. Neuropathic pain: redefinition and a grading system for clinical and research purposes. *Neurology* **70**(18):1630–1635, 2008.
12. Finnerup NB, Jensen TS. Mechanisms of disease: mechanism-based classification of neuropathic pain: a critical analysis. *Nat Clin Pract Neurol* **2**(2):107–115, 2006.
13. Bennett MI, Attal N, Backonja MM, et al. Using screening tools to identify neuropathic pain. *Pain* **127**(3):199–203, 2007.
14. Foley KM. Acute and chronic pain syndromes. In: Doyle D, Hanks G, Cherny NI, Calman K, eds. *Oxford Textbook of Palliative Medicine.* New York: Oxford University Press, 2004:298–316.
15. Windebank AJ, Grisold W. Chemotherapy-induced neuropathy. *J Peripher Nerv Syst* **13**(1):27–46, 2008.
16. Henry NL, Giles JT, Ang D, et al. Prospective characterization of musculoskeletal symptoms in early stage breast cancer patients treated with aromatase inhibitors. *Breast Cancer Res Treat* **111**(2):365–372, 2008.
17. Jensen MP. The validity and reliability of pain measures in adults with cancer. *J Pain* **4**(1):2–21, 2003.
18. Patrick DL, Ferketich SL, Frame PS, et al. National Institutes of Health State-of-the-Science Conference statement: symptom management in cancer: pain, depression, and fatigue, July 15–17, 2002. *J Natl Cancer Inst* **95**(15):1110–1117, 2003.
19. Fairclough DL, Wang XS. Understanding the correlations between biologic and symptom measures over time. In: Lenderking WR, Revicki DA, eds. *Advancing Health Outcomes Research Methods and Clinical Applications.* McLean, VA: Degnon Associates, 2005:177–190.
20. Hjermstad MJ, Gibbins J, Haugen DF, Caraceni A, Loge JH, Kaasa S. Pain assessment tools in palliative care: an urgent need for consensus. *Palliat Med* **22**(8):895–903, 2008.
21. Knudsen AK, Aass N, Fainsinger R, et al. Classification of pain in cancer patients: a systematic literature review. *Palliat Med* **23**(4):295–308, 2009.
22. Lai JS, Dineen K, Reeve BB, et al. An item response theory-based pain item bank can enhance measurement precision. *J Pain Symptom Manage* **30**(3):278–288, 2005.
23. Patient-Reported Outcomes Measurement Information System. Welcome to PROMIS. Available from: URL: http://www.nihpromis.org. Accessed Oct 30, 2009.
24. Gendreau M, Hufford MR, Stone AA. Measuring clinical pain in chronic widespread pain: selected methodological issues. *Best Pract Res Clin Rheumatol* **17**(4):575–592, 2003.
25. Hansson P, Backonja M, Bouhassira D. Usefulness and limitations of quantitative sensory testing: clinical and research application in neuropathic pain states. *Pain* **129**(3):256–259, 2007.
26. Mogil JS, Max MB. The genetics of pain. In: McMahon SB, Koltzenburg M, eds. *Wall and Melzack's Textbook of Pain.* Philadelphia: Elsevier/Churchill Livingstone, 2006:159–174.
27. Zaza C, Baine N. Cancer pain and psychosocial factors: a critical review of the literature. *J Pain Symptom Manage* **24**(5):526–542, 2002.
28. Langford DJ, Crager SE, Shehzad Z, et al. Social modulation of pain as evidence for empathy in mice. *Science* **312**(5782):1967–1970, 2006.
29. Arcangeli G, Giovinazzo G, Saracino B, et al. Radiation therapy in the management of symptomatic bone metastases: the effect of total dose and histology on pain relief and response duration. *Int J Radiat Oncol Biol Phys* **42**(5):1119–1126, 1998.
30. Delaney A, Fleetwood-Walker SM, Colvin LA, Fallon M. Translational medicine: cancer pain mechanisms and management. *Br J Anaesth* **101**(1):87–94, 2008.
31. Patchell RA, Tibbs PA, Regine WF, et al. Direct decompressive surgical resection in the treatment of spinal cord compression caused by metastatic cancer: a randomised trial. *Lancet* **366**(9486):643–648, 2005.
32. Dworkin RH, Barbano RL, Tyring SK, et al. A randomized, placebo-controlled trial of oxycodone and of gabapentin for acute pain in herpes zoster. *Pain* **142**(3):209–217, 2009.
33. Gilron I, Coderre TJ. Emerging drugs in neuropathic pain. *Expert Opin Emerg Drugs* **12**(1):113–126, 2007.
34. Exner HJ, Peters J, Eikermann M. Epidural analgesia at end of life: facing empirical contraindications. *Anesth Analg* **97**(6):1740–1742, 2003.
35. Smith TJ, Staats PS, Deer T, et al. Randomized clinical trial of an implantable drug delivery system compared

with comprehensive medical management for refractory cancer pain: impact on pain, drug-related toxicity, and survival. *J Clin Oncol* **20**(19):4040–4049, 2002.

36. Walker SM, Goudas LC, Cousins MJ, Carr DB. Combination spinal analgesic chemotherapy: a systematic review. *Anesth Analg* **95**(3):674–715, 2002.
37. Wong GY, Schroeder DR, Carns PE, et al. Effect of neurolytic celiac plexus block on pain relief, quality of life, and survival in patients with unresectable pancreatic cancer: a randomized controlled trial. *JAMA* **291**(9):1092–1099, 2004.
38. Goudas L, Carr DB, Bloch R, et al. *Evidence Report/Technology Assessment No. 35: Management of Cancer Pain*. Rockville MD: Agency for Healthcare Research and Quality, 2001. AHRQ publication 02–E002.
39. Carr DB, Goudas LC, Balk EM, Bloch R, Ioannidis JP, Lau J. Evidence report on the treatment of pain in cancer patients. *J Natl Cancer Inst Monogr* **32**:23–31, 2004.
40. Chow E, Harris K, Fan G, Tsao M, Sze WM. Palliative radiotherapy trials for bone metastases: a systematic review. *J Clin Oncol* **25**(11):1423–1436, 2007.
41. Erickson MH. Hypnosis in painful terminal illness. *J Ark Med Soc* **56**(2):67–71, 1959.
42. Rajasekaran M, Edmonds PM, Higginson IL. Systematic review of hypnotherapy for treating symptoms in terminally ill adult cancer patients. *Palliat Med* **19**(5):418–426, 2005.
43. Tatrow K, Montgomery GH. Cognitive behavioral therapy techniques for distress and pain in breast cancer patients: a meta-analysis. *J Behav Med* **29**(1):17–27, 2006.
44. Keefe FJ, Abernethy AP, Campbell C. Psychological approaches to understanding and treating disease-related pain. *Annu Rev Psychol* **56**:601–630, 2005.
45. Carr DB, Loeser JD, Morris DB. *Narrative, Pain, and Suffering*. Seattle WA: IASP Press, 2005. Progress in Pain Research and Management; vol. 34.
46. Dy SM, Asch SM, Naeim A, Sanati H, Walling A, Lorenz KA. Evidence-based standards for cancer pain management. *J Clin Oncol* **26**(23):3879–3885, 2008.
47. Basbaum AI, Bushnell MC. *Science of Pain*. Oxford: Elsevier /Academic Press, 2009.
48. Pacharinsak C, Beitz A. Animal models of cancer pain. *Comp Med* **58**(3):220–233, 2008.
49. Basbaum AI. The future of pain therapy: something old, something new, something borrowed, and something blue. In: Merskey H, Loeser JD, Dubner R, eds. *The Paths of Pain, 1975–2005*. Seattle WA: IASP Press, 2005:513–532.
50. Rice AS, Cimino-Brown D, Eisenach JC, et al. Animal models and the prediction of efficacy in clinical trials of analgesic drugs: a critical appraisal and call for uniform reporting standards. *Pain* **139**(2):243–247, 2008.
51. Apolone G, Corli O, Caraceni A, et al. Pattern and quality of care of cancer pain management: results from the Cancer Pain Outcome Research Study Group. *Br J Cancer* **100**(10):1566–1574, 2009.
52. Klungel OH, Martens EP, Psaty BM, et al. Methods to assess intended effects of drug treatment in observational studies are reviewed. *J Clin Epidemiol* **57**(12):1223–1231, 2004.
53. D'Agostino RB, Jr. Propensity score methods for bias reduction in the comparison of a treatment to a non-randomized control group. *Stat Med* **17**(19):2265–2281, 1998.
54. Maida V, Ennis M, Irani S, Corbo M, Dolzhykov M. Adjunctive nabilone in cancer pain and symptom management: a prospective observational study using propensity scoring. *J Support Oncol* **6**(3):119–124, 2008.
55. Penrod JD, Goldstein NE, Deb P. When and how to use instrumental variables in palliative care research. *J Palliat Med* **12**(5):471–474, 2009.
56. Lorenz KA, Dy SM, Naeim A, et al. Quality measures for supportive cancer care: the Cancer Quality-ASSIST Project. *J Pain Symptom Manage* **37**(6):943–964, 2009.
57. Fleming TR. Current issues in non-inferiority trials. *Stat Med* **27**(3):317–332, 2008.
58. Williams RL, Chen ML, Hauck WW. Equivalence approaches. *Clin Pharmacol Ther* **72**(3):229–237, 2002.
59. Haythornthwaite JA. Clinical trials studying pharmacotherapy and psychological treatments alone and together. *Neurology* **65**(12 Suppl 4):S20–S31, 2005.
60. Russell PB, Aveyard SC, Oxenham DR. An assessment of methods used to evaluate the adequacy of cancer pain management. *J Pain Symptom Manage* **32**(6): 581–588, 2006.
61. Max M, Portenoy RK, Laska EM. The Design of Analgesic Clinical Trials. New York: Raven Press, 1991. *Advances in Pain Research and Therapy*; vol. **18**.
62. Farrar JT, Young JP, Jr., LaMoreaux L, Werth JL, Poole RM. Clinical importance of changes in chronic pain intensity measured on an 11-point numerical pain rating scale. *Pain* **94**(2):149–158, 2001.
63. Chow E, Wu JS, Hoskin P, Coia LR, Bentzen SM, Blitzer PH. International consensus on palliative radiotherapy endpoints for future clinical trials in bone metastases. *Radiother Oncol* **64**(3):275–280, 2002.
64. Dworkin RH, Turk DC, Farrar JT, et al. Core outcome measures for chronic pain clinical trials: IMMPACT recommendations. *Pain* **113**(1–2):9–19, 2005.
65. Turk DC, Dworkin RH, Allen RR, et al. Core outcome domains for chronic pain clinical trials: IMMPACT recommendations. *Pain* **106**(3):337–345, 2003.
66. Turk DC, Dworkin RH, McDermott MP, et al. Analyzing multiple endpoints in clinical trials of pain treatments: IMMPACT recommendations. Initiative

on Methods, Measurement, and Pain Assessment in Clinical Trials. *Pain* **139**(3):485–493, 2008.

67. Revicki D, Hays RD, Cella D, Sloan J. Recommended methods for determining responsiveness and minimally important differences for patient-reported outcomes. *J Clin Epidemiol* **61**(2):102–109, 2008.
68. US Food and Drug Administration, Center for Drug Evaluation and Research, Center for Biologics Evaluation and Research, Center for Devices and Radiological Health. Guidance for industry. Patient-reported outcome measures: use in medical product development to support labeling claims. Available from: URL: http://www.fda.gov/downloads/Drugs/GuidanceComplianceRegulatoryInformation/Guidances/UCM071975.pdf. Accessed Dec 18, 2009.
69. Farrar JT, Dworkin RH, Max MB. Use of the cumulative proportion of responders analysis graph to present pain data over a range of cut-off points: making clinical trial data more understandable. *J Pain Symptom Manage* **31**(4):369–377, 2006.
70. Gilron I, Max MB. Combination pharmacotherapy for neuropathic pain: current evidence and future directions. *Expert Rev Neurother* **5**(6):823–830, 2005.
71. Gilron I, Bailey JM, Tu D, Holden RR, Weaver DF, Houlden RL. Morphine, gabapentin, or their combination for neuropathic pain. *N Engl J Med* **352**(13):1324–1334, 2005.
72. Tallarida RJ. Drug synergism: its detection and applications. *J Pharmacol Exp Ther* **298**(3):865–872, 2001.
73. Tallarida RJ. An overview of drug combination analysis with isobolograms. *J Pharmacol Exp Ther* **319**(1):1–7, 2006.
74. Black DR, Sang CN. Advances and limitations in the evaluation of analgesic combination therapy. *Neurology* **65**(12 Suppl 4):S3–S6, 2005.
75. Minto CF, Schnider TW, Short TG, Gregg KM, Gentilini A, Shafer SL. Response surface model for anesthetic drug interactions. *Anesthesiology* **92**(6):1603–1616, 2000.
76. Sveticic G, Gentilini A, Eichenberger U, et al. Combinations of bupivacaine, fentanyl, and clonidine for lumbar epidural postoperative analgesia: a novel optimization procedure. *Anesthesiology* **101**(6): 1381–1393, 2004.
77. Reyes-Gibby CC, Wu X, Spitz M, et al. Molecular epidemiology, cancer-related symptoms, and cytokines pathway. *Lancet Oncol* **9**(8):777–785, 2008.
78. Houde RW. Pain and the patient with cancer. *Med Clin North Am* **40**(3):687–703, 1956.
79. Bell R, Kalso E, Paice J, Soyannwo O. A Global Problem: Cancer Pain From the Laboratory to the Bedside. Seattle WA: IASP Press, 2010.

Section 2 Chapter 5

Cancer Symptom Mechanisms and Models: Clinical and Basic Science

Pain: basic science

Unfortunately, pain comes in many sizes and shapes for the patient with cancer. Not only is pain caused by tissue destruction or transformation produced by the cancer itself, but it also may be a long lasting or even late effect of cancer treatment. Cancer can destroy bone and other tissue, can distort viscera, and can impinge on neural structures, all with the potential for causing pain. Cancer therapies can also result in painful neuropathy, produced by toxic or traumatic damage to peripheral and central neural structures. The two sections of this chapter report on the status of research in two common types of pain that patients with cancer may experience.

In the first section, Juan Miguel Jimenez-Andrade and Patrick Mantyh address the issue of disease-related pain, focusing primarily on pain that is the result of changes in bone produced by the cancer itself. In the second section, Haijun Zhang and Patrick Dougherty focus on pain produced as a side effect of neural destruction. Whereas pain from either source can be extremely disabling, the mechanisms causing these two types of pain are distinct, and call for differences in approaches to treatment as well as in research for developing new target agents for pain management.

Cancer Symptom Science: Measurement, Mechanisms, and Management, eds. Charles S. Cleeland, Michael J. Fisch, and Adrian J. Dunn.
Published by Cambridge University Press.

Mechanisms of disease-related pain in cancer: insights from the study of bone tumors

Juan Miguel Jimenez-Andrade and Patrick W. Mantyh

More than 10 million people are diagnosed with cancer (other than skin cancer) every year, and this number is expected to increase to 15 million per year by 2020.[1] In 2005, cancer caused 7.6 million deaths worldwide.[2] Cancer is a major health problem in the United States: 25% of US mortalities are related to cancer,[3] making it the second leading cause of death.

Despite the increasing prevalence of cancer, improvements in the detection and treatment of most types of cancers have resulted in significantly increased survival rates.[4] Pain is the first sign of cancer for many patients, most of whom will experience moderate to severe pain during the course of their disease and even into survivorship.[5,6] Cancer-associated pain can be present at any time during the course of the disease, but the frequency and intensity of cancer pain tends to increase as the disease progresses, such that 62% to 86% of patients with advanced-stage cancer experience significant amounts of cancer-induced pain.[7] If cancer patients and survivors, given their increasing life spans, are to remain functional, integrated, and contributing members of society, novel mechanism-based therapies will need to be developed to reduce cancer-related pain.[8]

Cancer pain may arise from different processes: by direct tumor infiltration or involvement, as a result of diagnostic or therapeutic surgical procedures (eg, biopsies, resection), or as a side effect or toxicity related to therapies used to treat cancer (eg, chemotherapy, radiation therapy). Until recently, the management of cancer pain has been largely empirical and based on scientific studies of painful conditions other than cancer. In this chapter, we will focus on recent insights provided by preclinical and clinical studies of cancer-induced pain. These studies have led to the beginnings of a mechanism-based understanding of the factors that generate and maintain cancer-induced pain.

Primary afferent neurons and cancer-induced pain

Primary afferent neurons are the gateway by which sensory information from peripheral tissues is transmitted to the spinal cord and brain (Figure 5.1). These sensory neurons innervate every organ of the body, with the exception of the brain. The cell bodies of sensory fibers that innervate the head and body are housed in the trigeminal and dorsal root ganglia (DRG), respectively, and can be divided into three major categories, large-diameter myelinated A-beta (Aβ) fibers, the small-diameter, thinly myelinated A-delta (Aδ) fibers, and unmyelinated C fibers.

Most small-diameter sensory fibers (finely myelinated Aδ fibers and unmyelinated C fibers) are sensory neurons known as nociceptors. Nociceptors express an extremely diverse repertoire of receptors and transduction molecules that can sense forms of noxious thermal, mechanical, and chemical stimuli, albeit with varying degrees of sensitivity.[9] These unmyelinated C fibers and finely myelinated Aδ sensory neurons are involved in generating the chronic pain that accompanies many cancers.[10] After tissue injury induced by the tumor or tumor-associated cells, many nociceptors alter their pattern of neurotransmitter, receptor, and growth factor expression and response properties (Figure 5.1). These changes underlie, in part, the development of peripheral sensitization, in which mild noxious sensory stimulation is perceived as highly noxious (hyperalgesia), and normally nonnoxious sensory stimulation is perceived as noxious (allodynia). Sensitization of the C-fiber nociceptors induced by tumors or tumor-associated cells leads to long-term changes in spinal excitability that may in turn lead to secondary hyperalgesia, represented by the increased response of Aδ fibers to mechanical stimulation outside of the site of direct injury. In contrast, large-diameter myelinated Aβ fibers originating in skin, joints, and muscles normally conduct only nonnoxious stimuli, including fine touch, vibration, and proprioception. In a normal noninjured

Cancer Symptom Science: Measurement, Mechanisms, and Management, eds. Charles S. Cleeland, Michael J. Fisch, and Adrian J. Dunn.
Published by Cambridge University Press.

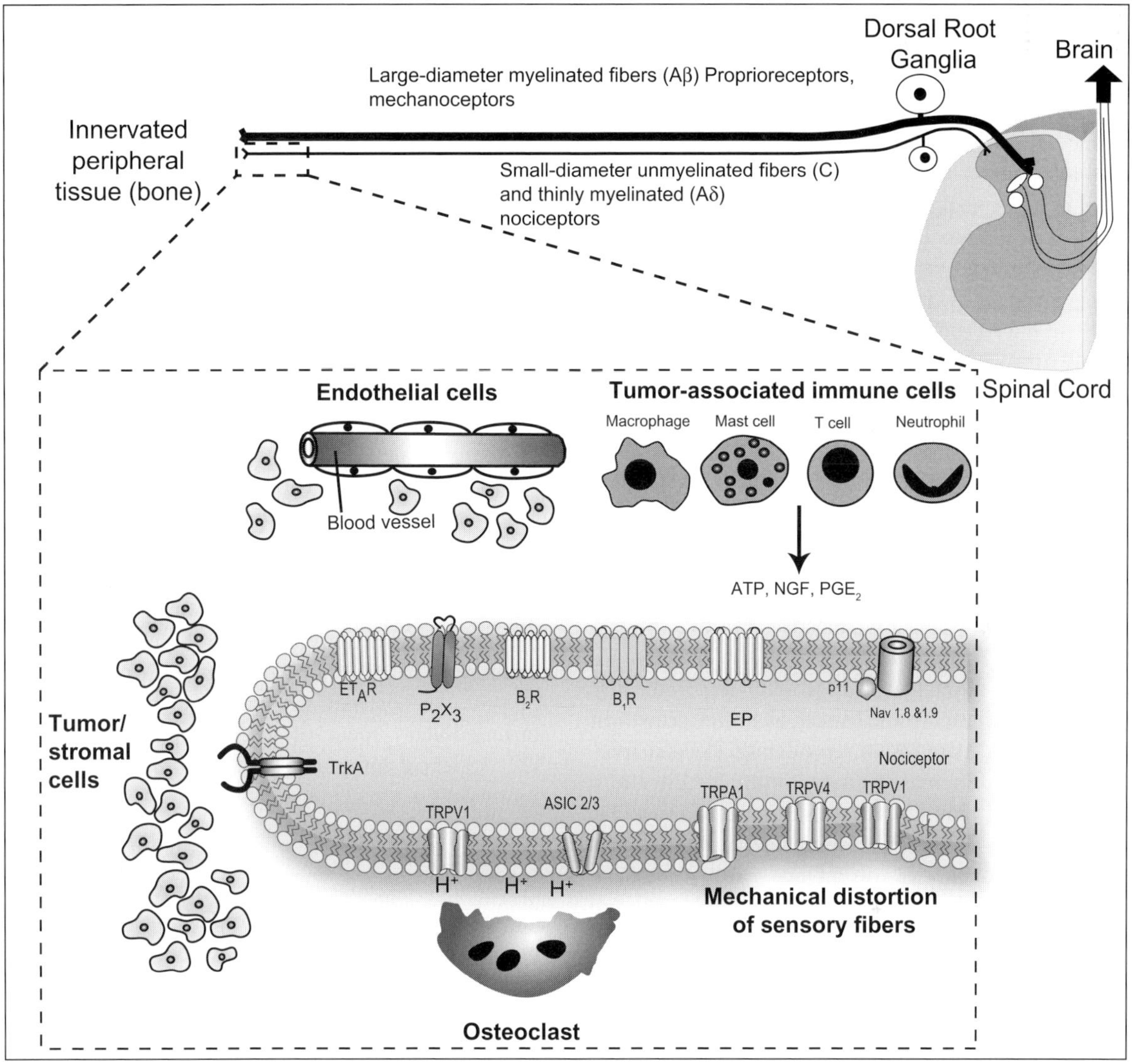

Figure 5.1. Primary afferent sensory nerve fibers involved in generating the cancer pain. Primary afferent neurons innervating the body have their cell bodies in the dorsal root ganglia (DRG) and transmit sensory information from the periphery to the spinal cord and brain. Myelinated A fibers (Aβ) containing large-diameter cell bodies, which project centrally to the dorsal column nuclei and deep spinal cord, are involved in detecting nonnoxious sensations including light touch, vibration, and proprioception. Unmyelinated C fibers and thinly myelinated Aδ fibers contain small-diameter cell bodies which project centrally to the superficial spinal cord. These fibers are involved in detecting multiple noxious stimuli (chemical, thermal, and mechanical). Box: Nociceptors use several different types of receptors to detect and transmit signals about noxious stimuli produced by cancer cells (yellow), tumor-associated immune cells (orange), or other aspects of the tumor microenvironment. Multiple factors may contribute to the pain associated with cancer. The transient receptor potential vanilloid receptor-1 (TRPV1) and acid-sensing ion channels (ASICs) detect extracellular protons produced by tumor-induced tissue damage or abnormal osteoclast-mediated bone resorption. Several mechanosensitive ion channels may be involved in detecting high-threshold mechanical stimuli that occur when distal aspects of sensory nerve fiber are distended from mechanical pressure due to the growing tumor or as a result of destabilization or fracture of bone. Tumor cells and associated inflammatory (immune) cells produce a variety of chemical mediators, including prostaglandins (PGE_2), nerve growth factor (NGF), endothelins, bradykinin, and extracellular ATP. Several of these proinflammatory mediators have receptors on peripheral terminals and can directly activate or sensitize nociceptors. NGF, together with its cognate receptor trkA, may serve as a master regulator of bone cancer pain by modulating the sensitivity of or increasing the expression of several receptors and ion channels contributing to increased excitability of nociceptors in the vicinity of the tumor. See plate section for color version.

condition, these large sensory neurons do not conduct noxious stimuli.

This review will focus on the involvement of sensory neurons in the generation and maintenance of bone tumor-induced pain. However, it should be stressed that, after cancer-induced injury to sensory neurons, areas of the spinal cord and central nervous system involved in the processing of somatosensory information also undergo various neurochemical and cellular changes known as central sensitization. These changes facilitate the transmission and conscious appreciation of both noxious and nonnoxious sensory information.

Tumor-induced cancer pain

Tumor-induced bone pain is the most common pain experienced by patients with advanced cancer. It is also the most common symptom indicating that tumor cells have metastasized to sites beyond the primary tumor.[11] Although bone is not a vital organ, most common tumors have a remarkable affinity to metastasize to bone. Tumor metastases to the skeleton are major contributors to the morbidity and mortality associated with metastatic cancer, as tumor growth in bone results in pain, bone remodeling, skeletal fractures, anemia, increased susceptibility to infection, and decreased mobility with resulting cardiovascular dysfunction – all of which compromise the patient's survival and quality of life.[12] Once tumor cells have metastasized to the skeleton, the tumor-induced bone pain is usually described as dull in character, constant in presentation, and gradually increasing in intensity with time.[11] As bone remodeling progresses, severe spontaneous pain frequently occurs,[11] and given that the onset of this pain is both acute and unpredictable, it can be particularly debilitating to the patient's functional status and quality of life.[11] Breakthrough pain, which is an intermittent episode of extreme pain, can occur spontaneously but more commonly is induced by movement of the tumor-bearing bone(s).[5]

The treatment of pain from bone metastases involves the use of multiple complementary approaches, including radiotherapy, chemotherapy, bisphosphonates, and analgesics.[11] However, bone cancer pain is one of the most difficult of all persistent pains to fully control, because the metastases are generally not limited to a single site and the analgesics most commonly used to treat bone cancer pain – the nonsteroidal anti-inflammatory drugs (NSAIDs)[11] and opioids[11,13] – are limited by significant adverse side effects. For example, nonselective NSAIDs can cause intestinal bleeding, whereas some selective cyclooxygenase (COX)-2 inhibitors cause less bleeding but may have cardiovascular safety issues.[14] Opioids are effective in attenuating bone cancer pain but are frequently accompanied by side effects, such as constipation, sedation, nausea, vomiting, and respiratory depression.[15]

Individuals with primary bone tumors (such as sarcomas) or with breast or prostate tumors (which metastasize primarily to bone as opposed to vital organs such as lung, liver, or brain) tend to live for a significant period of time beyond their initial diagnosis. For example, patients with prostate cancer live for 55 months, on average.[16] As the length of survival continues to increase for patients with cancer, it is essential that any new therapies be administrable over a period of years to control bone pain without the side effects commonly encountered with the currently available analgesics.

Animal models of cancer pain have been developed to facilitate the creation of mechanism-based therapies to treat cancer pain. In these models, bone cancer pain is induced by injecting murine osteolytic sarcoma or osteoblastic prostate cells into the intramedullary space of the murine femur (Figure 5.2). A critical component of these models is that the tumor cells are confined within the marrow space of the injected femur and do not invade adjacent soft tissues. After the tumor cells proliferate, both ongoing and movement-evoked pain-related behaviors develop and increase in severity with time. These pain behaviors correlate with progressive tumor-induced bone destruction or bone formation, and they appear to mimic the condition in humans with primary or metastatic bone cancer. These models will allow us to gain mechanistic insights into how cancer pain is generated and how the sensory information it initiates is processed as it moves from sense organ to the cerebral cortex under a constantly changing molecular architecture. As detailed below, these insights promise to fundamentally change the way cancer pain is controlled.

Acidosis in bone cancer pain

Recent reports from studies of both murine and human bone cancer pain have suggested that osteoclasts play an essential role in cancer-induced bone loss and contribute to the etiology of bone cancer pain.[17,18] Osteoclasts are terminally differentiated, multinucleated, monocyte lineage cells that resorb bone by maintaining an extracellular microenvironment of

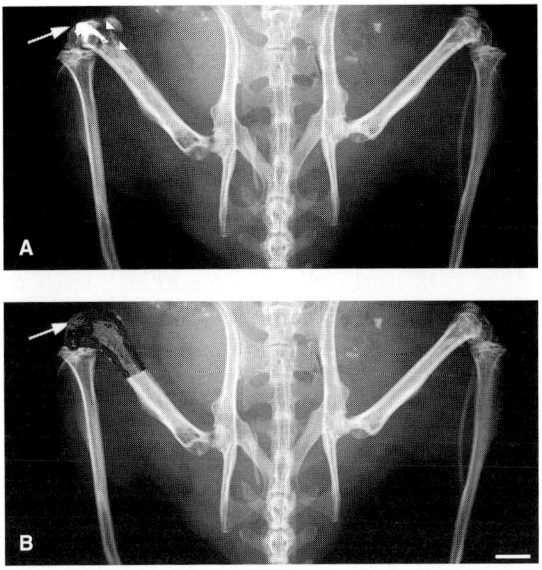

Figure 5.2. Development of a murine bone-cancer pain model. A. Low power anterior–posterior radiograph of mouse pelvis and hind limbs after a unilatereal injection of sarcoma cells into the distal part of the femur and closure of the injection site with an amalgam plug (arrow), which prevents the tumor cells from growing outside the bone. Extensive bone destruction occurs as tumor progression continues, characterized by multifocal radiolucencies and complete loss of trabecular bone regions as compared with contralateral hind limb (arrowheads). B. Tumor burden may be visualized and quantified using sarcoma cancer cells genetically manipulated to express enhanced green fluorescent protein (GFP), as in shown in the overlapping confocal immunofluorescence picture. By day 14 postinjection, GFP-expressing tumor cells (green) had completely filled the intramedullary space. Scale bar 3 mm. See plate section for color version.

acidic (4.0–5.0) pH at the osteoclast-mineralized bone interface.[19] Both osteolytic (primarily bone destroying) and osteoblastic (primarily bone forming) cancers are characterized by osteoclast proliferation and hypertrophy.[20]

Bisphosphonates, a class of antiresorptive compounds that induce osteoclast apoptosis, have also been reported to reduce pain in patients with osteolytic and/or osteoblastic skeletal metastases.[21,22] Bisphosphonates are pyrophosphate analogues that display high affinity for calcium ions, causing them to rapidly target the mineralized matrix of bone.[23] These drugs have been reported to act directly on osteoclasts, inducing their apoptosis by impairing either the synthesis of adenosine triphosphate or cholesterol, both of which are necessary for cell survival.[24] Studies in both clinical[21,22] and animal[25,26] models of bone cancer have reported antiresorptive effects of bisphosphonate therapy. The effect of bisphosphonates on tumor growth and long-term survival rates remains controversial.

In a recent study of the bisphosphonate alendronate in the murine 2472 sarcoma model, Sevcik et al[27] noted a reduction in the number of osteoclasts and in osteoclast activity, evidenced by the reduction in tumor-induced bone resorption. Alendronate treatment also resulted in a reduction in the number of osteoclasts displaying the clear zone at the basal bone resorbing surface, which is characteristic of highly active osteoclasts. In this model, alendronate also attenuated ongoing and movement-evoked bone cancer pain and the neurochemical reorganization of the peripheral and central nervous system, while at the same time promoting both tumor growth and tumor necrosis. These results suggest that in bone cancer, alendronate can simultaneously modulate pain, bone destruction, tumor growth, and tumor necrosis, and that administration of alendronate along with a tumoricidal agent may synergistically improve the survival and quality of life of patients with bone cancer pain. In recent human studies, ibandronate, a novel nitrogen-containing bisphosphonate, has shown remarkable effects in being able to rapidly induce long-lasting relief of bone cancer pain.[28]

Along with the current use of bisphosphonates to reduce bone destruction and bone cancer pain induced by osteolytic and osteoblastic tumors, the use of osteoprotegerin (OPG) or antibodies with OPG-like activities holds significant promise for alleviating bone cancer pain. OPG is a secreted soluble receptor that is a member of the tumor necrosis factor receptor family.[29] This decoy receptor prevents the activation and proliferation of osteoclasts by binding to and sequestering OPG ligand (OPGL; also known as receptor for activator of nuclear factor kappa B ligand, RANKL).[29,30] OPG has been shown to decrease pain behaviors in the murine sarcoma model of bone cancer.[17] A monoclonal antibody (AMG-162) that also blocks the interaction of OPGL and RANKL is also being developed for use in treating skeletal pain. These results suggest that a substantial part of the actions of OPG results from inhibition of tumor-induced bone destruction via a reduction in osteoclast function.

The finding that sensory neurons (Figure 5.1) can be directly excited by protons or acid originating from cells such as osteoclasts in bone has generated intense clinical interest in pain research. Studies have shown that subsets of sensory neurons express various acid-sensing ion channels.[9] Two acid-sensing ion channels expressed by nociceptors are the transient receptor potential vanilloid-1 (TRPV1)[31] and the acid-sensing ion channel-3 (ASIC-3).[32] Both of these channels are sensitized and excited by a decrease in pH. Tumor stroma[33] and areas of tumor necrosis such as those observed in bone cancer typically exhibit lower extracellular pH than do surrounding normal tissues. As inflammatory and immune cells invade the tumor stroma, they also release protons that generate a local acidosis.

It has been shown that TRPV1 is expressed by a subset of sensory neuron fibers that innervate the mouse femur, and that in an *in vivo* model of bone cancer pain, acute or chronic administration of a TRPV1 antagonist or disruption of the TRPV1 gene results in a significant attenuation of both ongoing and movement-evoked nocifensive behaviors.[34] In addition, previous studies have shown that in a sarcoma model of bone cancer pain, administration of a TRPV1 antagonist retains its efficacy at early, middle, and late stages of tumor growth.[34] These results suggest that the TRPV1 channel plays a role in the integration of nociceptive signaling in a severe pain state, and that antagonists of TRPV1 may be effective in attenuating difficult-to-treat, mixed chronic-pain states, such as those encountered in patients with bone cancer pain.

Another major source of bone pain is mechanical distortion of the periosteum.[11,35] Thus, after fracture caused by tumor-induced bone remodeling, the pain associated with the fracture is partially relieved if the bone and periosteum are repositioned and stabilized to their normal orientation.[36]

Tumor-derived products and bone cancer pain

The tumor stroma is made up of many different cell types apart from cancer cells, including immune cells such as macrophages, neutrophils, and T-lymphocytes. These secrete a variety of factors, such as prostaglandins, endothelins, kinins, tumor necrosis factor (TNF)-α, interleukin (IL)-1 and IL-6, nerve growth factor, epidermal growth factor, transforming growth factor-beta, and platelet-derived growth factor,[10] that have been shown to sensitize or directly excite primary afferent neurons. Receptors for many of these factors are expressed by primary afferent neurons, as discussed below.

Prostaglandins

Prostaglandins are lipid-derived eicosanoids that are synthesized from arachidonic acid by COX isoenzymes COX-1 and COX-2. Cancer cells and tumor-associated macrophages have both been shown to express high levels of COX isoenzymes, leading to high levels of prostaglandins.[37,38] Studies in the murine sarcoma model of bone cancer pain have shown that chronic inhibition of COX-2 activity with selective COX-2 inhibitors results in significant attenuation of bone cancer pain behaviors as well as many of the neurochemical changes suggestive of both peripheral and central sensitization.[18] In addition, prostaglandins have been shown to be involved in tumor growth, survival, and angiogenesis.[39–41] Therefore, COX-2 inhibitors are capable of blocking cancer pain and retarding tumor growth within bone.[18] Chronic administration of a selective COX-2 inhibitor significantly reduces tumor burden in sarcoma-bearing bones, which may, in turn, reduce factors released by tumor cells capable of exciting primary afferent fibers.[42] Both acute and chronic administration of a selective COX-2 inhibitor significantly attenuated both ongoing and movement-evoked pain.[18] Whereas acute administration of a COX-2 inhibitor presumably reduces prostaglandins capable of activating sensory or spinal cord neurons, chronic inhibition of COX-2 appears to simultaneously reduce osteoclastogenesis, bone resorption, and tumor burden. Together, suppression of prostaglandin synthesis and release at multiple sites by selective inhibition of COX-2 may synergistically improve the survival and quality of life of patients with bone cancer pain.

Endothelins

Endothelins (endothelin-1, -2, and -3) are a family of vasoactive peptides that are expressed at high levels by several types of tumors, including those that arise from the prostate.[43] Clinical studies have shown a correlation between the severity of pain and the plasma levels of endothelins in patients with prostate cancer.[44] Endothelins may contribute to cancer pain by directly sensitizing or exciting nociceptors, as a subset of small unmyelinated primary afferent neurons express endothelin type-A receptors.[45] Furthermore, direct application of endothelin to peripheral nerves induces activation of primary afferent fibers and an induction of pain-related behaviors.[46] These findings suggest that endothelin antagonists may be useful in inhibiting bone cancer pain. In the sarcoma model of bone cancer pain, acute or chronic administration of an endothelin A receptor (ET_AR)-selective antagonist significantly attenuated ongoing and movement-evoked bone cancer pain. Chronic administration of this drug also reduced several neurochemical indices of peripheral and central sensitization without influencing tumor growth or bone destruction.[47]

Kinins

Previous studies have shown that bradykinin and related kinins are released in response to tissue injury and that they play a significant role in driving acute and chronic inflammatory pain.[48] The action of bradykinin is mediated by two receptors termed B_1 and B_2. Whereas B_2 receptors are constitutively expressed at high levels by sensory neurons, B_1 receptors are normally expressed at low but detectable levels by sensory neurons and are significantly upregulated after peripheral inflammation or tissue injury.[49] Tumor metastases to the skeleton induce significant bone remodeling with accompanying tissue injury, which presumably induces the release of bradykinin. After pharmacological blockade of the B_1 receptor, both bone-cancer-induced ongoing and movement-evoked nocifensive behaviors were reduced and the therapeutic efficacy was retained, even in advanced bone cancer.[50]

Nerve growth factor

Nerve growth factor (NGF) is a small secreted protein that induces the differentiation and survival of particular target neurons. NGF can directly activate sensory neurons, and it also modulates expression and function of a wide variety of molecules and proteins expressed by sensory neurons that express the trkA or p75 receptor. Some of these molecules and proteins are: neurotransmitters (substance P and calcitonin gene-related peptide), receptors (bradykinin R), channels (P2X3, TRPV1, ASIC-3, and sodium channels), transcription factors (ATF-3), and structural molecules (neurofilaments and the sodium channel anchoring molecule p11).[51] Additionally, NGF has been shown to modulate the trafficking and insertion of sodium channels, such as Nav 1.8 and TRPV1, in the sensory neurons, and to modulate the expression profile of supporting cells, such as nonmyelinating Schwann cells and macrophages, in the DRG and peripheral nerve.[52]

In light of the potential role that NGF may play in driving bone cancer pain, anti-NGF therapy was examined in primarily osteolytic sarcoma and osteoblastic prostate models of bone cancer pain. In both models of bone cancer pain, it was demonstrated that administration of anti-NGF therapy was not only highly efficacious in reducing both early-stage and late-stage bone cancer pain-related behaviors, but that this reduction was greater than that achieved with acute administration of 10 or 30mg/kg of morphine sulfate.[53,54] Given that the bone is primarily innervated by calcitonin gene-related peptide/trkA-expressing sensory fibers,[10] NGF-sequestering therapies may be uniquely efficacious in attenuating the pain and improving the quality of life and function of patients with significant skeletal pain.

Neuropathic component of bone cancer pain

To examine the interface of tumor cells and sensory nerve fibers as tumor cells invade the bone, Peters et al.[55] injected osteosarcoma cells into the intramedullary space of the mouse femur. Using this model, the investigators noted that tumor cells grew within the bone and came into contact with, injured, and then destroyed the very distal processes of sensory fibers that innervate the bone marrow and the mineralized bone. Thus, the sensory nerve fibers observed at and within the leading edge of the tumor's deep stromal regions displayed a discontinuous and fragmented appearance, suggesting that after initial activation by the osteolytic tumor cells, the distal processes of the sensory fibers ultimately were injured by the invading tumor cells. Tumor-induced injury to sensory fibers that normally innervate the tumor-bearing femur resulted in the expression of ATF-3 (which is upregulated after peripheral nerve injury) in the nucleus of those sensory neurons.

Tumor-induced injury of sensory nerve fibers by the invading sarcoma cells was also accompanied by an increase in ongoing and movement-evoked pain behaviors, an upregulation of galanin by sensory neurons that innervate the tumor-bearing femur, upregulation of glial fibrillary acidic protein (GFAP) and hypertrophy of satellite cells surrounding sensory neuron cell bodies within the ipsilateral DRG, and macrophage infiltration of the DRG ipsilateral to the tumor-bearing femur.[55]

Similar neurochemical changes after peripheral nerve injury and in other noncancerous neuropathic pain states have been described.[56,57] Chronic treatment with gabapentin in this model of bone cancer pain attenuated both ongoing and movement-evoked bone cancer-related pain behaviors, although it did not influence tumor growth, tumor-induced bone destruction, or the tumor-induced neurochemical reorganization that occurs in sensory neurons or the spinal cord.[55] These results suggest that even when the tumor is confined within the bone, a component of bone cancer pain appears to be neuropathic in origin, as tumor cells clearly induce injury or remodeling of the primary afferent nerve fibers that normally innervate the tumor-bearing bone.

Conclusions and future perspectives

Advances in cancer detection and therapies have dramatically increased the survival rates of patients with most cancers. With this increased survival there is an ever-developing need to focus on cancer-associated pain and the impact it has on the patient, from initial diagnosis through therapy to survivorship. Pain can have a significant impact on the quality of life of both the cancer patient and cancer survivor. Animal models now available merge pain research with cancer research, and by working closely with clinicians who treat patients with cancer, translational researchers will be able to capitalize on significant synergies occurring at the interface of these two previously separate disciplines. By focusing and incorporating both preclinical and clinical pain research into mainstream cancer research and therapies, we have the opportunity to target and affect not only the tumor, but also the overall health, quality of life, and survival of the patient with cancer.

References

1. Stewart BW, Kleihues P. *International Agency for Research on Cancer. World Cancer Report.* Lyon: IARC Press, 2003.
2. World Health Organization. Cancer: quick cancer facts. Available from: URL: http://www.who.int/cancer. Accessed Aug 12, 2008.
3. Jemal A, Siegel R, Ward E, Murray T, Xu J, Thun MJ. Cancer statistics, 2007. *CA Cancer J Clin* **57**(1):43–66, 2007.
4. Edwards BK, Brown ML, Wingo PA, et al. Annual report to the nation on the status of cancer, 1975–2002, featuring population-based trends in cancer treatment. *J Natl Cancer Inst* **97**(19):1407–1427, 2005.
5. Mercadante S, Arcuri E. Breakthrough pain in cancer patients: pathophysiology and treatment. *Cancer Treat Rev* **24**(6):425–432, 1998.
6. Portenoy RK, Payne D, Jacobsen P. Breakthrough pain: characteristics and impact in patients with cancer pain. *Pain* **81**(1–2):129–134, 1999.
7. van den Beuken-van Everdingen MH, de Rijke JM, Kessels AG, Schouten HC, van Kleef M, Patijn J. Prevalence of pain in patients with cancer: a systematic review of the past 40 years. *Ann Oncol* **18**(9):1437–1449, 2007.
8. Aalto Y, Forsgren S, Kjörell U, Bergh J, Franzén L, Henriksson R. Enhanced expression of neuropeptides in human breast cancer cell lines following irradiation. *Peptides* **19**(2):231–239, 1998.
9. Julius D, Basbaum AI. Molecular mechanisms of nociception. *Nature* **413**(6852):203–210, 2001.
10. Mantyh PW. Cancer pain and its impact on diagnosis, survival and quality of life. *Nat Rev Neurosci* **7**(10):797–809, 2006.
11. Mercadante S. Malignant bone pain: pathophysiology and treatment. *Pain* **69**(1–2):1–18, 1997.
12. Coleman RE. Metastatic bone disease: clinical features, pathophysiology and treatment strategies. *Cancer Treat Rev* **27**(3):165–176, 2001.
13. Portenoy RK, Lesage P. Management of cancer pain. *Lancet* **353**(9165):1695–1700, 1999.
14. Mukherjee D, Nissen SE, Topol EJ. Risk of cardiovascular events associated with selective COX-2 inhibitors. *JAMA* **286**(8):954–959, 2001.
15. Mercadante S. Problems of long-term spinal opioid treatment in advanced cancer patients. *Pain* **79**(1): 1–13, 1999.
16. Jemal A, Siegel R, Ward E, et al. Cancer statistics, 2006. *CA Cancer J Clin* **56**(2):106–130, 2006.
17. Honore P, Luger NM, Sabino MA, et al. Osteoprotegerin blocks bone cancer-induced skeletal destruction, skeletal pain and pain-related neurochemical reorganization of the spinal cord. *Nat Med* **6**(5):521–528, 2000.
18. Sabino MA, Ghilardi JR, Jongen JL, et al. Simultaneous reduction in cancer pain, bone destruction, and tumor growth by selective inhibition of cyclooxygenase-2. *Cancer Res* **62**(24):7343–7349, 2002.
19. Delaissé JM, Vaes G. Mechanism of mineral solubilization and matrix degradation in osteoclastic bone resorption. In: Rifkin BR, Gay CV, eds. *Biology and Physiology of the Osteoclast.* Boca Raton: CRC Press, 1992:289–314.

20. Clohisy DR, Perkins SL, Ramnaraine ML. Review of cellular mechanisms of tumor osteolysis. *Clin Orthop Relat Res* **373**:104–114, 2000.
21. Fulfaro F, Casuccio A, Ticozzi C, Ripamonti C. The role of bisphosphonates in the treatment of painful metastatic bone disease: a review of phase III trials. *Pain* **78**(3):157–169, 1998.
22. Major PP, Lipton A, Berenson J, Hortobagyi G. Oral bisphosphonates: a review of clinical use in patients with bone metastases. *Cancer* **88**(1):6–14, 2000.
23. Rogers MJ, Gordon S, Benford HL, et al. Cellular and molecular mechanisms of action of bisphosphonates. *Cancer* **88**(12 Suppl):2961–2978, 2000.
24. Rodan GA, Martin TJ. Therapeutic approaches to bone diseases. *Science* **289**(5484):1508–1514, 2000.
25. Hiraga T, Tanaka S, Yamamoto M, Nakajima T, Ozawa H. Inhibitory effects of bisphosphonate (YM175) on bone resorption induced by a metastatic bone tumor. *Bone* **18**(1):1–7, 1996.
26. Sasaki A, Boyce BF, Story B, et al. Bisphosphonate risedronate reduces metastatic human breast cancer burden in bone in nude mice. *Cancer Res* **55**(16):3551–3557, 1995.
27. Sevcik MA, Luger NM, Mach DB, et al. Bone cancer pain: the effects of the bisphosphonate alendronate on pain, skeletal remodeling, tumor growth and tumor necrosis. *Pain* **111**(1–2):169–180, 2004.
28. Tripathy D, Body JJ, Bergström B. Review of ibandronate in the treatment of metastatic bone disease: experience from phase III trials. *Clin Ther* **26**(12):1947–1959, 2004.
29. Simonet WS, Lacey DL, Dunstan CR, et al. Osteoprotegerin: a novel secreted protein involved in the regulation of bone density. *Cell* **89**(2):309–319, 1997.
30. Yasuda H, Shima N, Nakagawa N, et al. Identity of osteoclastogenesis inhibitory factor (OCIF) and osteoprotegerin (OPG): a mechanism by which OPG/OCIF inhibits osteoclastogenesis in vitro. *Endocrinology* **139**(3):1329–1337, 1998.
31. Tominaga M, Caterina MJ, Malmberg AB, et al. The cloned capsaicin receptor integrates multiple pain-producing stimuli. *Neuron* **21**(3):531–543, 1998.
32. Alvarez de la Rosa D, Zhang P, Shao D, White F, Canessa CM. Functional implications of the localization and activity of acid-sensitive channels in rat peripheral nervous system. *Proc Natl Acad Sci U S A* **99**(4):2326–2331, 2002.
33. Griffiths JR. Are cancer cells acidic? *Br J Cancer* **64**(3):425–427, 1991.
34. Ghilardi JR, Röhrich H, Lindsay TH, et al. Selective blockade of the capsaicin receptor TRPV1 attenuates bone cancer pain. *J Neurosci* **25**(12):3126–3131, 2005.
35. Mundy GR. *Bone Remodeling and its Disorders*, 2nd ed. London: Martin Dunitz, 1999.
36. Rubert CK, Henshaw RM, Malawer MM. Orthopedic management of skeletal metastases. In: Body JJ, ed. *Tumor Bone Diseases and Osteoporosis in Cancer Patients: Pathophysiology, Diagnosis, and Therapy*. New York: Marcel Dekker, 2000:305–356.
37. Kundu N, Yang Q, Dorsey R, Fulton AM. Increased cyclooxygenase-2 (cox-2) expression and activity in a murine model of metastatic breast cancer. *Int J Cancer* **93**(5):681–686, 2001.
38. Molina MA, Sitja-Arnau M, Lemoine MG, Frazier ML, Sinicrope FA. Increased cyclooxygenase-2 expression in human pancreatic carcinomas and cell lines: growth inhibition by nonsteroidal anti-inflammatory drugs. *Cancer Res* **59**(17):4356–4362, 1999.
39. Iñiguez MA, Rodriguez A, Volpert OV, Fresno M, Redondo JM. Cyclooxygenase-2: a therapeutic target in angiogenesis. *Trends Mol Med* **9**(2):73–78, 2003.
40. Masferrer JL, Leahy KM, Koki AT, et al. Antiangiogenic and antitumor activities of cyclooxygenase-2 inhibitors. *Cancer Res* **60**(5):1306–1311, 2000.
41. Williams CS, Tsujii M, Reese J, Dey SK, DuBois RN. Host cyclooxygenase-2 modulates carcinoma growth. *J Clin Invest* **105**(11):1589–1594, 2000.
42. Davar G. Endothelin-1 and metastatic cancer pain. *Pain Med* **2**(1):24–27, 2001.
43. Nelson JB, Carducci MA. The role of endothelin-1 and endothelin receptor antagonists in prostate cancer. *BJU Int* **85**(Suppl 2):45–48, 2000.
44. Nelson JB, Hedican SP, George DJ, et al. Identification of endothelin-1 in the pathophysiology of metastatic adenocarcinoma of the prostate. *Nat Med* **1**(9):944–949, 1995.
45. Pomonis JD, Rogers SD, Peters CM, Ghilardi JR, Mantyh PW. Expression and localization of endothelin receptors: implications for the involvement of peripheral glia in nociception. *J Neurosci* **21**(3):999–1006, 2001.
46. Davar G, Hans G, Fareed MU, Sinnott C, Strichartz G. Behavioral signs of acute pain produced by application of endothelin-1 to rat sciatic nerve. *Neuroreport* **9**(10):2279–2283, 1998.
47. Peters CM, Lindsay TH, Pomonis JD, et al. Endothelin and the tumorigenic component of bone cancer pain. *Neuroscience* **126**(4):1043–1052, 2004.
48. Couture R, Harrisson M, Vianna RM, Cloutier F. Kinin receptors in pain and inflammation. *Eur J Pharmacol* **429**(1–3):161–176, 2001.
49. Fox A, Wotherspoon G, McNair K, et al. Regulation and function of spinal and peripheral neuronal B1

bradykinin receptors in inflammatory mechanical hyperalgesia. *Pain* **104**(3):683–691, 2003.

50. Sevcik MA, Ghilardi JR, Halvorson KG, Lindsay TH, Kubota K, Mantyh PW. Analgesic efficacy of bradykinin B1 antagonists in a murine bone cancer pain model. *J Pain* **6**(11):771–775, 2005.
51. Pezet S, McMahon SB. Neurotrophins: mediators and modulators of pain. *Annu Rev Neurosci* **29**:507–538, 2006.
52. Heumann R, Korsching S, Bandtlow C, Thoenen H. Changes of nerve growth factor synthesis in nonneuronal cells in response to sciatic nerve transection. *J Cell Biol* **104**(6):1623–1631, 1987.
53. Halvorson KG, Kubota K, Sevcik MA, et al. A blocking antibody to nerve growth factor attenuates skeletal pain induced by prostate tumor cells growing in bone. *Cancer Res* **65**(20):9426–9435, 2005.
54. Sevcik MA, Ghilardi JR, Peters CM, et al. Anti-NGF therapy profoundly reduces bone cancer pain and the accompanying increase in markers of peripheral and central sensitization. *Pain* **115**(1–2):128–141, 2005.
55. Peters CM, Ghilardi JR, Keyser CP, et al. Tumor-induced injury of primary afferent sensory nerve fibers in bone cancer pain. *Exp Neurol* **193**(1):85–100, 2005.
56. Hu P, McLachlan EM. Macrophage and lymphocyte invasion of dorsal root ganglia after peripheral nerve lesions in the rat. *Neuroscience* **112**(1):23–38, 2002.
57. Woodham P, Anderson PN, Nadim W, Turmaine M. Satellite cells surrounding axotomised rat dorsal root ganglion cells increase expression of a GFAP-like protein. *Neurosci Lett* **98**(1):8–12, 1989.

Section 2 Chapter 5b

Cancer Symptom Mechanisms and Models: Clinical and Basic Science

The physiology of neuropathic pain

Haijun Zhang and Patrick M. Dougherty

The International Association for the Study of Pain (IASP) defines pain as "an unpleasant, sensory and emotional experience associated with actual or potential tissue damage, or described in terms of such damage."[1] The pain that is commonly experienced by people with cancer may be caused by the disease itself or by cancer treatment. The three most common causes for cancer pain are: (1) tumors metastasizing to the bone; (2) tumors infiltrating the nerve and hollow viscus; and (3) cancer treatments such as chemotherapy, radiation, and surgery. Cancer pain thus involves multiple mechanisms, including inflammation and primary and secondary hyperalgesia after tissue or nerve injury.

In this chapter, we will describe the basic physiology of pain signal processing, including peripheral nociceptors that sense stimuli in multiple energy forms (eg, heat, mechanical, chemical) and central stations involved in coding pain sensibility. We will describe the mechanisms of primary and secondary hyperalgesia wherein normally innocuous stimuli become painful. Finally, we will discuss some of the alterations in the functions of neurons and nonneuronal cells when the nervous system itself is damaged.

Peripheral and central mechanisms of nociception

Peripheral nociceptors

Nociception – the ability to feel pain – is caused by activation of peripheral receptors known as nociceptors. Nociceptors respond selectively to a variety of noxious stimuli, such as heat, pinch, and chemicals, and provide information about the location and intensity of such stimuli. Nociceptors can be categorized into three classes according to their structural and functional properties.

A-fiber nociceptors transmit signals quickly and are responsible for pricking and sharp pain. A-fiber nociceptors are polymodal nociceptors, which means that they respond to mechanical, thermal, and chemical stimuli. A-fiber nociceptors have a myelin sheath formed by Schwann cells.

Two types of A-fiber nociceptors have been identified on the basis of their responses to heat stimuli. Type I A-fiber nociceptors have high mechanical thresholds and respond well to intense short-duration heat stimuli (typically > 53°C). In monkeys, the mean conduction velocity for Type I A-fiber nociceptors is 25 m/s, but can reach a maximum of 55 m/s. Type I nociceptors are mostly localized to hairy and glabrous skin. Type II nociceptors have a lower heat threshold and lower conduction velocity (15 m/s) than Type I nociceptors. Type II nociceptors respond to the application of a stepped-heat stimulus with an initial burst of activity that parallels to a fast-onset, sharp, pricking sensation, and thus are ideally suited for signaling initial pain.[2] Most Type II nociceptors do not respond to mechanical stimuli but are similar to Type I A-fiber nociceptors in their responses to chemical stimuli. Type II A-fiber nociceptors are found exclusively on hairy skin.

Unmyelinated C-fiber nociceptors have a relatively slow conduction velocity (<2 m/s) and are primarily responsible for producing the sensation of burning pain. Because most C-fiber nociceptors respond to mechanical and chemical stimuli, they also are considered polymodal nociceptors. C-fiber nociceptors exhibit a monotonical increase in discharge frequency with stimulus intensity, which resembles that of Type II nociceptors.[3,4] Because the depth of C-fiber terminals varies widely under the skin, the heat threshold to activate C-fiber nociceptors varies as well.

A third class of cutaneous afferents either do not respond to mechanical stimuli at all or have exceedingly high thresholds. These are referred to as mechanically insensitive afferents. They have been found in about 50% of A-fiber nociceptors and 30% of C-fiber

Cancer Symptom Science: Measurement, Mechanisms, and Management, eds. Charles S. Cleeland, Michael J. Fisch, and Adrian J. Dunn.

nociceptors, as well as in afferent fibers innervating the knee joint, viscera, and cornea.

Central neural mechanisms in pain signaling

Figure 5.3 shows a schematic diagram of the flow of somatosensory information through the neuraxis. Nociceptive information flows from the peripheral afferents to the central nervous system. The spinal dorsal horn, and to a much lesser extent the dorsal column nuclei, provide the first link in the central nociceptive pathways. From here, nociceptive information is distributed to sites in the brainstem, midbrain, hypothalamus, thalamus, and finally the sensory and limbic cortices.[5–7]

The spinal dorsal horn

In 1952, the Swedish neuroscientist Bror Rexed schematized the cells of the spinal cord into ten layers, or laminae, represented by Roman numerals – a system that is still in use today.[8] In Rexed's schema, the laminae are defined by their neuronal cytoarchitecture,

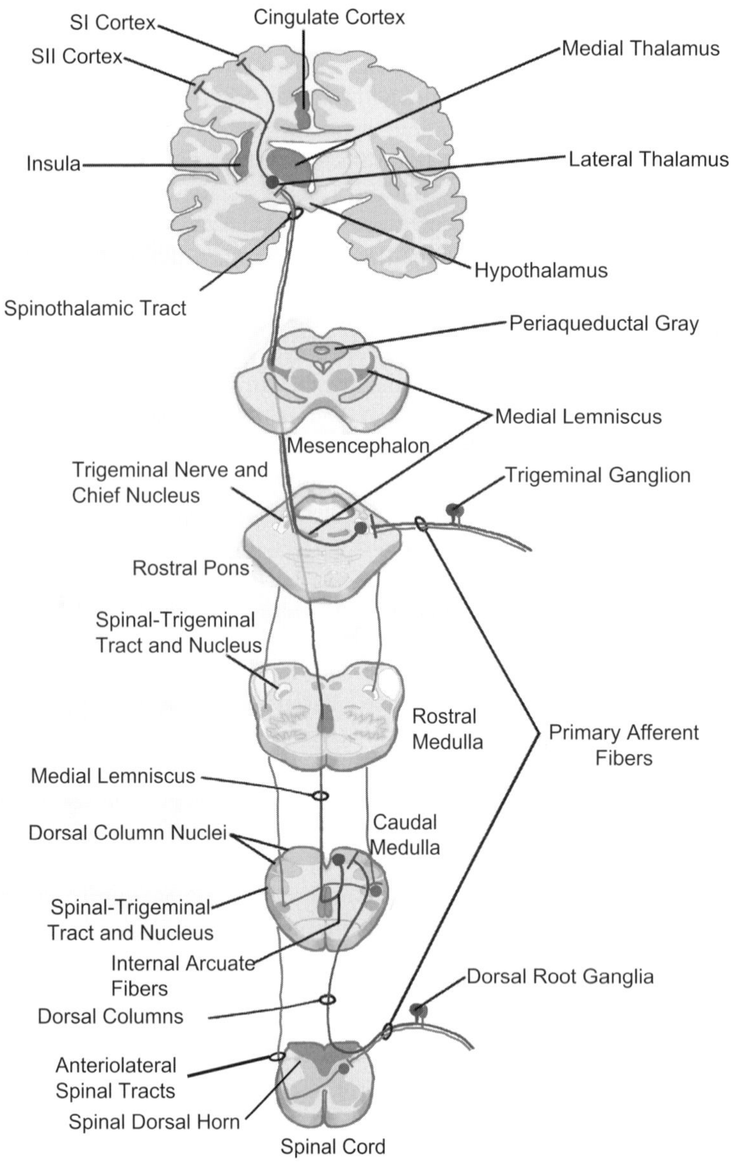

Figure 5.3. The central nociceptive pathways. Primary afferent fibers enter the neuraxis via spinal nerves with cell bodies in the dorsal root ganglia, or via the trigeminal nerve with cell bodies in the trigeminal ganglion. In anteriolateral spinal nociceptive pathway (gray lines), primary afferents from the dorsal root ganglia form synapses on the secondary-order neurons in spinal dorsal horn. The secondary-order axons then cross the midline in the anterior white commissure and gather into the anteriolateral spinal columns. Primary afferent fibers from trigeminal ganglia descend in the spinal-trigeminal tract and form synapses on the secondary-order neurons in the spinal-trigeminal nucleus. The secondary-order axons from spinal-trigeminal nucleus cross the midline to join in the anteriolateral tract. The axons in anteriolateral tract send collaterals to the reticular formation, midbrain, and hypothalamus while ascending and finally terminating in the lateral or medial thalamus. The third-order neurons in the thalamus project to various cortical areas. In the dorsal column-medial lemniscal sensory pathway (medial lemniscus: black line), primary afferents from dorsal root ganglia ascend in the dorsal spinal columns and form synapses on the secondary-order neurons in the dorsal column nuclei. The axons from the secondary-order neurons cross the midline in the internal arcuate fibers and gather to form the medial lemniscus. The primary afferents from trigeminal ganglia enter and synapse in the chief (main) sensory trigeminal nucleus, and axons from the secondary-order neurons cross the midline and join in the medial lemniscus. The secondary-order axons then ascend and terminate in the lateral thalamus. Finally, the third-order neurons in thalamus project to cortical areas. See plate section for color version.

which also generally describes their location within the spinal cord. The spinal dorsal horn contains layers I to VI, where primary afferent fibers make stereotyped connections with dorsal horn neurons. Aδ and C afferents primarily terminate in layers I and II outer, whereas Aβ afferents terminate in layer II inner to layer V after they enter spinal cord.

Neurons in the spinal cord have physiological properties that mirror this pattern of primary afferent fiber termination. Many of the neurons in the superficial layers of the dorsal horn are often called nociceptive-specific (NS) or high-threshold (HT) neurons because they respond exclusively to noxious inputs. NS neurons tend to have ongoing background activity and relatively small-sized excitatory somatic receptive fields. Many NS cells exhibit polymodal characteristics by responding to mechanical, heat, chemical, and sometimes cooling stimuli applied to their somatic receptive fields.

Two other classes of cells are found in the dorsal horn. Low-threshold (LT) cells respond only to nonnoxious stimuli[6]; wide-dynamic-range (WDR) or multireceptive cells respond to both noxious and nonnoxious stimuli.[9,10] LT and WDR cells have a higher level of spontaneous activity than NS neurons and a larger excitatory receptive field.[9,10] LT cells are mostly inhibitory interneurons and are especially prevalent in laminae II. Most LT tract neurons project from the spinal cord to the dorsal column nuclei; only a few of them project to the brainstem, midbrain, or diencephalon. WDR cells are found in laminae I to VI and are both intrinsic and projection neurons. They receive inputs from nociceptors either via contacts from more superficial intrinsic cells or via direct contacts of afferents penetrating into the superficial layers. WDR neurons found in layer I may be essential for the transmission of cooling and warm (nonnoxious thermal) stimuli.[11,12] WDR cells in layers III to V respond to both cutaneous mechanical and heat stimuli; WDR cells in layers VI and VII tend especially to show responses from deep tissue and visceral receptors.

The dorsal column nuclei

In addition to the primary afferent input, the dorsal column nuclei receive input from at least two groupings of dorsal horn projection neurons: the postsynaptic dorsal column pathway and the spinocervical tract.[6,7] The cells of the dorsal column nuclei largely respond to innocuous stimuli alone, receiving information primarily from hair follicle receptors, Pacinian corpuscles, muscle spindles, golgi tendon organs, and Types I and II slowly adapting mechanoreceptors that belong to Type I A-fibers.[5,6] However, several lines of evidence suggest a role of the dorsal column nuclei in nociceptive transmission. It has been shown that dorsal column nuclei consist of a small number of nociceptive neurons and that they receive inputs from unmyelinated afferents.[13]

Rostral areas of the central nervous system

As they ascend rostrally, axons of dorsal horn neurons project to the medullary reticular formation (spinoreticular tract), the mesencephalic periaqueductal gray and neighboring area (spinomesencephalic tract), and the hypothalamus (spinohypothalamic tract) before they finally reach the sensory regions of thalamus (spinothalamic tract).[5,7] Although the specific functions of these pathways remain poorly defined, they are suggested to include the affective/motivational and vegetative (autonomic and neuroendocrine) aspects of nociception. Among the higher nociceptive centers, neurons of the spinothalamic tract encode stimuli in a way that matches best with the perceptions of humans to noxious stimuli. Some neurons in the other spinal pathways (eg, the spinoreticular, spinomesencephalic, and spinohypothalamic tracts) also show responses similar to those of the spinothalamic cells.

The dorsal column nuclei project via the medial lemniscus to the ventral posterior thalamus anterior to the termination of the spinothalamic tract. Neurons in the thalamus receiving lemniscal inputs project to the more rostral areas of the sensory cortex, and neurons receiving spinothalamic input project to the posterior-inferior retroinsular cortex. The neurons in the brainstem reticular formation, the mesencephalic gray, and the hypothalamus diffusely project to some rostral areas and also send input to the spinal cord via descending pathways.

Neurochemistry of somatosensory transmission

As illustrated in Figure 5.4, multiple neurotransmitters and neuropeptides are involved in somatosensory neurotransmission.[7] Glutamate and aspartate are the two main excitatory neurotransmitters in the somatosensory system and mediate transmission at various

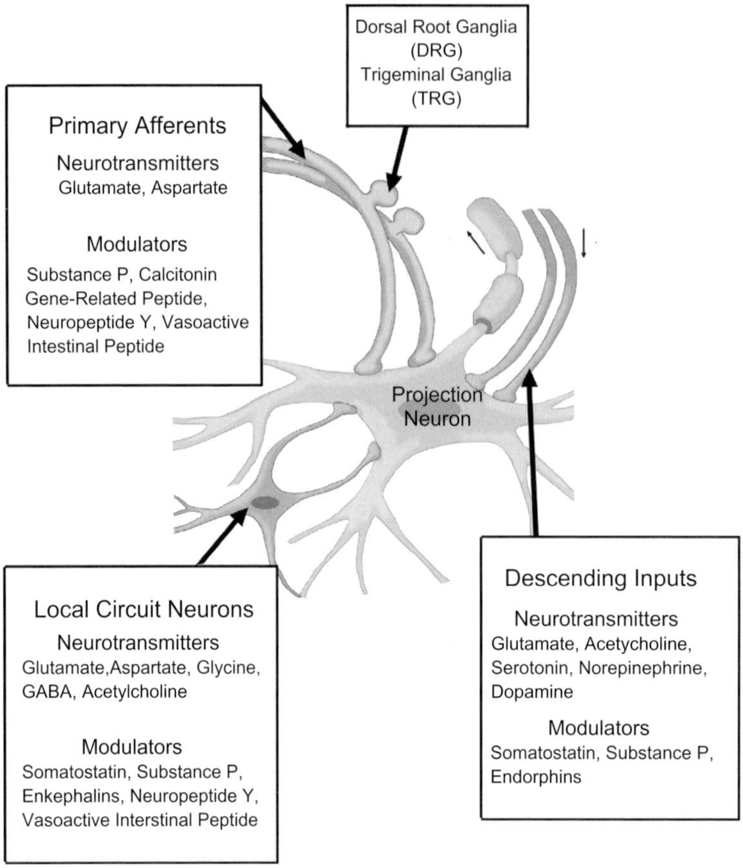

Figure 5.4. Neurotransmission in the spinal dorsal horn. This schematic summarizes the neurochemical pathways involved in somatosensory neurotransmission in the dorsal horn. Intrinsic sources of each transmitter are indicated by the labeled boxes. See plate section for color version.

levels of the afferent connections in the somatosensory system. The physiological functions of these excitatory amino acids largely depend on their combination with different receptor types or subtypes localized at various sites of the nervous system. Adenosine triphosphate (ATP) has been observed to excite dorsal horn neurons and thus may play a transmitter role in the somatosensory system.

Glycine and gamma-aminobutyric acid (GABA) are two primary inhibitory neurotransmitters of the somatosensory system. It has been shown that alterations in the functions of the inhibitory neurotransmitters may be particularly important in the development of neuropathic pain.[14] Several other molecules, such as norepinephrine, purine adenosine, acetylcholine, and serotonin, are considered to be inhibitory neurotransmitters under various conditions.

Neuropeptides also contribute to the signaling of somatosensory information by exerting excitatory and inhibitory effects. Substance P and neurokinin A are the excitatory neuropeptides in the somatosensory system. These peptides are especially concentrated in primary afferent fibers but are also present in intrinsic neurons of the spinal dorsal horn and thalamus. At the spinal level, only sustained activation of C-fiber nociceptors can induce the release of these peptides. The inhibitory neuropeptides, including somatostatin, enkephalin, and dynorphin, are present in both intrinsic neurons of the dorsal horn and in the descending fibers that connect the brainstem nuclei to the dorsal horn.

Hyperalgesia after tissue injury and inflammation

Hyperalgesia after injury or inflammation of cutaneous or deep tissue is characterized by a decrease in pain threshold, an increase in the painful response to suprathreshold stimuli, and ongoing pain. Hyperalgesia occurs not only at the site of injury (primary hyperalgesia) but also in the surrounding uninjured area (secondary hyperalgesia).[15]

Primary hyperalgesia and primary afferent sensitization

Primary hyperalgesia is mediated by sensitization of nociceptors,[16,17] characterized by a decrease in the pain threshold, an augmented response to suprathreshold stimuli, and ongoing spontaneous activity. Electrophysiological studies[17] have shown that C-fiber nociceptors displayed a decreased response after burn injury to glabrous skin, whereas Type I A-fiber nociceptors were markedly sensitized. In contrast, both C-fiber and A-fiber nociceptors in hairy skin are sensitized after injury.[18] In addition, mechanically insensitive afferents also play an important role in the mechanical hyperalgesia that occurs after either cutaneous or deep-tissue injury, as evidenced by their onset response to mechanical stimuli after inflammation.[19–21]

Secondary hyperalgesia and spinal neuron sensitization

Neurophysiological investigations have shown that the characteristics of secondary hyperalgesia are well explained by properties of dorsal horn neurons after injury.[10,22,23] The responses of spinothalamic cells to noxious stimuli correlate well with the pain ratings of humans to the same stimuli before and after the development of secondary hyperalgesia postinjury.[22,24] Most WDR neurons are sensitized by a variety of peripheral injuries, suggesting that this subtype of neurons is important for the detection of and response to tissue-damaging stimuli and in the generation of secondary hyperalgesia (Figure 5.5). NS cells may play a role in secondary hyperalgesia, although they sensitize less frequently than WDR neurons after peripheral injury.[7]

Neurons in higher central nervous system (CNS) areas also show enhanced response after injury. This may simply reflect changes that have taken place in the primary afferents and spinal cord neurons, but it is possible that a third or even fourth component contributes to secondary hyperalgesia.

Neurochemistry of primary afferent and central sensitization

Inflammatory mediators released from damaged tissues or activated immune and inflammatory cells result in sensitization of primary afferents.[25] Many of these mediators – such as bradykinin, serotonin, and histamine – can directly cause pain. Interestingly, specific primary afferent fibers are often sensitized by only one or a few of these substances, and specific substances often produce hyperalgesia to only a specific modality of sensation. For example, bradykinin produces thermal hyperalgesia only when injected to human skin,[25] whereas prostaglandins themselves do not cause pain or hyperalgesia but sensitize some fibers to other mediators.[26] Nevertheless, most mediators share a final common biochemical pathway (activation of adenyl cyclase) in their effects on primary afferent fibers.

Sensitization in the spinal dorsal horn is influenced by many of these chemical mediators that regulate sensory neurotransmission. However, the essential event in spinal sensitization is the facilitation of excitatory amino acid neurotransmission between primary afferent fibers and dorsal horn neurons by co-released neuropeptides.[10] For example, substance P and neurokinin A released from C-fibers in response to noxious stimulation can enhance the postsynaptic effects of glutamate and aspartate. Facilitation of responses at α-amino-3-hydroxyl-5-methyl-4-isoxazole-propionate (AMPA)-type glutamate receptors by tachykinin requires continuous activation of tachykinin receptors. This provides a neurochemical mechanism for the secondary hyperalgesia reversed by anesthesia at the site of injury. Conversely, facilitation of responses at *N*-methyl-D-aspartic acid (NMDA)-type glutamate receptors by tachykinins often lasts much longer after even a single coordinated coactivation of these receptors, thus providing a neurochemical mechanism for the secondary hyperalgesia not reversed by anesthesia of the injury site, such as punctuate hyperalgesia.

Hyperalgesia after nerve injury: neuropathic pain

Traumatic injury to nerve sometimes leads to neuropathic pain, a chronic pain state characterized by ongoing pain and hyperalgesia. In patients with neuropathic pain, pain is commonly evoked by activation of low-threshold mechanoreceptors (eg, light touch). Because central neurons develop an enhanced response to input from nonnociceptive afferents such as low-threshold mechanoreceptors, hyperalgesia after nerve injury is thought to result primarily from central sensitization. Intriguingly, in some patients the pain and hyperalgesia are dependent on sympathetic innervation of the affected area (sympathetically maintained pain),[27] whereas in others the pain is independent of the sympathetics.[28,29] Clinically, both of these conditions often present with similar signs and symptoms.

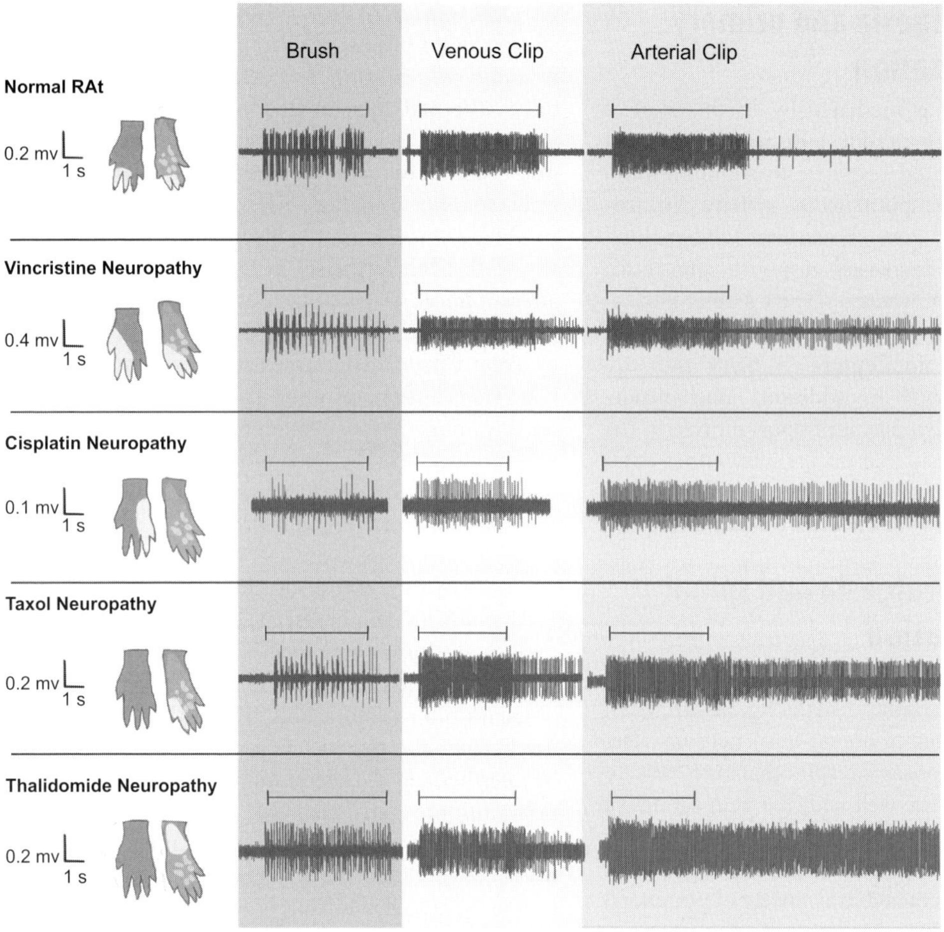

Figure 5.5. Analogue recordings of neuronal activity from the spinal cord. Hyperalgesic rats that had been treated for three to five days with vincristine or cisplatin exhibited excess neuronal after discharge in response to cutaneous stimuli. The times of each stimulus application are indicted by the lines over each trace, and the receptive field locations are shown in the drawings at the left. See plate section for color version.

Physiological changes after nerve injury

Peripheral nerves show an initial but transient bursting discharge after injury. This injury discharge appears to be a pivotal event that triggers many of the sequelae of nerve injury. Application of anesthetics or other neural blockers prior to nerve injury – which in laboratory studies includes ligation and transection – reduces the duration and intensity of the injury-induced hyperalgesia. After the initial injury discharges, the injured axons become quiet for a short period. Three to five days after nerve injury, spontaneous discharges develop mostly in small myelinated and some unmyelinated fibers, reaching a peak frequency approximately 14 days after injury and then slowly tapering to a low level that is sustained for many weeks. Spontaneous discharges arise from sites both in the neuroma at the cut ends of fibers and near the soma in the dorsal root ganglia.

Like primary afferents, CNS neurons discharge robustly after peripheral nerve transection, having a similar time course to that of primary afferents but with a three-to-five-day lag in the CNS. Most of the CNS cells that show functional changes after nerve transection are in the center of a deafferented zone without a defined peripheral receptive field. However, some of the cells at the margins of the deafferented zones show enhanced responses only to noxious stimuli. Similar changes in the spontaneous activity of dorsal horn cells was also shown after partial nerve injury, although most dorsal horn cells retained receptive fields.[30,31] Altered spontaneous discharges develop in the dorsal horn and dorsal column nuclei a week after peripheral nerve injury, whereas similar changes in the thalamus and cortex occur later.[32]

Approximately one to two weeks after injury, dorsal horn neurons that were originally deafferented regain some receptive fields, but these new fields typically have unusual sizes, varying from very large to very small, and are often split. The neurons with these new receptive fields respond only to low-intensity mechanical stimuli. In addition, many of the fields are somatotopically inappropriate, usually located in dermatomes neighboring the deafferented areas. The development of inappropriate somatotopy has also been reported to take place in the human thalamus after nerve injury[33] and in the cortex of experimental animals.[34–36]

Neurochemistry of neuropathic pain

The neurochemistry underlying neuropathic pain shares much in common with that underlying acute primary and secondary hyperalgesia, as reviewed above. Because damage to the nervous system is involved, degenerative and regenerative processes in both primary afferent and central neurons contribute to the altered neurochemistry underlying neuropathic pain.

The most obvious degenerative change in response to peripheral nerve damage is the loss of primary afferent drive to the spinal dorsal horn. The gate theory of pain control posits that inputs in large-diameter fibers inhibit spinal processing of signals from small-diameter nociceptors.[37] A disinhibition of pain signaling in cells that normally have convergent input could be envisaged as a consequence of nerve damage that preferentially affects large fiber inputs to the targeted cells. It has been thought that the transsynaptic loss of inhibitory neurons in the spinal cord after peripheral nerve injury also contribute to neuropathic pain.[38] A similar loss of inhibitory neurons in the thalamus may contribute to central pain in response to spinal cord injury.[39]

Subsequent to axonal or neuronal degeneration induced by injury, the surviving injured axons and neurons regrow and proliferate, respectively, to reconnect the deafferented neurons and peripheral targets. Because both injured and uninjured neurons will attempt to restore the lost connectivity to an original innervation target, competition between these two sets of growing neurons usually results in inappropriate connectivity within the CNS and their peripheral innervations targets. In addition, the spontaneous discharges in neurons when they grow increase signal traffic throughout the somatosensory axis. As a consequence of the altered gene expression inside the cells, changes occur in the phenotypes of neurons, including ion channels, neurotransmitter and neuropeptide receptors, surface growth-associated proteins, neurotransmitters, neuropeptides, and synaptic release.

Cytokines play important roles in the pathogenesis of neuropathic and inflammatory pain in several preclinical models. During the development of neuropathic pain, inflammatory cells infiltrate the site and release various cytokines (eg, interleukin [IL]-1 and tumor necrosis factor [TNF]-α), inducing altered neuronal function and neuropathic pain. Cytokines might produce pain through various functions, such as directly activating nociceptors, altering the trafficking of growth factors along nerve fibers, altering the function of glial cells, or inducing the degeneration of neurons and the retraction of cell processes.

Chemotherapy-induced neuropathy may be highly related to the induction of proinflammatory cytokines around nerve endings or in the CNS. Cytokines are released by macrophages, monocytes, tumor and endothelial cells, neurons, and glial cells in response to chemotherapy drugs. For example, cisplatin, paclitaxel, and both ionizing and ultraviolet radiation increase the levels of the cytokines interferon (IFN)-α, IFN-γ, TNF-α, IL-1, and IL-6 *in vitro.*[40] The pattern of cytokine gene induction, synthesis, and release induced by paclitaxel is identical to that induced by the endotoxin lipopolysaccharide. Paclitaxel, cisplatin, and vincristine directly activate the signaling pathway for nuclear factor kappa B (NF-κB), a key player in the inflammatory response and a common downstream factor after activation of lipopolysaccharide, IL-1, IL-6, IFN, or TNF-α.

Glial cells and neuropathic pain

Recently, glial cells – particularly microglia and astrocytes – have been recognized as playing an important role in the development of chronic pain. It is now firmly established that injury to peripheral nerve causes rapid and significant activation first of microglia and then of astrocytes in the spinal dorsal horn on the side of the injury.[41] Mechanical allodynia may be prevented or decreased by metabolic inhibitors specific to glial cells, such as fluorocitrate.[42,43] Further studies have revealed that glial cells express various types of neurotransmitter receptors, including ionotropic NMDA and non-NMDA receptors, metabotropic glutamate receptors, purinergic receptors, and substance P receptors. These receptors enable them to respond to neuronal signals. Activated microglia in the spinal cord express pain-related signaling molecules, such as chemokine receptor CX3CR1 and P2X4 purinoreceptors. Stimulation of microglia by activation of these receptors results in mechanical allodynia in animals. Conversely, pharmacological inhibition of CX3CR1 or P2X4 receptors reverses mechanical allodynia after peripheral nerve injury in animals.[44,45] Similarly important is microglial p38 mitogen-activated protein kinase (MAPK), which is rapidly activated after nerve injury, possibly through activation of the CX3CR1 receptor. Pharmacological inhibition of p38 MAPK attenuates neuropathic pain symptoms.[46,47] Glial cells also synthetize various inflammatory mediators, including proinflammatory cytokines (IL-1β, IL-6, and TNF-α), prostaglandin E2, nitric oxide, and nerve growth factor. It has been found that the proinflammatory cytokines are upregulated in the spinal cord in chronic pain conditions. Functional inhibition of these cytokines can attenuate persistent pain and enhance opioid analgesia.[48–50]

Most synapses in the CNS are ensheathed by astroglial processes. It has now been demonstrated that astrocytes release at least some neurotransmitters, such as glutamate, ATP, aspartate, and D-serine.[51] Astrocytes also express transporters to remove and sequester synaptically released neurotransmitters from the extracellular space. Synaptic transmission can thus be modified by manipulating the dynamics between the releasing and uptaking of neurotransmitters by astrocytes. Persistent activation of astrocytes has been found in numerous pain models. Pharmacological intervention with an astrocyte-specific toxin has shown a dose-dependent attenuation of mechanical allodynia.[52] Although the exact method by which astrocytes influence pain behavior is still unclear, it appears that activation of spinal astrocytes predominantly contributes to the maintenance of neuropathic pain, possibly involving the activation of c-Jun N-terminal kinase.[52]

Both myelinating and non-myelinating Schwann cells express receptors for certain cytokines, such as TNF, IFN, IL-1, and IL-6. Activation of these receptors triggers NF-κB and c-Jun pathways inside the cells, which in turn result in a cascade of downstream reactions that include downregulation of myelin synthesis, increased expression of the p75 NGF receptor, dedifferentiation, and proliferation.[53,54] The activated Schwann cells then begin to synthesize and release proinflammatory cytokines, affecting neighboring Schwann cells and thus closing a positive feedback loop that can sustain the neuropathy.

Conclusion

The physiological basis of pain sensation from skin can be summarized as a series of neuronal linkages that run from the skin to the spinal cord and then on to a number of more rostral centers located in the brainstem, midbrain, diencephalon, and cortex. Hyperalgesia after tissue or nerve damage occurs as a result of alterations in the usual manners in which both noxious and nonnoxious stimuli are processed by the networks of neurons and nonneuronal cells. It involves the routine processing of acute nociceptive stimuli and short-term and long-term sensitization of peripheral and central neurons. Each of these pain processes share signaling pathways but also have unique neurochemical and physiological components.

References

1. Merskey H, Bogduk N. *Classification of Chronic Pain: Descriptions of Chronic Pain Syndromes and Definitions of Pain Terms*, 2nd ed. Seattle: IASP Press, 1994.
2. Campbell JN, LaMotte RH. Latency to detection of first pain. *Brain Res* **266**(2):203–208, 1983.
3. Meyer RA, Campbell JN. Peripheral neural coding of pain sensation. *J H A P L Tech Digest* **2**:164–171, 1981.
4. Torebjörk HE, LaMotte RH, Robinson CJ. Peripheral neural correlates of magnitude of cutaneous pain and hyperalgesia: simultaneous recordings in humans of sensory judgments of pain and evoked responses in nociceptors with C-fibers. *J Neurophysiol* **51**(2): 325–339, 1984.
5. Willis WD. *The Pain System: the Neural Basis of Nociceptive Transmission in the Mammalian Nervous System*. Basel: Karger, 1985. Pain and Headache; vol. 8.
6. Willis WD, Coggeshall RE. *Sensory Mechanisms of the Spinal Cord*, 2nd ed. New York: Plenum Press, 1991.
7. Cata JP, Weng HR, Dougherty PM. Basic neurobiology of cancer pain. In: Fisch MJ, Burton AW, eds. *Cancer Pain Management*. New York: McGraw-Hill, Medical Pub. Division, 2007:57–74.
8. Rexed B. The cytoarchitectonic organization of the spinal cord in the cat. *J Comp Neurol* **96**(3):414–495, 1952.

9. Dougherty PM, Palecek J, Palecková V, Sorkin LS, Willis WD. The role of NMDA and non-NMDA excitatory amino acid receptors in the excitation of primate spinothalamic tract neurons by mechanical, thermal, chemical, and electrical stimuli. *J Neurosci* **12**:3025–3041, 1992.

10. Dougherty PM, Willis WD. Enhanced responses of spinothalamic tract neurons to excitatory amino acids accompany capsaicin-induced sensitization in the monkey. *J Neurosci* **12**(3):883–894, 1992.

11. Craig AD, Hunsley SJ. Morphine enhances the activity of thermoreceptive cold-specific lamina I spinothalamic neurons in the cat. *Brain Res* **558**(1):93–97, 1991.

12. Handwerker HO, Kobal G. Psychophysiology of experimentally induced pain. *Physiol Rev* **73**(3): 639–671, 1993.

13. Al-Chaer ED, Feng Y, Willis WD. A role for the dorsal column in nociceptive visceral input into the thalamus of primates. *J Neurophysiol* **79**(6):3143–3150, 1998.

14. Woolf CJ, Salter MW. Neuronal plasticity: increasing the gain in pain. *Science* **288**(5472):1765–1769, 2000.

15. Lewis T. *Pain*. New York: The Macmillan Company, 1942.

16. LaMotte RH, Thalhammer JG, Torebjörk HE, Robinson CJ. Peripheral neural mechanisms of cutaneous hyperalgesia following mild injury by heat. *J Neurosci* **2**(6):765–781, 1982.

17. Meyer RA, Campbell JN. Myelinated nociceptive afferents account for the hyperalgesia that follows a burn to the hand. *Science* **213**(4515):1527–1529, 1981.

18. LaMotte RH, Thalhammer JG, Robinson CJ. Peripheral neural correlates of magnitude of cutaneous pain and hyperalgesia: a comparison of neural events in monkey with sensory judgments in human. *J Neurophysiol* **50**(1):1–26, 1983.

19. Grigg P, Schaible HG, Schmidt RF. Mechanical sensitivity of group III and IV afferents from posterior articular nerve in normal and inflamed cat knee. *J Neurophysiol* **55**(4):635–643, 1986.

20. Davis KD, Meyer RA, Campbell JN. Chemosensitivity and sensitization of nociceptive afferents that innervate the hairy skin of monkey. *J Neurophysiol* **69**(4):1071–1081, 1993.

21. Schmelz M, Schmidt R, Ringkamp M, Handwerker HO, Torebjörk HE. Sensitization of insensitive branches of C nociceptors in human skin. *J Physiol* **480**(Pt 2):389–394, 1994.

22. Simone DA, Sorkin LS, Oh U, et al. Neurogenic hyperalgesia: central neural correlates in responses of spinothalamic tract neurons. *J Neurophysiol* **66**(1):228–246, 1991.

23. Woolf CJ. Evidence for a central component of post-injury pain hypersensitivity. *Nature* **306**(5944):686–688, 1983.

24. Dougherty PM, Willis WD, Lenz FA. Transient inhibition of responses to thermal stimuli of spinal sensory tract neurons in monkeys during sensitization by intradermal capsaicin. *Pain* **77**(2):129–136, 1998.

25. Meyer RA, Raja SN, Campbell JN. Neural mechanisms of primary hyperalgesia. In: Belmonte C, Cervero F, eds. *Neurobiology of Nociceptors*. Oxford: Oxford University Press, 1996:370–389.

26. Kress M, Reeh RW. Chemical excitation and sensitization in nociceptors. In: Belmonte C, Cervero F, eds. *Neurobiology of Nociceptors*. Oxford: Oxford University Press, 1996:258–297.

27. Roberts WJ, Elardo SM. Sympathetic activation of unmyelinated mechanoreceptors in cat skin. *Brain Res* **339**(1):123–125, 1985.

28. Campbell JN, Khan AA, Meyer RA, Raja SN. Responses to heat of C-fiber nociceptors in monkey are altered by injury in the receptive field but not by adjacent injury. *Pain* **32**(3):327–332, 1988.

29. Campbell JN, Raja SN, Meyer RA, Mackinnon SE. Myelinated afferents signal the hyperalgesia associated with nerve injury. *Pain* **32**(1):89–94, 1988.

30. Laird JM, Bennett GJ. An electrophysiological study of dorsal horn neurons in the spinal cord of rats with an experimental peripheral neuropathy. *J Neurophysiol* **69**(6):2072–2085, 1993.

31. Palecek J, Dougherty PM, Kim SH, et al. Responses of spinothalamic tract neurons to mechanical and thermal stimuli in an experimental model of peripheral neuropathy in primates. *J Neurophysiol* **68**(6):1951–1966, 1992.

32. Albe-Fessard DA, Rampin O. Neurophysiological studies in rats deafferented by dorsal root section. In: Nashold BS, Ovelmen-Levitt J, eds. *Deafferentation Pain Syndromes: Pathophysiology and Treatment*. New York: Raven Press, 1991:125–139. Advances in Pain Research and Therapy; vol. 19.

33. Lenz FA, Gracely RH, Baker FH, Richardson RT, Dougherty PM. Reorganization of sensory modalities evoked by microstimulation in region of the thalamic principal sensory nucleus in patients with pain due to nervous system injury. *J Comp Neurol* **399**(1):125–138, 1998.

34. Kaas JH, Merzenich MM, Killackey HP. The reorganization of somatosensory cortex following peripheral nerve damage in adult and developing mammals. *Annu Rev Neurosci* **6**:325–356, 1983.

35. Pons TP, Garraghty PE, Ommaya AK, Kaas JH, Taub E, Mishkin M. Massive cortical reorganization after sensory deafferentation in adult macaques. *Science* **252**(5014):1857–1860, 1991.

36. Wall JT, Cusick CG. Cutaneous responsiveness in primary somatosensory (S-I) hindpaw cortex before and after partial hindpaw deafferentation in adult rats. *J Neurosci* **4**(6):1499–1515, 1984.

37. Melzack R, Wall PD. Pain mechanisms: a new theory. *Science* **150**(699):971–979, 1965.

38. Bennett GJ, Kajander KC, Sahara Y, Iadarola MJ, Sugimoto T. Neurochemical and anatomical changes in the dorsal horn of rats with an experimental painful peripheral neuropathy. In: Cervero F, Bennett GJ, Headley PM, eds. *Processing of Sensory Information in the Superficial Dorsal Horn of the Spinal Cord.* New York: Plenum Press, 1989:1–23. NATO ASI Series: Series A, Life Sciences; vol. 176.

39. Ralston DD, Dougherty PM, Lenz FA, Weng HR, Vierck CJ, Ralston HJ. Plasticity of the inhibitory circuits of the primate ventrobasal thalamus following lesions of the somatosensory pathways. In: Devor M, Rowbotham MC, Wiesenfeld-Hallin Z, eds. *Proceedings of the 9th World Congress on Pain.* Seattle: IASP Press, 2000:427–434. Progress in Pain Research and Management; vol. 16.

40. Watkins LR, Maier SF. Glia: a novel drug discovery target for clinical pain. *Nat Rev Drug Discov* **2**(12):973–985, 2003.

41. Zhuang ZY, Gerner P, Woolf CJ, Ji RR. ERK is sequentially activated in neurons, microglia, and astrocytes by spinal nerve ligation and contributes to mechanical allodynia in this neuropathic pain model. *Pain* **114**(1–2):149–159, 2005.

42. Meller ST, Dykstra C, Grzybycki D, Murphy S, Gebhart GF. The possible role of glia in nociceptive processing and hyperalgesia in the spinal cord of the rat. *Neuropharmacology* **33**(11):1471–1478, 1994.

43. Watkins LR, Martin D, Ulrich P, Tracey KJ, Maier SF. Evidence for the involvement of spinal cord glia in subcutaneous formalin induced hyperalgesia in the rat. *Pain* **71**(3):225–235, 1997.

44. Inoue K, Tsuda M, Koizumi S. ATP receptors in pain sensation: involvement of spinal microglia and P2X(4) receptors. *Purinergic Signal* **1**(2):95–100, 2005.

45. Zhuang ZY, Kawasaki Y, Tan PH, Wen YR, Huang J, Ji RR. Role of the CX3CR1/p38 MAPK pathway in spinal microglia for the development of neuropathic pain following nerve injury-induced cleavage of fractalkine. *Brain Behav Immun* **21**(5):642–651, 2007.

46. Jin SX, Zhuang ZY, Woolf CJ, Ji RR. p38 mitogen-activated protein kinase is activated after a spinal nerve ligation in spinal cord microglia and dorsal root ganglion neurons and contributes to the generation of neuropathic pain. *J Neurosci* **23**(10):4017–4022, 2003.

47. Tsuda M, Mizokoshi A, Shigemoto-Mogami Y, Koizumi S, Inoue K. Activation of p38 mitogen-activated protein kinase in spinal hyperactive microglia contributes to pain hypersensitivity following peripheral nerve injury. *Glia* **45**(1):89–95, 2004.

48. Sweitzer S, Martin D, DeLeo JA. Intrathecal interleukin-1 receptor antagonist in combination with soluble tumor necrosis factor receptor exhibits an anti-allodynic action in a rat model of neuropathic pain. *Neuroscience* **103**(2):529–539, 2001.

49. Watkins LR, Hutchinson MR, Johnston IN, Maier SF. Glia: novel counter-regulators of opioid analgesia. *Trends Neurosci* **28**(12):661–669, 2005.

50. Milligan ED, Twining C, Chacur M, et al. Spinal glia and proinflammatory cytokines mediate mirror-image neuropathic pain in rats. *J Neurosci* **23**(3):1026–1040, 2003.

51. Milligan ED, Watkins LR. Pathological and protective roles of glia in chronic pain. *Nat Rev Neurosci* **10**(1):23–36, 2009.

52. Zhuang ZY, Wen YR, Zhang DR, et al. A peptide c-Jun N-terminal kinase (JNK) inhibitor blocks mechanical allodynia after spinal nerve ligation: respective roles of JNK activation in primary sensory neurons and spinal astrocytes for neuropathic pain development and maintenance. *J Neurosci* **26**(13):3551–3560, 2006.

53. Conti G, De Pol A, Scarpini E, et al. Interleukin-1 beta and interferon-gamma induce proliferation and apoptosis in cultured Schwann cells. *J Neuroimmunol* **124**(1–2):29–35, 2002.

54. Shubayev VI, Myers RR. Endoneurial remodeling by TNFalph- and TNFalpha-releasing proteases: A spatial and temporal co-localization study in painful neuropathy. *J Peripher Nerv Syst* 7(1):28–36, 2002.

Section 2 Chapter 6

Cancer Symptom Mechanisms and Models: Clinical and Basic Science

Cognitive dysfunction: is chemobrain real?

Christina A. Meyers and Jeffrey S. Wefel

Cognitive dysfunction is ubiquitous in patients with cancer. It can be caused by various factors, including: (1) cancer in the central nervous system (CNS); (2) cancers outside the CNS that have remote effects on brain function; (3) cancer treatment; (4) adjuvant medication(s); and/or (5) neurological disorders unrelated to cancer. Long seen as a problem in the pediatric population,[1,2] cognitive difficulties related to chemotherapy treatment are becoming recognized as a real phenomenon in adults as well.[3–5]

Clinical research studies have used various definitions of cognitive impairment and different methodologies for assessment and statistical analysis which contributes to the variability in findings across studies.[6] This chapter discusses both the preclinical and human studies that are advancing our knowledge of the effects of cancer and cancer treatment on brain function.

Chemobrain: a pattern of cognitive dysfunction

Adult patients with cancer who complain of "chemobrain" or "chemofog" typically report cognitive symptoms soon after they begin chemotherapy treatment. The most commonly described cognitive problems include difficulties with memory, attention, information-processing speed, and organization (ie, executive dysfunction). In patients with chemotherapy-related cognitive dysfunction, neuropsychological evaluation frequently uncovers difficulties sustaining focused attention that substantiate patient reports of episodes during which they have "spaced out" and lost their concentration. Deficits in working memory and executive function are also common and may correspond to patient reports of disorganization and difficulty multitasking. Measures of information-processing speed and fine motor function suggest further inefficiencies in cognitive and motor functioning. Memory testing is generally consistent with reduced learning efficiency and deficits in memory retrieval but not memory storage. This pattern of cognitive performance suggests an adverse effect on frontal subcortical networks.

For many patients, these symptoms persist even after therapy is finished. Unfortunately, it is not uncommon for patients and providers to treat these acute symptoms as an expected, and likely untreatable, side effect of treatment. Persistent cognitive symptoms are also a cause of considerable distress for individuals who are unable to return to their previous scholastic, occupational, or social activities, or who are able to do so only with significant additional mental effort. There is further concern that cancer and cancer therapies may increase an individual's susceptibility to late-emerging cognitive dysfunction.[7] Although this theory has yet to be conclusively established,[8,9] some preclinical animal studies have shown delayed effects of chemotherapy on brain anatomy and function.[10]

Studies of chemotherapy-related cognitive dysfunction

Although there is rich anecdotal and clinical evidence for the existence of chemobrain, the cognitive and neurobehavioral sequelae associated with chemotherapeutic agents have rarely been systematically studied. An emerging body of literature is beginning to characterize the cognitive and neurobehavioral sequelae of chemotherapeutic agents, suggesting that the incidence of chemotherapy-related cognitive dysfunction ranges from 15% to 70%.[5,11,12] However, few methodologically rigorous studies exist to guide clinical practice: most are retrospective, fail to incorporate assessments of pretreatment cognitive and neurobehavioral function, consist of small and heterogeneous patient samples that often received various chemotherapeutic regimens, lack appropriate control groups, and suffer from poor measurement selection. Further studies are warranted to address both the acute and long-term effects of these treatments.

Cancer Symptom Science: Measurement, Mechanisms, and Management, eds. Charles S. Cleeland, Michael J. Fisch, and Adrian J. Dunn. Published by Cambridge University Press.

Descriptive studies based on patient self-report

Most studies that have assessed self-report of cognitive function have shown little to no relationship with tested cognitive performance.[13–17] Self-reported cognitive impairment has tended to be correlated with depression and anxiety in these studies; however, findings that self-reported cognitive disturbance is related to fatigue or overall quality of life have been inconsistent, with some studies not finding a relationship[16] while others do find such a relationship.[14]

Imaging and electrophysiological studies

Recent functional imaging studies have revealed alterations in brain activity in long-term survivors of cancer compared with healthy controls. Using positron emission tomography (PET) during a memory-activation paradigm, Silverman et al.[18] found alterations in resting metabolism and cerebral blood flow in the basal ganglia, inferior frontal gyri, and cerebellums of women who had received chemotherapy 5–10 years earlier.

Anatomical studies have also found changes in cancer survivors treated with chemotherapy. Inagaki et al.[19] used magnetic resonance imaging (MRI) to compare the brains of breast cancer survivors who had been treated with adjuvant chemotherapy with the brains of healthy controls. One year after treatment, the cancer survivors were found to have smaller volumes of gray and white matter in multiple brain regions compared with the controls. This effect was not observed three years after treatment. The reduced brain volumes at one year correlated with poor cognitive performance. The loss of gray and white matter and atrophy of the hippocampus have also been reported in association with chemotherapeutic treatments.[20–22] However, these findings have not been replicated consistently,[23] suggesting the need for further investigation.

Electroencephalography was employed to study aspects of information processing in female breast cancer survivors who had been treated with chemotherapy four years earlier.[24] Survivors who received high-dose chemotherapy demonstrated decreased event-related potential P3 amplitudes relative to untreated controls, but P3 amplitudes were not significantly different from survivors treated with standard-dose chemotherapy.

Preclinical and animal studies

A number of studies have utilized preclinical and functional animal models of cognitive function to better understand the effects of antineoplastic treatment on the brain.

Radiation therapy

The cognitive decline seen in patients treated with brain irradiation has been hypothesized to be related to hippocampal dysfunction resulting from decreased hippocampal neurogenesis and proliferation, as well as to increased cell death.[25] Radiation has been shown to induce a defect in the proliferative capacity of the neural progenitor-cell population, while the remaining neural precursors adopt a nonneuronal glial fate.[26]

When grafted stem or precursor cells are implanted into an irradiated animal hippocampus, there is a marked reduction in the differentiation of these cells into neurons, indicating that the microenvironment affects neurogenesis. Interestingly, irradiation results in a marked increase in the number of activated microglia within these neurogenic zones.[25] This increase in activated microglia indicates chronic inflammation in response to cranial radiation exposure. The activated microglia secrete cytokines that negatively affect neural precursor cell proliferation and fate. Co-culture of activated microglia with neuronal precursors decrease *in vitro* neurogenesis. The key component mediating this effect is interleukin (IL)-6, which is produced by microglia.[27]

IL-6 induces both a decrease in cell survival and a decrease in the accumulation of neurons, likely due to reduced neuronal differentiation. Thus, IL-6 is a potent regulator of hippocampal neurogenesis by specifically promoting the development of astrocytes and oligodendrocytes at the expense of neurogenesis.

Chemotherapy

Winocur et al.[28] found that a combination of methotrexate and 5-fluorouracil (agents widely used to treat breast and colon cancers) induced impairments in tests of spatial memory and other cognitive tasks in mice. Reiriz et al.[29] reported transient acute memory impairment in mice treated with a single dose of cyclophosphamide. Crandall et al.[30] reported that long-term exposure to 13-cis-retinoic acid was associated with decreased neurogenesis and cell proliferation in the hippocampus and subventricular zone of young adult mice, as well as impaired spatial learning and memory.

Adriamycin has been demonstrated to increase oxidative stress in the brain, which may lead to cell dysfunction or death and thus may contribute to the symptoms of chemobrain.[31] Dietrich et al.[32] found that three widely used chemotherapy agents (carmustine, cisplatin, and cytosine arabinoside) were more toxic to CNS progenitor cells and nondividing oligodendrocytes than to multiple cancer cell lines *in vitro*. They also found that the agents caused increased cell death and decreased cell division in the subventricular zone, the dentate gyrus of the hippocampus, and the corpus callosum in mice. These effects were observed for weeks after completion of drug administration.

In contrast to these neurotoxic effects of chemotherapeutic agents, Lee et al.[33] found transient improvement in memory and synaptic plasticity in rats treated with cyclophosphamide or 5-fluorouracil eight weeks after administration, but not 29–42 weeks later, when the treated rats performed no differently than controls. Even so, enhanced long-term potentiation was seen in hippocampal slices obtained eight and 53 weeks after cyclophosphamide treatment, whereas slices taken during treatment showed impaired long-term potentiation. The variability in the results of these studies may be related to the time points of toxicity evaluation (acute vs. chronic), the agents under study, and the specific animal or preclinical model utilized.

A recent preclinical study showed that mice receiving therapeutic doses of methotrexate and 5-fluorouracil had altered whole-brain event-related potentials during a sensory gating task, as well as a hyperactive response to fear conditioning and reduced adaptation to novel objects, suggesting an additional component of emotional dysregulation.[34]

Most of the preclinical studies cited above involve investigations of hippocampal function and associated deficits in learning and memory. However, clinical studies of patients indicate that memory *retrieval*, not memory *consolidation*, is the primary deficit on formal neuropsychological assessments. This deficit suggests an effect on frontal-subcortical white matter.

In a ground-breaking preclinical study, Han et al.[10] found that therapeutic levels of 5-fluorouracil produced delayed damage to myelin associated with altered transcriptional regulation in oligodendrocytes and extensive myelin pathology. In contrast, CNS inflammation and vascular damage was acute and did not appear to be related to the delayed effects on myelin. Further, myelin damage was associated with increased latency of the auditory brainstem response *in vivo*. These findings support the notion of delayed white matter injury as a result of exposure to chemotherapy, consistent with the clinical syndrome observed in patients.

Risk factors and mechanisms of chemotherapy-induced cognitive dysfunction

Several factors appear to increase the risk of developing neurotoxicity associated with chemotherapy, including dose-intensive regimens, high concentrations of the agent or its metabolites resulting from impaired systemic clearance or pharmacogenetic modulation of drug pharmacokinetics,[35] and the additive or synergistic effects of multiagent chemotherapy. For patients with CNS malignancies, increased neurotoxicity may be related to the additive or synergistic effect of chemotherapy concurrent with or subsequent to cerebral irradiation,[36,37] intra-arterial administration with blood–brain barrier disruption after radiation therapy,[38] or intrathecal administration.[36,39–43] The mechanisms by which these chemotherapeutic agents affect CNS function have been reported to occur through both direct and indirect pathways. It is also likely that specific mechanisms are influential at various time points in the course of an emerging neurotoxicity.

Metabolic abnormalities

Many chemotherapeutic agents can cause systemic metabolic perturbations that may contribute to alterations in cognitive and neurobehavioral function. Both high and intermediate doses of 5-fluorouracil have been reported to cause encephalopathy in association with hyperammonemia. With normalization of ammonia levels, the encephalopathy resolves.[44]

Methotrexate, a folate antagonist, has been reported to decrease dihydrofolate reductase, leading to deficiency in *S*-adenosylmethionine (SAM). SAM deficiency has been associated with demyelination,[45] and polymorphisms of genes involved in methionine metabolism appear to place individuals at greater risk for this neurotoxicity.[46] Methotrexate has also been reported to lead to hyperhomocysteinemia, a metabolic syndrome of high levels of neurotransmitters, homocysteic acid, cysteine sulfinic acid, homocysteine sulfonic acid, and toxic levels of adenosine. These abnormalities may lead to mineralizing microangiopathy in the white matter, *N*-methyl-D-aspartate-mediated excitotoxicity, and alterations in brain monoamines (ie, norepinephrine, dopamine, serotonin).[22,47,48]

Encephalopathy has also been reported in association with the syndrome of inappropriate antidiuretic hormone secretion secondary to intrathecal vincristine or cyclophosphamide treatment,[49] hyperglycemia secondary to L-asparaginase, streptozoscin, or corticosteroid use, and salt-wasting nephropathy due to cisplatin.[50]

Hormonal abnormalities

Chemotherapy-induced menopause[51,52] and hormone ablation therapy for both women[53,54] and men[55,56] have been implicated in the development of cognitive dysfunction. In women, the incidence of ovarian failure due to chemotherapy is variable (20% to 100%) and depends upon patient age, dosage, type of therapy, and prior or concurrent use of radiation therapy.[52]

Estrogen receptors have been found in the hypothalamus, anterior pituitary, amygdala, and CA1 region of the hippocampus.[57] The mechanisms by which estrogen benefits cognitive function include: (1) increasing cholinergic activity through its actions on choline acetyltransferase; (2) maintaining dendritic spine density on CA1 pyramidal cells of the hippocampus; (3) facilitating the induction of long-term potentiation in the hippocampus; (4) increasing serotonergic and cholinergic activity; (5) altering lipoprotein levels; and (6) decreasing the risk of cerebral ischemia.[58] It remains unclear whether the cognitive and neurobehavioral effects of hormonal manipulations arise through the estrogen receptors (including aromatization of androgens to estradiol in men) or via androgen receptors.

Inflammatory response

Inflammatory cytokine activation may contribute to the cognitive and neurobehavioral sequelae associated with chemotherapy. Several studies have reported increases in IL-1β, IL-6, IL-8, IL-10, interferon (IFN)-γ, tumor necrosis factor (TNF)-α, and granulocyte–monocyte colony-stimulating factor, all of which are associated with various schedules of paclitaxel, docetaxel, etoposide, and carboplatin.[59–61] The ability of distinct chemotherapeutic agents to induce similar inflammatory cytokine activity has been hypothesized to occur through the common activation of p38 mitogen-activated protein kinase.[62] The appearance of cancer-related symptom clusters after exposure to various cytokines has also been attributed to activation of nuclear factor κB.[63] Cytokines such as IFN-α are themselves given therapeutically for certain cancers and other diseases. The neurotoxicities associated with these agents, including cognitive dysfunction, depression, and fatigue, are considerable and often dose-limiting.[64,65]

Anemia and fatigue

Across all classes of chemotherapeutic agents, anemia has been estimated to occur in up to 80% of patients[66] and is a well-known side effect of myelosuppressive chemotherapies. Anemia may cause cerebral hypoxia due to diminished circulating erythrocyte levels and hemoglobin concentrations[67] and is associated with patient reports of reduced quality of life, fatigue, and cognitive dysfunction.[68,69]

Secondary malignancies and organ toxicities

Other late-emerging side effects that may be associated with cognitive and neurobehavioral dysfunction include the development of secondary malignancies that require further cancer treatment (eg, leukemia and myelodysplastic syndrome).[70] In addition, treatment-related late injury to essential organs such as the heart (eg, myopericarditis, arrhythmia, pericardial effusion, cardiomyopathy, congestive heart failure)[71–74] and lungs[75] are increasingly of concern for long-term survivors.

Pharmacogenetic factors

Clinically, and in most research studies to date, cognitive and neurobehavioral dysfunction has been found to occur only in a subgroup of patients. This finding has provoked interest in clarifying the pharmacogenetic differences that may underlie an individual's vulnerability to these side effects. Polymorphisms that alter the pharmacodynamics of chemotherapeutic agents may place individuals at greater risk through increased exposure to potentially toxic agents secondary to reduced detoxification and/or increased permeability of agents across the blood–brain barrier.[76–78] In children with leukemia treated with methotrexate regimens with or without cranial radiation, polymorphisms of genes modulating the folate pathway have been associated with diminished intelligence.[79] The relationship between polymorphisms in genes responsible for various repair processes (eg, apolipoprotein E) and the development of cognitive dysfunction also are receiving attention.[80,81] Recent studies have examined the relationship between brain-derived neurotrophic factor and memory[82] and between catechol-*O*-methyltransferase and executive function.[83] There is evidence that polymorphisms in these genes are related to differences in cognitive function in healthy individuals. It is unknown whether these same polymorphisms confer an additional risk to an individual exposed to a potentially neurotoxic treatment.

Interventions

Chemotherapy and immunotherapy are necessary components in the management and eradication of many types of cancer. Although not all patients will experience treatment-related neurotoxicity, a subpopulation of patients will suffer from cognitive symptoms that are both distressing and disruptive. There is opportunity and a very real need to explore therapies that may prevent negative side effects or minimize the impact and extent of symptoms that are already present. Ideally, these interventions should be tailored to the symptom (eg, anemia, durable fatigue, memory retrieval deficit) and based on the hypothesized mechanism. Whereas determining the nature of the symptom is often feasible, our understanding of the etiological mechanisms underlying these symptoms is frequently limited.

Clinical experience and research has informed clinicians about the risks involved with certain regimens and administration schedules, as outlined above, such that the occurrence of neurotoxicities has been reduced even as adequate cancer control is maintained.[41,49] In cases where a specific mechanism underlying the neurotoxicity has been characterized, targeted treatment strategies have been explored. For example, treatment with naltrexone (a μ-opioid receptor antagonist) was effective in relieving neurotoxic side effects in seven of nine patients undergoing interferon treatment for hematological malignancies.[84] Musselman et al.[85] demonstrated the benefit of pretreatment with paroxetine (eg, selective serotonin reuptake inhibitor) in minimizing depression in melanoma patients receiving interferon treatment.

Despite such findings, empirically supported therapies for persistent cognitive and neurobehavioral dysfunction are limited. Stimulant therapies have proven effective in treating the cognitive dysfunction that is common in cancer patients.[86] Various pharmacological interventions commonly used to treat non-cancer diseases affecting cognitive function are being explored.[87] Cognitive and behavioral intervention strategies used as part of traditional rehabilitation with stroke and traumatic brain injury survivors may also be employed. These interventions often focus on compensatory strategy training, stress management, energy conservation, and psychoeducation.

Future directions

As our understanding of the pathogenesis of cognitive dysfunction in cancer patients advances, targeted interventions based upon those mechanisms will be developed. For instance, as suggested above, there is growing evidence that cognitive dysfunction and other adverse cancer-related symptoms may result in part from a cancer-induced or cancer treatment-induced inflammatory response (ie, the induction of inflammatory cytokines).[63,88] Thus, modulating cytokines and their receptors may ameliorate or protect against the development of these symptoms. Research into the potential benefit of anti-inflammatory agents or specific cytokine antagonists in conjunction with standard rehabilitative approaches is just beginning and may hold great promise. In fact, a recent preclinical study found that rats given chemotherapy with adriamycin and cytoxan showed a significant decline in memory as assessed by a passive avoidance test, but that the memory dysfunction could be completely prevented by concomitant administration of an antioxidant.[89]

Another potential treatment approach would be to stimulate neurogenesis for stem cells normally residing in the CNS. A recent study of tissue from patients undergoing tumor resection provided exciting evidence of stem cells in the subventricular zone.[90] This work has potential implications for developing neuroregenerative approaches. However, it is not known how the functionality of neural stem cells is affected by cancer treatment to the brain, as this may negatively affect the microenvironment as described above.[25] Efforts to prevent delayed demyelination associated with certain chemotherapy agents may be a tenable neuroprotective strategy.[10]

As primary therapy becomes more effective and more patients experience long-term remissions, assessment of neurobehavioral function and symptoms and establishing effective treatment strategies will gain even greater importance.

References

1. Butler RW, Haser JK. Neurocognitive effects of treatment for childhood cancer. *Ment Retard Dev Disabil Res Rev* **12**(3):184–191, 2006.
2. Alvarez JA, Scully RE, Miller TL, et al. Long-term effects of treatments for childhood cancers. *Curr Opin Pediatr* **19**(1):23–31, 2007.

3. Hurria A, Rosen C, Hudis C, et al. Cognitive function of older patients receiving adjuvant chemotherapy for breast cancer: a pilot prospective longitudinal study. *J Am Geriatr Soc* **54**(6):925–931, 2006.
4. Schagen SB, Muller MJ, Boogerd W, Mellenbergh GJ, van Dam FSAM. Change in cognitive function after chemotherapy: a prospective longitudinal study in breast cancer patients. *J Natl Cancer Inst* **98**(23):1742–1745, 2006.
5. Wefel JS, Lenzi R, Theriault RL, Davis RN, Meyers CA. The cognitive sequelae of standard-dose adjuvant chemotherapy in women with breast carcinoma: results of a prospective, randomized, longitudinal trial. *Cancer* **100**(11):2292–2299, 2004.
6. Vardy J, Wefel JS, Ahles T, Tannock IF, Schagen SB. Cancer and cancer-therapy related cognitive dysfunction: an international perspective from the Venice cognitive workshop. *Ann Oncol* **19**(4):623–629, 2008.
7. Heflin LH, Meyerowitz BE, Hall P, et al. Cancer as a risk factor for long-term cognitive deficits and dementia. *J Natl Cancer Inst* **97**(11):854–856, 2005.
8. Roe CM, Behrens MI, Xiong C, Miller JP, Morris JC. Alzheimer disease and cancer. *Neurology* **64**(5): 895–898, 2005.
9. Wefel JS, Meyers CA. Cancer as a risk factor for dementia: a house built on shifting sand. *J Natl Cancer Inst* **97**(11):788–789, 2005.
10. Han R, Yang YM, Dietrich J, Luebke A, Mayer-Pröschel M, Noble M. Systemic 5-fluorouracil treatment causes a syndrome of delayed myelin destruction in the central nervous system. *J Biol* 7(4):12.1–12.22, 2008.
11. Shilling V, Jenkins V, Morris R, Deutsch G, Bloomfield D. The effects of adjuvant chemotherapy on cognition in women with breast cancer: preliminary results of an observational longitudinal study. *Breast* **14**(2): 142–150, 2005.
12. Moleski M. Neuropsychological, neuroanatomical, and neurophysiological consequences of CNS chemotherapy for acute lymphoblastic leukemia. *Arch Clin Neuropsychol* **15**(7):603–630, 2000.
13. Hermelink K, Untch M, Lux MP, et al. Cognitive function during neoadjuvant chemotherapy for breast cancer: results of a prospective, multicenter, longitudinal study. *Cancer* **109**(9):1905–1913, 2007.
14. Jacobs SR, Jacobsen PB, Booth-Jones M, Wagner LI, Anasetti C. Evaluation of the functional assessment of cancer therapy cognitive scale with hematopoietic stem cell transplant patients. *J Pain Symptom Manage* **33**(1):13–23, 2007.
15. Vardy J, Wong K, Yi QL, et al. Assessing cognitive function in cancer patients. *Support Care Cancer* **14**(11):1111–1118, 2006.
16. Mehnert A, Scherwath A, Schirmer L, et al. The association between neuropsychological impairment, self-perceived cognitive deficits, fatigue and health related quality of life in breast cancer survivors following standard adjuvant versus high-dose chemotherapy. *Patient Educ Couns* **66**(1):108–118, 2007.
17. Jenkins V, Shilling V, Deutsch G, et al. A 3-year prospective study of the effects of adjuvant treatments on cognition in women with early stage breast cancer. *Br J Cancer* **94**(6):828–834, 2006.
18. Silverman DH, Dy CJ, Castellon SA, et al. Altered frontocortical, cerebellar, and basal ganglia activity in adjuvant-treated breast cancer survivors 5–10 years after chemotherapy. *Breast Cancer Res Treat* **103**(3):303–311, 2007.
19. Inagaki M, Yoshikawa E, Matsuoka Y, et al. Smaller regional volumes of brain gray and white matter demonstrated in breast cancer survivors exposed to adjuvant chemotherapy. *Cancer* **109**(1):146–156, 2007.
20. Schneiderman B. Hippocampal volumes smaller in chemotherapy patients. *Lancet Oncol* **5**(4):202, 2004.
21. Saykin AJ, Ahles TA, McDonald BC. Mechanisms of chemotherapy-induced cognitive disorders: neuropsychological, pathophysiological, and neuroimaging perspectives. *Semin Clin Neuropsychiatry* **8**(4):201–216, 2003.
22. Madhyastha S, Somayaji SN, Rao MS, Nalini K, Bairy KL. Hippocampal brain amines in methotrexate-induced learning and memory deficit. *Can J Physiol Pharmacol* **80**(11):1076–1084, 2002.
23. Yoshikawa E, Matsuoka Y, Inagaki M, et al. No adverse effects of adjuvant chemotherapy on hippocampal volume in Japanese breast cancer survivors. *Breast Cancer Res Treat* **92**(1):81–84, 2005.
24. Kreukels BP, Schagen SB, Ridderinkhof KR, et al. Effects of high-dose and conventional-dose adjuvant chemotherapy on long-term cognitive sequelae in patients with breast cancer: an electrophysiologic study. *Clin Breast Cancer* **7**(1):67–78, 2006.
25. Monje ML, Mizumatsu S, Fike JR, Palmer TD. Irradiation induces neural precursor-cell dysfunction. *Nat Med* **8**(9):955–962, 2002.
26. Dietrich J, Monje M, Wefel J, Meyers C. Clinical patterns and biological correlates of cognitive dysfunction associated with cancer therapy. *Oncologist* **13**(12):1285–1295, 2008.
27. Monje ML, Toda H, Palmer TD. Inflammatory blockade restores adult hippocampal neurogenesis. *Science* **302**(5651):1760–1765, 2003.
28. Winocur G, Vardy J, Binns MA, Kerr L, Tannock I. The effects of the anti-cancer drugs, methotrexate and 5-fluorouracil, on cognitive function in mice. *Pharmacol Biochem Behav* **85**(1):66–75, 2006.

29. Reiriz AB, Reolon GK, Preissler T, et al. Cancer chemotherapy and cognitive function in rodent models: memory impairment induced by cyclophosphamide in mice [letter]. *Clin Cancer Res* **12**(16):5000–5001, 2006.

30. Crandall J, Sakai Y, Zhang J, et al. 13-cis-retinoic acid suppresses hippocampal cell division and hippocampal-dependent learning in mice. *Proc Natl Acad Sci U S A* **101**(14):5111–5116, 2004.

31. Joshi G, Sultana R, Tangpong J, et al. Free radical mediated oxidative stress and toxic side effects in brain induced by the anti cancer drug adriamycin: insight into chemobrain. *Free Radic Res* **39**(11):1147–1154, 2005.

32. Dietrich J, Han R, Yang Y, Mayer-Pröschel M, Noble M. CNS progenitor cells and oligodendrocytes are targets of chemotherapeutic agents in vitro and in vivo. *J Biol* **5**(7):22.1–22.23, 2006.

33. Lee GD, Longo DL, Wang Y, et al. Transient improvement in cognitive function and synaptic plasticity in rats following cancer chemotherapy. *Clin Cancer Res* **12**(1):198–205, 2006.

34. Gandal MJ, Ehrlichman RS, Rudnick ND, Siegel SJ. A novel electrophysiological model of chemotherapy-induced cognitive impairments in mice. *Neuroscience* **157**(1):95–104, 2008.

35. Shah RR. Mechanistic basis of adverse drug reactions: the perils of inappropriate dose schedules. *Expert Opin Drug Saf* **4**(1):103–128, 2005.

36. Sul JK, DeAngelis LM. Neurologic complications of cancer chemotherapy. *Semin Oncol* **33**(3):324–332, 2006.

37. Sheline GE, Wara WM, Smith V. Therapeutic irradiation and brain injury. *Int J Radiat Oncol Biol Phys* **6**(9):1215–1228, 1980.

38. Jahnke K, Kraemer DF, Knight KR, et al. Intraarterial chemotherapy and osmotic blood-brain barrier disruption for patients with embryonal and germ cell tumors of the central nervous system. *Cancer* **112**(3):581–588, 2008.

39. Jansen C, Miaskowski C, Dodd M, Dowling G, Kramer J. Potential mechanisms for chemotherapy-induced impairments in cognitive function. *Oncol Nurs Forum* **32**(6):1151–1163, 2005.

40. Taphoorn MJB, Klein M. Cognitive deficits in adult patients with brain tumours. *Lancet Neurol* **3**(3): 159–168, 2004.

41. Keime-Guibert F, Napolitano M, Delattre JY. Neurological complications of radiotherapy and chemotherapy. *J Neurol* **245**(11):695–708, 1998.

42. Delattre JY, Posner JB. Neurological complications of chemotherapy and radiation therapy. In: Aminoff MJ, ed. *Neurology and General Medicine: the Neurological Aspects of Medical Disorders*. New York: Churchill Livingstone, 1995:421–445.

43. Weiss RB, Vogelzang NJ. Miscellaneous toxicities. In: DeVita VT, Hellman S, Rosenberg SA, eds. *Cancer, Principles & Practice of Oncology*. Philadelphia: J. B. Lippincott Company, 1993:2349–2358.

44. Kim YA, Chung HC, Choi HJ, Rha SY, Seong JS, Jeung HC. Intermediate dose 5-fluorouracil-induced encephalopathy. *Jpn J Clin Oncol* **36**(1):55–59, 2006.

45. Shuper A, Stark B, Kornreich L, et al. Methotrexate treatment protocols and the central nervous system: significant cure with significant neurotoxicity. *J Child Neurol* **15**(9):573–580, 2000.

46. Linnebank M, Pels H, Kleczar N, et al. MTX-induced white matter changes are associated with polymorphisms of methionine metabolism. *Neurology* **64**(5):912–913, 2005.

47. Haykin ME, Gorman M, van Hoff J, Fulbright RK, Baehring JM. Diffusion-weighted MRI correlates of subacute methotrexate-related neurotoxicity. *J Neurooncol* **76**(2):153–157, 2006.

48. Quinn CT, Kamen BA. A biochemical perspective of methotrexate neurotoxicity with insight on nonfolate rescue modalities. *J Investig Med* **44**(9):522–530, 1996.

49. Forman AD, Meyers CA, Levin VA. Neurotoxic effects of pharmaceutical agents IV: cancer chemotherapeutic agents. In: Dobbs MR, ed. *Clinical Neurotoxicology: Syndromes, Substances, Environments*. Philadelphia PA: Saunders/Elsevier, 2009:372–381.

50. Gilbert MR, Armstrong TS. Neurotoxicities. In: Kirkwood JM, Lotze MT, Yasko JM, eds. *Current Cancer Therapeutics*. Philadelphia: Current Medicine, 1996:364–371.

51. Knobf MT. Reproductive and hormonal sequelae of chemotherapy in women: Premature menopause and impaired fertility can result, effects that are especially disturbing to young women. *Am J Nurs* **106** (3 Suppl):60–65, 2006.

52. Molina JR, Barton DL, Loprinzi CL. Chemotherapy-induced ovarian failure: manifestations and management. *Drug Saf* **28**(5):401–416, 2005.

53. Eberling JL, Wu C, Tong-Turnbeaugh R, Jagust WJ. Estrogen- and tamoxifen-associated effects on brain structure and function. *Neuroimage* **21**(1):364–371, 2004.

54. Jenkins V, Shilling V, Fallowfield L, Howell A, Hutton S. Does hormone therapy for the treatment of breast cancer have a detrimental effect on memory and cognition? A pilot study. *Psychooncology* **13**(1):61–66, 2004.

55. Mottet N, Prayer-Galetti T, Hammerer P, Kattan MW, Tunn U. Optimizing outcomes and quality of life in the hormonal treatment of prostate cancer. *BJU Int* **98**(1):20–27, 2006.

56. Green HJ, Pakenham KI, Headley BC, et al. Altered cognitive function in men treated for prostate cancer

with luteinizing hormone-releasing hormone analogues and cyproterone acetate: a randomized controlled trial. *BJU Int* **90**(4):427–432, 2002.

57. McEwen BS, Alves SE. Estrogen actions in the central nervous system. *Endocr Rev* **20**(3):279–307, 1999.
58. Yaffe K, Sawaya G, Lieberburg I, Grady D. Estrogen therapy in postmenopausal women: effects on cognitive function and dementia. *JAMA* **279**(9): 688–695, 1998.
59. Pusztai L, Mendoza TR, Reuben JM, et al. Changes in plasma levels of inflammatory cytokines in response to paclitaxel chemotherapy. *Cytokine* **25**(3):94–102, 2004.
60. Tsavaris N, Kosmas C, Vadiaka M, Kanelopoulos P, Boulamatsis D. Immune changes in patients with advanced breast cancer undergoing chemotherapy with taxanes. *Br J Cancer* **87**(1):21–27, 2002.
61. Penson RT, Kronish K, Duan Z, et al. Cytokines IL-1beta, IL-2, IL-6, IL-8, MCP-1, GM-CSF and TNFalpha in patients with epithelial ovarian cancer and their relationship to treatment with paclitaxel. *Int J Gynecol Cancer* **10**(1):33–41, 2000.
62. Wood LJ, Nail LM, Gilster A, Winters KA, Elsea CR. Cancer chemotherapy-related symptoms: evidence to suggest a role for proinflammatory cytokines. *Oncol Nurs Forum* **33**(3):535–542, 2006.
63. Lee BN, Dantzer R, Langley KE, et al. A cytokine-based neuroimmunologic mechanism of cancer-related symptoms. *Neuroimmunomodulation* **11**(5):279–292, 2004.
64. Scheibel RS, Valentine AD, O'Brien S, Meyers CA. Cognitive dysfunction and depression during treatment with interferon-alpha and chemotherapy. *J Neuropsychiatry Clin Neurosci* **16**(2):185–191, 2004.
65. Valentine AD, Meyers CA, Kling MA, Richelson E, Hauser P. Mood and cognitive side effects of interferon-alpha therapy. *Semin Oncol* **25** (1 Suppl 1):39–47, 1998.
66. Cunningham RS. Anemia in the oncology patient: cognitive function and cancer. *Cancer Nurs* **26** (6 Suppl):38S–42S, 2003.
67. Birgegård G, Aapro MS, Bokemeyer C, et al. Cancer-related anemia: pathogenesis, prevalence and treatment. *Oncology***68**(Suppl 1):3–11, 2005.
68. O'Shaughnessy JA, Vukelja SJ, Holmes FA, et al. Feasibility of quantifying the effects of epoetin alfa therapy on cognitive function in women with breast cancer undergoing adjuvant or neoadjuvant chemotherapy. *Clin Breast Cancer* **5**(6):439–446, 2005.
69. Groopman JE, Itri LM. Chemotherapy-induced anemia in adults: incidence and treatment. *J Natl Cancer Inst* **91**(19):1616–1634, 1999.
70. Shapiro CL, Recht A. Side effects of adjuvant treatment of breast cancer. *N Engl J Med* **344**(26):1997–2008, 2001.
71. Jensen BV. Cardiotoxic consequences of anthracycline-containing therapy in patients with breast cancer. *Semin Oncol* **33**(3 Suppl 8):S15–S21, 2006.
72. Johnson SA. Anthracycline-induced cardiotoxicity in adult hematologic malignancies. *Semin Oncol* **33** (3 Suppl 8):S22–S27, 2006.
73. Lipshultz SE. Exposure to anthracyclines during childhood causes cardiac injury. *Semin Oncol* **33** (3 Suppl 8):S8–S14, 2006.
74. Yahalom J, Portlock CS. Cardiac toxicity. In: DeVita VT, Lawrence TS, Rosenberg SA, eds. *DeVita, Hellman, and Rosenberg's Cancer: Principles & Practice of Oncology*. Philadelphia: Wolters Kluwer/Lippincott Williams & Wilkins, 2008:2678–2688.
75. Abratt RP, Morgan GW, Silvestri G, Willcox P. Pulmonary complications of radiation therapy. *Clin Chest Med* **25**(1):167–177, 2004.
76. Largillier R, Etienne-Grimaldi MC, Formento JL, et al. Pharmacogenetics of capecitabine in advanced breast cancer patients. *Clin Cancer Res* **12**(18):5496–5502, 2006.
77. McAllister TW, Ahles TA, Saykin AJ, et al. Cognitive effects of cytotoxic cancer chemotherapy: predisposing risk factors and potential treatments. *Curr Psychiatry Rep* **6**(5):364–371, 2004.
78. Okcu MF, Selvan M, Wang LE, et al. Glutathione S-transferase polymorphisms and survival in primary malignant glioma. *Clin Cancer Res* **10**(8):2618–2625, 2004.
79. Krajinovic M, Robaey P, Chiasson S, et al. Polymorphisms of genes controlling homocysteine levels and IQ score following the treatment for childhood ALL. *Pharmacogenomics* **6**(3):293–302, 2005.
80. Ahles TA, Saykin AJ, Noll WW, et al. The relationship of APOE genotype to neuropsychological performance in long-term cancer survivors treated with standard dose chemotherapy. *Psychooncology* **12**(6):612–619, 2003.
81. Chen Y, Lomnitski L, Michaelson DM, Shohami E. Motor and cognitive deficits in apolipoprotein E-deficient mice after closed head injury. *Neuroscience* **80**(4):1255–1262, 1997.
82. Egan MF, Kojima M, Callicott JH, et al. The BDNF val66met polymorphism affects activity-dependent secretion of BDNF and human memory and hippocampal function. *Cell* **112**(2):257–269, 2003.
83. Egan MF, Goldberg TE, Kolachana BS, et al. Effect of COMT Val108/158 Met genotype on frontal lobe

function and risk for schizophrenia. *Proc Natl Acad Sci U S A* **98**(12):6917–6922, 2001.

84. Valentine AD, Meyers CA, Talpaz M. Treatment of neurotoxic side effects of interferon-alpha with naltrexone. *Cancer Invest* **13**(6):561–566, 1995.

85. Musselman DL, Lawson DH, Gumnick JF, et al. Paroxetine for the prevention of depression induced by high-dose interferon alfa. *N Engl J Med* **344**(13):961–966, 2001.

86. Meyers CA, Weitzner MA, Valentine AD, Levin VA. Methylphenidate therapy improves cognition, mood, and function of brain tumor patients. *J Clin Oncol* **16**(7):2522–2527, 1998.

87. Barton D, Loprinzi C. Novel approaches to preventing chemotherapy-induced cognitive dysfunction in breast cancer: the art of the possible. *Clin Breast Cancer***3**(Suppl 3):S121–S127, 2002.

88. Meyers CA, Albitar M, Estey E. Cognitive impairment, fatigue, and cytokine levels in patients with acute myelogenous leukemia or myelodysplastic syndrome. *Cancer* **104**(4):788–793, 2005.

89. Konat GW, Kraszpulski M, James I, Zhang HT, Abraham J. Cognitive dysfunction induced by chronic administration of common cancer chemotherapeutics in rats. *Metab Brain Dis* **23**(3):325–333, 2008.

90. Sanai N, Tramontin AD, Quiñones-Hinojosa A, et al. Unique astrocyte ribbon in adult human brain contains neural stem cells but lacks chain migration. *Nature* **427**(6976):740–744, 2004.

Section 2 Chapter 7

Cancer Symptom Mechanisms and Models: Clinical and Basic Science

Cognitive impairment: basic science

Perry N. Fuchs, Jessica A. Boyette-Davis, and Adrian J. Dunn

Cognitive dysfunction is increasingly recognized by practitioners and researchers as one of the symptoms that cause great distress for patients with cancer, their families, and their health care providers. The prevalence of cognitive impairment varies and is based on several factors, including the amount of time the patient has had cancer, the type of cancer, the length of treatment, and the treatment used, and is estimated to affect anywhere between 17% and 75% of patients with cancer.[1] In a series of experiments, Wefel et al.[2,3] noted signs of cognitive impairment in 33% to 35% of cancer patients prior to treatment with chemotherapy and in approximately 61% of patients after chemotherapeutic treatment.

Findings such as these, coupled with the fact that treatment for cancer begins soon after diagnosis, has led to the characterization of chemotherapy-related cognitive impairments as "chemofog" or "chemobrain." Although the nature of the impairment seems to vary among patients, those who experience chemobrain generally report subtle changes in the ability to maintain focus and engage in routine daily activities. Some investigations performed before and after the initiation of chemotherapeutic treatment find that memory, motor dexterity, and executive function (frontal subcortical components) tend to be impaired, with attention and psychomotor speed remaining unimpaired. Other studies have shown that working memory, or the ability to process information and do multiple tasks, is often impaired, whereas hippocampal components of memory, such as retention and consolidation, frequently are not.

Cytokines and cognitive impairment

The cause of the cognitive impairment is not fully understood, but one line of research provides evidence that cytokines may contribute significantly.[4–6] Cytokines are proteinaceous signaling compounds that are extensively involved in cell-to-cell communication (see Chapters 2 and 3). As naturally occurring biological-response modifiers, cytokines are released by cells of the immune system, such as macrophages and T-helper cells, in response to illness, threat, injury, age, and stress.[6] Cytokines are involved in various immune-system activities, including the activation and production of monocytes, the secretion of antibodies, chemotaxis, and phagocytosis.[7] Interleukin (IL)-1 has been shown to induce the "sickness behavior" often associated with cancer, including decreases in locomotor activity, eating, exploratory behavior, sexual behavior, and other social interactions. The sickness response requires immune-to-brain communication and can be elicited in animal models and in humans by bacterial infections and by administration of pathological components of bacteria, such as lipopolysaccharide. Lipopolysaccharide initiates the release of a cascade of cytokines (IL-1, IL-6, and tumor necrosis factor-α) and the activation of other immune cells (B cells and T cells).[8]

Chapter 16 provides a complete discussion of cytokines; here, we provide a brief synopsis of those cytokines related specifically to cognitive impairment in animal models. Three major classes of cytokines are particularly relevant to chemotherapy, and each contributes to cognitive impairment.

The interleukins are the largest class of cytokines and have been shown to have many noxious side effects to the body, including neurodegeneration. Specifically, IL-1 has been found to lead to increased calcium influx in hippocampal neurons.[6,9] This finding has been supported by research showing that animals exposed to exogenous IL-1 exhibit deficits in tasks requiring uncompromised spatial abilities, such as the Morris water maze, discussed below.[10] Similar results have been found with IL-2.[6] Heyser et al.[11] showed that IL-6 may lead to excitotoxicity, which in turn produces hippocampal interneuron damage and degeneration of neurons in the frontal cortex that lead to poor performance on a task of avoidance learning. However,

Cancer Symptom Science: Measurement, Mechanisms, and Management, eds. Charles S. Cleeland, Michael J. Fisch, and Adrian J. Dunn.

other studies examining exogenous administration of IL-6 have found little effect in the Morris water maze.[12]

Aside from these cognitive effects, peripheral administration of IL-1 causes classic sickness behaviors such as decreases in general activity,[13] eating,[13] exploration of the environment,[14] and social interactions,[15] decreased sexual behavior in females,[16] and increased sleep.[17] One study using IL-6 knockout mice reported increased emotionality in the elevated plus maze and hole board tests,[18] and another study found increased aggression in these knockout mice. [19]However, such findings were not observed in a subsequent study.[20]

Interferons (IFNs) also have been associated with cognitive impairment. Valentine et al.[21] proposed a model by which chronic administration of IFN-α may lead to neurotoxicity, producing cognitive effects including memory loss and slowed reaction times via alterations in dopamine and serotonin levels. Similar cognitive impairments, and other impairments such as thought blockade and confusion, have been cited by other researchers using IFN therapy.[22]

The tumor necrosis factors (TNFs), a third major class of cytokines, have also been shown to contribute to cognitive impairment. Increased levels of TNF-α have been found in patients with HIV-associated dementia[23] and in close temporal proximity to traumatic brain injury.[24] Further, Suzuki et al.[25] recently conducted a study on elderly patients with diabetes mellitus and found that higher TNF-α levels were observed in relation to declines on the WAIS-R digit symbol test and a test of delayed recall. Plasma levels of TNF-α have further been found to correlate with the degree of cognitive impairment, depression, and pain in cancer patients and with emotional behavior in mice.[26] Research indicates that TNF-α may exert its cognitive effects by leading to demyelination and to oligodendrocyte apoptosis throughout the central nervous system.[27]

Chemotherapeutic agents have been shown to lead to increases in cytokines.[28] For instance, the proinflammatory cytokines IFN-γ, TNF-α, and IL-1 are increased by cisplatin[29] and paclitaxel.[28,30] In researching paclitaxel, Dina et al.[31] showed that an increase in cytokines may be the result of activation of second messenger systems, especially protein kinase C and protein kinase A. Activation of these systems leads to expression of immunomodulatory genes, which then increases production of cytokines via macrophages and T cells.[30]

Models of cognitive impairment

The approach of current research should be to measure cognitive function in rodents and then to use what is learned from the animal models to determine the impact of cancer and cancer treatment on normal cognitive functioning in humans. Modeling cognitive impairment in animals allows researchers to study cognition in controlled circumstances and to perform specific and precisely controlled manipulations targeted at the underlying biological mechanisms of cancer-related and cancer treatment-related cognitive impairment. Appropriate animal models of cancer-related cognitive impairment are thus needed to more fully understand the mechanisms involved in this impairment and to better test potential treatments for cancer. For example, little is known about the extent of cortical and subcortical damage that may be related to cognitive impairment; a useful animal model would allow for identification of impairment and testing of potential brain damage. Specific tests – based on findings that cancer and its treatment are especially damaging to memory, attention, information processing speeds, visuospatial abilities, and hippocampal function in general – may be used to investigate cancer-related cognitive impairments. A number of such tests exist,[32] and some may be beneficial in contributing to the goal of current research.

The Morris water maze

The Morris water maze is used extensively to study different aspects of spatial and working memory. The behavioral paradigm is an open-field water-maze procedure during which rats learn to escape from opaque water onto a hidden platform using extramaze cues.[33] Typically, the swim chamber is divided into several regions: an outer boundary that circles the perimeter of the chamber, a central area, and four quadrants dividing the swim chamber into equal areas (Figure 7.1). The hidden platform is placed into one of these quadrants. In the basic paradigm, the hidden platform remains in the same location of the pool across test days and rats learn the location of the platform by the use of extramaze cues. Variants of the typical procedure have been developed, such as the movement of the platform to a different location on each test day, or after a period of initial training. At the end of training, the platform can be removed from the tank and a probe test can be performed. The animals typically show a preference for the quadrant in which the platform had been located, and the

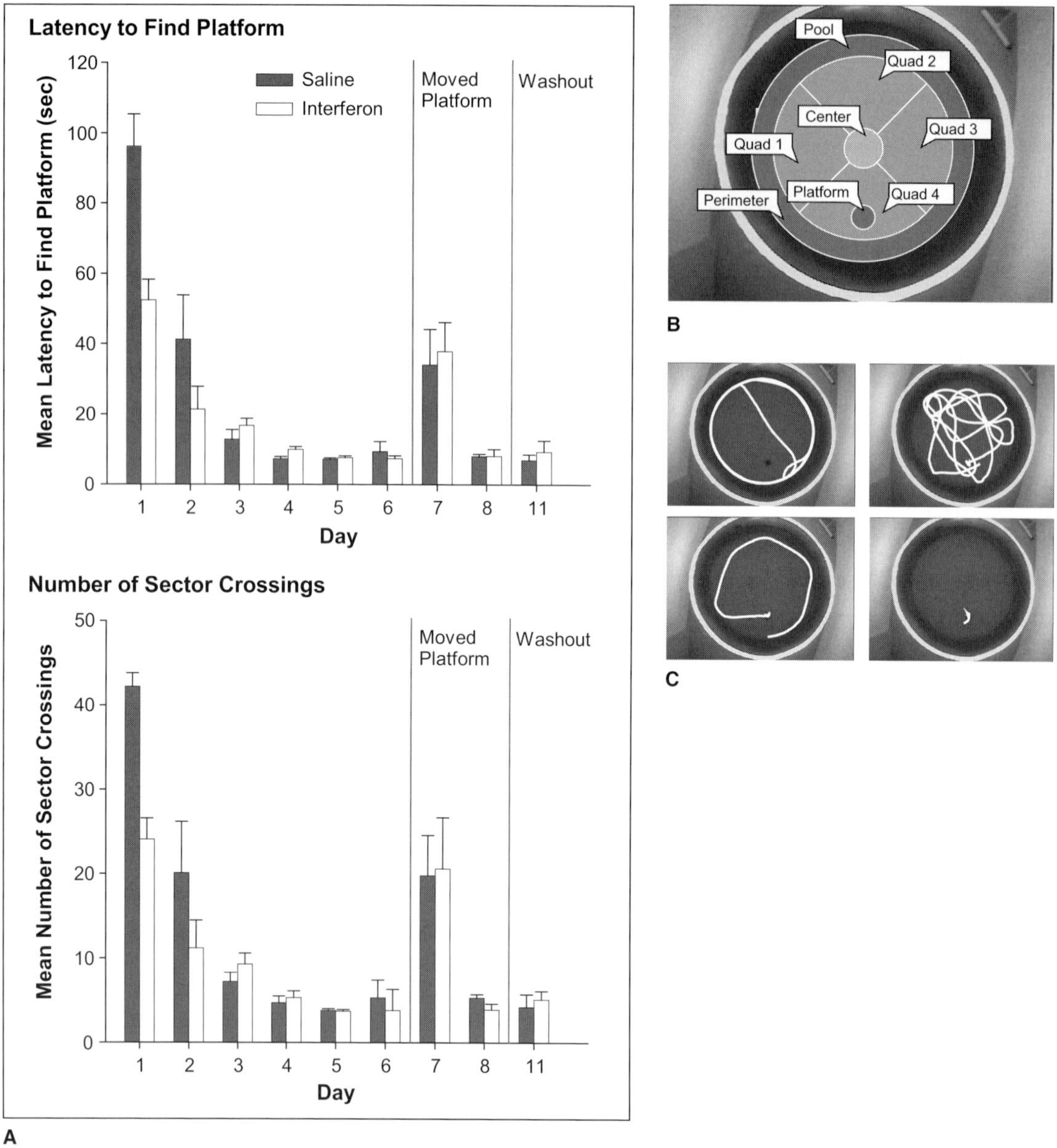

Figure 7.1. Cognitive testing with the Morris water maze. A. Mean (±SEM) latency for finding the hidden platform and number of sector crossings across an 11-day test period for animals treated with saline or interferon (IFN)-α. Both groups of animals quickly learned the location of the hidden platform, as indicated by a rapid decrease in the latency to find the platform during the first 3–4 days of testing. More time was spent finding the platform during the probe phase (after the platform was moved). B. The sector organization of the swim chamber. C. Typical swim patterns across the test days. The top left panel shows the swim path during the initial period of training, when the animal spent almost the entire time swimming along the perimeter of the chamber. As training continued (top right, bottom left, bottom right), the swim paths became more precise and consequently the latency in finding the platform and the number of sector crossings decreased.

measurement of time spent in the goal quadrant of the tank is thought to reflect spatial memory.[34] The usual dependent measures are the animal's latency in climbing onto the hidden platform, the total distance traveled, and the number of quadrant entrances during the test.

The Morris water maze is frequently used to study the underlying neurobiology of learning and memory (for review, see D'Hooge and De Deyn[35]); for example, a recent study examined the effects of chronic unpredictable stress on performance in the Morris water maze.[36] Sparkman et al[37] recently reported that administration of lipopolysaccharide caused a significant alteration in the performance of C57BL/6J mice performing the Morris water maze test, primarily in swim speed but also in learning. Exogenous administration of IL-1β has also been demonstrated to block the acquisition of spatial learning, suggesting that cognitive impairment might be a component of cytokine-mediated sickness behavior.[10]

We administered the cytokine IFN-α to rats and measured their performance in the Morris water maze (Figure 7.1, unpublished data). Test results showed no impact from interferon treatment on the development of spatial memory and, after six days of training, no impact on a modified probe test. Additional studies are required to examine the effect of various dosing regimens and chemotherapeutic agents in spatial/working memory function in normal and tumor-bearing animals.

Pre-pulse inhibition

Pre-pulse inhibition is a measurement of sensorimotor gating and is used to assess the inhibition and gating of sensory and cognitive information. In this paradigm, the response to an auditory stimulus is blunted by pre-exposure to a priming stimulus presented a brief time (ie, 50–300 milliseconds) earlier. The blunting response is thought to result from an inhibitory control that modulates the processing of intense sensory input.[38] Attenuation of the inhibitory response is thought to reflect an impairment of attentional mechanisms.

We tested pre-pulse inhibition in animals treated with vincristine.[39] Figure 7.2 shows that these animals displayed characteristic peripheral neuropathy as a result of vincristine treatment, indicating that the drug had reached efficacy at the time of prepulse inhibition testing. During the pre-pulse testing, animals were exposed to various stimuli: (1) a 118 dB, 40-millisecond noise burst presented alone ("Pulse"); (2) the same pulse preceded 60 milliseconds earlier by a 20-millisecond noise burst ("Pre-pulse") that was 4, 8, or 16 dB above the 65 dB background noise; or (3) no stimulus ("Nostim"). As shown in Figure 7.2, vincristine did not significantly alter pre-pulse inhibition responses, indicating that chemotherapy treatment does not modify attentional mechanisms as measured by a test of pre-pulse inhibition.[39] Of particular interest

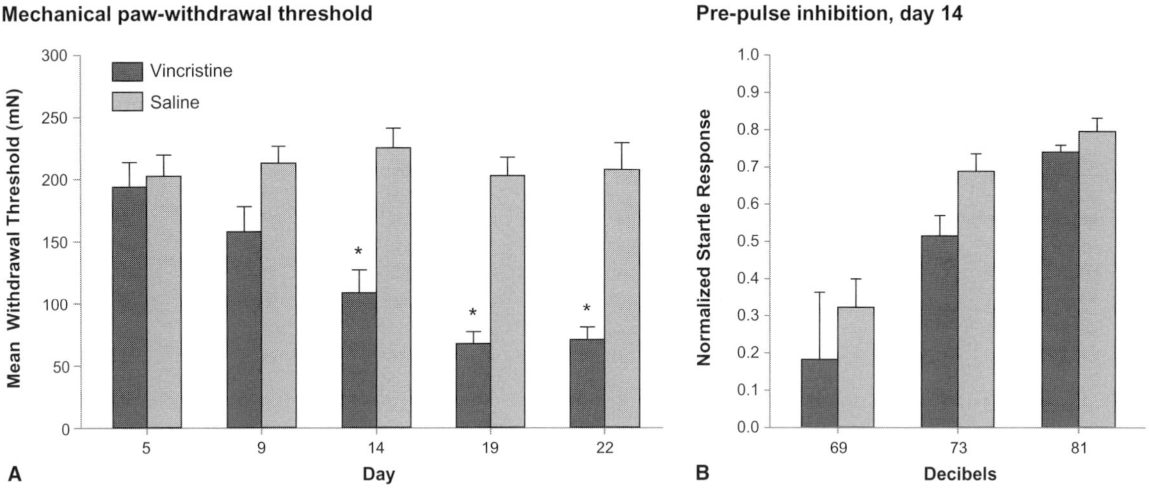

Figure 7.2. Effect of chronic vincristine treatment on mechanical paw withdrawal and pre-pulse inhibition. A. Mean (±SEM) mechanical paw-withdrawal threshold for animals treated with vincristine (0.1mg/kg) or vehicle. During testing, calibrated von Frey monofilaments were applied to the plantar surface of the hindpaw. Compared with vehicle, vincristine treatment produced a significant decrease in mechanical paw-withdrawal threshold (hyperalgesia) at days 14, 19, and 22 of treatment. B. Normalized startle response for animals treated with vincristine (0.1mg/kg) or vehicle. During testing, animals were exposed to random presentations of different decibel levels of the pre-pulse tone. For each pre-pulse intensity, the data was converted to a ratio of startle response relative to the 118 dB pulse using the formula ((response to 118 dB – response to pre-pulse)/response to 118 dB) and averaged across the test session. Pre-pulse inhibition to the 118 dB pulse increases as the amplitude of the pre-pulse tone increases. Compared with vehicle, vincristine treatment failed to significantly alter pre-pulse inhibition.
Source: Reprinted from Neuroscience Letters, vol. 364, Jasenka Borzan, Stacey C. LaGraize, and Perry N. Fuchs, Effect of chronic vincristine treatment on mechanical withdrawal response and pre-pulse inhibition in the rat, Pages 110–113, Copyright 2004, with permission from Elsevier.

is the lack of relationship between pre-pulse inhibition and the onset of peripheral neuropathy. At days 9–22, when vincristine-treated animals were displaying significant mechanical allodynia, pre-pulse inhibition was not altered compared with control animals.

Unlike the somatosensory system, in which chemotherapeutic treatment results in abnormal sensory processing and mechanical hypersensitivity, the finding of normal pre-pulse inhibition strongly suggests that the auditory system is relatively unaffected by chemotherapeutic treatment. Additional studies using pre-pulse inhibition to measure sensorimotor gating are required to examine the potential interaction of chemotherapeutic treatment with other pharmacotherapies in normal and tumor-bearing animals.

Classical conditioning

On the basis of evidence that certain chemotherapeutic agents used for the treatment of childhood cancers have neurocognitive side effects, Yanovski et al[40] utilized a simple classical conditioning paradigm in neonatal rats to detect the potential neuropsychological toxicity of anticancer agents. Treatment with methotrexate was found to interfere significantly with an animal's subsequent ability to learn about environmental stimuli as assessed by two classical conditioning techniques: conditioned emotional response and conditioned taste aversion (Figure 7.3). The results suggested that the effect of methotrexate was not related to altered perceptual abilities, but rather to alterations in neural systems involved in acquisition, retention, or recall. Stock et al.[41] used Pavlovian conditioning tasks and a conditioned taste-aversion paradigm to examine the generality of methotrexate-induced cognitive impairments in rats. In contrast with the study of Yanovski et al.,[40] Stock et al. failed to find any impairment after methotrexate exposure.

The outcomes of these two studies indicate that classical conditioning methodologies can be used to study cognitive function in tumor-bearing animals and cancer-treated animals and then to further explore the underlying mechanisms associated with the cognitive impairments. The discrepant findings highlight the difficulty of developing behavioral tests to model

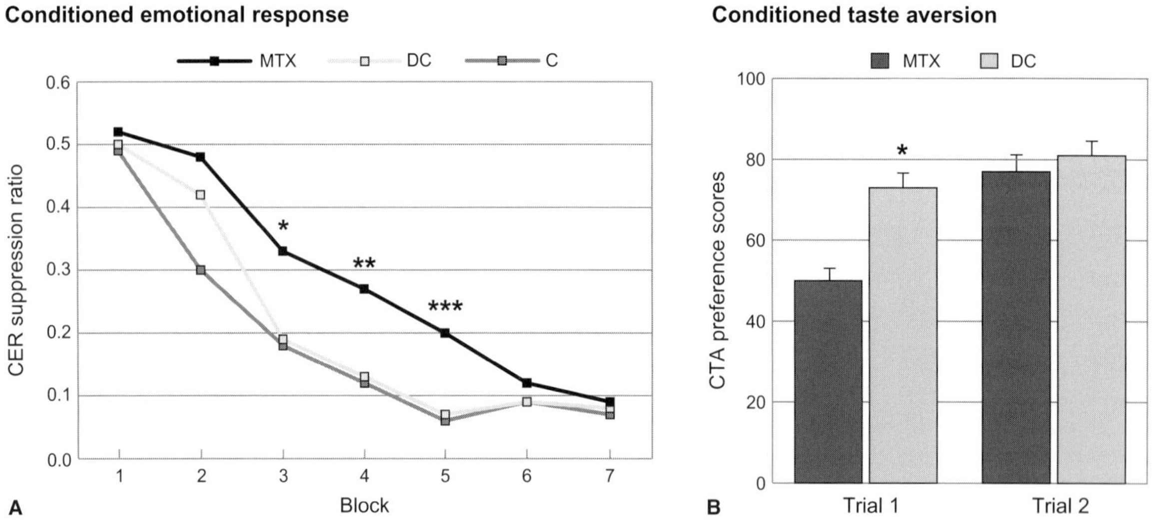

Figure 7.3. Classical conditioning to detect the neuropsychological toxicity of anticancer agents. Animals were treated with methotrexate (MTX) or saline at 16–17 days of age. Because the animals in the treatment group exhibited MTX-induced illness, half of the control animals were food deprived to more closely mirror the undernourishment in the MTX group (DC), and half were treated normally (C). Testing then occurred at 12–14 weeks of age. A. The mean (±SEM) suppression ratio of lever pressing during a test for acquisition of a conditioned emotional response (CER). During training, a 60 dB white noise was paired with a 0.4 mA shock. Animals were then tested for suppression of lever pressing during presentation of the white noise. The MTX-treated animals were significantly impaired in their ability to acquire the conditioned emotional response. B. Mean (±SEM) preference scores during a test of conditioned taste aversion (CTA). MTX and DC groups were offered sucrose or sodium chloride followed by lithium chloride to induce illness. On the test day, preference for the liquid paired with lithium chloride was measured. MTX animals were delayed in the acquisition of the conditioned taste aversion, as can be seen by the failed preference during Trial 1 and the acquired aversion during Trial 2.
Source: An animal model to detect the neuropsychological toxicity of anticancer agents, vol. 17, No. 3, 1989, 216–221. Copyright 1989 Medical and Pediatric Oncology. Reprinted with permission of John Wiley & Sons. Inc.

chemotherapy-induced cognitive impairment. Future studies using context conditioning, which examines unified representations of contexts and how reinforcement contingencies encourage the grouping of elements in configurable cues, are an intriguing experimental approach. The performance in context conditioning tasks is sensitive to the normal functioning of the temporal lobes, suggesting that these tests are a model of human declarative memory.[42] It is this neural system that might be significantly impaired by chemotherapeutic treatment in normal and tumor-bearing animals.

Operant paradigms

Operant behavioral techniques vary in complexity and are thought to model different aspects of complex brain function. The ability to make versatile modifications to operant procedures to study general cognitive function is almost limitless. This section will review some of the procedures that are appropriate for studying cancer-related cognitive impairment.

Fixed and progressive schedule for operant behavior

One operant paradigm that is used to study discrimination of environmental stimuli involves the concurrent fixed and progressive schedule. Specifically, this paradigm is thought to measure an organism's adaptive response to consequences that follow choices, and it has been used to evaluate decision making deficits following brain injury in humans. The use of concurrent schedules of reinforcement requires the organism to attend to the discriminated operants. A second paradigm utilizes a fixed schedule of reinforcement in the absence of external cues. This paradigm is thought to measure attentional mechanisms in the absence of external cues and has been extensively used to explore properties of many pharmacological agents.[43] The use of a fixed interval schedule requires the organism to maintain an internal representation of reinforcement contingencies. The rationale for the use of operant paradigms is that impairment in operant behavior would strongly indicate a decrease in the ability of the organism to attend to environmentally significant stimuli.

We conducted a study to look at the pattern of operant responding during a fixed-interval, 30-second schedule of reinforcement in animals treated with paclitaxel. This paradigm is relatively straightforward, requiring the animal to make a response after a fixed interval to receive reinforcement. Responses made before the 30-second interval are not reinforced. After a period of training, control animals learn to inhibit responses early in the interval, and then as the 30-second interval approaches, begin a gradual increase in the number of operant responses made. Paclitaxel did not alter performance on the fixed-interval schedule of reinforcement, even though the dose regimen resulted in significant peripheral neuropathy as indicated by significant mechanical hypersensitivity. This outcome is important because it demonstrates that an animal's ability to acquire relatively simple associations and the ability to keep track of this information over relatively prolonged periods of time is not compromised by chemotherapeutic treatment.

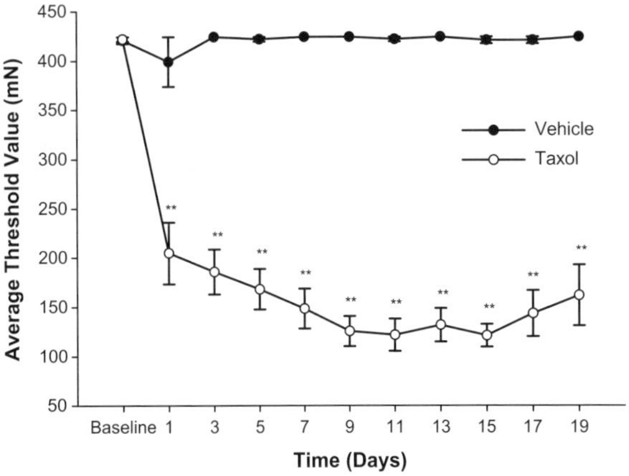

Figure 7.4. Average mechanical paw withdrawal thresholds for animals treated with paclitaxel or vehicle. Animals treated with paclitaxel showed mechanical hypersensitivity as revealed by a decrease in mechanical threshold values. Compared with vehicle-treated animals, the paclitaxel-treated animals exhibit significantly lower threshold values by day 1, with maximal differences seen by day 9 (all $P < 0.01$).
Source: Reprinted from Neuroscience Letters, vol. 453, Jessica A. Boyette-Davis and Perry N. Fuchs, Differential effects of paclitaxel treatment on cognitive functioning and mechanical sensitivity, Pages 170–174, Copyright 2009, with permission from Elsevier.

The 5-choice serial reaction time task

The 5-choice serial reaction time task (5CSRTT) is an established test of attentional mechanisms that is commonly used in rodents and primates and that could serve as a potential means to study postchemotherapy cognitive impairment in an animal model.[44] This paradigm uses a modified operant chamber with five nosepoke wells along the back wall of the chamber. The animal must attend and respond to randomly presented visual stimuli to receive a reward. The duration of the presentation of the visual stimulus can be varied

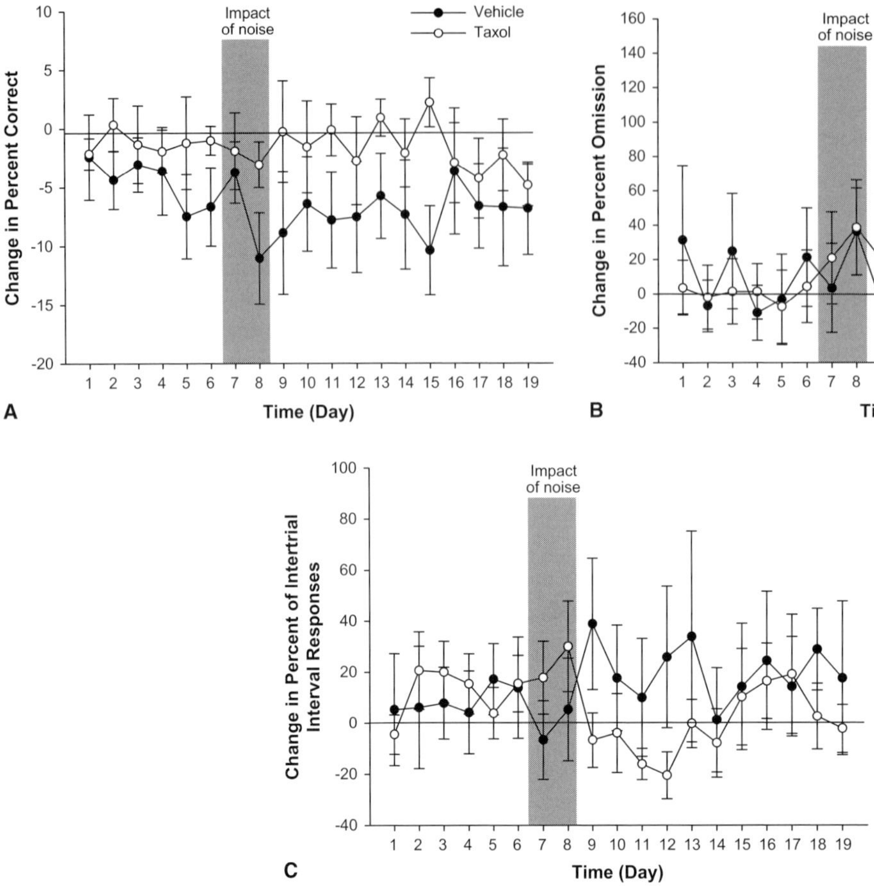

Figure 7.5. Cognitive data from the 5-choice serial reaction time task. A. Average percentage of correct responses for paclitaxel-treated and vehicle-treated animals in the 5CSRTT. Overall, there were no decrements in percent correct for paclitaxel-treated animals relative to vehicle-treated animals. B. Average percentage of omissions for paclitaxel-treated and vehicle-treated animals in the 5CSRTT. The analysis for percent omission indicate paclitaxel-treated animals were not making fewer responses than vehicle-treated animals. C. Average percentage of intertrial interval responses for paclitaxel-treated and vehicle-treated animals in the 5CSRTT. The analysis for percentage of intertrial interval responses show that paclitaxel-treated animals were not more impulsive than vehicle-treated animals.
Source: Reprinted from Neuroscience Letters, vol. 453, Jessica A. Boyette-Davis and Perry N. Fuchs, Differential effects of paclitaxel treatment on cognitive functioning and mechanical sensitivity, Pages 170–174, Copyright 2009, with permission from Elsevier.

to increase the difficulty of the task, but is most commonly set at 0.5–1.0 second. If the animal responds correctly via a nose-poke response to the lit well, a food pellet is dispensed and a correct response is recorded. If the animal responds to a nose-poke well that was not lit for that trial (incorrect response), or if the animal fails to make a response for that trial (omission), no food is earned and the house light is extinguished for a time-out period.

Deficits in attention can be detected by failures to respond (omissions), increased latencies to respond, and decreases in correct responses. The parameters of the test can be varied greatly, and many variables can be recorded for any one session. As a result, the test is sensitive to various types of attention. For instance, sustained attention, or the ability of the subject to maintain task commitment, is necessary to accurately perform the task. Inglis et al.[45] observed that bilateral lesions to the pedunculopontine tegmental nucleus, an area of the brain associated with sustained attention, result in a decrease in the percentage of correct responses, an increase in the number of omissions, and increases in the latencies to make correct responses.

In our laboratory, we have shown that the task is also sensitive to divided attention. Animals were exposed to an acute inflammatory condition and then tested by 5CSRTT, which forced them to either attend to the task or attend to the pain. We found no alterations in the percentage of correct responses or the latencies to obtain earned food rewards, but animals experiencing pain exhibited significant increases in the percentage of omissions.[46] Carli et al.[47] showed that the task can also be used to measure aspects of selective attention by introducing a burst of noise randomly during the session or by varying the intensity of the stimulus light. Overall, the versatility and sensitivity of this task makes it a very viable means for studying chemotherapy-related cognitive impairment.

We recently conducted a study using the 5CSRTT in an attempt to detect these impairments.[48] Animals receiving the chemotherapeutic agent paclitaxel were tested for signs of peripheral neuropathy (Figure 7.4) and were also tested in the 5CSRTT (Figure 7.5). The animals showed rapid and significant development of neuropathy subsequent to the commencement of paclitaxel treatment, validating the biological effects of the paclitaxel. Of primary interest is the finding that, relative to control animals, paclitaxel-treated animals did not exhibit alterations in cognitive function in the 5CSRTT.

Conclusions

In this chapter we have briefly summarized the current state of knowledge regarding cancer-related and cancer treatment-related cognitive impairment in patients and have proposed an approach for modeling impairments in animals. The use of animal behavioral methodology to assess cognition, and the impact of manipulations of neural substrates on normal cognitive function, have been an important aspect in many areas of biomedical research. Indeed, the literature reflects a significant increase in the number of experiments involving tests of cognitive function in animals. However, the validity (face, construct, predictive ability) of animal models of cognition – and preclinical models of disease in general – must always be questioned. It remains to be determined whether the various animal models of cognition, although strong in face validity, truly measure the aspects of cognitive impairment that should be modeled, and whether the results from studies based on these models can be used to predict the nature of the impairment and to identify positive therapeutic outcomes.

Animal models of chemofog, or chemobrain – subtle changes in the ability to focus and engage in routine daily activities – are most urgently needed to study the role of chemotherapeutic regimens in producing cognitive impairment. At this time, the underlying mechanism(s) of cognitive impairment remains unknown, but most likely involves a significant contribution of cytokines and other closely related biological systems. A number of animal behavioral test paradigms can be used to model various aspects of cognitive function. We have summarized a few of these tests, such as the Morris water maze for spatial/working memory, pre-pulse inhibition for sensorimotor gating, and classical/operant (eg, fixed and progressive schedules of reinforcement, 5-choice serial reaction time task) for testing complex environmental associations.

The optimal behavioral paradigms for modeling cognitive impairment in patients with cancer remain to be determined. Ultimately, such paradigms will be useful for exploring the underlying mechanisms of cognitive impairment, and may provide a means to study novel therapeutic approaches to prevent and alleviate such impairments and to improve the quality of life.

References

1. Wieneke MH, Dienst ER. Neuropsychological assessment of cognitive functioning following chemotherapy for breast cancer. *Psychooncology* **4**(1):61–66, 1995.
2. Wefel JS, Lenzi R, Theriault R, Buzdar AU, Cruickshank S, Meyers CA. 'Chemobrain' in breast carcinoma? A prologue. *Cancer* **101**(3):466–475, 2004.
3. Wefel JS, Lenzi R, Theriault RL, Davis RN, Meyers CA. The cognitive sequelae of standard-dose adjuvant chemotherapy in women with breast carcinoma: results of a prospective, randomized, longitudinal trial. *Cancer* **100**(11):2292–2299, 2004.
4. Cleeland CS. Cancer-related symptoms. *Semin Radiat Oncol* **10**(3):175–190, 2000.
5. Meyers CA, Albitar M, Estey E. Cognitive impairment, fatigue, and cytokine levels in patients with acute myelogenous leukemia or myelodysplastic syndrome. *Cancer* **104**(4):788–793, 2005.
6. Wilson CJ, Finch CE, Cohen HJ. Cytokines and cognition: the case for a head-to-toe inflammatory paradigm. *J Am Geriatr Soc* **50**(12):2041–2056, 2002.
7. Miller GE, Cohen S, Ritchey AK. Chronic psychological stress and the regulation of pro-inflammatory cytokines: a glucocorticoid-resistance model. *Health Psychol* **21**(6):531–541, 2002.

8. Aubert A, Goodall G, Dantzer R, Gheusi G. Differential effects of lipopolysaccharide on pup retrieving and nest building in lactating mice. *Brain Behav Immun* **11**(2):107–118, 1997.
9. Larson SJ, Dunn AJ. Behavioral effects of cytokines. *Brain Behav Immun* **15**(4):371–387, 2001.
10. Gibertini M, Newton C, Friedman H, Klein TW. Spatial learning impairment in mice infected with *Legionella pneumophila* or administered exogenous interleukin-1-beta. *Brain Behav Immun* **9**(2):113–128, 1995.
11. Heyser CJ, Masliah E, Samimi A, Campbell IL, Gold LH. Progressive decline in avoidance learning paralleled by inflammatory neurodegeneration in transgenic mice expressing interleukin 6 in the brain. *Proc Natl Acad Sci U S A* **94**(4):1500–1505, 1997.
12. Oitzl MS, van Oers H, Schöbitz B, De Kloet ER. Interleukin-1 beta, but not interleukin-6, impairs spatial navigation learning. *Brain Res* **613**(1):160–163, 1993.
13. Otterness IG, Seymour PA, Golden HW, Reynolds JA, Daumy GO. The effects of continuous administration of murine interleukin-1 alpha in the rat. *Physiol Behav* **43**(6):797–804, 1988.
14. Dunn AJ, Chapman Y, Antoon M. Endotoxin-induced behavioral changes of mice in the multicompartment chamber are distinct from those of interleukin-1. *Neurosci Res Commun* **10**:63–69, 1992.
15. Dantzer R. Cytokine-induced sickness behavior: where do we stand? *Brain Behav Immun* **15**(1):7–24, 2001.
16. Avitsur R, Donchin O, Barak O, Cohen E, Yirmiya R. Behavioral effects of interleukin-1 beta: modulation by gender, estrus cycle, and progesterone. *Brain Behav Immun* **9**(3):234–241, 1995.
17. Krueger JM, Majde JA. Microbial products and cytokines in sleep and fever regulation. *Crit Rev Immunol* **14**(3–4):355–379, 1994.
18. Armario A, Hernández J, Bluethmann H, Hidalgo J. IL-6 deficiency leads to increased emotionality in mice: evidence in transgenic mice carrying a null mutation for IL-6. *J Neuroimmunol* **92**(1–2):160–169, 1998.
19. Alleva E, Cirulli F, Bianchi M, et al. Behavioural characterization of interleukin-6 overexpressing or deficient mice during agonistic encounters. *Eur J Neurosci* **10**(12):3664–3672, 1998.
20. Swiergiel AH, Dunn AJ. Feeding, exploratory, anxiety- and depression-related behaviors are not altered in interleukin-6-deficient male mice. *Behav Brain Res* **171**(1):94–108, 2006.
21. Valentine AD, Meyers CA, Kling MA, Richelson E, Hauser P. Mood and cognitive side effects of interferon-alpha therapy. *Semin Oncol* **25**(1 Suppl 1):39–47, 1998.
22. Licinio J, Kling MA, Hauser P. Cytokines and brain function: relevance to interferon-alpha-induced mood and cognitive changes. *Semin Oncol* **25**(1 Suppl 1):30–38, 1998.
23. Glass JD, Wesselingh SL, Selnes OA, McArthur JC. Clinical-neuropathologic correlation in HIV-associated dementia. *Neurology* **43**(11):2230–2237, 1993.
24. Knoblach SM, Fan L, Faden AI. Early neuronal expression of tumor necrosis factor-alpha after experimental brain injury contributes to neurological impairment. *J Neuroimmunol* **95**(1–2):115–125, 1999.
25. Suzuki M, Umegaki H, Ieda S, Mogi N, Iguchi A. Factors associated with cognitive impairment in elderly patients with diabetes mellitus. *J Am Geriatr Soc* **54**(3):558–559, 2006.
26. Yamada K, Iida R, Miyamoto Y, et al. Neurobehavioral alterations in mice with a targeted deletion of the tumor necrosis factor-alpha gene: implications for emotional behavior. *J Neuroimmunol* **111**(1–2):131–138, 2000.
27. Magnano MD, Robinson WH, Genovese MC. Demyelination and inhibition of tumor necrosis factor (TNF). *Clin Exp Rheumatol* **22**(5 Suppl 35):S134–S140, 2004.
28. O'Brien JM, Jr., Wewers MD, Moore SA, Allen JN. Taxol and colchicine increase LPS-induced pro-IL-1 beta production, but do not increase IL-1 beta secretion: a role for microtubules in the regulation of IL-1 beta production. *J Immunol* **154**(8):4113–4122, 1995.
29. Gan XH, Jewett A, Bonavida B. Activation of human peripheral-blood-derived monocytes by cis-diamminedichloroplatinum: enhanced tumoricidal activity and secretion of tumor necrosis factor-alpha. *Nat Immun* **11**(3):144–155, 1992.
30. Zaks-Zilberman M, Zaks TZ, Vogel SN. Induction of proinflammatory and chemokine genes by lipopolysaccharide and paclitaxel (Taxol) in murine and human breast cancer cell lines. *Cytokine* **15**(3):156–165, 2001.
31. Dina OA, Chen X, Reichling D, Levine JD. Role of protein kinase Cepsilon and protein kinase A in a model of paclitaxel-induced painful peripheral neuropathy in the rat. *Neuroscience* **108**(3):507–515, 2001.
32. Dudchenko PA. An overview of the tasks used to test working memory in rodents. *Neurosci Biobehav Rev* **28**(7):699–709, 2004.
33. Morris R. Developments of a water-maze procedure for studying spatial learning in the rat. *J Neurosci Methods* **11**(1):47–60, 1984.

34. Baldi E, Efoudebe M, Lorenzini CA, Bucherelli C. Spatial navigation in the Morris water maze: working and long lasting reference memories. *Neurosci Lett* **378**(3):176–180, 2005.

35. D'Hooge R, De Deyn PP. Applications of the Morris water maze in the study of learning and memory. *Brain Res Brain Res Rev* **36**(1):60–90, 2001.

36. Gouirand AM, Matuszewich L. The effects of chronic unpredictable stress on male rats in the water maze. *Physiol Behav* **86**(1–2):21–31, 2005.

37. Sparkman NL, Kohman RA, Scott VJ, Boehm GW. Bacterial endotoxin-induced behavioral alterations in two variations of the Morris water maze. *Physiol Behav* **86**(1–2):244–251, 2005.

38. Martin RS, Secchi RL, Sung E, et al. Effects of cannabinoid receptor ligands on psychosis-relevant behavior models in the rat. *Psychopharmacology (Berl)* **165**(2):128–135, 2003.

39. Borzan J, LaGraize SC, Fuchs PN. Effect of chronic vincristine treatment on mechanical withdrawal response and pre-pulse inhibition in the rat. *Neurosci Lett* **364**(2):110–113, 2004.

40. Yanovski JA, Packer RJ, Levine JD, Davidson TL, Micalizzi M, D'Angio G. An animal model to detect the neuropsychological toxicity of anticancer agents. *Med Pediatr Oncol* **17**(3):216–221, 1989.

41. Stock HS, Rosellini RA, Abrahamsen GC, McCaffrey RJ, Ruckdeschel JC. Methotrexate does not interfere with an appetitive Pavlovian conditioning task in Sprague-Dawley rats. *Physiol Behav* **58**(5):969–973, 1995.

42. Pickens CL, Holland PC. Conditioning and cognition. *Neurosci Biobehav Rev* **28**(7):651–661, 2004.

43. Lejeune H, Hermans I, Mocaër E, Rettori MC, Poignant JC, Richelle M. Amineptine, response timing, and time discrimination in the albino rat. *Pharmacol Biochem Behav* **51**(2–3):165–173, 1995.

44. Robbins TW. The 5-choice serial reaction time task: behavioural pharmacology and functional neurochemistry. *Psychopharmacology (Berl)* **163**(3–4):362–380, 2002.

45. Inglis WL, Olmstead MC, Robbins TW. Selective deficits in attentional performance on the 5-choice serial reaction time task following pedunculopontine tegmental nucleus lesions. *Behav Brain Res* **123**(2):117–131, 2001.

46. Boyette-Davis JA, Thompson CD, Fuchs PN. Alterations in attentional mechanisms in response to acute inflammatory pain and morphine administration. *Neuroscience* **151**(2):558–563, 2008.

47. Carli M, Robbins TW, Evenden JL, Everitt BJ. Effects of lesions to ascending noradrenergic neurones on performance of a 5-choice serial reaction task in rats; implications for theories of dorsal noradrenergic bundle function based on selective attention and arousal. *Behav Brain Res* **9**(3):361–380, 1983.

48. Boyette-Davis JA, Fuchs PN. Differential effects of paclitaxel treatment on cognitive functioning and mechanical sensitivity. *Neurosci Lett* **453**(3):170–174, 2009.

Section 2 Chapter 8

Cancer symptom mechanisms and models: clinical and basic science

Depression in cancer: pathophysiology at the mind-body interface

Michael A. Burke, Charles L. Raison, and Andrew H. Miller

Undergoing the challenges of cancer and its treatment is an exceedingly daunting task. From a psychological standpoint, the road traveled is fraught with uncertainty, fear, frustration, and anger. On the physical side, there can be multiple bodily assaults, including surgery, chemotherapy, and radiation. Not uncommonly, these psychological and physical traumas become overwhelming and conspire to create an ever-widening sense of despair that invades virtually every aspect of one's being. Symptoms that can emerge include a profound loss of interest in usually pleasurable activities (often including social isolation), depressed mood, anxiety, impaired sleep, anorexia, fatigue, problems with memory and concentration, and, in some cases, severe desperation accompanied by suicidal ideation and even suicide attempts. This constellation of symptoms represents the syndrome of depression, and given its potentially damaging effects on quality of life, treatment adherence, and ultimately morbidity and mortality, understanding the pathophysiological pathways involved is of paramount importance for early identification, treatment, and prevention of this psychiatric disease.

Recent developments in our understanding of stress neurobiology and the contributions of the immune system to behavioral alterations have led to the recognition that the patient with cancer may be especially vulnerable to the convergence of psychological and biological forces that collude to create the substrates for depression. More specifically, data indicate that psychological stress as well as cancer and its treatment are associated with activation of innate immune responses and the release of relevant soluble proteins called cytokines, which in turn can access the brain and have powerful influences on pathways known to be involved in the pathophysiology of depression, including neuroendocrine function, neurotransmitter metabolism, synaptic plasticity, and information processing.

In this chapter we will review what is known about depression in patients with cancer and will emphasize a consideration of new knowledge that integrates the pathophysiological contributions with the psychological and biological components associated with having and being treated for cancer. Translational implications of this work also will be explored.

Depression in cancer: prevalence, predictors, and consequences

Prevalence

Results from point-prevalence and cross-sectional studies indicate that depression as a comorbid condition in cancer occurs in approximately 15% to 30% of patients, a rate roughly three-to-five-times greater than in the general population (Table 8.1).[1,2] Nevertheless, few longitudinal studies have been conducted, and it is unknown whether there are critical periods of risk (eg, immediately after diagnosis, at recurrence, or during or immediately after specific cancer therapies) that may be missed by cross-sectional and point-prevalence study designs. Thus, the true incidence of depression in cancer may be significantly underestimated.

Predictors

There are a number of known risk factors for the development of depression in cancer patients (Table 8.2). Some of these are cancer-specific, including advanced stage, pancreatic cancer, poorly controlled pain, high levels of physical impairment or discomfort, or treatment with certain chemotherapy agents such as procarbazine, amphotericin-B, L-asparaginase, or corticosteroids.[3] Other risk factors are related to psychosocial characteristics, such as past history of depression or suicide attempts, family history of depression or suicide, history of alcoholism or drug abuse, concurrent illnesses that are associated with

Cancer Symptom Science: Measurement, Mechanisms, and Management, eds. Charles S. Cleeland, Michael J. Fisch, and Adrian J. Dunn.

Table 8.1. Rates of depression in representative cancers

Cancer site	Prevalence (%)
Pancreas	50
Oropharyngeal	40
Colon	13 to 25
Breast	18 to 25
Gynecological	23
Hodgkin's and non-Hodgkin's lymphoma	17
Gastric	11
General population	3 to 5

Table 8.2. Risk factors for depression in patients with cancer

Cancer-related risk factors:
• Depression at time of cancer diagnosis
• Poorly controlled pain
• Advanced-stage cancer
• Additional concurrent life stressors
• Increased physical impairment or discomfort
• Pancreatic cancer
• Being unmarried and having head and neck cancer
• Treatment with certain chemotherapeutic agents:
o Corticosteroids
o Procarbazine
o L-Asparaginase
o Amphotericin-B
Noncancer-related risk factors:
• History of depression:
o Two or more episodes in a lifetime
o First episode early or late in life
• Lack of family support
• Family history of depression or suicide
• Previous suicide attempts
• History of alcoholism or drug abuse
• Concurrent illnesses that produce depressive symptoms (ie, stroke or myocardial infarction)
• Past treatment for psychological problems

depressive symptoms (eg, stroke, myocardial infarction), and a lack of social support.[3]

Consequences

The consequences of depression can be devastating. Cancer patients with comorbid depression have reduced quality of life, including increased cancer-associated symptoms (especially pain)[4] and increased functional impairment.[5] In addition, comorbid depression is a likely contributor to the elevation in suicide rates in cancer patients.[6] Untreated depression has been noted in seven of 10 patients with prostate cancer who committed suicide.[7]

Depressed patients with cancer also tend to utilize health care resources at a high rate. For example, a large study of Medicare patients indicated that cancer patients with comorbid depression were approximately three times more likely than nondepressed cancer patients to access emergency department services or require inpatient hospitalization.[8] Even so, cancer patients who are depressed have been found to have reduced optimism about the effectiveness of medical treatment[4] and therefore may be less likely to adhere to complex treatment regimens or to pursue alternative options when initial treatment efforts have failed. Emotional distress also may interfere with the patient's seeking and participating in appropriate diagnostic procedures.[5]

Lastly, data increasingly indicate that depression may be a risk factor for cancer onset or progression and increased morbidity or mortality. For example, large population studies suggest that depressed mood or stressful life events may increase the risk of cancer development.[9,10] However, the literature in this area has been inconsistent, and effect sizes have been relatively small when compared with other illnesses such as cardiovascular disease.[4] More reliable is the association of comorbid depression with increased morbidity and mortality in patients with cancer that has already been diagnosed.[2,4] For example, Onitilo and colleagues[11] examined a large database of subjects from the National Health and Nutrition Examination Survey (NHANES). Almost uniformly, mortality rates were higher in cancer patients with comorbid depression than in cancer patients without depression. Depressed patients with breast cancer in the Surveillance Epidemiology and End Results (SEER) database also exhibited a higher risk of death independently from other survival factors.[12]

Diagnosing depression

Despite the detrimental consequences, depression in patients with cancer is often missed. In a study conducted in Great Britain, oncologists and nurses diagnosed depression in only half of the patients with cancer who had been identified as having depression using a standardized psychiatric interview.[13] In another study, physicians were less able to identify depression as the severity of symptoms increased.[14] The physicians correctly identified four of five nondepressed individuals, but identified only one of three patients with mild to moderate depression and fewer than one in eight who had severe depression. As discussed below, a critical reason that depression may be missed in oncology patients is the overlap of symptoms of depression with symptoms of "sickness" that are often attributed to the cancer itself or its treatment.

As shown in Table 8.3, depression is diagnosed as a syndrome using standardized criteria that include the symptom domains of mood, cognition, and neurovegetative function.[15] For a patient to meet diagnostic criteria, not only do the appropriate number and type of symptoms need to be present, but they must also be persistent over a two-week period and must interfere with the patient's function. Of note, however, is that the symptoms used to make a diagnosis of depression – anhedonia, insomnia, anorexia, fatigue, and cognitive dysfunction – significantly overlap with sickness symptoms that are frequently attributed to the cancer or its treatment.[16] Nevertheless, antidepressants have demonstrated efficacy in the treatment of a number of these symptoms as well as pain, suggesting that shared pathophysiological pathways between the symptoms of sickness and depression may be involved.[16,17] Therefore, although there is some controversy regarding the approach that should be taken when diagnosing depression in patients with cancer (in light of the shared symptoms between depression and sickness), given their potentially shared pathophysiology and treatment, it seems prudent both from a clinical and research standpoint to be inclusive of all symptoms that are traditionally used to make a diagnosis of depression.

Mechanisms and mediators

Whereas prevalence rates of depression are high in patients with cancer, depression is not universal, indicating that the vulnerability to depression in patients with cancer may be due to a complex interplay of multiple factors. Promising avenues of research include the relatively recent understanding that psychosocial stress and the biological effects of cancer and its treatments may converge. This convergence can lead to exaggerated inflammatory responses, which, in turn, may directly influence central nervous system (CNS) pathways that are implicated in depression and other behavioral comorbidities, including fatigue and cognitive dysfunction (Figure 8.1).

Psychological stress

The marked disruption of social and family relationships and the challenges to the enduring integrity of one's own body make being diagnosed and treated for cancer one of life's major stressors. An extensive body of literature has repeatedly shown that stressful life events, including illness, are associated with an increased risk of major depression. It is generally believed that the relationship between stress and depression is largely causal.[18]

Regarding factors that may influence the effects of stress on emotional and physiological status, stress early in life may be especially relevant as it appears to sensitize an individual to subsequent stressors, representing

Table 8.3. Criteria for DSM IV diagnosis of major depression

• Depressed mood and/or loss of interest that persists for at least two weeks	
• Four of the following associated symptoms (three if both depressed mood and loss of interest are present)	
Neurovegetative	**Psychological/cognitive**
Appetite and/or weight loss or overeating and weight gain	Feelings of guilt, worthlessness, helplessness
Insomnia, early-morning awakening, or oversleeping	Feelings of hopelessness, pessimism
Decreased energy, fatigue, being "slowed down"	Thoughts of death or suicide; suicide attempts
Difficulty concentrating, remembering, or making decisions	
Physical agitation or lack of movement	

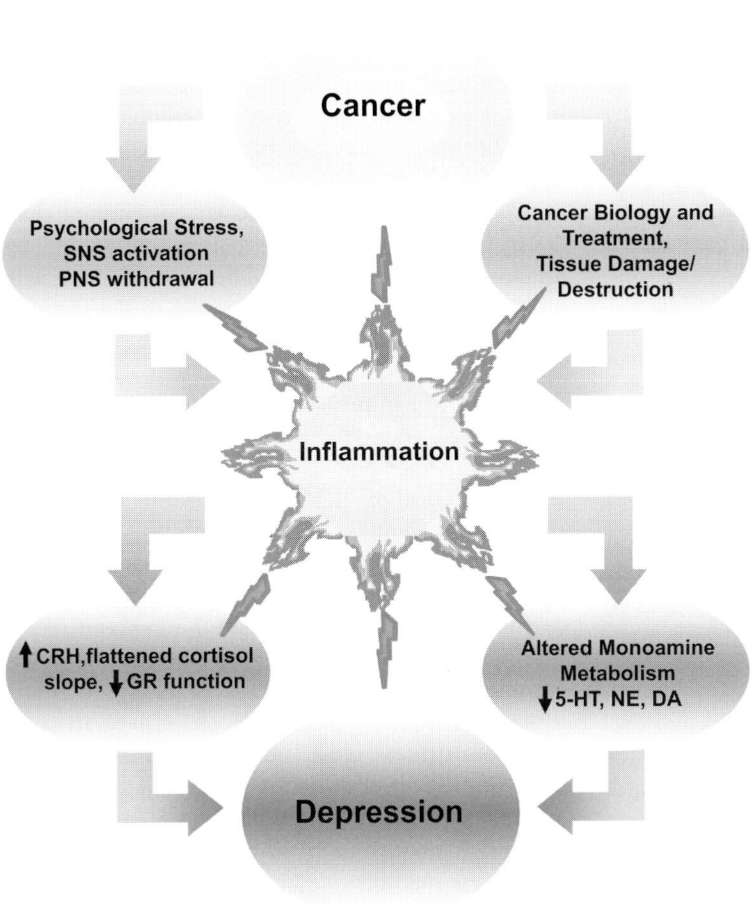

Figure 8.1. Cancer and depression: psychological and biological influences on inflammation and the brain. Receiving a cancer diagnosis frequently causes significant psychological stress, and being treated for cancer is associated with tissue damage and destruction. Together, these processes are potent activators of the innate immune response and inflammation. In the context of psychological stress, sympathetic nervous system (SNS) pathways can activate inflammatory responses, whereas parasympathetic nervous system (PNS) responses can inhibit inflammation. Stress can also sensitize the immune system to the activation of inflammatory pathways by cancer and its treatment. In turn, activation of innate immune responses and inflammation can alter neuroendocrine function by increasing corticotropin-releasing hormone (CRH), flattening the diurnal cortisol curve and disrupting glucocorticoid receptor (GR) function, all of which have been associated with the development of depression. Activation of inflammation and innate immune cytokines can also disrupt monoamine metabolism, leading to reductions in serotonin (5-hydroxytryptophan [5-HT]), norepinephrine (NE), and dopamine (DA). Reduced availability of these neurotransmitters is believed to play an important role in mood regulation. See plate section for color version.

an additional long-term risk factor for the development of depression.[19] For example, prospective animal data and retrospective studies in humans with early-life stress demonstrate persistent alterations in the hypothalamic-pituitary-adrenal (HPA) axis and hyperactivity of corticotropin-releasing hormone (CRH) pathways. These perturbations are consistent with the pathophysiological changes found in patients with depression.[19] The mechanism underlying these events is believed to involve changes in glucocorticoid receptor (GR) gene expression in the hippocampus and frontal cortex, regions that have been strongly implicated as sites involved with the negative-feedback regulation of CRH. In addition, there is increasing evidence of an interaction between early-life stress leading to depression and a polymorphism in the serotonin transporter gene. This finding may be especially important to the impact of innate immune cytokines on serotonin availability.[20]

These data suggest that the stress of having and being treated for cancer in the context of early-life stress may be a critical factor in determining why some patients experience only transient distress during a cancer encounter, whereas others develop a clinically significant depressive disorder. This notion is supported by the data of Felitti et al.,[21] who found that an increased number of adverse childhood experiences were associated with an increased relative risk of depression (eg, four or more childhood events we associated with a 4.6 relative risk of depression for two weeks in the past year). Interestingly, they also found that early adverse events were associated with an increased risk of cancer, which is consistent with the notion of a convergence of stress-induced pathology and the pathophysiology of cancer (1.9 relative risk of having cancer [all types]).

Stress and the immune response

Although current life stress and early life stress have been studied extensively, as reflected in the literature on both depression and cancer, recent research into the neurobiology of stress has begun to reveal some interesting developments that suggest there may be some convergence of pathologies relevant to both stress and cancer. This association involves the immune system in general and, more specifically, activation of innate immune inflammatory responses.

Recent data from laboratory animals and humans suggest that a wide variety of stressors can activate inflammatory pathways, including the release of innate immune cytokines and the induction of DNA-binding activity of relevant inflammatory signaling molecules such as nuclear factor kappa B (NF-κB), a lynchpin in the initiation of the inflammatory response. For example, normal human volunteers exposed to a public speaking task and mental arithmetic stressor were found to exhibit significant increases in NF-κB–DNA binding within 10 minutes after exposure to the stressor.[22] Interestingly, this stress response appears to be exaggerated in individuals with early-life stress and depression. Using the same public speaking/mental arithmetic task, patients with early-life stress and depression exhibited increased plasma concentrations of the inflammatory cytokine interleukin (IL)-6 in response to stressor exposure and also exhibited a much greater induction of activated NF-κB.[23]

Relevant to the relationship between stress and depression, stress-induced activation of innate immune responses may have profound influences on neurobiological substrates related to brain function. For example, the capacity of isolation stress to inhibit the expression of brain-derived neurotrophic factor in the hippocampus was completely reversed by pretreatment with an IL-1 receptor antagonist, suggesting that stress-induced activation of the inflammatory response may disrupt growth factors central to neuronal plasticity.[24] Brain-derived neurotrophic factor is believed to play an important role in neurogenesis and may be an essential element in the efficacy of antidepressants in relieving depression.[25]

Finally, data suggest that prior stressor exposure may enhance the innate immune response to a subsequent inflammatory stimulus. For example, rats exposed to inescapable tailshock exhibited markedly exaggerated IL-1 responses when exposed to bacterial endotoxin for up to four days after stressor exposure, compared with nonstressed control animals. This effect appears to be mediated by stress-induced activation of brain microglia.[26] Taken together, these data suggest that stress (especially in combination with early-life stress) activates inflammatory pathways in the absence of an immune challenge and sensitizes the innate immune response to subsequent immune challenge. Given the capacity of innate immune cytokines to influence neurobiology and behavior, patients with cancer may be especially vulnerable to the combination of intense psychosocial stress combined with the immune challenges inherent in the tissue damage and destruction (and subsequent inflammation) secondary to cancer and its treatment with surgery, radiation, or chemotherapy.

A great deal of attention has been focused on the autonomic nervous system and the pathways by which psychosocial stress influences the innate immune response. Stress-induced elevations in catecholamines acting through α-adrenergic and β-adrenergic receptors have been shown to mediate activation of innate immune responses. For example, β-adrenergic antagonists blocked stress-induced increases in IL-1β in the brain of rats, and α-adrenergic antagonists reduced stress-induced elevations of IL-1β and IL-6 in the peripheral blood.[27] In humans, the induction of increased concentrations of circulating IL-6 by altitude stress was abrogated by the α-adrenergic antagonist prazosin.[28] Of note, activation of parasympathetic pathways via simulation of the efferent portion of the vagus nerve has been shown to inhibit lethality in mice after administration of endotoxin; an effect mediated by acetylcholine binding to the α_7 subunit of the nicotinic acetylcholine receptor.[29]

Taken together, these data suggest that the effects of stress on the innate immune response may represent a "yin-yang" influence of excitatory sympathetic and inhibitory parasympathetic nervous system pathways. Thus, therapeutic interventions (eg, exercise and certain meditative techniques) targeting the relative balance of these pathways may be especially relevant in managing the impact of stress on the immune response. Pharmacological strategies targeting sympathetic and parasympathetic signaling pathways also warrant consideration.

Inflammation

An increasing body of literature supports the hypothesis that activation of the innate immune response and the release of innate immune cytokines represent a risk factor for the development of depression and other symptoms associated with cancer, including fatigue and cognitive dysfunction. As indicated above, this activation can result from psychosocial stress and from the tissue damage and destruction that is often a consequence of cancer or its treatment. Aside from behavioral disturbances, there is also evidence that inflammatory signaling pathways may play a pivotal role in all three stages of tumor development: initiation, progression, and metastasis.[30] For example, a recent study by Greten et al.[31] found that the inactivation of the gene IKKβ, which activates NF-κB, decreased incidence and tumor growth in mice by nearly 80%.

Inflammation and depression

Compelling evidence indicates a role for activation of the innate immune response and inflammation in the etiology of depression.[32] Whether medically ill or healthy, depressed patients demonstrate all of the cardinal features of inflammation, including: (1) increased plasma and cerebrospinal concentrations of innate immune cytokines (IL-6 being the most reliable); (2) increased acute-phase proteins (C-reactive protein being the most reliable); (3) increased chemokines; and (4) increased cellular adhesion molecules.[32] Of further relevance to depression, the administration or induction of innate immune cytokines such as tumor necrosis factor (TNF)-α, IL-1, IL-6, and interferon (IFN)-α can induce behavioral changes often referred to as "sickness behavior."[16] These behavioral manifestations extensively overlap with the symptoms used to make a diagnosis of major depression, including anhedonia, fatigue, anorexia, impaired sleep, and cognitive dysfunction.[32] For example, patients being treated with IFN-α for malignant melanoma exhibit rates of major depression approaching 50%. In a double-blind placebo-controlled trial, the antidepressant paroxetine, a serotonin reuptake inhibitor, was found to reduce this rate of depression to slightly more than 10%,[33] emphasizing the responsiveness of cytokine-induced behavioral changes to drugs that influence the availability of serotonin.

Of further relevance to the role of inflammation in the development of depression in patients with cancer, plasma concentrations of the innate immune cytokine IL-6 are greater in cancer patients with depression than in cancer patients without depression and medically healthy controls.[17] In addition, elevations in plasma or serum concentrations of a number of innate immune cytokines (and their soluble receptors) have been found in patients with cancer in conjunction with other depressive symptoms, including fatigue, impaired sleep, and cognitive dysfunction.[34,35] Given the impact of innate immune cytokines on the brain and behavior, such elevations in inflammatory markers in patients with cancer may actively contribute to the onset of these diverse behavioral symptoms.

Because cytokines are relatively large molecules that do not freely pass through the blood–brain barrier, much attention has been paid to the mechanism by which cytokine signals reach the brain. Three major pathways have been described, including: (1) passage of cytokines through "leaky" regions in the blood–brain barrier (eg, through the circumventricular organs), a pathway especially relevant when circulating cytokine concentrations are high; (2) active transport via transport molecules with specific binding affinity for relevant cytokines; and (3) binding to local nerve fibers, where cytokine signals are relayed to the brain through afferent parasympathetic nerves to the nucleus of the solitary tract.[32,36] Once in the brain, the signals encounter a cytokine network that includes local expression and production of cytokines by glia (microglia being the richest source of cytokines in the brain) and neurons, both of which produce cytokines and express cytokine receptors.[32,36]

Mechanisms by which cytokines may contribute to depression

Once cytokine signals reach the brain, innate immune cytokines can have profound effects on pathophysiological pathways involved in the development of depressive symptoms, including neuroendocrine (HPA axis and CRH) function and neurotransmitter metabolism.[32]

Depression, innate immune cytokines, and the HPA axis

Dysregulation of the HPA axis has been studied as one of the mechanisms responsible for the association between cancer and depression and other depressive symptoms, including fatigue. One of the most consistent observations concerning HPA axis dysregulation in cancer patients is flattening of the diurnal cortisol curve with increased cortisol production during the evening, normally a quiescent period of HPA axis activity.[4] Flattened cortisol rhythm has most often been associated with fatigue in survivors of breast cancer, although in a seminal study on women with metastatic breast cancer, flattened cortisol rhythm was also associated with increased mortality.[37] In addition, women who experienced lack of spousal support as a function of being divorced or widowed also had flattened diurnal cortisol rhythms,[4] indicating that psychosocial factors may play a role in cancer morbidity and mortality. Depressed patients with cancer have also exhibited abnormalities in the dexamethasone suppression test, indicative of impaired regulation of HPA-axis function by glucocorticoids acting through their receptors.[17]

Innate immune cytokines may contribute to the HPA axis alterations found in patients with cancer, both through their effects on the release of HPA-axis hormones and their impact on GR function. Innate immune cytokines stimulate the HPA axis largely through their activation of CRH. Increased CRH mRNA and protein are noted in multiple relevant brain regions after administration of the innate immune cytokines IL-1β, IL-6, TNF-α, and IFN-α.[2,38] Depressed patients have been found to exhibit CRH hypersecretion, as manifested by increased cerebrospinal CRH and increased CRH mRNA and protein in the paraventricular nucleus in postmortem samples. Moreover, administration of CRH in the ventricles of laboratory animals leads to behavioral changes consistent with depression.[39]

Innate immune cytokines also have the capacity to further activate the HPA axis via direct stimulation of the anterior pituitary to release adrenocorticotropic hormone and of the adrenal cortex to release cortisol.[40] Interestingly, activation of the HPA axis by the first dose of IFN-α was significantly higher in patients with malignant melanoma who subsequently developed depression during IFN-α therapy, compared with those who did not.[41] These data suggest that sensitization of HPA axis responsivity, including CRH pathways, such as may occur during chronic stress exposure or early-life stress, may leave some cancer patients especially vulnerable to the effects of innate immune cytokines on the neuroendocrine system and behavior. Such interactions exemplify the collaboration between psychosocial and biological factors in the development of behavioral changes in the context of cancer and its treatment.

In addition to stimulating CRH production, innate immune cytokines disrupt GR function. These effects appear to be largely mediated through the interaction of innate immune cytokine signaling pathways with GR signaling pathways. Induction of cytokine signaling pathways, including both p38 mitogen-activated protein kinase (MAPK) and signal transducer and activator of transcription-5 (STAT5), have been shown to alter the ability of the GR to translocate from the cytoplasm to the nucleus and to bind GR-responsive elements on DNA.[42] These influences may, in turn, lead to glucocorticoid resistance and may contribute to the dexamethasone nonsuppression found in depressed patients with cancer and to hypersecretion of CRH, which is negatively regulated by glucocorticoids.

Given the role of glucocorticoids in inhibiting innate immune inflammatory responses, disruption of GR function may further exacerbate already exaggerated inflammatory responses, leading to a feed-forward inflammatory cascade. Abnormal responses in the dexamethasone suppression test (a measure of glucocorticoid resistance) have been associated with increased mitogen-induced production of IL-1 by peripheral blood mononuclear cells in healthy depressed subjects.[43] Interestingly, inflammatory cytokines also have been associated with flattening of the diurnal cortisol curve in a cross-sectional study of patients with colorectal cancer.[44] Nevertheless, the directionality of this association and the mechanisms involved remain unclear and require further study.

Monoamine metabolism alteration

Aside from the HPA axis, a number of studies have demonstrated that monoamine pathways play a critical role in the development of depression. Most currently available antidepressant drugs increase the availability of the monoamines serotonin, norepinephrine, and dopamine as a primary mechanism of action. Innate immune cytokines have been shown to have a profound effect on monoamine neurotransmitters, which are implicated in the pathogenesis of depression. After administration of innate immune cytokines, increased metabolism and turnover of all of the monoamines have been found in multiple brain regions affecting mood and cognition, including the hypothalamus, hippocampus, and amygdala.[38]

Among the mechanisms by which innate immune cytokines might influence neurotransmitter metabolism and turnover, probably the best studied are the effects of cytokines on serotonin. For example, IFN-α and other cytokines have potent stimulatory effects on the activity of the enzyme indolamine 2,3 dioxygenase (IDO).[41] IDO is responsible for breaking down tryptophan into kyurenine and quinolinic acid. Therefore, increased IDO activity reduces tryptophan, the primary amino acid precursor of serotonin, and increases quinolinic acid, which has neurotoxic properties of its own. Through activation of p38 MAPK signaling pathways, innate immune cytokines, including TNF-α, IL-1, and IFN-α, can also reduce the synaptic availability of serotonin by increasing the function and expression of the serotonin transporter, which serves as a reuptake pump to remove serotonin from the synapse.[45]

Taken together, these mechanisms (ie, reduced serotonin synthesis through breakdown of tryptophan and increased serotonin reuptake) represent a "double hit" on serotonin availability. A correlation between activation of p38 MAPK pathways and decreased cerebrospinal 5-hydroxyindole acetic acid (a major serotonin metabolite) has been found in rhesus monkeys exposed to poor maternal care, again suggesting an interaction between stress, activation of innate immune responses, and the expression of pathophysiological changes relevant to depression.[46]

There is also evidence that innate immune cytokines may target dopamine pathways. For example, IFN-α has been associated with the development of psychomotor slowing and other motor symptoms (eg, akathisia) similar to those seen in Parkinson disease, which have been relieved by the dopamine precursor, levodopa. In addition, recent data using positron emission tomography have demonstrated IFN-α-induced alterations in basal ganglia metabolism that were associated with symptoms of fatigue.[47] The basal ganglia contain a number of dopamine-rich pathways, and disruption of basal ganglia function has been invoked as a mechanism involved in the development of central fatigue.[48]

Alterations in basal ganglia circuits may also contribute to or be associated with other pathologies in brain circuitry that are observed after administration of innate immune cytokines. After administration of IFN-α, increased activation of the dorsal anterior cingulate cortex was associated with a task of visuospatial attention.[49] The dorsal anterior cingulate cortex plays a fundamental role in resource allocation in demanding tasks and is intimately interconnected with frontal cortex and basal ganglia circuits. Increased activity in the dorsal anterior cingulate cortex has been found in patients with high trait anxiety, neuroticism, and obsessive compulsive disorder, suggesting that cytokine effects on neural circuitry involving the dorsal anterior cingulate cortex (and the basal ganglia) may play a role in cytokine effects on vulnerability to mood disorders.[49]

Translational implications

Given that psychological and biological factors inherent to cancer conspire to cause an increased activation of innate immune inflammatory responses (which in turn interact with pathways known to be involved in depression), there are multiple opportunities for translational developments that target the multiple pathways involved (Figure 8.1). Two such targets are psychological stress and inflammation.

Psychological stress

Social support is one of the foremost factors buffering an individual from stressful life events, thus potentially decreasing the effects of stress on inflammatory responses. Social support has been directly and indirectly associated with a decreased incidence of cancer and increased cancer survival in patients with breast or prostate cancer.[4,50,51] Lack of social support is a predictor of the development of depression.[52]

The ability to make attachments is a fundamental component of a person's ease in accessing social support. Attachment theory posits that "an individual will have certain beliefs and feelings about themselves and others that have been guided by early caretaking environments. These beliefs, in turn, can affect [the individual's] expectations about social responsiveness and availability, as well as the importance of self-care and attention."[53] An organized pattern of attachment behavior or "attachment style" develops early in life. Thus, early-life stress such as abuse, neglect, or early loss often leads to insecure attachment styles.[54] A recent longitudinal study indicated that attachment style may be a critical mediator between adverse childhood experiences and their consequences on behavioral (and possibly biological) outcomes, including depression.[55] Taken together, the data suggest that therapeutic strategies targeting social support (eg, support groups, group therapy) coupled with cognitive behavioral approaches to improve stress management (eg, relaxation, exercise, meditation) and coping styles may be most relevant for dealing with the influences of psychological stress on the development of depression. Given the primary role played by attachment style in the ability to access social support resources, special attention should be paid to individuals with insecure or ambivalent attachments (especially those with early-life stress or a lack of family support), who may be at greatest risk.

Inflammation

There are several points at which therapies might target the impact of an activated innate immune inflammatory response on behavior. The most upstream of these targets are the cytokines themselves. Commercially available drugs can be used to neutralize TNF-α and IL-1: the TNF-α blocker etanercept has been shown to improve depressive symptoms in patients with psoriasis.[56] Etanercept also improved the tolerability of chemotherapy for advanced-stage cancer by significantly reducing fatigue.[57] Nonetheless, determining which specific cytokine to target is a continuing challenge. Alternative strategies, such as the antagonism of relevant inflammatory signaling pathways (including NF-kB and p38 MAPK), are becoming increasingly appealing. These strategies may have a broader spectrum of activity and have more far-reaching effects than targeting individual cytokines.

Other potential targets further downstream are those that are already being addressed by ongoing developments in the treatment of depression in medically healthy individuals. These targets include CRH, the GR, and the monoamines. Monoamine reuptake inhibitors and monoamine agonists remain viable objectives for addressing the contribution of inflammation to behavior. In a double-blind, placebo-controlled study of patients receiving IFN-α for the treatment of depression, pretreatment with the serotonin reuptake inhibitor paroxetine was found to reduce rates of major depression more than fourfold compared with placebo.[33] Stimulants such as methylphenidate that enhance dopamine pathways also have been a mainstay in the treatment of psychomotor slowing and fatigue in patients with cancer.[2]

Conclusions

The data presented herein suggest that cancer patients may be especially vulnerable to depression secondary to a combination of psychological stress and the biological processes inherent to cancer treatment that involve tissue damage and destruction. Together, these factors conspire to lead to exaggerated innate immune inflammatory responses which, in turn, have the capacity to interact with pathophysiological pathways in the brain that are inherent to the development of depression. Treatment strategies targeting the contributions of psychological stress and inflammation to behavioral change are already available, and new approaches based on an increasing appreciation of stress neurobiology and its interaction with the immune system represent an exciting direction for future drug discovery and development.

References

1. McDaniel JS, Musselman DL, Porter MR, Reed DA, Nemeroff CB. Depression in patients with cancer: diagnosis, biology, and treatment. *Arch Gen Psychiatry* **52**(2):89–99, 1995.
2. Raison CL, Miller AH. Depression in cancer: new developments regarding diagnosis and treatment. *Biol Psychiatry* **54**(3):283–294, 2003.
3. National Cancer Institute. Depression (PDQ®): assessment and diagnosis. Available from: URL: http://www.cancer.gov/cancertopics/pdq/supportivecare/depression/HealthProfessional/page3. Accessed Oct 15, 2008.
4. Spiegel D, Giese-Davis J. Depression and cancer: mechanisms and disease progression. *Biol Psychiatry* **54**(3):269–282, 2003.
5. Burke MA, Lowrance W, Perczek R. Emotional and cognitive burden of prostate cancer. *Urol Clin North Am* **30**(2):295–304, 2003.
6. Kendal W. Suicide and cancer: a gender-comparative study. *Ann Oncol* **18**(2):381–387, 2007.
7. Llorente MD, Burke M, Gregory GR, et al. Prostate cancer: a significant risk factor for late-life suicide. *Am J Geriatr Psychiatry* **13**(3):195–201, 2005.
8. Himelhoch S, Weller WE, Wu AW, Anderson GF, Cooper LA. Chronic medical illness, depression, and use of acute medical services among Medicare beneficiaries. *Med Care* **42**(6):512–521, 2004.
9. Lillberg K, Verkasalo PK, Kaprio J, Teppo L, Helenius H, Koskenvuo M. Stressful life events and risk of breast cancer in 10,808 women: a cohort study. *Am J Epidemiol* **157**(5):415–423, 2003.
10. Penninx BW, Guralnik JM, Pahor M, et al. Chronically depressed mood and cancer risk in older persons. *J Natl Cancer Inst* **90**(24):1888–1893, 1998.
11. Onitilo AA, Nietert PJ, Egede LE. Effect of depression on all-cause mortality in adults with cancer and differential effects by cancer site. *Gen Hosp Psychiatry* **28**(5):396–402, 2006.
12. Goodwin JS, Zhang DD, Ostir GV. Effect of depression on diagnosis, treatment, and survival of older women

with breast cancer. *J Am Geriatr Soc* **52**(1):106–111, 2004.

13. Hardman A, Maguire P, Crowther D. The recognition of psychiatric morbidity on a medical oncology ward. *J Psychosom Res* **33**(2):235–239, 1989.
14. Passik SD, Dugan W, McDonald MV, Rosenfeld B, Theobald DE, Edgerton S. Oncologists' recognition of depression in their patients with cancer. *J Clin Oncol* **16**(4):1594–1600, 1998.
15. American Psychiatric Association. *Diagnostic and Statistical Manual of Mental Disorders: DSM-IV*, 4th ed. Washington DC: American Psychiatric Association, 1994.
16. Dantzer R, Kelley KW. Twenty years of research on cytokine-induced sickness behavior. *Brain Behav Immun* **21**(2):153–160, 2007.
17. Musselman DL, Miller AH, Porter MR, et al. Higher than normal plasma interleukin-6 concentrations in cancer patients with depression: preliminary findings. *Am J Psychiatry* **158**(8):1252–1257, 2001.
18. Kendler KS, Thornton LM, Gardner CO. Stressful life events and previous episodes in the etiology of major depression in women: an evaluation of the "kindling" hypothesis. *Am J Psychiatry* **157**(8):1243–1251, 2000.
19. Heim C, Plotsky PM, Nemeroff CB. Importance of studying the contributions of early adverse experience to neurobiological findings in depression. *Neuropsychopharmacology* **29**(4):641–648, 2004.
20. Caspi A, Sugden K, Moffitt TE, et al. Influence of life stress on depression: moderation by a polymorphism in the 5-HTT gene. *Science* **301**(5631):386–389, 2003.
21. Felitti VJ, Anda RF, Nordenberg D, et al. Relationship of childhood abuse and household dysfunction to many of the leading causes of death in adults. The Adverse Childhood Experiences (ACE) Study. *Am J Prev Med* **14**(4):245–258, 1998.
22. Bierhaus A, Humpert PM, Nawroth PP. NF-kappaB as a molecular link between psychosocial stress and organ dysfunction. *Pediatr Nephrol* **19**(11):1189–1191, 2004.
23. Pace TW, Mletzko TC, Alagbe O, et al. Increased stress-induced inflammatory responses in male patients with major depression and increased early life stress. *Am J Psychiatry* **163**(9):1630–1633, 2006.
24. Barrientos RM, Sprunger DB, Campeau S, et al. Brain-derived neurotrophic factor mRNA downregulation produced by social isolation is blocked by intrahippocampal interleukin-1 receptor antagonist. *Neuroscience* **121**(4):847–853, 2003.
25. Duman RS, Monteggia LM. A neurotrophic model for stress-related mood disorders. *Biol Psychiatry* **59**(12):1116–1127, 2006.
26. Frank MG, Baratta MV, Sprunger DB, Watkins LR, Maier SF. Microglia serve as a neuroimmune substrate for stress-induced potentiation of CNS pro-inflammatory cytokine responses. *Brain Behav Immun* **21**(1):47–59, 2007.
27. Johnson JD, Campisi J, Sharkey CM, et al. Catecholamines mediate stress-induced increases in peripheral and central inflammatory cytokines. *Neuroscience* **135**(4):1295–1307, 2005.
28. Mazzeo SE, Slof-Op't Landt MC, Jones I, et al. Associations among postpartum depression, eating disorders, and perfectionism in a population-based sample of adult women. *Int J Eat Disord* **39**(3):202–211, 2006.
29. Wang H, Yu M, Ochani M, et al. Nicotinic acetylcholine receptor alpha7 subunit is an essential regulator of inflammation. *Nature* **421**(6921):384–388, 2003.
30. Coussens LM, Werb Z. Inflammation and cancer. *Nature* **420**(6917):860–867, 2002.
31. Greten FR, Eckmann L, Greten TF, et al. IKKbeta links inflammation and tumorigenesis in a mouse model of colitis-associated cancer. *Cell* **118**(3):285–296, 2004.
32. Raison CL, Capuron L, Miller AH. Cytokines sing the blues: inflammation and the pathogenesis of depression. *Trends Immunol* **27**(1):24–31, 2006.
33. Musselman DL, Lawson DH, Gumnick JF, et al. Paroxetine for the prevention of depression induced by high-dose interferon alfa. *N Engl J Med* **344**(13):961–966, 2001.
34. Bower JE, Ganz PA, Aziz N, Fahey JL. Fatigue and proinflammatory cytokine activity in breast cancer survivors. *Psychosom Med* **64**(4):604–611, 2002.
35. Meyers CA, Albitar M, Estey E. Cognitive impairment, fatigue, and cytokine levels in patients with acute myelogenous leukemia or myelodysplastic syndrome. *Cancer* **104**(4):788–793, 2005.
36. Kelley KW, Bluthé RM, Dantzer R, et al. Cytokine-induced sickness behavior. *Brain Behav Immun* **17**(Suppl 1):S112–S118, 2003.
37. Turner-Cobb JM, Sephton SE, Koopman C, Blake-Mortimer J, Spiegel D. Social support and salivary cortisol in women with metastatic breast cancer. *Psychosom Med* **62**(3):337–345, 2000.
38. Hayley S, Poulter MO, Merali Z, Anisman H. The pathogenesis of clinical depression: stressor- and cytokine-induced alterations of neuroplasticity. *Neuroscience* **135**(3):659–678, 2005.
39. Owens MJ, Nemeroff CB. Physiology and pharmacology of corticotropin-releasing factor. *Pharmacol Rev* **43**(4):425–473, 1991.
40. Silverman MN, Miller AH, Biron CA, Pearce BD. Characterization of an interleukin-6- and adrenocorticotropin-dependent, immune-to-adrenal

pathway during viral infection. *Endocrinology* **145**(8):3580–3589, 2004.

41. Capuron L, Neurauter G, Musselman DL, et al. Interferon-alpha-induced changes in tryptophan metabolism: relationship to depression and paroxetine treatment. *Biol Psychiatry* **54**(9):906–914, 2003.
42. Pace TW, Hu F, Miller AH. Cytokine-effects on glucocorticoid receptor function: relevance to glucocorticoid resistance and the pathophysiology and treatment of major depression. *Brain Behav Immun* **21**(1):9–19, 2007.
43. Maes M, Bosmans E, Meltzer HY, Scharpé S, Suy E. Interleukin-1 beta: a putative mediator of HPA axis hyperactivity in major depression? *Am J Psychiatry* **150**(8):1189–1193, 1993.
44. Rich T, Innominato PF, Boerner J, et al. Elevated serum cytokines correlated with altered behavior, serum cortisol rhythm, and dampened 24-hour rest-activity patterns in patients with metastatic colorectal cancer. *Clin Cancer Res* **11**(5):1757–1764, 2005.
45. Zhu CB, Carneiro AM, Dostmann WR, Hewlett WA, Blakely RD. p38 MAPK activation elevates serotonin transport activity via a trafficking-independent, protein phosphatase 2A-dependent process. *J Biol Chem* **280**(16):15649–15658, 2005.
46. Sanchez MM, Alagbe O, Felger JC, et al. Activated p38 MAPK is associated with decreased CSF 5-HIAA and increased maternal rejection during infancy in rhesus monkeys. *Mol Psychiatry* **12**(10):895–897, 2007.
47. Capuron L, Pagnoni G, Demetrashvili MF, et al. Basal ganglia hypermetabolism and symptoms of fatigue during interferon-alpha therapy. *Neuropsychopharmacology* **32**(11):2384–2392, 2007.
48. Chaudhuri A, Behan PO. Fatigue and basal ganglia. *J Neurol Sci* **179**(S 1–2):34–42, 2000.
49. Capuron L, Pagnoni G, Demetrashvili M, et al. Anterior cingulate activation and error processing during interferon-alpha treatment. *Biol Psychiatry* **58**:190–196, 2005.
50. Krongrad A, Lai H, Burke MA, Goodkin K, Lai S. Marriage and mortality in prostate cancer. *J Urol* **156**(5):1696–1670, 1996.
51. Price MA, Tennant CC, Butow PN, et al. The role of psychosocial factors in the development of breast carcinoma: Part II. Life event stressors, social support, defense style, and emotional control and their interactions. *Cancer* **91**(4):686–697, 2001.
52. Walker MS, Zona DM, Fisher EB. Depressive symptoms after lung cancer surgery: Their relation to coping style and social support. *Psychooncology* **15**(8):684–693, 2006.
53. Kaati G, Vester M, Sjöström M, Bygren LO. Patients' attachment patterns and response to a program for alleviating cardiovascular risk factors: a 1-year follow-up of patients in a patient education program. *Patient Educ Couns* **44**(3):235–241, 2001.
54. Pearlman LA, Courtois CA. Clinical applications of the attachment framework: relational treatment of complex trauma. *J Trauma Stress* **18**(5):449–459, 2005.
55. Bifulco A, Kwon J, Jacobs C, Moran PM, Bunn A, Beer N. Adult attachment style as mediator between childhood neglect/abuse and adult depression and anxiety. *Soc Psychiatry Psychiatr Epidemiol* **41**(10): 796–805, 2006.
56. Tyring S, Gottlieb A, Papp K, et al. Etanercept and clinical outcomes, fatigue, and depression in psoriasis: double-blind placebo-controlled randomised Phase III trial. *Lancet* **367**(9504): 29–35, 2006.
57. Monk JP, Phillips G, Waite R, et al. Assessment of tumor necrosis factor alpha blockade as an intervention to improve tolerability of dose-intensive chemotherapy in cancer patients. *J Clin Oncol* **24**(12):1852–1859, 2006.

Section 2 Chapter 9

Cancer Symptom Mechanisms and Models: Clinical and Basic Science

Depressive illness: basic science

The two sections of this chapter provide complementary expositions of our complex, and as yet incomplete, understanding of the biology of depression. In the first section, Adrian Dunn offers a brief historical overview of antidepressant treatments to introduce the need for conducting more extensive animal-based pharmacological validation studies of new antidepressant drugs. He describes with vivid clarity the most important behavioral tests available today to measure depressive-like symptoms in animals, such as the forced-swim test, tail-suspension test, and sucrose preference test. In addition, he discusses important biological processes that are potential markers or inducers of depression, such as the enhanced metabolism of brain tryptophan and serotonin, the inhibition of nerve regeneration in the hippocampus, and the sickness behavior induced by tumor burden and inflammatory cytokines. In the second section, Robert Dantzer and Keith Kelley offer a detailed account of the possible neuroimmune mechanisms of sickness and depression that are induced by inflammatory cytokines. They begin by describing some of the cellular changes in the brain that follow infection and inflammation in the periphery, with particular emphasis on the role of interleukin (IL)-1 and lipopolysaccharide (LPS) in the induction of neuroimmune pathways of communication. Motivational changes triggered by sensory pathways and their involvement in sickness and depression are discussed, along with the difficult task of discriminating between the two phenotypes. A detailed description is given of the possible role of indoleamine 2,3 dioxygenase (IDO) and tryptophan metabolism as one of the key molecular mechanisms that may link inflammation with depression.

Predictably, the authors' views on the biological basis of depression and its treatment are broadly corresponding but not without some disagreement. For instance, whereas Dantzer and Kelley attribute to peripherally induced IL-1 and other proinflammatory cytokines a crucial role in the induction of depression and sickness-related symptoms, Dunn points out that there is not yet enough evidence linking elevated plasma levels of IL-1, and only limited evidence linking elevated plasma IL-6 and tumor necrosis factor (TNF)-α, to the development of major depressive illness. As these authors indicate, the answer may rely on the actual cytokines produced in the brain as a result of peripheral insults. Future research and discussion are thus needed to clearly define the role of inflammation and other neuroendocrine mechanisms in the development of depression in patients with cancer.

Cancer Symptom Science: Measurement, Mechanisms, and Management, eds. Charles S. Cleeland, Michael J. Fisch, and Adrian J. Dunn.

Section 2 Chapter 9a

Cancer Symptom Mechanisms and Models: Clinical and Basic Science

Animal models of depressive illness and sickness behavior

Adrian J. Dunn

For many patients with cancer, becoming depressed is frequently associated with both the cancer and its treatments. In a recent state-of-the-science conference,[1] depression was highlighted as one of the most important symptoms facing patients with cancer, along with fatigue and pain. Only a small proportion of patients with cancer present with major depression as defined by the revised fourth version of the *Diagnostic and Statistical Manual of Mental Disorders* (DSM-IVR),[2] but depression-like symptoms, including reduced interest in previously pleasurable activities, lack of motivation, and sadness are frequently reported by patients with cancer in various stages of the disease.

It is easy to attribute these changes in affect to the patient learning that they have a potentially fatal disease. However, the degree of disturbance reported by patients is typically only modestly correlated with the severity of their disease or their prognosis. Only recently has there been interest in the association between the biological insults caused by cancer and its treatment, and the changes in affect and the other symptoms that patients report. Having a greater understanding of the biology contributing to cancer-related changes in affect should lead to better control or prevention of this source of distress.

Animal models of depressed affect related to disease burden or treatment toxicities may be important for developing a mechanistic understanding of why these changes occur. Currently, animal models of depressed affect related to cancer are relatively unexplored (but see below). However, there are animal models of depression, and these can provide a framework for studying depression-like symptoms related to both cancer and its therapy. In this chapter, we briefly review the history of antidepressant treatments, discuss available animal models and tests for depressive illness, and examine several possible mechanisms of cancer-related depression.

Depression and antidepressant treatment

Depressive illness is by far the most common psychiatric disorder and as such has been the subject of extensive research. Depression in humans can be unipolar (only depressed signs and symptoms occur), or bipolar (swinging between depression and mania, as with the phases of the moon). According to the DSM-IVR,[2] a major depressive episode is defined as either depressed mood or anhedonia, plus any four of the following symptoms: significant loss of weight or appetite; insomnia; psychomotor agitation or retardation; fatigue or loss of energy; feelings of worthlessness; diminished ability to think or concentrate, or indecisiveness; and recurrent thoughts of death or suicidal ideation for a two-week period. Atypical depression can involve weight gain, hypersomnia, or both. Several of these criteria are difficult, if not impossible, to apply to laboratory animals. Moreover, psychiatrists distinguish between depression and dysthymia, which is considered a type of low-grade depression that has fewer or less-serious symptoms than major depression but lasts longer. Dysthymia is very difficult to detect in animals.

The first major breakthrough in the pharmacological treatment of depressive illness was the discovery in the late 1950s that the tricyclic drug imipramine, synthesized at CIBA-Geigy, had the ability to ameliorate depressive illness. Imipramine was shown to be an inhibitor of monoamine oxidase,[3] an enzyme important for the degradation of amines, especially amine neurotransmitters. However, imipramine also inhibited the uptake (and reuptake) of catecholamines, such as dopamine and noradrenaline (norepinephrine), as well as the indoleamine 5-hydroxytryptamine (5-HT, serotonin). Inhibition of these selective uptake systems prolongs the extracellular existence of these biogenic amines. Thus imipramine acts acutely as a potent dopamine, norepinephrine, and serotonin agonist,

Cancer Symptom Science: Measurement, Mechanisms, and Management, eds. Charles S. Cleeland, Michael J. Fisch, and Adrian J. Dunn.

significantly potentiating the effects of these neurotransmitters by prolonging their time in the extracellular space. Catecholamines and catecholamine agonists elevate mood, potentially inducing mania, which is commonly associated with hyperactivity of a number of different amines (dopamine, norepinephrine, serotonin, and glutamate). Blocking the reuptake of catecholamines may reverse depression and may even induce mania. Imipramine is still regarded as a most potent and effective antidepressant, although its side effects limit its prescription.

A number of other compounds that inhibit catecholamine and/or serotonin reuptake were subsequently synthesized (eg, amitriptyline, desmethylimipramine), and many of these drugs are still used effectively today to treat depressive illness. However, like imipramine, many of the first-generation antidepressants have significant side effects, such as orthostatic hypertension (faintness associated with standing upright caused by antagonism of the α_1-adrenergic reflex, which drives blood from the lower limbs upwards to the trunk and the brain). These drugs also have undesirable anticholinergic effects, such as dry mouth, constipation, dizziness, blurred vision, urinary retention, and insomnia.

Building on these initial breakthroughs, the pharmaceutical companies explored the serotonin reuptake-blocking abilities of antidepressants and, in 1970, the first serotonin-selective reuptake inhibitor (SSRI), fluoxetine (Prozac®), was introduced. The SSRIs were a significant breakthrough because they lacked many of the side effects of the first-generation antidepressant drugs. However, SSRIs are not without their problems. For example, fluoxetine, the "breakthrough" drug, induces sexual dysfunction in a significant proportion of patients (both males and females), not a particularly desirable property in an antidepressant. Fortunately, most of the more-recently developed SSRIs lack this detrimental effect. More recently, a number of new related drugs, most notably the serotonin-norepinephrine reuptake inhibitors (SNRIs, such as venlafaxine and duloxetine), which inhibit both norepinephrine and serotonin reuptake, were introduced. Although imipramine, desmethylimipramine, and amitriptyline are also SNRIs, the newly developed SNRIs lack the side effects of these first-generation drugs.

Because psychiatrists have noted that depression is comorbid with anxiety in as many as half of their patients with depressive illness, many physicians often prescribe anxiolytic drugs along with the antidepressants to treat depression. In general, the comorbid disease is harder to treat than depression alone.

Finally, it is important to recognize that chronic treatment with antidepressant drugs is required to exert their antidepressant effects. Typically, significant antidepressant responses do not occur before two weeks, and maximal effects may not be achieved for six months or more. Thus, the long-term effects of antidepressants may involve downregulation of the effects of adrenergic and/or serotonergic systems.

Animal models of depression

Depressive disorders are relatively common; approximately 17% of the US population suffers at least one clinically diagnosable depressive episode in their lifetime. Such episodes are substantially more frequent in women than in men. Similar statistics exist for many other countries. Even so, only about 70% of depressed patients are effectively treated by current antidepressant drugs (although the placebo effect may be as high as 60%). For this reason, numerous efforts have been devoted to using animal models to develop new and better therapies (Table 9.1). Several classic articles have described the genesis of animal models of depressive illness, most notably those of McKinney[4,5] and, more recently, Kalueff and Tuohimaa[6] and McArthur and Borsini.[7] For an excellent account of the relationship between human problems and animal models, see Anisman and Matheson.[8]

Table 9.1. Animal models of depressive illness

Animal	Model
Rats	Chronic electric footshock[9,99]
	Chronic restraint[99]
	Learned helplessness[100]
	Chronic mild stress (CMS)[16]
Rat genetic models	Flinders sensitive (FSL) and resistant (FSR) lines [19]
	Congenitally learned helpless[20]
	Footshock (FS) high and low activity[21]
Mice	Chronic electric footshock[99]
	Chronic restraint[99]
Mouse genetic models	H/Rouen[22]
	Elevated plus maze (EPM) high and low activity[23]

It is not at all clear that the animals commonly used in research laboratories experience depression as humans do. Thus, reliance has been placed on pharmacological validation, ie, that drugs and other treatments that are effective in depressed humans should also be effective in the animal models. One of the earliest models was so-called "learned helplessness."[9–11] In this model, the animals (dogs, in the initial experiments) are exposed to inescapable electric footshock. The animals soon learn that escape is not possible and they give up, no longer even attempting to escape. In some of the early experiments, the shock was controlled by another dog, so the subject once again had no control over the shock. This paradigm was subsequently extended to rats, and then to mice.[9] Learned helplessness can be reversed by chronic treatment with antidepressant drugs, thus providing a pharmacological validation for the procedure.[11,12]

Because life stress frequently precedes depressive illness in humans, often following bereavement, divorce, and the like,[11,13–15] the focus of the animal studies has been on models of depression induced by chronic stress.[7,13,15] The simplest models use the stressors most commonly employed with rodents in the laboratory, namely electric footshock and restraint, which are rarely applied to humans. Typical treatments involve administering footshock or restraint to rats or mice daily for short periods of time, from several days to several weeks. More sophisticated models involve the use of multiple stressors over time, such as the chronic mild stress (CMS) model in which rats are subjected to an alternating series of moderate stressors (eg, wet bedding, constant lighting, or food deprivation) over a relatively long time period.[16] Unlike the preceding models, the depression-like manifestations of this latter procedure are prevented only by chronic (not acute) administration of antidepressant medications, and the effects are long-lasting. This procedure thus has more face validity than the simpler chronic-stress models. A similar procedure has been used effectively in mice.[17,18]

There are also a number of genetic models. For example, the Flinders Sensitive Line (FSL) of rats was developed at Flinders University in Adelaide by Overstreet et al.,[19] who selectively bred Sprague-Dawley rats for their sensitivity to cholinesterase inhibitors. Comparisons are made in parallel with the Flinders Resistant Line (FRL). There are also congenitally learned helpless rats,[20] and rats selectively bred for high or low activity in the forced-swim test.[21] Vaugeois et al.[22] selectively bred CD-1 mice for high and low activity in the tail-suspension test (H/Rouen mice), and Krömer et al.[23] selectively bred CD-1 mice for high anxiety in the elevated plus-maze test. For a more detailed review of these genetic models, see El Yacoubi and Vaugeois.[24]

Alternative models that have yet to be explored adequately are the stress of natural predators (eg, cats as natural enemies of rats, rats as natural enemies of mice, etc.) and of aggressive conspecifics, such as in social hierarchies.

For a more detailed analysis of the various forms of depressive illness, and the appropriate animal models and assessments, see the studied review by Anisman and Matheson.[8]

Animal tests of depression

Another important issue with the animal models is how to test for depression-like illness. The most commonly used behavioral tests are the forced-swim test developed by Porsolt[25–27] and the tail-suspension test pioneered by Steru et al.[28] (Table 9.2). Tests that examine biological indicators of depression parallel findings in humans and may also be instructive.

Behavioral tests

As Porsolt described originally for rats, the forced-swim test involves placing the rat in a tall cylinder partially filled with lukewarm water (25°C) such that it must swim to breathe. After 15 minutes, the rat is removed from the cylinder, partially dried with a towel, and allowed to dry out in a heated enclosure for 15 minutes. Twenty-four hours later the rat is replaced in the cylinder of water, and the total duration of immobility is measured during a five-minute test. Candidate antidepressant treatments are administered immediately after the first session or at selected intervals between the first and second swims. On the second day of the test, untreated rats typically remain

Table 9.2. Animal tests of depression-like illness

Animal	Test
Rats	Forced-swim test[25,27]
	Ingestion of palatable fluids[101]
Mice	Forced-swim test[29]
	Tail-suspension test[28]
	Ingestion of sweetened milk[102]

immobile for 75% of the time,[27,29] whereas rats treated with different antidepressant drugs exhibit reduced immobility times that vary depending on the drug administered. Electroconvulsive shock treatment, the animal equivalent of the electroconvulsive therapy used to treat depressive illness in humans (most often as a last resort), also reduces immobility.[27] However, a major shortcoming of the original version of the forced-swim test is its failure to show positive results with the SSRIs.[30]

The forced-swim test was modified significantly for mice: they were placed in the cylinder on only one day, and for only six minutes.[26] As with rats, the time for which the mouse remained immobile was scored as an index of depression. Because the mice typically exhibited little immobility in the first two minutes, only the last four minutes were scored. As in rats, antidepressant treatments decreased the time spent immobile.[26]

Other researchers have made many minor modifications to these tests. For example, Lucki[31] modified the test slightly by increasing the water depth to 30 cm from the traditional depth of 15–18 cm, so that the rat cannot gain support from its hind paws touching the bottom of the cylinder. They also used a time-sampling technique to rate the predominant behavior over each five-second interval. These alterations enabled distinction of specific components of the active behaviors, namely: (1) climbing behavior (thrashing), defined as upward-directed movements of the forepaws along the side of the swim chamber; (2) swimming, defined as horizontal movement through the chamber; and (3) immobility, defined as in the traditional Porsolt test. Most importantly, these modifications rendered the test sensitive to the serotonin-selective SSRIs in a distinct pattern.[30,32,33] The revised scoring system suggested that the action of the SSRI fluoxetine involved 5-HT_{2c} receptors.[33] For a more detailed review of the various modifications of the forced-swim test, see McArthur and Borsini.[7]

In the tail-suspension test,[28] the mouse is suspended by its tail with adhesive tape attached to the tail 2 cm from its extremity. At first, the mouse attempts to climb its own tail, but it soon gives up and hangs immobile. As in the Porsolt test, the time spent immobile is scored as the index of despair (ie, depression). Many researchers have found this test to be more reliable than the forced-swim test in mice. Although there are a few reports using a tail-suspension test in rats,[34] most researchers have not found it to be useful, largely because the rats tend to spin when suspended and consequently often sever their own tails.

An alternative strategy is to assess the anhedonic symptoms of depression. This can readily be assessed in rats and mice by scoring their propensity to drink sucrose or saccharin solutions in preference to pure water.[35] Sweetened milk is particularly palatable for both rats and mice.[36] Chronically stressed rats and mice have a decreased propensity to consume the sweet fluids. Decreased milk consumption is also induced by peripheral or central injections of endotoxin (lipopolysaccharide) and the cytokine interleukin (IL)-1[36]; see also Chapter 3.

Biological assessments

A surprising aspect of basic research on depression is the relative lack of attention to impairment of reward mechanisms, which would seem an obvious target for treatment.[37] Current thinking is that reward systems largely involve dopaminergic systems, primarily the mesolimbic and mesocortical systems. However, endogenous opiates may also be involved, and there are multiple interactions between opiatergic (ie, various of the endorphins, including the enkephalins and dynorphins) and both dopaminergic and noradrenergic systems. There is less evidence for the involvement of serotonergic systems and opiates, although interactions between serotonergic and opiatergic systems occur in the brain stem and spinal cord in regions associated with pain.

Tryptophan is an essential amino acid that is critical not only for the synthesis of proteins, but also for the synthesis of serotonin (as well as melatonin). If the SSRIs exert their antidepressant action by inhibiting the reuptake of serotonin, this may result in a net loss of serotonin from the brain, and thus increase the body's need for tryptophan. In fact, dietary supplementation with tryptophan has been used by some physicians to treat depression successfully.[38] Acute tryptophan depletion has been reported to lower mood, but overall the results have been somewhat variable. One study indicated that tryptophan depletion impaired long-term memory formation and interfered with the consolidation of memory, while it improved attention.[39] Most studies have failed to show an exacerbation of depressive symptoms subsequent to tryptophan depletion.[40]

Serotonin also has a complex role in sleep. It changes the architecture of sleep, and this could explain some of the abnormalities observed in the sleep patterns of depressed patients. However, the literature does not indicate simple relationships between tryptophan depletion and the sleep abnormalities of depressed patients.[40]

The association of depression with the cerebral activity of serotonin and catecholamines is not a simple one. In an elegant series of studies, Delgado et al.[41] examined the effects of tryptophan depletion and catecholamine depletion on depressed patients who had been treated successfully with SSRIs or tricyclic antidepressants. When brain tryptophan was depleted by administering a cocktail of amino acids that compete for the same brain uptake system used by tryptophan (thus limiting serotonin synthesis), the patients whose depression had been alleviated by SSRIs became depressed again. However, when the tryptophan depletion was performed in patients that had been successfully treated with tricyclic antidepressants, the depression did not return. Conversely, when depressed patients that had been treated successfully with catecholamine uptake inhibitors were treated with α-methyl-*p*-tyrosine, an inhibitor of catecholamine synthesis (thus depleting brain dopamine and norepinephrine), the depressive symptoms returned. However, tryptophan depletion in such patients did not alter their depression scores. Thus, the effect of the posttreatment manipulations depended on the mechanism used to alleviate the depression, rather than on any underlying abnormality in the depressed patient. This suggests that the depression is not associated in a simple way with deficiencies in catecholamine or serotonin metabolism or function.

Potential mechanisms of depression in the patient with cancer

The occurrence of depression in patients with cancer is undoubtedly multifaceted. Learning that one has cancer is stressful in and of itself and could induce depression. The patient's own physiology, including brain processes and the direct effects of the cancer cells, may also play a part in causing depression. Even the treatments prescribed for the patient's cancer might be responsible for the depression.

Inhibition of hippocampal neurogenesis

The hippocampus is a brain structure that has long been associated with the formation of memory. Animal studies have identified a chain of events suggesting that the diminishment of neurogenesis in the hippocampus is a precipitating factor in the development of clinical depression.[42] Conversely, the generation of neurons in the hippocampus appears to be required for the antidepressant-like behavioral effects of imipramine and fluoxetine,[43] suggesting a role for neurogenesis in recovery from depression.

In most mammals, new neurons are generated until the animal reaches sexual maturity. A long-standing dogma in the field of neuroscience has been that, once sexual maturity is achieved, the generation of new neurons does not occur in the mammalian brain. However, studies have shown that this is not the case. In a classical study, Altman and Das[44] showed that the incorporation of radiolabeled [^{3}H]thymidine into the DNA of neurons (indicative of DNA synthesis and, presumably, of cell division) occurred to a limited extent in the olfactory bulb and the hippocampus of adult rats. (Current techniques employ administration of the nonradioactive tracer bromodeoxyuridine, which can readily be detected histologically in the DNA without the use of radioisotopes.) More recent studies have indicated a continual generation of new neurons in the hippocampus, primarily granule cells.[45,46]

Building on Sapolsky's observation that high concentrations of glucocorticoid hormones appeared to kill hippocampal neurons,[47] Gould et al.[48] showed that it was the generation of new neurons (largely granule cells) in the adult hippocampus that was inhibited by adrenal glucocorticoids and thus, indirectly, by stress.[49] Animals lacking a functional adrenal cortex (adrenalectomized animals) did not display the apparent loss of neurons. Jacobs et al.[45] proposed that "stress-induced decreases in dentate gyrus neurogenesis are an important causal factor in precipitating episodes of depression," and that "therapeutic interventions for depression that increase serotonergic neurotransmission act, at least in part, by augmenting dentate gyrus neurogenesis and thereby promoting recovery from depression."

The precise mechanisms are not yet fully understood. However, a current hypothesis is that the generation of new neurons appears to be stimulated by serotonin and by brain-derived neurotrophic factor (BDNF).[42] BDNF promotes the conversion of progenitor cells to new hippocampal neurons. BDNF also promotes the survival and differentiation of serotonergic neurons.[50] SSRIs enhance the expression of BDNF, thus serotonin promotes the synthesis of

BDNF; 5-HT_{1A} receptors appear to be involved in these effects. Abnormalities in 5-HT_{1A} receptors have been observed in depressed patients.[51] Thus there are mutual stimulatory effects between serotonin and BDNF. Serotonin stimulates BDNF synthesis, and BDNF appears to play a role in the generation or growth of serotonergic neurons.

Neuronal cell division is inhibited by corticosteroids (corticosterone in rodents, cortisol in most other mammals), whose secretion is stimulated under stressful conditions. A substantial proportion of depressed patients exhibit elevated plasma or salivary concentrations of cortisol, the predominant corticosteroid in humans, which may explain the apparent hippocampal neuronal cell death that is associated with depression. There have also been reports that circulating concentrations of BDNF were lower in depressed patients, and that BDNF concentrations increased as patients improved on treatment.[51–53] Nevertheless, it appears unlikely that the loss of granule cells alone accounts for observed decreases in hippocampal volume[43]; the loss of other types of cells may play a part.

In a recent review of the structural magnetic resonance imaging (MRI) findings published between 2000 and 2007 and collected in patients with major depressive disorders, the authors concluded that volumetric reductions of the hippocampus, basal ganglia, orbitofrontal cortex, and subgenual prefrontal cortex are more likely to be found in patients with more persistent forms of depression (eg, multiple episodes or repeated relapses, longer illness duration) than in patients with less-severe forms of the disease.[54] Corticosteroid-induced inhibition of the generation of new neurons could account for the slightly shrunken hippocampus and the consequent enlargement of the lateral ventricles that occur in many depressed patients.

Behavioral, neurochemical, and endocrine effects of tumors

The depression frequently observed in patients with cancer is echoed in animal data indicating depression-like activity after tumor inoculation. We have studied neurochemical, endocrine, and behavioral responses to infection in mice with a leukemia cell line and have found that leukemic mice exhibit neurobehavioral disturbances that resemble the responses observed in humans. DBA2 mice were inoculated intraperitoneally with L1210 mouse leukemia cells at doses of 5000 or 50 000 cells per mouse.[53] The behavioral activity of the mice was assessed at various times in the tail-suspension test and the forced-swim test, as well as in the open field. No consistent differences from controls were observed in the behavior of these animals on days 8 or 11 after inoculation. However, on day 15, the mice inoculated with either 5000 or 50 000 L1210 cells exhibited statistically significant increases in immobility in the tail-suspension test and the forced swim test; in the open field, the mice injected with 50 000 L1210 cells showed statistically significant decreases in activity, whereas those that received only 5000 cells did not. This suggests that the depression-like activity was not attributable simply to a general reduction in activity. Both doses of L1210 cells increased plasma corticosterone concentrations, indicating the stressful nature of the leukemia. These mice also exhibited statistically significant increases in the metabolism of norepinephrine, but not dopamine, in the hypothalamus, and increases in tryptophan and serotonin metabolism in the cortex and hypothalamus. These indications of activation in the hypothalamic-pituitary-adrenal (HPA) axis and brain noradrenergic and serotonergic systems are characteristic of stress and replicate our earlier observations with the murine lymphoma cell line AW5E.[55]

These results are supported by a recent report on the depression-like behavioral activity of rats bearing mammary tumors.[56] In this study, mammary tumors were induced in female rats by the carcinogen *N*-nitroso-*N*-methylurea. Females were tested 8–10 weeks later, after the tumors had developed. Rats with tumors displayed increased floating behavior in the forced-swim test and decreased consumption of 0.1%, but not 1.0%, sucrose solution. Such rats also showed increased marble-burying behavior but did not differ from controls in the more usual measures of anxiety-like behavior in the elevated plus maze and open-field tests. The observed behavioral alterations were independent of any sign of sickness and were associated with an increase in concentrations of IL-1β, tumor necrosis factor (TNF)-α, IL-6, and IL-10 in the hippocampus but not in the hypothalamus. Rats with tumors had a decreased peak corticosterone response to a 30-minute swim stressor compared with control rats, despite a similar baseline. They also displayed significant increases in the genes expressing both mineralocorticoid and glucocorticoid receptors in the hippocampus, indicating a possible increased sensitivity of the negative feedback effect exerted by glucocorticoids on the stress response.

Overall, despite the weaknesses in the animal models and tests for depression, the few existing data indicate that tumors induce depression-like behavior in the animal models, lending credence to the validity of using antidepressants to treat patients with cancer. Needless to say, this has already been introduced into clinical practice, with significant success in some, but certainly not all, cases.

Cytokine-induced sickness behavior

Cytokines are relatively large polypeptides (some of which may be glycosylated) that are produced and released by immune cells and act as autocrine and paracrine messengers within the immune system; in other words, they are the hormones of the immune system. Recently there has been a flurry of speculation on the possible role of proinflammatory cytokines in depressive illness.[57–59] This may be relevant to cancer because many tumoral processes are inflammatory.[60] In addition, surgery and adjunctive cancer treatments, including chemotherapy and radiotherapy, can induce inflammation.[61]

The primary impetus for the theory that cytokines can cause depression is that IL-1, which is a critical cytokine synthesized and released early in the response to invading pathogens, has the ability to induce a behavioral pattern known as sickness behavior. Sickness behavior is a term that was coined by Hart[62] to describe the physiological and behavioral responses to illness and infections commonly observed in most species. In Hart's words: "The behavior of a sick individual is not a maladaptive and undesirable effect of illness, but rather a highly organized strategy that is at times critical to the survival of the individual if it were living in the wild state." According to Kent et al.,[63] "Sick individuals experience weakness, malaise, listlessness and inability to concentrate. They also show hypersomnia, anorexia, depressed activity and loss of interest in usual activities, including social contacts." The evidence cited for a cytokine hypothesis of depression includes:

- Administration of IL-1 to animals induces sickness behavior, a behavioral pattern that resembles depression. It includes reduced activity, decreased interest in exploring the environment and reinforcing stimuli. Because administration of lipopolysaccharide (LPS) rapidly induces IL-1,[63] LPS has been used to induce sickness behavior; however, LPS induces a cascade of other cytokines after binding to receptors that are ubiquitous in the body and prevalent on blood vessels.
- Administration of certain cytokines (IL-1, and some forms of interferon [IFN]-α) to humans induces responses characteristic of depression and flu-like symptoms.
- Elevated plasma concentrations of certain cytokines – primarily IL-6, IL-1-receptor antagonist (IL-1RA), and C-reactive protein, an acute-phase protein produced in the liver considered to be a marker of immune activation – have been observed in patients with depression.
- Depression is often observed in patients with peripheral inflammation.
- Cytokines (especially IL-1, and to a lesser extent, IL-6 and TNF-α) can activate the HPA axis, thus elevating plasma concentrations of adrenocorticotropic hormone and glucocorticoids.[64]
- Peripheral IL-1 administration potently activates brain noradrenergic systems,[65] which occurs commonly in depressed patients. TNF-α has a similar effect but is much less potent.[66]

Cytokines in animal studies of depression

IL-1 is the only cytokine whose administration to animals reliably induces sickness behavior. Both forms, IL-1α and IL-1β, are essentially equally potent, and both act on the same IL-1 receptor,[67,68] although some interferons, primarily IFN-α, can induce symptoms in humans. IL-6 does not induce sickness behavior in mice or rats,[69,70] although peripherally administered IL-6 does increase brain tryptophan concentrations and serotonin metabolism in mice.[70] Mice lacking the gene for IL-6 (IL-6 knockout mice) exhibited normal behavioral responses to IL-1 and LPS in the forced-swim and tail-suspension tests.[69] However, the sickness behavior in response to peripheral or central LPS or IL-1β is somewhat attenuated.[71,72] IL-6-deficient (knockout) mice showed normal HPA axis responses to IL-1 and LPS, but lacked the changes in tryptophan and serotonin metabolism.[69] TNF-α administration induces small increases in norepinephrine metabolism and brain tryptophan, but only at relatively high doses.[66,72]

Because of the close similarity between some aspects of sickness behavior and symptoms of depression, Yirmiya et al.[73] reasoned that antidepressant treatment should abrogate the behavioral and neuroendocrine effects of cytokines. In agreement with this prediction, they found that chronic treatment of rats with fluoxetine significantly attenuated LPS-induced anorexia and loss of body weight, depletion of corticotropin-releasing hormone 41 from the median eminence, and elevation of serum corticosterone concentrations, and also prevented the initial hypothermia observed after LPS administration to rats and mice. Chronic treatment with imipramine also attenuated the LPS-induced adrenocortical activation. However, in a subsequent study, no attenuation in the sickness behavior responses of mice to intraperitoneal LPS administration after chronic treatment with imipramine or venlafaxine was observed.[36] R. Yirmiya (personal communication, 2003) confirmed that antidepressants were not effective in this paradigm in mice. Chronic administration of the atypical antidepressant drug tianeptine attenuated sickness behavior caused by peripheral but not central administration of LPS or IL-1.[74] This was associated with a reduced HPA response to LPS, which paralleled the decrease in c-fos activation of the paraventricular nucleus of the hypothalamus.[75]

Cytokines in depressed patients

If cytokines play a causal role in depression, they should be elevated in depressed patients. Accordingly, there have been a significant number of studies on the circulating concentrations of cytokines in patients with depression. The initial reports emanated from Maes' laboratory, but these researchers measured only the production of IL-1 when immune cells isolated from depressed patients were stimulated *in vitro* with mitogens.[76,77] These results have been replicated by others,[78] but not consistently; Weizman et al.[79] observed a decrease of *in vitro* IL-1 production by macrophages from depressed patients in response to LPS. Because of the normally extremely low circulating concentrations of IL-1, the practice of using mitogen stimulation of isolated cells has been followed in many other studies; however, some reviewers of the published data on the presence of cytokines in depressed patients have failed to note this, perhaps because it was not always clearly indicated in the abstracts of some of the publications.

Although a small number of reports have indicated significant elevations of plasma concentrations of IL-1 in patients with major depression, most have not.[80] Results from a recent study revealed a significant elevation of serum IL-1 in late-life depression.[81] Owen et al[82] reported a significant elevation of circulating IL-1β in a group of 20 patients suffering from postviral depression; however, the elevation may have been induced by the viral infection itself, and thus does not necessarily implicate IL-1 in the depressive symptoms. A recent New Zealand study of 33 unmedicated patients found elevations of IL-6 and TNF-α, but not of IL-1β, linked to major depressive disorder.[83] In contrast to these studies, Brambilla and Maggioni[84] observed no difference in circulating IL-1β in depressed elderly women and age-matched controls. Subsequently, Brambilla et al.[85] reported an association of circulating IL-1β with dysthymia, but no association with major depressive disorder. Other studies have failed to find elevations of IL-1 in patients with depression.[86–92] Importantly, a recent large study in Finland revealed overall decreases in plasma IL-1, accompanied by increase in IL-1 receptor antagonist (IL1-RA), in male depressed patients.[91]

There are only a few meta-analyses of the clinical data. In 2001, Zorrilla et al.[93] noted the clear correlation between depression and elevation of circulating concentrations of IL-6, but they did not assess the relationship between circulating IL-1 and depression because there were too few data (E. P. Zorrilla, personal communication, November 2008). A recent thorough meta-analysis reinforced the existence of elevated IL-6 and of IL-1RA in depressed patients, and also noted a highly significant increase in C-reactive protein.[94] This study indicated an association of plasma IL-1 with depression that just met statistical significance ($P = 0.03$), whereas the other parameters associated with depression were highly statistically significant. In a 2009 meta-analysis, Dowlati et al.[95] concluded that circulating concentrations of both IL-6 and TNF-α were significantly elevated in depressed patients, whereas those of IL-1β were not.

Overall, the evidence for a ubiquitous elevation of plasma concentrations of IL-1 in depressed patients is unconvincing and is insufficient to support the hypothesis that an elevated circulating concentration of IL-1 is a major cause of depressive illness. Moreover, despite the fact that an endogenous IL-1 antagonist (IL-1RA) was identified and synthesized more than 20 years ago, there have been no reports that the use of this antagonist, or any other (for example, antibodies to IL-1) have antidepressant effects in humans.

Proponents of an IL-1 hypothesis of depression have subsequently argued that it is the appearance of IL-1 within the brain that causes depressive illness.[57,58] Such a hypothesis is tenable, because intracerebral administration of IL-1β in low doses can induce sickness behavior.[96] Thus, it would not be surprising if the appearance of IL-1 in the brain were to be associated with depression-like symptoms. It is known that strong immune challenges (for example, large doses of LPS injected peripherally) can result in the appearance of IL-1 and other proinflammatory cytokines in microglia and macrophage-like cells in the brain.[97] This would be expected to induce a fever and engender sickness behavior, which as discussed above resembles depressive illness.

In support of this, Levine et al.[98] reported a small study (13 subjects; 10 controls) in which cerebrospinal fluid concentrations of IL-1β were measured in unmedicated patients with acute severe depression. CSF concentrations of IL-1 were significantly elevated, whereas concentrations of IL-6 and TNF-α were not altered. Interestingly, plasma concentrations of IL-1β in the same patients were not elevated. More studies need to be performed to determine whether elevated CSF concentrations of IL-1β occur in a substantially larger population of depressed patients, and not just those suffering from severe acute depression, before we can conclude that elevated brain IL-1β is responsible for depressive illness.

It is likely that induction of IL-1 in the brain may be responsible for depressive illness in some patients. However, whether or not this is a common mechanism underlying depressive illness remains to be demonstrated.

Conclusion

The foregoing review has indicated the many problems associated with using animals to model the complexities associated with the human nervous system. Whereas, many of the challenges and frustrations that humans experience in modern life resemble those of other mammals, it is not at all clear that animals respond similarly to them, although they may. The truth is that the lack of a sophisticated means of communication in nonhuman animals renders difficult the modeling of the human conditions associated with cancer and its treatment. The problem is essentially the same one that confronts researchers seeking cures for depressive illness. Although depression is far and away the most common psychiatric illness, the currently available treatments fall far short of our expectations for many other medical conditions. Perhaps the best hope for the future is an expansion of the work on animal models involving tumors, such as the leukemia and mammary tumor models reviewed above.

Despite the various problems with the existing animal models and tests for depression, animal studies may provide some useful insights for the treatment of patients with cancer. Relatively new data indicating that cancer in animals can induce behavioral and physiological responses that match those observed in cancer patients are encouraging. It will be especially interesting to test the effects of antidepressant drugs and other antidepressant treatments in these models, which may provide insights into potential therapies for human patients.

References

1. Patrick DL, Ferketich SL, Frame PS, et al. National Institutes of Health State-of-the-Science Conference statement: symptom management in cancer: pain, depression, and fatigue, July 15–17, 2002. *J Natl Cancer Inst* **95**(15):1110–1117, 2003.
2. American Psychiatric Association. *Diagnostic and Statistical Manual of Mental Disorders: DSM-IV-TR*, revised 4th ed. Washington DC: American Psychiatric Association, 2000.
3. Granata AR, Numao Y, Kumada M, Reis DJ. A1 noradrenergic neurons tonically inhibit sympathoexcitatory neurons of C1 area in rat brainstem. *Brain Res* **377**(1):127–146, 1986.
4. McKinney WT. Overview of the past contributions of animal models and their changing place in psychiatry. *Semin Clin Neuropsychiatry* **6**(1): 68–78, 2001.
5. McKinney WT. Animal models of depression: an overview. *Psychiatr Dev* **2**(2):77–96, 1984.
6. Kalueff AV, Tuohimaa P. Experimental modeling of anxiety and depression. *Acta Neurobiol Exp (Wars)* **64**(4):439–448, 2004.
7. McArthur R, Borsini F. Animal models of depression in drug discovery: a historical perspective. *Pharmacol Biochem Behav* **84**(3):436–452, 2006.
8. Anisman H, Matheson K. Stress, depression, and anhedonia: caveats concerning animal models. *Neurosci Biobehav Rev* **29**(4–5):525–546, 2005.
9. Maier SF. Learned helplessness and animal models of depression. *Prog Neuropsychopharmacol Biol Psychiatry* **8**(3):435–446, 1984.

10. Seligman ME, Maier SF. Failure to escape traumatic shock. *J Exp Psychol* **74**(1):1–9, 1967.
11. Sherman AD, Sacquitne JL, Petty F. Specificity of the learned helplessness model of depression. *Pharmacol Biochem Behav* **16**(3):449–454, 1982.
12. Henn FA, Vollmayr B. Stress models of depression: forming genetically vulnerable strains. *Neurosci Biobehav Rev* **29**(4–5):799–804, 2005.
13. Anisman H, Zacharko RM. Depression: the predisposing influence of stress. *Behav Brain Sci* **5**(1):89–99, 1982.
14. van Praag HM. Can stress cause depression? *Prog Neuropsychopharmacol Biol Psychiatry* **28**(5):891–907, 2004.
15. Willner P. The validity of animal models of depression. *Psychopharmacology (Berl)* **83**(1):1–16, 1984.
16. Willner P. Validity, reliability and utility of the chronic mild stress model of depression: a 10-year review and evaluation. *Psychopharmacology (Berl)* **134**(4):319–329, 1997.
17. Ducottet C, Griebel G, Belzung C. Effects of the selective nonpeptide corticotropin-releasing factor receptor 1 antagonist antalarmin in the chronic mild stress model of depression in mice. *Prog Neuropsychopharmacol Biol Psychiatry* **27**(4):625–631, 2003.
18. Griebel G, Simiand J, Serradeil-Le Gal C, et al. Anxiolytic- and antidepressant-like effects of the non-peptide vasopressin V1b receptor antagonist, SSR149415, suggest an innovative approach for the treatment of stress-related disorders. *Proc Natl Acad Sci U S A* **99**(9):6370–6375, 2002.
19. Overstreet DH, Pucilowski O, Rezvani AH, Janowsky DS. Administration of antidepressants, diazepam and psychomotor stimulants further confirms the utility of Flinders Sensitive Line rats as an animal model of depression. *Psychopharmacology (Berl)* **121**(1):27–37, 1995.
20. Lachman HM, Papolos DF, Weiner ED, et al. Hippocampal neuropeptide Y mRNA is reduced in a strain of learned helpless resistant rats. *Brain Res Mol Brain Res* **14**(1–2):94–100, 1992.
21. Weiss JM, Kilts CD. Animal models of depression and schizophrenia. In: Schatzberg AF, Nemeroff CB, eds. *The American Psychiatric Press Textbook of Psychopharmacology*. Washington DC: American Psychiatric Press, 1998:89–131.
22. Vaugeois JM, Passera G, Zuccaro F, Costentin J. Individual differences in response to imipramine in the mouse tail suspension test. *Psychopharmacology (Berl)* **134**(4):387–391, 1997.
23. Krömer SA, Kessler MS, Milfay D, et al. Identification of glyoxalase-I as a protein marker in a mouse model of extremes in trait anxiety. *J Neurosci* **25**(17):4375–4384, 2005.
24. El Yacoubi M, Vaugeois JM. Genetic rodent models of depression. *Curr Opin Pharmacol* **7**(1):3–7, 2007.
25. Porsolt RD, Anton G, Blavet N, Jalfre M. Behavioural despair in rats: a new model sensitive to antidepressant treatments. *Eur J Pharmacol* **47**(4):379–391, 1978.
26. Porsolt RD, Bertin A, Jalfre M. Behavioral despair in mice: a primary screening test for antidepressants. *Arch Int Pharmacodyn Ther* **229**(2):327–336, 1977.
27. Porsolt RD, Le Pichon M, Jalfre M. Depression: a new animal model sensitive to antidepressant treatments. *Nature* **266**(5604):730–732, 1977.
28. Steru L, Chermat R, Thierry B, Simon P. The tail suspension test: a new method for screening antidepressants in mice. *Psychopharmacology (Berl)* **85**(3):367–370, 1985.
29. Porsolt RD, Bertin A, Jalfre M. "Behavioural despair" in rats and mice: strain differences and the effects of imipramine. *Eur J Pharmacol* **51**(3):291–294, 1978.
30. Cryan JF, Markou A, Lucki I. Assessing antidepressant activity in rodents: recent developments and future needs. *Trends Pharmacol Sci* **23**(5):238–245, 2002.
31. Lucki I. The forced swimming test as a model for core and component behavioral effects of antidepressant drugs. *Behav Pharmacol* **8**(6–7):523–532, 1997.
32. Cryan JF, Holmes A. The ascent of mouse: advances in modelling human depression and anxiety. *Nat Rev Drug Discov* **4**(9):775–790, 2005.
33. Cryan JF, Valentino RJ, Lucki I. Assessing substrates underlying the behavioral effects of antidepressants using the modified rat forced swimming test. *Neurosci Biobehav Rev* **29**(4–5):547–569, 2005.
34. Chermat R, Thierry B, Mico JA, Steru L, Simon P. Adaptation of the tail suspension test to the rat. *J Pharmacol* **17**(3):348–350, 1986.
35. Harkin A, Houlihan DD, Kelly JP. Reduction in preference for saccharin by repeated unpredictable stress in mice and its prevention by imipramine. *J Psychopharmacol* **16**(2):115–123, 2002.
36. Dunn AJ, Swiergiel AH. The reductions in sweetened milk intake induced by interleukin-1 and endotoxin are not prevented by chronic antidepressant treatment. *Neuroimmunomodulation* **9**(3):163–169, 2001.
37. Forbes EE. Where's the fun in that? Broadening the focus on reward function in depression. *Biol Psychiatry* **66**(3):199–200, 2009.
38. van Praag HM. Serotonin precursors in the treatment of depression. *Adv Biochem Psychopharmacol* **34**:259–286, 1982.

39. Schmitt JA, Jorissen BL, Sobczak S, et al. Tryptophan depletion impairs memory consolidation but improves focussed attention in healthy young volunteers. *J Psychopharmacol* **14**(1):21–29, 2000.

40. Bell C, Abrams J, Nutt D. Tryptophan depletion and its implications for psychiatry. *Br J Psychiatry* **178**:399–405, 2001.

41. Delgado PL, Miller HL, Salomon RM, et al. Tryptophan-depletion challenge in depressed patients treated with desipramine or fluoxetine: implications for the role of serotonin in the mechanism of antidepressant action. *Biol Psychiatry* **46**(2): 212–220, 1999.

42. Jacobs BL. Adult brain neurogenesis and depression. *Brain Behav Immun* **16**(5):602–609, 2002.

43. Sahay A, Hen R. Adult hippocampal neurogenesis in depression. *Nat Neurosci* **10**(9):1110–1115, 2007.

44. Altman J, Das GD. Post-natal origin of microneurones in the rat brain. *Nature* **207**(5000):953–956, 1965.

45. Jacobs BL, van Praag H, Gage FH. Adult brain neurogenesis and psychiatry: a novel theory of depression. *Mol Psychiatry* **5**(3):262–269, 2000.

46. Ming GL, Song H. Adult neurogenesis in the mammalian central nervous system. *Annu Rev Neurosci* **28**:223–250, 2005.

47. Sapolsky RM, Krey LC, McEwen BS. Glucocorticoid-sensitive hippocampal neurons are involved in terminating the adrenocortical stress response. *Proc Natl Acad Sci U S A* **81**(19):6174–6177, 1984.

48. Gould E, Cameron HA, Daniels DC, Woolley CS, McEwen BS. Adrenal hormones suppress cell division in the adult rat dentate gyrus. *J Neurosci* **12**(9):3642–3650, 1992.

49. Gould E, Tanapat P, McEwen BS, Flügge G, Fuchs E. Proliferation of granule cell precursors in the dentate gyrus of adult monkeys is diminished by stress. *Proc Natl Acad Sci U S A* **95**(6):3168–3171, 1998.

50. Martinowich K, Lu B. Interaction between BDNF and serotonin: role in mood disorders. *Neuropsychopharmacology* **33**(1):73–83, 2008.

51. Sargent PA, Kjaer KH, Bench CJ, et al. Brain serotonin1A receptor binding measured by positron emission tomography with [11C]WAY-100635: effects of depression and antidepressant treatment. *Arch Gen Psychiatry* **57**(2):174–180, 2000.

52. Yoshimura R, Mitoma M, Sugita A, et al. Effects of paroxetine or milnacipran on serum brain-derived neurotrophic factor in depressed patients. *Prog Neuropsychopharmacol Biol Psychiatry* **31**(5):1034–1037, 2007.

53. Dunn AJ, Swiergiel AH, Cork R, Newman RA. Behavioral, neurochemical and neuroendocrine responses to leukemia in mice [abstract]. *Society for Neuroscience 2004* Annual Meeting, San Diego CA, Oct 23–27, 2004. Abstract 462.13.

54. Lorenzetti V, Allen NB, Fornito A, Yücel M. Structural brain abnormalities in major depressive disorder: a selective review of recent MRI studies. *J Affect Disord* **117**(1–2):1–17, 2009.

55. Chuluyan HE, Wolcott RM, Chervenak R, Dunn AJ. Catecholamine, indoleamine and corticosteroid responses in mice bearing tumors. *Neuroimmunomodulation* **8**(3):107–113, 2000.

56. Pyter LM, Pineros V, Galang JA, McClintock MK, Prendergast BJ. Peripheral tumors induce depressive-like behaviors and cytokine production and alter hypothalamic-pituitary-adrenal axis regulation. *Proc Natl Acad Sci U S A* **106**(22): 9069–9074, 2009.

57. Dantzer R, O'Connor JC, Freund GG, Johnson RW, Kelley KW. From inflammation to sickness and depression: when the immune system subjugates the brain. *Nat Rev Neurosci* **9**(1):46–56, 2008.

58. Miller AH, Maletic V, Raison CL. Inflammation and its discontents: the role of cytokines in the pathophysiology of major depression. *Biol Psychiatry* **65**(9):732–741, 2009.

59. Miller AH. Mechanisms of cytokine-induced behavioral changes: Psychoneuroimmunology at the translational interface. *Brain Behav Immun* **23**(2): 149–158, 2009.

60. Coussens LM, Werb Z. Inflammation and cancer. *Nature* **420**(6917):860–867, 2002.

61. Williams J, Chen Y, Rubin P, Finkelstein J, Okunieff P. The biological basis of a comprehensive grading system for the adverse effects of cancer treatment. *Semin Radiat Oncol* **13**(3):182–188, 2003.

62. Hart BL. Biological basis of the behavior of sick animals. *Neurosci Biobehav Rev* **12**(2):123–137, 1988.

63. Kent S, Bluthé RM, Kelley KW, Dantzer R. Sickness behavior as a new target for drug development. *Trends Pharmacol Sci* **13**(1):24–28, 1992.

64. Dunn AJ. Cytokine activation of the HPA axis. *Ann N Y Acad Sci* **917**:608–617, 2000.

65. Dunn AJ, Wang J, Ando T. Effects of cytokines on cerebral neurotransmission. Comparison with the effects of stress. *Adv Exp Med Biol* **461**:117–127, 1999.

66. Ando T, Dunn AJ. Mouse tumor necrosis factor-alpha increases brain tryptophan concentrations and norepinephrine metabolism while activating the HPA axis in mice. *Neuroimmunomodulation* **6**(5):319–329, 1999.

67. Larson SJ, Dunn AJ. Behavioral effects of cytokines. *Brain Behav Immun* **15**(4):371–387, 2001.

68. Dantzer R, Bluthé RM, Castanon N, et al. Cytokine effects on behavior. In: Ader R, Felten DL, Cohen N, eds. *Psychoneuroimmunology*. San Diego, CA: Academic Press, 2001:703–727.

69. Swiergiel AH, Dunn AJ. Feeding, exploratory, anxiety- and depression-related behaviors are not altered in interleukin-6-deficient male mice. *Behav Brain Res* **171**(1):94–108, 2006.

70. Wang J, Dunn AJ. Mouse interleukin-6 stimulates the HPA axis and increases brain tryptophan and serotonin metabolism. *Neurochem Int* **33**(2):143–154, 1998.

71. Bluthé RM, Michaud B, Poli V, Dantzer R. Role of IL-6 in cytokine-induced sickness behavior: a study with IL-6 deficient mice. *Physiol Behav* **70**(3–4):367–373, 2000.

72. Bluthé RM, Layé S, Michaud B, Combe C, Dantzer R, Parnet P. Role of interleukin-1beta and tumour necrosis factor-alpha in lipopolysaccharide-induced sickness behaviour: a study with interleukin-1 type I receptor-deficient mice. *Eur J Neurosci* **12**(12): 4447–4456, 2000.

73. Yirmiya R, Pollak Y, Barak O, et al. Effects of antidepressant drugs on the behavioral and physiological responses to lipopolysaccharide (LPS) in rodents. *Neuropsychopharmacology* **24**(5):531–544, 2001.

74. Castanon N, Bluthé RM, Dantzer R. Chronic treatment with the atypical antidepressant tianeptine attenuates sickness behavior induced by peripheral but not central lipopolysaccharide and interleukin-1beta in the rat. *Psychopharmacology (Berl)* **154**(1):50–60, 2001.

75. Castanon N, Konsman JP, Médina C, Chauvet N, Dantzer R. Chronic treatment with the antidepressant tianeptine attenuates lipopolysaccharide-induced Fos expression in the rat paraventricular nucleus and HPA axis activation. *Psychoneuroendocrinology* **28**(1): 19–34, 2003.

76. Maes M. A review on the acute phase response in major depression. *Rev Neurosci* **4**(4):407–416, 1993.

77. Maes M, Bosmans E, Suy E, Vandervorst C, DeJonckheere C, Raus J. Depression-related disturbances in mitogen-induced lymphocyte responses and interleukin-1 beta and soluble interleukin-2 receptor production. *Acta Psychiatr Scand* **84**(4):379–386, 1991.

78. Schlatter J, Ortuño F, Cervera-Enguix S. Lymphocyte subsets and lymphokine production in patients with melancholic versus nonmelancholic depression. *Psychiatry Res* **128**(3):259–265, 2004.

79. Weizman R, Laor N, Podliszewski E, Notti I, Djaldetti M, Bessler H. Cytokine production in major depressed patients before and after clomipramine treatment. *Biol Psychiatry* **35**(1):42–47, 1994.

80. Anisman H, Ravindran AV, Griffiths J, Merali Z. Endocrine and cytokine correlates of major depression and dysthymia with typical or atypical features. *Mol Psychiatry* **4**(2):182–188, 1999.

81. Thomas AJ, Davis S, Morris C, Jackson E, Harrison R, O'Brien JT. Increase in interleukin-1beta in late-life depression. *Am J Psychiatry* **162**(1):175–177, 2005.

82. Owen BM, Eccleston D, Ferrier IN, Young AH. Raised levels of plasma interleukin-1beta in major and postviral depression. *Acta Psychiatr Scand* **103**(3): 226–228, 2001.

83. Yang K, Xie G, Zhang Z, et al. Levels of serum interleukin (IL)-6, IL-1beta, tumour necrosis factor-alpha and leptin and their correlation in depression. *Aust N Z J Psychiatry***41**(3):266–273, 2007.

84. Brambilla F, Maggioni M. Blood levels of cytokines in elderly patients with major depressive disorder. *Acta Psychiatr Scand* **97**(4):309–313, 1998.

85. Brambilla F, Monteleone P, Maj M. Interleukin-1beta and tumor necrosis factor-alpha in children with major depressive disorder or dysthymia. *J Affect Disord* **78**(3):273–277, 2004.

86. Kagaya A, Kugaya A, Takebayashi M, et al. Plasma concentrations of interleukin-1beta, interleukin-6, soluble interleukin-2 receptor and tumor necrosis factor alpha of depressed patients in Japan. *Neuropsychobiology* **43**(2):59–62, 2001.

87. Huang TL, Lee CT. T-helper 1/T-helper 2 cytokine imbalance and clinical phenotypes of acute-phase major depression. *Psychiatry Clin Neurosci* **61**(4):415–420, 2007.

88. Rothermundt M, Arolt V, Fenker J, Gutbrodt H, Peters M, Kirchner H. Different immune patterns in melancholic and non-melancholic major depression. *Eur Arch Psychiatry Clin Neurosci* **251**(2):90–97, 2001.

89. Rothermundt M, Arolt V, Peters M, et al. Inflammatory markers in major depression and melancholia. *J Affect Disord* **63**(1–3):93–102, 2001.

90. Milaneschi Y, Corsi AM, Penninx BW, Bandinelli S, Guralnik JM, Ferrucci L. Interleukin-1 receptor antagonist and incident depressive symptoms over 6 years in older persons: the InCHIANTI study. *Biol Psychiatry* **65**(11):973–978, 2009.

91. Ovaskainen Y, Koponen H, Jokelainen J, Keinänen-Kiukaanniemi S, Kumpusalo E, Vanhala M. Depressive symptomatology is associated with decreased interleukin-1 beta and increased interleukin-1 receptor antagonist levels in males. *Psychiatry Res* **167**(1–2):73–79, 2009.

92. Rothermundt M, Arolt V, Bayer TA. Review of immunological and immunopathological findings in

schizophrenia. *Brain Behav Immun* **15**(4):319–339, 2001.

93. Zorrilla EP, Luborsky L, McKay JR, et al. The relationship of depression and stressors to immunological assays: a meta-analytic review. *Brain Behav Immun* **15**(3):199–226, 2001.
94. Howren MB, Lamkin DM, Suls J. Associations of depression with C-reactive protein, IL-1, and IL-6: a meta-analysis. *Psychosom Med* **71**(2):171–186, 2009.
95. Dowlati Y, Herrmann N, Swardfager W, et al. A meta-analysis of cytokines in major depression. *Biol Psychiatry:*e-pub ahead of print, 2009.
96. Dunn AJ, Swiergiel AH. Cytokines and stress: neurochemistry, endocrinology and behavior. In: McCarty R, Aguilera G, Sabban E, Kvetnanský R, eds. *Stress: Neural, Endocrine, and Molecular Studies.* London: Taylor & Francis, 2002:163–166.
97. Quan N, Banks WA. Brain-immune communication pathways. *Brain Behav Immun* **21**(6):727–735, 2007.
98. Levine J, Barak Y, Chengappa KN, Rapoport A, Rebey M, Barak V. Cerebrospinal cytokine levels in patients with acute depression. *Neuropsychobiology* **40**(4):171–176, 1999.
99. Dunn AJ, Swiergiel AH. Effects of acute and chronic stressors and CRF in rat and mouse tests for depression. *Ann N Y Acad Sci* **1148**:118–126, 2008.
100. Maier SF, Seligman MEP. Learned helplessness: theory and evidence. *J Exp Psychol Gen* **105**(1):3–46, 1976.
101. Yirmiya R, Pollak Y, Morag M, et al. Illness, cytokines, and depression. *Ann N Y Acad Sci* **917**:478–487, 2000.
102. Swiergiel AH, Dunn AJ. The roles of IL-1, IL-6, and TNFalpha in the feeding responses to endotoxin and influenza virus infection in mice. *Brain Behav Immun* **13**(3):252–265, 1999.

Section 2 Chapter 9b

Cancer Symptom Mechanisms and Models: Clinical and Basic Science

From inflammation to sickness and depression: the cytokine connection

Robert Dantzer and Keith W. Kelley

The possibility that inflammation plays a major role in the symptoms of sickness and depression experienced by cancer patients was initially proposed by a group of investigators led by Charles Cleeland, one of the editors of this book.[1] The authors' reasoning was based on analogies. Laboratory animals injected with proinflammatory cytokines, or with cytokine inducers such as lipopolysaccharide, develop striking signs of sickness characterized by pain, wasting, cognitive impairment, anxiety, and fatigue. The same symptoms are observed in many patients with cancer and are exacerbated during inflammation-inducing cancer treatments, such as chemotherapy and radiotherapy. In addition, cancer patients subjected to long-term immunotherapy with interferon (IFN)-α and/or interleukin (IL)-2 for the treatment of metastatic kidney cancer or metastatic melanoma rapidly develop symptoms of sickness that can culminate in true depressive disorders. Since Cleeland's seminal paper was published, many studies have confirmed that nonspecific symptoms such as fatigue, even in long-term cancer survivors, are associated with inflammatory biomarkers and cannot be explained away solely as psychological difficulties related to coping with a diagnosis of cancer or living with the disease. A recent review paper confirmed the plausibility of the relationship between inflammation and the behavioral comorbidities experienced by patients with cancer and pointed to the pivotal role of neuroendocrine-immune mechanisms in this relationship.[2]

The objective of this chapter is to discuss the neuroimmune mechanisms that are likely to be responsible for the development of symptoms of sickness and depression in patients with cancer. In doing so, we will not examine the epidemiological evidence that points to a very high prevalence of symptoms of sickness and depression in cancer patients nor consider the limiting role that symptom burden plays in the acceptability of aggressive cancer therapies, as these issues are covered elsewhere in this book.

Inflammation induces behavioral alterations that are characteristic of sickness

In the mid 1960s, the experimental psychologist Neal Miller observed that systemic administration of endotoxin to rats inhibited lever pressing for water and food reward. Because the effect developed only after 30 minutes postinjection and lasted as long as 24 hours, he proposed that studying the behavioral effects of endotoxin could "provide a way of analyzing mechanisms involved in the behavioral phenomena of feeling sick."[3] He and his collaborators subsequently conducted several experiments on the generality of these phenomena and found that endotoxin did not simply decrease motivated behaviors in a nonspecific manner. He trained rats to press a lever to stop a constantly moving running wheel so that they could rest. He found that the trained rats actually pressed the lever more often when they were injected with endotoxin than when they were injected with physiological saline. This is exactly what one would expect from a sick organism: the motivation to rest after strenuous exercise should replace all other motivations, including searching for food and water.

It took a little more than two decades after this pioneering work to discover the exact mechanisms responsible for endotoxin-induced motivational changes. This discovery was made possible by the identification and characterization of the signaling molecules that are produced by the organism in response to endotoxin, as well as the subsequent cloning and expression of the recombinant forms of these proteins so they could be injected directly into experimental animals. As its name indicates, IL-1 was the first proinflammatory cytokine to be identified in this manner. IL-1 actually exists in two distinct molecular forms, IL-1α and IL-1β, that are the products of two separate genes but act on the same receptors, the type I and type II IL-1

Cancer Symptom Science: Measurement, Mechanisms, and Management, eds. Charles S. Cleeland, Michael J. Fisch, and Adrian J. Dunn.

receptors. The former (IL-1RI) is a signaling receptor that, upon binding its ligand, forms a dimer with the IL-1 receptor accessory protein. The type II IL-1 receptor (IL-1RII) functions as a nonsignaling decoy. Shortly after its characterization, IL-1β was shown to be able to induce fever and activation of the hypothalamic-pituitary-adrenal axis when injected systemically or directly into the brain. The demonstration of its ability to induce behavioral changes that are characteristic of sickness took place a few years later. The observation that administration of IL-1β in the brain mimicked the effects of peripherally administered IL-1β was a strong piece of evidence for the functionality of the brain's IL-1 receptors, of which the existence had already been demonstrated by biochemical and neuroanatomical techniques.

Another important step in the elucidation of the sickness-inducing activity of IL-1β and other proinflammatory cytokines was the demonstration that both peripherally injected cytokines and cytokines produced in the periphery in response to lipopolysaccharide (LPS), the active fragment of endotoxin, did not act directly on the brain. Instead, endotoxin was shown to induce expression of proinflammatory cytokines in the brain directly, pointing to the existence of an inducible brain compartment of proinflammatory cytokines that mirrors systemic immune activation. This was made possible by the use of polymerase chain reaction after reverse transcription of RNA to reveal the relatively small number of cytokine transcripts produced in the brain. The expression of cytokines at the protein level was later confirmed by the use of specific antibodies raised against individual cytokines. These antibodies are able to recognize the corresponding cytokine in very sensitive immunoassays carried out on biological fluids or tissue homogenates (enzyme-linked immunosorbent assay, or ELISA) or on brain sections (immunohistochemistry). The latter technique, coupled with *in situ* hybridization, identified the cellular sources of brain IL-1β to be meningeal and perivascular macrophages and microglia (the equivalent of macrophages in the brain parenchyma).

The immune message propagates from the periphery to the brain

A brain cytokine response that mirrors the peripheral cytokine response is dependent of some form of immune-to-brain communication. The concept that leukocytes inform the brain of peripheral immune events, constituting a sensory system that forms our "sixth sense," had already been formulated in the mid-1980s. Eric Smith and colleagues showed that immune cells and neurons share several communication signals and receptors. They illustrated this notion by the illuminating example of production of adrenocorticotrophic hormone (ACTH) and endorphins by stimulated lymphocytes.[4] Around the same time, Hugo Besedovsky observed that an antibody response is associated with activation of both the pituitary-adrenal axis and the sympathetic nervous system, which necessarily requires an immunoregulatory signal to act on the brain.[5,6] However, Dwight Nance is credited with setting the stage for identification of the immune-to-brain pathway that is critical for sickness behavior. He initially showed that intraperitoneal administration of LPS to rats activates specific brain areas that correspond to the primary and secondary projections of the vagus nerves, using immunohistochemistry to identify brain areas that expressed the immediate early gene c-fos.[7] In a subsequent experiment, he sectioned the vagus nerve underneath the diaphragm, which resulted in the complete disappearance of c-fos labeling in the same brain areas in response to LPS.[8]

The idea that sensory nerves convey information from the immune system to the brain is consistent with the fact that two of the four cardinal signs of inflammation are sensory in nature, *dolor* (pain) and *calor* (heat). Therefore, it did not take long for other groups to study the impact of subdiaphragmatic vagotomy on the brain actions of cytokines, including pain and sickness. As expected, subdiaphragmatic vagotomy abrogated LPS-induced hyperalgia[9] and LPS-induced sickness behavior in rats.[10] This effect was site specific for the inflammatory stimulus, as subdiaphragmatic vagotomy did not alter the behavioral response to subcutaneous, intravenous, or intracerebroventricular injections of IL-1β.[11,12] Further, sectioning of the vagus nerve also blocked induction of IL-1β mRNA in the hypothalamus in response to intraperitoneal LPS.[13] In a similar approach, bilateral transection of the glossopharyngeal nerves was found to block the febrile response to intrapalate but not to intraperitoneal injection of lipopolysaccharide and IL-1β.[14] However, the same nerve sectioning had no effect on the corticosterone and hypothalamic cytokine response to intrapalate injection of lipopolysaccharide.[15]

The demonstration of a neural pathway of communication from the immune system to the brain was an important step forward. However, it remained necessary to specify the importance of this pathway relative to other communication pathways. As indicated by the experiments of Romeo cited above, afferent nerves are necessary but not sufficient, because some of the brain actions of cytokines can take place even when specific nerves are severed. Luheshi et al[16] compared behavioral and febrile responses to LPS and IL-1β in the same rats. They observed that subdiaphragmatic vagotomy blocked sickness behavior but had no effect on the development of fever, indicating that neural afferents are more important for behavior than fever.

A problem with surgical transection of nerves is that this procedure eliminates both afferent and efferent fibers. That afferent fibers are critical for LPS-induced sickness behavior was demonstrated in an elegant experiment in which elective interruption of afferent fibers was achieved by injection of the local anesthetic bupivacaine into the nucleus tractus solitarius of the rat brain, where the afferent fibers of the vagus nerves project. The rats that were treated in this manner did not display c-fos activation in the primary and secondary projection areas of the vagus nerves when injected with LPS intraperitoneally, and this was accompanied by a full blockade of LPS-induced social withdrawal.[17]

The observation that interruption of the neural afferent pathway is not sufficient to block some of the effects of peripheral immune activation on the brain implies that other communication pathways are involved. The concept of a humoral pathway of communication from the immune system to the brain was originally built upon the results of experiments carried out for several decades on the febrile response to intravenous administration of LPS. Circulating endogenous pyrogens (now known as proinflammatory cytokines) were supposed to enter the brain via fenestrated capillaries of blood vessels in the circumventricular organs. This action would be relayed by the induction of the type 2 cyclo-oxgenase enzyme (COX-2), leading to synthesis of prostaglandins of the E2 series (PGE2) by astrocytes. PGE2 would then freely diffuse into the brain parenchyma to reach their target structures, in this case the preoptic anterior hypothalamus.[18]

The discovery of an inducible compartment of brain cytokines and the observation that cytokines act mainly on endothelial cells to induce the synthesis of prostaglandins required a revision of humoral pathway of communication from the periphery to the brain.[19] Macrophages in circumventricular organs respond to circulating pathogen-associated molecular patterns by producing and releasing proinflammatory cytokines that propagate by volume diffusion into the brain parenchyma. The cytokines reach their targets probably after they have actively recruited resident microglia and perivascular macrophages *en passant*.[20] The next step in the process would depend very much on the anatomical location of the various circumventricular organs. Cytokines produced at the level of the organum vasculosum of the lamina terminalis would preferentially reach the ventromedial preoptic area to increase the thermoregulatory set point, possibly via an endothelial cell relay involving the synthesis of PGE2. Cytokines produced at the level of the median eminence would act directly or indirectly via PGE2 on the adjacent arcuate nucleus of the hypothalamus to modulate food intake.[21] Cytokines produced in other circumventricular organs and the choroid plexus would propagate to limbic structures where they would be at the origin of sickness behavior, probably in a prostaglandin-independent manner, although this is disputed.[22,23]

What is missing in this account of immune-to-brain communication pathways, at least in the case of fever, is the fact that the relatively long latency of the brain cytokine signaling response to peripheral immune events and the subsequent induction of COX-2 leading to the synthesis of PGE2 cannot account for the rapid fever response that develops after intravenous injection of LPS. It has therefore been proposed that the peripheral immune message, in this case the intravenous injection of LPS, is first conveyed to the ventromedial portion of the anterior hypothalamus via the vagal pathway.[24,25] This pathway would be activated as a result of the direct action of LPS on liver macrophages known as Kupffer cells, which would result in the activation of the complement cascade leading to the production of C5a, an anaphylatoxin. C5a can directly stimulate PGE2 production via activation of constitutive COX-1 and inducible COX-2. PGE2 would then activate the hepatic vagal afferents that transmit the signal to the preoptic anterior hypothalamus via the nucleus tractus solitarius. The ventral noradrenergic bundle would then relay the signal to the hypothalamus via a fast PGE2-independent α1-adrenoreceptor-mediated response followed by a slower COX-2/PGE2-dependent α2-adrenoreceptor-mediated response. This last response would be accompanied and intensified by the local production of cytokines.

It is tempting to speculate that the same temporal succession of events takes place in the case of sickness behavior. Hyperalgesia is probably the first component of sickness in terms of onset. The fact that hyperalgesia is blocked by sectioning of the hepatic vagal afferents[9] would be in agreement with a peripherally initiated phenomenon. Sickness behavior itself, as measured by social withdrawal or decreases in food intake, takes longer to develop and could be more dependent on the progressive brain cytokine signaling response to peripheral immune activation, amplified by the earlier neural response.[26] Although this hypothesis is attractive and not necessarily incompatible with the existence of various doors of entry of the humoral cytokine message at the level of circumventricular organs, its predictions remain to be tested. This would require a very precise temporal dissection of the various components of sickness behavior since sickness behavior, in contrast to body temperature, cannot be easily measured continuously.

From sickness to depression

Sickness as a form of depression

To feel sick and behave in a sick way is something that is familiar to anyone who has experienced an infection. In addition to feeling feverish, one loses appetite and interest in one's usual social and nonsocial activities. Fatigue, nausea, and aching in the joints and muscles are common. Slow-wave sleep is increased to the detriment of rapid eye movement sleep, and this is usually accompanied by sleep fragmentation that leads to impaired quality of sleep. Attention span is somewhat limited. Food and water consumption are decreased, locomotion is reduced, and social contacts disappear. In rodents, a huddled posture with piloerection and disheveled fur dominates the scene. It is therefore relatively easy to measure sickness behavior in animals by assessing alterations in usual social and nonsocial behavioral activities.

The many different facets of sickness have been intensively explored over the last 20 years in laboratory animals injected with LPS or recombinant cytokines or inoculated with various pathogens, including influenza virus.[19] All of these treatments induce the same set of behavioral alterations. For instance, influenza virus infection decreases food intake and locomotor activity in mice, and the same response is observed in response to systemic LPS and IL-1β.[27] However, this does not mean that IL-1 is the common denominator among all these conditions. Neutralization of IL-1 receptor activation by administration of the specific IL-1 receptor antagonist IL-1RA blocked the effect of IL-1β but only attenuated the effects of LPS, and had little effect on the behavioral alterations induced by influenza virus infection. This result may be related to the fact that proinflammatory cytokines seldom act independently of each other. They are part of a network of cytokines in which every member is able to stimulate the production of other cytokines and has synergistic or antagonistic interactions with others. When one cytokine is missing, other cytokines with redundant activities can take over. For instance, such is the case with IL-1 and another proinflammatory cytokine known as tumor necrosis factor (TNF)-α. Mice that lack IL-1 signaling because their IL-1RI has been genetically deleted are no longer sensitive to the sickness-inducing effects of IL-1β. However, they still develop a full-blown sickness response to LPS that apparently is mediated by TNF-α, as it is abrogated by inhibition of TNF-α activity using the recombinant TNF binding protein (TNFbp).[28] Administration of TNFbp has no effect on LPS-induced sickness behavior in normal wild-type mice.

In terms of behavioral activity, proinflammatory cytokines attenuate not only locomotor activity, food intake, and social exploration, but they also impair normally rewarding behavior, such as sexually motivated behavior,[29] preference for a sweet taste,[30] and electrical self-stimulation of the so-called reward areas in the brain.[31] The decline in responses for reward has been interpreted as evidence for anhedonia, which refers to the absence of pleasure or the inability to experience it and is a key symptom of clinical depression.[30,31] Raz Yirmiya was among the first scientists to draw a parallel between clinical signs of sickness and the symptoms of depression.[30] Yirmiya's hypothesis was not very different from the macrophage theory of depression proposed earlier by Ronald Smith,[32] which inspired Michael Maes' quest for clinical evidence of the association between depression and chronic inflammation.[33–35] Yirmiya proposed that if cytokine-induced sickness behavior is equivalent to depression, it should be alleviated by clinically effective antidepressant drugs. He showed that this is indeed the case, as chronic but not acute treatment with the tricyclic antidepressant imipramine abrogated the suppressive effects of LPS on saccharin preference and attenuated

LPS-induced loss of body weight, reduction in food intake, and decrease in social exploration.[30] Fluoxetine was subsequently shown to act in the same manner as imipramine, but with much less potency.[36]

In the first international meeting on cytokines and depression that took place in Roscoff, France in 1999, the consensus was that there were enough convergent data to support the hypothesis of an association between cytokines and depression. This was based on five categories of evidence: (1) cytokines administered to patients and laboratory animals induce some signs of depression; (2) some depressed patients display enhanced biomarkers of inflammation; (3) depressive disorders frequently occur in patients afflicted with diseases, such as those associated with the heart and vasculature, that have an important inflammatory component; (4) some stressors stimulate expression of cytokines in both the periphery and the brain; and (5) some antidepressant drugs have anti-inflammatory properties and attenuate the behavioral effects of immune challenge.[37] Preclinical studies have since confirmed that proinflammatory cytokines are involved in the pathogenesis of depression in response to both immune and nonimmune factors. Depressive-like behavior is usually measured in rodents by decreased preference for sucrose or decreased self-stimulation of the lateral hypothalamus (conditions that mimic anhedonia), or increased duration of immobility in the forced-swim and tail-suspension tests (which assess resignation or helplessness in a situation that cannot be controlled). Administration of LPS or proinflammatory cytokines induces depressive-like behavior, although it is difficult to separate it from sickness behavior.[38] The involvement of cytokines in depression does not apparently require any immune stimulation, as suggested by healthy TNF receptor knockout mice that display an antidepressant-like phenotype.[39] In the same manner, blockade of IL-1 receptor signaling abrogates the anhedonic behavior caused by exposure to chronic mild stress.[40,41]

There is not necessarily any equivalence between sickness and depression. The research that was carried out on symptoms of depression in patients who received massive doses of IFN-α and/or IL-2 for treatment of kidney cancer or melanoma with metastasis revealed that depression actually developed relatively late (a few days to a few weeks) after initiation of cytokine immunotherapy, and did so on a background of an early sickness response. Furthermore, depression was observed only in about one third of the patients, whereas all patients displayed sickness in response to the treatment. Last but not least, pretreatment with the specific serotonin reuptake inhibitor paroxetine in patients with malignant melanoma scheduled to undergo IFN-α therapy prevented only symptoms of depressed mood and anxiety, cognitive dysfunction, and pain, whereas symptoms of sickness, including fatigue and anorexia, were not altered. These clinical observations have been instrumental in allowing the separation of depression from sicknesss.[42]

Depression as distinct from sickness

It must be recognized that the distinction between sickness and depression could have been anticipated on the basis of the adaptive nature of the sickness response and its motivational aspects. Sickness is very much related to fever, but they can be readily separated because they occur via different mechanisms.[43] Fever is the result of an increased set point in thermoregulation that translates into increased heat production and decreased heat loss. The higher body temperature associated with fever promotes resistance of the host to pathogens. Redistribution of energy expenditure is necessary to mount a fever response and to promote clonal expansion of lymphocytes that will enable development of an adaptive immune response to pathogens. This means that the organism cannot waste energy in useless behavioral activities. The decrease in food intake appears somewhat paradoxical in this context in the sense that it should normally help the organism to obtain exogenous sources of energy. However, the energy obtained from food is compromised by the amount of energy that is necessary to find food plus the energy needed to digest it. In addition, food itself can be at the origin of the infection.

On the basis of these considerations, sickness behavior should be an integral part of the fever response and as such should contribute positively to pathogen resistance. Benjamin Hart made use of the available literature on the adaptive value of fever and the various forms that sickness behavior can present during infection in vertebrates and invertebrates to specifically propose this concept.[44] The concept that sickness is the expression of a motivational state corresponding to a reorganization of the organism's priorities to cope with infection was tested in a series of experiments.[45–47] In a typical experiment using the paradigm of motivational conflict developed many years earlier by Neal Miller, sickness behavior was placed in competition with maternal behavior in lactating mice injected with LPS.[46] Sick mice did not pay attention to their pups in the usual environment of their home cage, yet they promptly exhibited normal maternal behavior by retrieving pups after their dispersal throughout the cage. When the nests the mothers had built were removed and replaced with cotton wool, the mothers did not rebuild the nests when tested at 24°C. However, they both rebuilt their nests and retrieved pups when they were tested at 6°C. In other words, the behavioral alterations that develop during sickness are not just dependent on the changes in internal states triggered by proinflammatory cytokines. They are a joint function of the intensity of these changes and the nature of the environmental factors that are present, and this environment-by-internal-state interaction is a basic feature of all motivated behaviors.

The concept of sickness as an expression of a motivational state has important theoretical implications. Just as fear is adaptive in the presence of a predator, sickness is adaptive when animals and humans are challenged with pathogens. Because microbial pathogens are everywhere and can affect the organism at any time, sickness should be an archetypical response independent of phylogeny. Like fear, however, the amplitude and duration of this response should be proportional to the threat to the organism. However, if sickness does not resolve quickly after the infectious episode, this response can be maladaptive. In this case, pathology replaces physiology.

It does not take long to realize that conditions of chronic and/or intense activation of the immune response are associated with a higher prevalence of mood disorders (eg, anxiety and depression) and other nonspecific symptoms of sickness (eg, fatigue, pain, cognitive alterations, and sleep disorders). The next question is whether the mechanisms that are responsible for the transition from physiology to pathology correspond solely to the exacerbation of the mechanisms of sickness or involve new biological processes.

Molecular mechanisms of inflammation-induced depression: the pivotal role of indoleamine 2,3 dioxygenase

Dietmar Fuchs was probably the first scientist to point to an association between clinical signs of inflammation, degradation of tryptophan, and the development of neuropsychiatric symptoms in medically ill patients. He first established that activation of macrophages is associated with the production of neopterin and the degradation of tryptophan into kynurenine in response to activation of the tryptophan-degrading enzyme indoleamine 2,3 dioxygenase (IDO) by IFN-γ.[48] IDO is a ubiquitous enzyme that is present not only in macrophages but also in other myeloid cells in the immune system, including dendritic cells. It is also present in a number of brain cells, including microglia, astrocytes, endothelial cells, and neurons. By depleting the local milieu of the essential amino acid tryptophan that is necessary for T cell proliferation and cytotoxicity, activation of this enzyme suppresses T cell responses and promotes immune tolerance. IDO-mediated immune tolerance plays a key role in mammalian pregnancy, tumor resistance, chronic infections, and autoimmune diseases.[49]

Fuchs documented the association between the action of IDO and neuropsychiatric symptoms in patients infected with HIV-1[50] before generalizing it to other medical illnesses, such as systemic lupus erythematosus,[51] colorectal cancer,[52] and coronary heart disease.[53] The association was not only qualitative but also quantitative. Cancer patients treated with IFN-α and/or IL-2 experienced a drastic decrease in tryptophan levels over the first four weeks of cytokine immunotherapy that was negatively correlated to increasing depression scores.[54] Among patients with coronary artery disease, the activation of IDO, as measured by the kynurenine/tryptophan ratio in the plasma, tended to be higher in depressed than in nondepressed individuals and was positively associated with the severity of depressive symptoms.[55]

The bioavailability of tryptophan is well known to modulate synthesis of serotonin,[56] whereas acute depletion of tryptophan induces depressed mood in subjects at risk for depression.[57] It is therefore logical to investigate whether depression associated with activation of IDO is mediated by a deficiency in brain serotonin. The problem with any type of preclinical research on the mechanisms of inflammation-induced depression, however, is that the usual behavioral measures of depression, whether they rely on decreased preference for a sweet taste or increased duration of immobility in the forced-swim and tail-suspension tests, are confounded by the decreased appetite and reduced locomotor activity associated with sickness. Nonetheless, on the basis of clinical data showing a temporal dissociation between early occurrence of sickness and the delayed emergence of depression in response to immune activation in patients receiving cytokine immunotherapy, it should be possible to measure depressive-like behavior after animals have recovered from their early episode of sickness.

This was verified in mice treated with LPS[58] and in mice inoculated with Bacillus Calmette-Guerin (BCG), an attenuated form of *Mycobacterium bovis*.[59] In the first case, LPS induced an increase in the duration of immobility in the forced-swim and tail-suspension tests at a time (24 hours post-LPS administration) at which the sickness response had already dissipated, as measured by locomotor activity and food intake. In the second case, BCG-treated mice displayed a transient episode of sickness for 2–5 days postinoculation; increased duration of immobility in the forced-swim and tail-suspension tests and reduced preference for sucrose were observed at 7 and 14 days after inoculation. In both cases, the occurrence of depressive-like behavior coincided with an increase in IDO expression.

Systemic administration of the specific IDO inhibitor 1-methyl tryptophan abrogated the increased duration of immobility in the forced-swim and tail-suspension tests in mice injected with LPS or inoculated with BCG.[60,61] The 1-methyl tryptophan treatment had no effect on the induction of brain cytokines in response to LPS or BCG and did not alter LPS-induced or BCG-induced sickness behavior. In contrast, administration of the anti-inflammatory tetracycline antibiotic minocycline abrogated induction of brain cytokines in response to BCG and blocked both sickness behavior and depressive-like behavior; the same effect was observed in LPS-treated mice.[62] These results were important because they demonstrated that IDO acts downstream of proinflammatory cytokines and mediates the depressogenic effects of inflammation. In a further series of experiments, IFN-γ receptor knockout mice administered the TNF-α antagonist TNF binding protein did not display any depressive-like behavior in response to BCG despite a normal sickness response, and this was associated with a lack of activation of IDO.[60,63] These results confirm that IDO activation is mediated by IFN-γ and TNF-α and that IDO is responsible for development of depressive-like behavior.

Because there is always the possibility that 1-methyl tryptophan has other pharmacological activities in addition to IDO antagonism, complementary genetic experiments were conducted on IDO knockout mice. These mice responded normally to BCG in terms of brain cytokine expression and sickness behavior but did not show any sign of depressive-like behavior, confirming the specificity of action of IDO in inflammation-induced depression.[60]

Degradation of tryptophan into kynurenine and kynurenine metabolites is mediated by both IDO and tryptophan 2,3 dioxygenase (TDO), with expression of the latter enzyme restricted to the liver. Another gene that encodes IDO was recently discovered, and the corresponding protein is termed “IDO2,” with “IDO1” referring to the originally identified IDO protein.[64] The IDO1 and IDO2 proteins share 43% identity at the amino acid level. However, the ability of IDO2 to degrade tryptophan is much less than that of IDO1. IDO2 is predominantly expressed in the kidney and sex organs, although its expression can also be detected in the brain. The IDO knockout mice mentioned above were only deficient in IDO1; no behavioral studies of IDO2 knockout mice have yet been reported. It is apparently possible to selectively inhibit IDO2 by the use of 1-methyl-D-tryptophan, with the L-racemer being specific of the IDO1 enzyme.[64] The O’Connor et al. experiments described previously used 1-methyl-D,L-tryptophan, which probably inhibits both IDO1 and IDO2.

TDO expression was initially thought to be restricted to the liver, but this enzyme is also present in the brain.[65] Genetic deletion of TDO is associated with a biochemical phenotype consisting of increased levels of tryptophan and kynurenine in plasma and increased levels of tryptophan, serotonin, and its metabolite 5-hydroxy indole-acetic acid in the brain. At the behavioral level, these TDO knockout mice display an anxiolytic phenotype in the plus-maze and open-field tests.[65] Although cytokines have no direct effect on TDO, they could activate this enzyme indirectly by increasing the synthesis of adrenal glucocorticoids. The possible relevance of this phenomenon to chronic inflammation is not straightforward. BCG-treated mice that had increased IDO activity actually displayed decreased TDO activity, perhaps as a compensatory mechanism.[66]

Despite a decrease in circulating levels of tryptophan, the brain does not appear to suffer from a deficiency in serotoninergic neurotransmission because tryptophan levels are actually increased in the brain in response to LPS and the turnover of serotonin is enhanced.[67,68] Brain serotonin turnover is unchanged in response to BCG.[69] However, it is important to note that these data do not completely discard the possibility of interference with brain serotonin by cytokines. The expression of presynaptic serotonin transporter can be increased by cytokines, which should result in a decrease in the amount of serotonin available for neurotransmission.[70–72] This mechanism has been proposed to account for inflammation-induced fatigue in rats[73] and for the negative association between IFN-γ and reduced serotonin transporter expression in leukocytes of depressed patients.[71]

IDO is expressed both at the periphery and in the brain, and its enzymatic activity, as measured by the ratio of kynurenine to tryptophan, is increased in both compartments in response to LPS and BCG.[66,74] Acute administration of kynurenine to naïve mice mimics the effect of LPS on duration of immobility in the forced-swim and tail-suspension tests.[61] It is therefore likely that kynurenine is catabolized further into bioactive kynurenine metabolites that ultimately affect brain functions. Kynurenine does not need to be produced *in situ* in the brain because peripheral kynurenine is transported into the brain via the same transporter as tryptophan.[75]

The degradation pathway of kynurenine in brain cells has been fully described.[76] Astrocytes transform kynurenine into kynurenic acid, which acts as an antagonist of the alpha-7-nicotinic receptor and an antagonist of *N*-methyl-D-aspartate (NMDA) receptors. In contrast, microglial cells produce 3-hydroxy kynurenine and quinolinic acid, which both act as free-radical donors and, in the case of quinolinic acid, as an NMDA receptor agonist. The predominance of one metabolic pathway over the other could shift the balance between these compounds and be at the origin of various neuropsychiatric disorders, as postulated by Müller and Schwarz.[77] Another aspect of brain kynurenine metabolism that has received much less attention is the observation that normally firing neurons are able to metabolize kynurenine to picolinic acid, which has neuroprotective properties, but that compromised neurons produce quinolinic acid, which is neurotoxic and could contribute to their elimination.[78] Although the properties of kynurenine metabolites have mainly been studied in the context of neurodegenerative disorders,[76] it is quite possible that they alter neuronal function when produced in lower quantities.

A limited number of clinical studies support the possibility of the contribution of macrophage/microglial kynurenine metabolism to clinical depression. Using total choline as a marker of membrane phospholipid turnover, which can be assayed *in vivo* by proton magnetic resonance spectroscopic imaging, Gabbay et al.[79] reported a positive correlation between plasma levels of kynurenine and 2-hydroxyanthralinic acid (an intermediate in the degradation pathway from kynurenine to quinolinic acid) on one hand and total choline in the striatum on the other hand in adolescents with melancholic depression. In adults with chronic hepatitis C treated with IFN-α, depression scores were positively correlated with the ratio of plasma kynurenine to kynurenic acid.[80] In another study with a similar clinical population, a high correlation was found between depression scores and cerebrospinal fluid concentrations of quinolinic acid, which themselves strongly correlated with plasma levels of quinolinic acid.[81]

Risk factors for inflammation-induced depression

If inflammation-induced depression does not develop in all patients who have chronic inflammation or are treated with cytokine immunotherapy, there must be risk factors for developing inflammation-induced depression. These risk factors have been studied in the context of cytokine immunotherapy. Although this is a very artificial situation, it has the advantage of permitting longitudinal time-course studies in patients and therefore of relating the occurrence and intensity of their depressive symptoms to specific treatments.

Prior or concurrent psychiatric disorders had already been recognized as a risk factor for the occurrence of mood and cognitive side effects of IFN-α in patients with cancer.[82] In a study of cancer patients treated with IFN-α and/or IL-2, patients with relatively high scores of depression but without any prior incidence of major depressive disorders were more likely to respond to cytokine immunotherapy by a worsening of their depression scores.[83] In a follow-up study of these patients, prior occurrence of sadness, pessimistic thoughts, and neurovegetative symptoms, including sleep disturbances, were identified as specific risk factors that add to the already-recognized adverse effect of low social support.[84]

At the neuroendocrine level, a retrospective assessment of an elevated response of the pituitary-adrenal axis to the first injection of IFN-α was found to predict the probability of developing major depression in response to the treatment in patients with malignant melanoma.[85] Interestingly, patients with enhanced pituitary-adrenal response to IFN-α also had higher depression scores at baseline. Since there was no systematic investigation of the hypothalamic-pituitary-adrenal axis in these patients, it is difficult to speculate on the possible involvement of intrinsic high glucocorticoid levels as a risk factor for inflammation-induced depression. Normally high glucocorticoid levels should have a moderating influence on inflammation in the absence of any sign of cortisol resistance.[86]

Knowing that inflammation-induced depression is the result of an interaction between responsiveness of the immune system to activation and sensitivity of the brain to depressogenic factors, development of inflammation-induced depression should be a joint function of these two factors. As predicted, patients who had the low IL-6-synthesizing genotype developed fewer symptoms of depression when they were chronically administered IFN-α for the treatment of hepatitis C. The same effect was observed in patients with the long version of the serotonin transporter gene polymorphism, although to a lesser extent.[87]

The observation that inflammation can play a key role in the development of major depressive disorders has been responsible for a reinvestigation of the classical risk factors for depression. In a birth cohort of 1000 individuals followed-up to 32 years of age in New Zealand, a history of childhood maltreatment (known to be a risk factor for depression) was found to be associated with elevated inflammation.[88] In the same manner, low socioeconomic status during early life, which is another risk factor for somatic disease and psychiatric disorders, is associated with resistance to glucocorticoid signaling, which in turn facilitates exaggerated adrenocortical and inflammatory responses.[89]

Neurobiological circuitry of inflammation-induced depression

On the basis of evidence for the role of inflammation in the development of depression, it can be predicted that inflammation-associated depression should be mediated by activation of the same neurobiological circuitry as that identified by brain imaging techniques in depressed patients. Major advances have taken place in this field during the last decade. Several abnormalities of regional blood flow and glucose metabolism – a marker of neuronal function – have been identified in the limbic cortex, prefrontral cortex, hypothalamus, amygdala, anterior cingulate cortex, and basal ganglia. It is now possible to refer to a true "neurobiological signature" of depression. Some of the structures that are part of this circuitry certainly play a causal role in the pathogenesis of depression, evidenced by the fact that stimulating them electrically can be curative.

Early work in this field was conducted in patients treated with IFN-α. In patients with malignant melanoma, administration of IFN-α was associated with increased glucose metabolism in the basal ganglia and cerebellum and with decreased glucose metabolism in the dorsal prefrontal cortex, as revealed by uptake of the radionuclide ^{18}F-fluorodeoxyglucose (FDG) imaged with positron emission tomography.[90] Alterations in the basal ganglia were positively correlated with self-reported fatigue. In patients with hepatitis C, administration of IFN-α was accompanied by greater activation of the dorsal portion of the anterior cingulate cortex, as revealed by functional magnetic resonance imaging (fMRI), which correlated highly with the number of task-related errors in a task of visuospatial attention.[91] These alterations likely reflect a higher sensitivity to emotionally negative stimuli.

The neuroimaging data obtained from patients receiving cytokine immunotherapy can easily be criticized on the basis of the rather extreme conditions of immune activation these subjects experience. However, similar neuroimaging data have been obtained in healthy subjects submitted to a very mild and transient activation of their immune response in the form of typhoid vaccination. At the peak of the innate immune response to immunization, when IL-6 levels are maximal, these subjects experience a slight but significant increase in their negative mood states. This was associated with slower reaction times to a color-word Stroop task and enhanced neural activation in the left substantia nigra, as revealed by fMRI, which was positively correlated with the IL-6 response to vaccination.[92] In addition, performance of the Stroop test in typhoid-vaccinated subjects activated brain regions implicated in processing of interoceptive information encoded by afferent autonomic nerves, in agreement with an immune-to-brain neural communication pathway.[93] In an implicit emotional-face perception task, typhoid-vaccinated subjects displayed an enhanced activation in their subgenual anterior cingulate cortex when asked to process the faces.[94]

Studies of normal subjects whose immune system was not activated by any exogenous stimulus indicate the existence of a functional coupling between inflammatory pathways and brain structures involved in the processing of emotional negative states. The best evidence of this functional coupling was provided by the results of an fMRI study in which female relatives of individuals deceased from breast cancer were presented with a photograph of the deceased person and words associated with the negative emotions experienced at the time, to invoke feelings of grief. During the experience of grief, the subjects displayed an enhanced activation of their subgenual anterior cingulate cortex that correlated positively with salivary IL-1β.[95]

From inflammation to depression and vice-versa

A plethora of evidence now supports the concept that inflammation can induce depression in vulnerable subjects. The reverse relationship also holds true: depression can enhance inflammation.[96] Indirect evidence for this relationship can be found in the results of a fully randomized biobehavioral intervention study in patients with breast cancer.[97] The psychological intervention, which was begun after surgery and before initiation of adjuvant treatment, included weekly 90-minute group sessions during the first 4 months of the study followed by eight monthly sessions, for a total of 12 months. Patients in both the intervention and control arms were assessed for symptoms, health behavior, and inflammation (measured by white blood cell count and T-helper:suppressor ratio at the start of the trial and then four, eight, and 12 months later). The psychological intervention alleviated depressive symptoms, including pain and fatigue, at eight months for patients newly diagnosed with breast cancer but lowered T cell and white blood cell counts (indicative of inflammation) only at 12 months.

In another prospective study carried out in healthy older men and women enrolled in the Pittsburgh Healthy Heart Project, depression measured by the Beck Depression Inventory was a predictor of 6-year changes in serum IL-6 independent of all other possible factors that were examined. These results indicate that depressive symptoms may precede and augment inflammatory processes.[98]

As pointed out by Thornton et al.,[97] the effect of depression on inflammation could be accounted for by the fact that depressed patients have altered physiological reactivity to daily stressors, in the form of activation of the sympathetic nervous system and cortisol tolerance, that would promote an inflammatory response.[99] This sensitization of the inflammatory response could be restricted to nonimmune stressors, as depressed patients with coronary heart disease did not show any alteration in the *in vitro* response of their white blood cells to LPS stimulation.[100] The sensitivity of systemic inflammatory activity to fluctuations in depressed mood has been confirmed in a number of independent studies, such as that conducted by Rohleder and Miller.[101] As discussed extensively in a recent review paper,[102] there is accumulating evidence that interpersonal conflict and low social support can effectively modulate proinflammatory cytokine production both directly, via central nervous system, neural, endocrine, and immune biobehavioral pathways, and indirectly, by promoting depression, emotional stress responses, and detrimental health behaviors.

It is generally much easier to study the influences of environmental stressors on immunity rather than those of emotions, despite the fact that in doing so one misses "the rich and varied ways in which people anticipate, perceive, and process events in their environment and even imagine events that are not present."[103] Dispositional optimism, defined as the general expectation that everything will turn out to be good rather than bad, was found to decrease the IL-6 response to two challenging mental tasks consisting of a Stroop test and a simulated public-speaking exercise.[104] Note that the effect of the two mental tasks on IL-6 levels confirms what is already known about the consequences of acute psychological stress on inflammation, ie, that there are robust effects for increased levels of circulating IL-6, whereas less consistent effects are observed for C-reactive protein and cytokine production by stimulated white blood cells *in vitro*.[105]

Conclusion

We have come full circle and shown that not only can inflammation affect mood, but also that mood can affect inflammation. Because the effects are going in the same direction, it is possible to imagine that there is a cascading series of interactions between inflammation and stress. This has already been pointed out by various authors,[106] although the importance of these cascades has not yet been fully appreciated in the clinic, probably because we are still accustomed to reasoning in a unidirectional rather than a bidirectional manner.

In the face of such pervading evidence for bilateral relationships between inflammation and depression, the question that ultimately needs to be asked is: What is the normal function of this relationship, particularly before the cascades lose control? In view of the high energy cost of innate and adaptive immunity, it certainly makes sense for the brain to function in an energy-conserving manner while maintaining its capacity to respond to any threatening environmental stimulus that further compromises the survival of the organism.[86] This hypothesis is supported by metabolic data showing that IL-1β resets glucose homeostasis at central levels.[107] In this context, the concomitant activation of inflammatory pathways would strengthen the first line of defense against any infection resulting from a breach in cutaneous and mucosal barriers. The mere existence of cascading interactions puts the organism at risk of dysfunction if one or several components of the normally tightly regulated cascade are not adequately controlled. Seen at its extreme, the pathophysiology of depressive disorders would be nothing other than the reflection of profound disturbances in metabolic networks, a hypothesis that has already been formulated with reference to neuroimmune interactions.[108]

References

1. Cleeland CS, Bennett GJ, Dantzer R, et al. Are the symptoms of cancer and cancer treatment due to a shared biologic mechanism? *Cancer* **97**(11):2919–2925, 2003.
2. Miller AH, Ancoli-Israel S, Bower JE, Capuron L, Irwin MR. Neuroendocrine-immune mechanisms of behavioral comorbidities in patients with cancer. *J Clin Oncol* **26**(6):971–982, 2008.
3. Miller NE, Gottesman KS, Holmes JE. Effects of chemostimulation of brain and of bacterial endotoxins on eating and drinking. *Science* **136**(3513):327–328, 1962.
4. Smith EM, Harbour-McMenamin D, Blalock JE. Lymphocyte production of endorphins and endorphin-mediated immunoregulatory activity. *J Immunol* **135**(2 Suppl):779s–782s, 1985.
5. Besedovsky HO, del Rey AE, Sorkin E. Immune-neuroendocrine interactions. *J Immunol* **135**(2 Suppl):750s–754s, 1985.
6. Besedovsky HO, del Rey A. Physiology of psychoneuroimmunology: a personal view. *Brain Behav Immun* **21**(1):34–44, 2007.
7. Wan W, Janz L, Vriend CY, Sorensen CM, Greenberg AH, Nance DM. Differential induction of c-Fos immunoreactivity in hypothalamus and brain stem nuclei following central and peripheral administration of endotoxin. *Brain Res Bull* **32**(6):581–587, 1993.
8. Wan W, Wetmore L, Sorensen CM, Greenberg AH, Nance DM. Neural and biochemical mediators of endotoxin and stress-induced c-fos expression in the rat brain. *Brain Res Bull* **34**(1):7–14, 1994.
9. Watkins LR, Wiertelak EP, Goehler LE, et al. Neurocircuitry of illness-induced hyperalgesia. *Brain Res* **639**(2):283–299, 1994.
10. Bluthé RM, Walter V, Parnet P, et al. Lipopolysaccharide induces sickness behaviour in rats by a vagal mediated mechanism. *C R Acad Sci III* **317**(6):499–503, 1994.
11. Bluthé RM, Michaud B, Kelley KW, Dantzer R. Vagotomy attenuates behavioural effects of interleukin-1 injected peripherally but not centrally. *Neuroreport* **7**(9):1485–1488, 1996.
12. Bluthé RM, Michaud B, Kelley KW, Dantzer R. Vagotomy blocks behavioural effects of interleukin-1 injected via the intraperitoneal route but not via other systemic routes. *Neuroreport* **7**(15–17):2823–2827, 1996.
13. Layé S, Bluthé RM, Kent S, et al. Subdiaphragmatic vagotomy blocks induction of IL-1 beta mRNA in mice brain in response to peripheral LPS. *Am J Physiol* **268**(5 Pt 2):R1327–R1331, 1995.
14. Romeo HE, Tio DL, Rahman SU, Chiappelli F, Taylor AN. The glossopharyngeal nerve as a novel pathway in immune-to-brain communication: relevance to neuroimmune surveillance of the oral cavity. *J Neuroimmunol* **115**(1–2):91–100, 2001.
15. Romeo HE, Tio DL, Taylor AN. Effects of glossopharyngeal nerve transection on central and peripheral cytokines and serum corticosterone induced by localized inflammation. *J Neuroimmunol* **136**(1–2):104–111, 2003.
16. Luheshi GN, Bluthé RM, Rushforth D, et al. Vagotomy attenuates the behavioural but not the pyrogenic effects of interleukin-1 in rats. *Auton Neurosci* **85**(1–3):127–132, 2000.
17. Marvel FA, Chen CC, Badr N, Gaykema RP, Goehler LE. Reversible inactivation of the dorsal vagal complex blocks lipopolysaccharide-induced social withdrawal and c-Fos expression in central autonomic nuclei. *Brain Behav Immun* **18**(2):123–134, 2004.
18. Saper CB, Breder CD. The neurologic basis of fever. *N Engl J Med* **330**(26):1880–1886, 1994.

19. Dantzer R, Kelley KW. Twenty years of research on cytokine-induced sickness behavior. *Brain Behav Immun* **21**(2):153–160, 2007.
20. Konsman JP, Parnet P, Dantzer R. Cytokine-induced sickness behaviour: mechanisms and implications. *Trends Neurosci* **25**(3):154–159, 2002.
21. Konsman JP, Dantzer R. How the immune and nervous systems interact during disease-associated anorexia. *Nutrition* **17**(7–8):664–668, 2001.
22. Konsman JP, Vigues S, Mackerlova L, Bristow A, Blomqvist A. Rat brain vascular distribution of interleukin-1 type-1 receptor immunoreactivity: relationship to patterns of inducible cyclooxygenase expression by peripheral inflammatory stimuli. *J Comp Neurol* **472**(1):113–129, 2004.
23. Konsman JP, Veeneman J, Combe C, Poole S, Luheshi GN, Dantzer R. Central nervous action of interleukin-1 mediates activation of limbic structures and behavioural depression in response to peripheral administration of bacterial lipopolysaccharide. *Eur J Neurosci* **28**(12):2499–2510, 2008.
24. Blatteis CM, Li S, Li Z, Feleder C, Perlik V. Cytokines, PGE2 and endotoxic fever: a re-assessment. *Prostaglandins Other Lipid Mediat* **76**(1–4):1–18, 2005.
25. Blatteis CM. The onset of fever: new insights into its mechanism. *Prog Brain Res* **162**:3–14, 2007.
26. Dantzer R, Konsman JP, Bluthé RM, Kelley KW. Neural and humoral pathways of communication from the immune system to the brain: parallel or convergent? *Auton Neurosci* **85**(1–3):60–65, 2000.
27. Dunn AJ, Swiergiel AH. The role of cytokines in infection-related behavior. *Ann N Y Acad Sci* **840**: 577–585, 1998.
28. Bluthé RM, Layé S, Michaud B, Combe C, Dantzer R, Parnet P. Role of interleukin-1beta and tumour necrosis factor-alpha in lipopolysaccharide-induced sickness behaviour: a study with interleukin-1 type I receptor-deficient mice. *Eur J Neurosci* **12**(12): 4447–4456, 2000.
29. Avitsur R, Yirmiya R. Cytokines inhibit sexual behavior in female rats: I. Synergistic effects of tumor necrosis factor alpha and interleukin-1. *Brain Behav Immun* **13**(1):14–32, 1999.
30. Yirmiya R. Endotoxin produces a depressive-like episode in rats. *Brain Res* **711**(1–2):163–174, 1996.
31. Borowski T, Kokkinidis L, Merali Z, Anisman H. Lipopolysaccharide, central in vivo biogenic amine variations, and anhedonia. *Neuroreport* **9**(17): 3797–3802, 1998.
32. Smith RS. The macrophage theory of depression. *Med Hypotheses* **35**(4):298–306, 1991.
33. Maes M. A review on the acute phase response in major depression. *Rev Neurosci* **4**(4):407–416, 1993.
34. Maes M, Smith R, Scharpé S. The monocyte-T-lymphocyte hypothesis of major depression. *Psychoneuroendocrinology* **20**(2):111–116, 1995.
35. Maes M. Major depression and activation of the inflammatory response system. *Adv Exp Med Biol* **461**:25–46, 1999.
36. Yirmiya R, Weidenfeld J, Pollak Y, et al. Cytokines, "depression due to a general medical condition," and antidepressant drugs. *Adv Exp Med Biol* **461**:283–316, 1999.
37. Dantzer R, Wollman E, Vitkovic L, Yirmiya R. Cytokines and depression: fortuitous or causative association? *Mol Psychiatry* **4**(4):328–332, 1999.
38. Dunn AJ, Swiergiel AH. Effects of interleukin-1 and endotoxin in the forced swim and tail suspension tests in mice. *Pharmacol Biochem Behav* **81**(3):688–693, 2005.
39. Simen BB, Duman CH, Simen AA, Duman RS. TNFalpha signaling in depression and anxiety: behavioral consequences of individual receptor targeting. *Biol Psychiatry* **59**(9):775–785, 2006.
40. Goshen I, Kreisel T, Ben-Menachem-Zidon O, et al. Brain interleukin-1 mediates chronic stress-induced depression in mice via adrenocortical activation and hippocampal neurogenesis suppression. *Mol Psychiatry* **13**(7):717–728, 2008.
41. Koo JW, Duman RS. IL-1beta is an essential mediator of the antineurogenic and anhedonic effects of stress. *Proc Natl Acad Sci U S A* **105**(2):751–756, 2008.
42. Capuron L, Gumnick JF, Musselman DL, et al. Neurobehavioral effects of interferon-alpha in cancer patients: phenomenology and paroxetine responsiveness of symptom dimensions. *Neuropsychopharmacology* **26**(5):643–652, 2002.
43. Kent S, Bluthé RM, Dantzer R, et al. Different receptor mechanisms mediate the pyrogenic and behavioral effects of interleukin 1. *Proc Natl Acad Sci U S A* **89**(19):9117–9120, 1992.
44. Hart BL. Biological basis of the behavior of sick animals. *Neurosci Biobehav Rev* **12**(2):123–137, 1988.
45. Aubert A, Goodall G, Dantzer R. Compared effects of cold ambient temperature and cytokines on macronutrient intake in rats. *Physiol Behav* **57**(5):869–873, 1995.
46. Aubert A, Goodall G, Dantzer R, Gheusi G. Differential effects of lipopolysaccharide on pup retrieving and nest building in lactating mice. *Brain Behav Immun* **11**(2):107–118, 1997.
47. Aubert A, Dantzer R. The taste of sickness: lipopolysaccharide-induced finickiness in rats. *Physiol Behav* **84**(3):437–444, 2005.

48. Werner ER, Werner-Felmayer G, Fuchs D, Hausen A, Reibnegger G, Wachter H. Parallel induction of tetrahydrobiopterin biosynthesis and indoleamine 2,3-dioxygenase activity in human cells and cell lines by interferon-gamma. *Biochem J* **262**(3):861–866, 1989.

49. Mellor AL, Munn DH. IDO expression by dendritic cells: tolerance and tryptophan catabolism. *Nat Rev Immunol* **4**(10):762–774, 2004.

50. Fuchs D, Möller AA, Reibnegger G, Stöckle E, Werner ER, Wachter H. Decreased serum tryptophan in patients with HIV-1 infection correlates with increased serum neopterin and with neurologic/psychiatric symptoms. *J Acquir Immune Defic Syndr* **3**(9):873–876, 1990.

51. Widner B, Sepp N, Kowald E, Kind S, Schmuth M, Fuchs D. Degradation of tryptophan in patients with systemic lupus erythematosus. *Adv Exp Med Biol* **467**:571–577, 1999.

52. Huang A, Fuchs D, Widner B, Glover C, Henderson DC, Allen-Mersh TG. Serum tryptophan decrease correlates with immune activation and impaired quality of life in colorectal cancer. *Br J Cancer* **86**(11):1691–1696, 2002.

53. Wirleitner B, Rudzite V, Neurauter G, et al. Immune activation and degradation of tryptophan in coronary heart disease. *Eur J Clin Invest* **33**(7):550–554, 2003.

54. Capuron L, Ravaud A, Neveu PJ, Miller AH, Maes M, Dantzer R. Association between decreased serum tryptophan concentrations and depressive symptoms in cancer patients undergoing cytokine therapy. *Mol Psychiatry* **7**(5):468–473, 2002.

55. Swardfager W, Herrmann N, Dowlati Y, et al. Indoleamine 2,3-dioxygenase activation and depressive symptoms in patients with coronary artery disease. *Psychoneuroendocrinology* **34**(10):1560–1566, 2009.

56. Wurtman RJ. Food consumption, neurotransmitter synthesis, and human behaviour. *Experientia Suppl* **44**:356–369, 1983.

57. Mendelsohn D, Riedel WJ, Sambeth A. Effects of acute tryptophan depletion on memory, attention and executive functions: a systematic review. *Neurosci Biobehav Rev* **33**(6):926–952, 2009.

58. Frenois F, Moreau M, O'Connor J, et al. Lipopolysaccharide induces delayed FosB/DeltaFosB immunostaining within the mouse extended amygdala, hippocampus and hypothalamus, that parallel the expression of depressive-like behavior. *Psychoneuroendocrinology* **32**(5):516–531, 2007.

59. Moreau M, André C, O'Connor JC, et al. Inoculation of Bacillus Calmette-Guerin to mice induces an acute episode of sickness behavior followed by chronic depressive-like behavior. *Brain Behav Immun* **22**(7):1087–1095, 2008.

60. O'Connor JC, Lawson MA, André C, et al. Induction of IDO by bacille Calmette-Guerin is responsible for development of murine depressive-like behavior. *J Immunol* **182**(5):3202–3212, 2009.

61. O'Connor JC, Lawson MA, André C, et al. Lipopolysaccharide-induced depressive-like behavior is mediated by indoleamine 2,3-dioxygenase activation in mice. *Mol Psychiatry* **14**(5):511–522, 2009.

62. Henry CJ, Huang Y, Wynne A, et al. Minocycline attenuates lipopolysaccharide (LPS)-induced neuroinflammation, sickness behavior, and anhedonia. *J Neuroinflammation* **5**:15, 2008.

63. O'Connor JC, André C, Wang Y, et al. Interferon-gamma and tumor necrosis factor-alpha mediate the upregulation of indoleamine 2,3-dioxygenase and the induction of depressive-like behavior in mice in response to bacillus Calmette-Guerin. *J Neurosci* **29**(13):4200–4209, 2009.

64. Ball HJ, Yuasa HJ, Austin CJ, Weiser S, Hunt NH. Indoleamine 2,3-dioxygenase-2; a new enzyme in the kynurenine pathway. *Int J Biochem Cell Biol* **41**(3): 467–471, 2009.

65. Kanai M, Nakamura T, Funakoshi H. Identification and characterization of novel variants of the tryptophan 2,3-dioxygenase gene: differential regulation in the mouse nervous system during development. *Neurosci Res* **64**(1):111–117, 2009.

66. Moreau M, Lestage J, Verrier D, et al. Bacille Calmette-Guerin inoculation induces chronic activation of peripheral and brain indoleamine 2,3-dioxygenase in mice. *J Infect Dis* **192**(3):537–544, 2005.

67. Dunn AJ, Wang J, Ando T. Effects of cytokines on cerebral neurotransmission: comparison with the effects of stress. *Adv Exp Med Biol* **461**:117–127, 1999.

68. Godbout JP, Moreau M, Lestage J, et al. Aging exacerbates depressive-like behavior in mice in response to activation of the peripheral innate immune system. *Neuropsychopharmacology* **33**(10):2341–2351, 2008.

69. Barneoud P, Rivet JM, Vitiello S, Le Moal M, Neveu PJ. Brain norepinephrine levels after BCG stimulation of the immune system. *Immunol Lett* **18**(3):201–204, 1988.

70. Mössner R, Heils A, Stöber G, Okladnova O, Daniel S, Lesch KP. Enhancement of serotonin transporter function by tumor necrosis factor alpha but not by interleukin-6. *Neurochem Int* **33**(3):251–254, 1998.

71. Tsao CW, Lin YS, Chen CC, Bai CH, Wu SR. Cytokines and serotonin transporter in patients with

major depression. *Prog Neuropsychopharmacol Biol Psychiatry* **30**(5):899–905, 2006.

72. Zhu CB, Blakely RD, Hewlett WA. The proinflammatory cytokines interleukin-1beta and tumor necrosis factor-alpha activate serotonin transporters. *Neuropsychopharmacology* **31**(10):2121–2131, 2006.

73. Katafuchi T, Kondo T, Take S, Yoshimura M. Brain cytokines and the 5-HT system during poly I: C-induced fatigue. *Ann N Y Acad Sci* **1088**:230–237, 2006.

74. Lestage J, Verrier D, Palin K, Dantzer R. The enzyme indoleamine 2,3-dioxygenase is induced in the mouse brain in response to peripheral administration of lipopolysaccharide and superantigen. *Brain Behav Immun* **16**(5):596–601, 2002.

75. Fukui S, Schwarcz R, Rapoport SI, Takada Y, Smith QR. Blood-brain barrier transport of kynurenines: implications for brain synthesis and metabolism. *J Neurochem* **56**(6):2007–2017, 1991.

76. Schwarcz R. The kynurenine pathway of tryptophan degradation as a drug target. *Curr Opin Pharmacol* **4**(1):12–17, 2004.

77. Müller N, Schwarz MJ. A psychoneuroimmunological perspective to Emil Kraepelins dichotomy: schizophrenia and major depression as inflammatory CNS disorders. *Eur Arch Psychiatry Clin Neurosci***258**(Suppl 2):97–106, 2008.

78. Guillemin GJ, Cullen KM, Lim CK, et al. Characterization of the kynurenine pathway in human neurons. *J Neurosci* **27**(47):12884–12892, 2007.

79. Gabbay V, Liebes L, Katz Y, et al. The kynurenine pathway in adolescent depression: preliminary findings from a proton MR spectroscopy study. *Prog Neuropsychopharmacol Biol Psychiatry* **34**(1):37–44, 2010.

80. Wichers MC, Koek GH, Robaeys G, Verkerk R, Scharpé S, Maes M. IDO and interferon-alpha-induced depressive symptoms: a shift in hypothesis from tryptophan depletion to neurotoxicity. *Mol Psychiatry* **10**(6):538–544, 2005.

81. Raison CL, Dantzer R, Kelley KW, et al. CSF concentrations of brain tryptophan and kynurenines during immune stimulation with IFN-alpha: relationship to CNS immune responses and depression. *Mol Psychiatry*:e-pub ahead of print, 2009.

82. Valentine AD, Meyers CA, Kling MA, Richelson E, Hauser P. Mood and cognitive side effects of interferon-alpha therapy. *Semin Oncol* **25**(1 Suppl 1):39–47, 1998.

83. Capuron L, Ravaud A. Prediction of the depressive effects of interferon alfa therapy by the patient's initial affective state. *N Engl J Med* **340**(17):1370, 1999.

84. Capuron L, Ravaud A, Miller AH, Dantzer R. Baseline mood and psychosocial characteristics of patients developing depressive symptoms during interleukin-2 and/or interferon-alpha cancer therapy. *Brain Behav Immun* **18**(3):205–213, 2004.

85. Capuron L, Raison CL, Musselman DL, Lawson DH, Nemeroff CB, Miller AH. Association of exaggerated HPA axis response to the initial injection of interferon-alpha with development of depression during interferon-alpha therapy. *Am J Psychiatry* **160**(7):1342–1345, 2003.

86. Miller AH. Norman Cousins Lecture. Mechanisms of cytokine-induced behavioral changes: psychoneuroimmunology at the translational interface. *Brain Behav Immun* **23**(2):149–158, 2009.

87. Bull SJ, Huezo-Diaz P, Binder EB, et al. Functional polymorphisms in the interleukin-6 and serotonin transporter genes, and depression and fatigue induced by interferon-alpha and ribavirin treatment. *Mol Psychiatry* **14**(12):1095–1104, 2009.

88. Danese A, Moffitt TE, Pariante CM, Ambler A, Poulton R, Caspi A. Elevated inflammation levels in depressed adults with a history of childhood maltreatment. *Arch Gen Psychiatry* **65**(4):409–415, 2008.

89. Miller GE, Chen E, Fok AK, et al. Low early-life social class leaves a biological residue manifested by decreased glucocorticoid and increased proinflammatory signaling. *Proc Natl Acad Sci U S A* **106**(34):14716–14721, 2009.

90. Capuron L, Pagnoni G, Demetrashvili MF, et al. Basal ganglia hypermetabolism and symptoms of fatigue during interferon-alpha therapy. *Neuropsychopharmacology* **32**(11):2384–2392, 2007.

91. Capuron L, Pagnoni G, Demetrashvili M, et al. Anterior cingulate activation and error processing during interferon-alpha treatment. *Biol Psychiatry* **58**:190–196, 2005.

92. Brydon L, Harrison NA, Walker C, Steptoe A, Critchley HD. Peripheral inflammation is associated with altered substantia nigra activity and psychomotor slowing in humans. *Biol Psychiatry* **63**(11):1022–1029, 2008.

93. Harrison NA, Brydon L, Walker C, et al. Neural origins of human sickness in interoceptive responses to inflammation. *Biol Psychiatry* **66**(5):415–422, 2009.

94. Harrison NA, Brydon L, Walker C, Gray MA, Steptoe A, Critchley HD. Inflammation causes mood changes through alterations in subgenual cingulate activity and mesolimbic connectivity. *Biol Psychiatry* **66**(5):407–414, 2009.

95. O'Connor MF, Irwin MR, Wellisch DK. When grief heats up: pro-inflammatory cytokines predict regional brain activation. *Neuroimage* **47**(3):891–896, 2009.

96. Irwin MR, Miller AH. Depressive disorders and immunity: 20 years of progress and discovery. *Brain Behav Immun* **21**(4):374–383, 2007.

97. Thornton LM, Andersen BL, Schuler TA, Carson WE, III. A psychological intervention reduces inflammatory markers by alleviating depressive symptoms: secondary analysis of a randomized controlled trial. *Psychosom Med* **71**(7):715–724, 2009.

98. Stewart JC, Rand KL, Muldoon MF, Kamarck TW. A prospective evaluation of the directionality of the depression-inflammation relationship. *Brain Behav Immun* **23**(7):936–944, 2009.

99. Miller GE, Rohleder N, Stetler C, Kirschbaum C. Clinical depression and regulation of the inflammatory response during acute stress. *Psychosom Med* **67**(5):679–687, 2005.

100. Miller GE, Freedland KE, Carney RM. Depressive symptoms and the regulation of proinflammatory cytokine expression in patients with coronary heart disease. *J Psychosom Res* **59**(4):231–236, 2005.

101. Rohleder N, Miller GE. Acute deviations from long-term trait depressive symptoms predict systemic inflammatory activity. *Brain Behav Immun* **22**(5):709–716, 2008.

102. Kiecolt-Glaser JK, Gouin JP, Hantsoo L. Close relationships, inflammation, and health. *Neurosci Biobehav Rev*: e-pub ahead of print, 2009.

103. Segerstrom SC, Kemeny ME. Worried to death? Stress, worry, and immune dysregulation in health and HIV. In: Plotnikoff NP, Faith RE, Murgo AJ, Good RA, eds. *Cytokines: Stress and Immunity*. Boca Raton FL: CRC Press, 2007:17–28.

104. Brydon L, Walker C, Wawrzyniak AJ, Chart H, Steptoe A. Dispositional optimism and stress-induced changes in immunity and negative mood. *Brain Behav Immun* **23**(6):810–816, 2009.

105. Steptoe A, Hamer M, Chida Y. The effects of acute psychological stress on circulating inflammatory factors in humans: a review and meta-analysis. *Brain Behav Immun* **21**(7):901–912, 2007.

106. Anisman H. Cascading effects of stressors and inflammatory immune system activation: implications for major depressive disorder. *J Psychiatry Neurosci* **34**(1):4–20, 2009.

107. del Rey A, Roggero E, Randolf A, et al. IL-1 resets glucose homeostasis at central levels. *Proc Natl Acad Sci U S A* **103**(43):16039–16044, 2006.

108. McIntyre RS, Soczynska JK, Konarski JZ, et al. Should depressive syndromes be reclassified as "Metabolic Syndrome Type II"? *Ann Clin Psychiatry* **19**(4): 257–264, 2007.

Cancer-related fatigue: clinical science

Xin Shelley Wang

Fatigue is one of the most common, yet complex, symptoms reported by cancer patients and survivors. When fatigue is severe, it can be disabling. Because of ongoing debate about the definition of fatigue, inconclusive evidence about underlying pathophysiological mechanisms, and lack of effective pharmacological therapies, fatigue is a controversial and challenging subject for both researchers and those who manage patient care.

In this chapter, we introduce current understanding of cancer-related fatigue (CRF) and research on the mechanisms underlying CRF, discuss methodological issues for measuring CRF and then interpreting fatigue assessment results, and review innovations in CRF intervention.

Why address cancer-related fatigue?

The high prevalence and significant burden of fatigue in patients with cancer indicate the importance of understanding and managing it. The various methods used to measure fatigue in population-based studies have shown it to be the most common symptom that patients with cancer experience.[1] In one study,[2] outpatients with a variety of cancers treated in a tertiary-care cancer center reported that "severe fatigue," "feeling weak," and "not getting things done" were the most severe of the 26 symptoms included in the study. The percentage of patients with severe fatigue (fatigue rated 7 or higher on a 0–10 scale) is significantly greater than the percentage of healthy individuals with fatigue (34% and 17%, respectively).[3] In a study of outpatients with hematological malignancies,[4] 50% of the respondents reported having severe fatigue. Persistent cancer-related fatigue may be present among a subset of cancer survivors who have no evidence of active disease.[5,6]

In 1996, a survey of more than 400 randomly selected US cancer patients was commissioned by the Fatigue Coalition, a group of medical practitioners, researchers, and patient advocates formed to develop educational and research initiatives that would help patients and health care providers better understand and treat fatigue. Their report[7] established that fatigue in patients with cancer is "both pervasive and profound." The survey revealed that 78% of patients with cancer experienced fatigue during the course of their disease and its treatment. Despite this fact, fatigue is rarely discussed in the clinical setting and is unlikely to be treated. Although some progress has been made in research and intervention in the past decade, most epidemiological studies of fatigue in general indicate that it still occurs more frequently than other symptoms in patients with cancer. Such findings indicate the importance of establishing a standardized method for assessing and managing fatigue in routine clinical oncology care.

Fatigue is also perceived to be a significant problem in children and young people who have a cancer diagnosis. In a multicenter survey in the United Kingdom,[8] 56% of health professionals reported that "most" or "all" of their child patients experienced moderate fatigue. Meeske et al.[9] found that 30% of 161 long-term survivors of acute lymphoblastic leukemia whose cancer was diagnosed before the age of 18 years reported having fatigue, and that fatigue was highly corrected with depression.

Defining cancer-related fatigue

Although fatigue is reported to be the most common symptom of cancer, its definition varies among researchers and clinicians and from study to study. However, many definitions of cancer-related fatigue share similar descriptors, such as subjective, behavioral, physical, emotional, cognitive, temporal, and unusual. The National Comprehensive Cancer Network (NCCN) defines CRF as "a persistent subjective sense of tiredness related to cancer or cancer treatment that interferes with usual functioning."[10]

In clinical documents, fatigue is generally described as malaise, discomfort, weariness, lassitude, weakness, impatience, exhaustion, or the inability to perform

Cancer Symptom Science: Measurement, Mechanisms, and Management, eds. Charles S. Cleeland, Michael J. Fisch, and Adrian J. Dunn.

aspects of normal functioning. Patients have described this subjective experience using a variety of negative phrases, such as, "I don't have any energy," "I can't get things done," "I am constantly exhausted," and "My legs are weak." In fact, patients with CRF characterize their experience as "suffering" from fatigue, as compared with healthy individuals' descriptions of typical fatigue. CRF may be present at all times, or may occur as a transient "fatigue attack," where its onset is more rapid than that of typical fatigue. CRF drains more energy, lasts longer and is more severe, and is unrelenting. CRF overlaps with multifactorial physical and psychological (eg, depression) disorders. It has a negative impact on patient daily functioning and can diminish quality of life. CRF can be so overwhelming that patients elect to discontinue treatment.

A quantitative study found that CRF-related interference with functioning, as measured by the Brief Fatigue Inventory (BFI),[3] helped to differentiate fatigue severity levels. In this study, increase in a patient's worst-fatigue rating was associated with increase in fatigue's interference with functioning. When the worst fatigue reached 6 or greater on the BFI's 0–10 scale, interference with all aspects of daily life was moderate to severe (4 or greater on the 0–10 scale).[11]

Consideration of data from qualitative studies could tease out a simplified approach to understanding CRF. For example, the results of one qualitative study,[12] which compared the key domains of adaptation for "tired," "fatigued," and "exhausted" in patients with cancer, suggest that behavioral changes in sleep quality, stamina, cognition, and emotional reactivity may serve as early markers of impending fatigue, and that decreased control over body processes and reduced social interaction may be signs that an individual has entered a state of fatigue.

Nonetheless, subjective measures of CRF present little specific diagnostic information, and objective measures of CRF based on physiological or behavioral markers are frustratingly absent. As a result of differences in definition and measurement and the lack of available treatments, CRF is often neglected and undertreated.

Current research on mechanisms underlying cancer-related fatigue

Clinical correlates of cancer-related fatigue

NCCN guidelines[10] describe the causes of CRF as both the cancer and the cancer therapy. CRF can occur during any phase of the disease and often results from a combination of disease progression and the body's acute or late response to cancer therapy (Figure 10.1).[13]

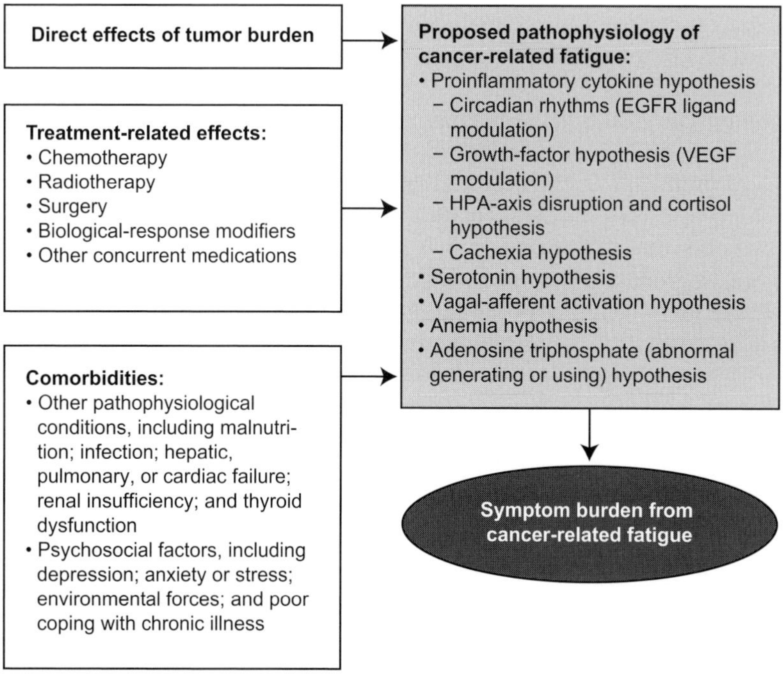

Figure 10.1. Proposed potential causes of cancer-related fatigue. EGFR indicates epidermal growth factor receptor; HPA, hypothalamic-pituitary-adrenal; VEGF, vascular endothelial growth factor.

Significant CRF related to the disease itself has been observed in patients with newly diagnosed cancer; in fact, unusual tiredness is frequently the first indicator that something is amiss.[13] In patients with advanced cancer, tumor progression affects multiple organ systems and causes neurological and physiological changes in skeletal muscles. Inflammatory processes responding to the tumor may cause abnormalities in energy metabolism and inhibit muscle function.

Cancer therapies, mainly chemotherapy, surgery, radiation therapy, bone marrow transplantation, and immunotherapy, can induce CRF outright and can exacerbate existing CRF. Gradual increases in levels of fatigue severity have been observed during chemotherapy and radiotherapy.[1,14–17] Chemotherapy-related nausea, vomiting, diarrhea, and neurotoxicity also may aggravate CRF severity, and CRF may be associated with chemotherapy-induced anemia and the end products of cell destruction. When high-dose chemotherapy is paired with stem cell transplantation, patients experience a posttransplantation dip in white blood cell count that has been associated with a peak in fatigue levels.[18,19] Chemotherapy combined with radiation treatment (combined modality therapy) is a known risk factor for persistent CRF. Radiation alone can induce anemia, diarrhea, anorexia, weight loss, and chronic pain, any of which may be associated with an increase in CRF. Radiation-induced fatigue may deepen over the course of treatment. Postoperative fatigue is often experienced by patients with cancer immediately after a curative surgical procedure, although increased analgesia has been shown to attenuate immediate postsurgical fatigue.[20]

Biological-response modifiers, such as proinflammatory cytokines and hormones, are known to produce CRF. Administration of interferon-α often causes a flu-like syndrome and has been shown to produce fatigue in 70% of patients.[21] Hormone treatment has been associated with lethargy and lack of energy in patients with breast cancer, equivalent in severity to the postradiotherapy fatigue experienced by patients with prostate cancer over a three-month course of hormone treatment.[22]

Finally, comorbidities that are also risk factors – such as acute or chronic medical conditions (eg, pain, sleep disturbance, decreased activity levels, infection, anemia, nutritional deficiencies, cardiac deconditioning, diabetes, and other medical conditions), psychosocial stress and emotional distress (eg, anxiety and depression), and sedating medications (eg, opioids) – may contribute to CRF in patients with cancer.

Translational research approaches

Establishing the causes of CRF presents numerous difficulties and challenges. We are not aware of any published research on the imaging of fatigue expression in the human brain, nor has an animal model representing CRF been established. Only a handful of human descriptive studies have carefully documented the development of fatigue and how it interacts with potential biological-mechanism targets in specific cohorts. Little progress has been made in identifying a reliable physiological marker as an objective measure of fatigue. CRF does not develop in all patients at risk for it, yet studies of genomic encoding for CRF that might explain this phenomenon have not been conducted.

In addition, patients with cancer rarely have severe fatigue alone; rather, individual patients, especially those who have accompanying medical comorbidities and/or psychological disorders, often experience a cluster of moderate to severe symptoms during active therapy or with advanced disease. This raises the question of whether CRF is caused by a constellation of risk factors or by a single factor. Complex interplay may be seen between the etiological agent (eg, cancer treatment, infections, use of central-acting drugs) and host susceptibility. A centrally mediated disorder, perhaps characterized by CRF, may underlie symptom clusters that currently lack clear pathophysiological explanations.

Although the underlying etiology of and risk factors for CRF are not fully resolved, potential mechanisms for this complex phenomenon are suggested by a number of working hypotheses (Figure 10.1),[13] chief of which is the proinflammatory cytokine hypothesis. Proinflammatory cytokines may act independently to produce CRF or may overlap or work synergistically with such mechanisms as vagal-afferent activation, hypothalamic-pituitary-adrenal (HPA) axis disruption, growth-factor activation, and circadian rhythm modulation. They many also act either directly or indirectly on the brain itself. Other proposed mechanisms include serotonin dysregulation, anemia, cachexia, and abnormalities in use of adenosine triphosphate. A similar proposal based on anatomical pathways for fatigue in central nervous system disorders suggests that such fatigue may result from a failure in the integration of limbic input and the motor functions within the basal ganglia affecting the striatal-thalamic-frontal cortical system.[23]

The proinflammatory cytokine hypothesis

The proinflammatory cytokine hypothesis offers one of the primary proposed mechanisms of CRF.[13,24] Fatigue, as a typical nonspecific symptom in patients with cancer, is similar to the sickness behavior (including general malaise, lack of motivation to eat, and reduced interest in activities) observed in studies of both central and behavioral effects of cytokine administration in animals.[25] The cytokine hypothesis suggests that dysregulated inflammation and its downstream toxic effects represent a significant biological basis for CRF and a cluster of other cancer-related symptoms.[18,26–28] In studies of persistent fatigue in survivors of breast cancer, certain inflammatory biomarkers (interleukin [IL]-6, tumor necrosis factor [TNF]-α) were identified *in vivo* and *in vitro*[29] and may be associated with the T-cell compartment.[30] Molecules that are downregulated by cytokines, such as albumin and C-reactive protein, are also highly correlated with the presence of CRF. In a quantitative review of 18 studies, Schubert et al.[31] showed positive association between CRF and circulating levels of IL-6, IL-1RA, and neopterin. Further, fatigue reduction was observed from a randomized clinical study of TNF-α blockade[32] as an intervention for improving tolerability of chemotherapy.

Cytokines have been shown to be highly correlated with physical and psychological symptoms in both humans and animal models. Clinical studies[18,33] have shown a temporal association between serum cytokines induced by aggressive cancer therapy and the development of multiple symptoms – particularly a cluster of symptoms that includes fatigue, pain, sleep disturbance, and poor appetite – that affect physical functioning in patients with cancer. The development of psychological symptoms, especially depression, in response to cytokines is well established in both animal models and in humans, specifically in relation to interferon-α-induced depressed mood and other sickness behaviors.[34–37]

Other hypotheses

The **vagal-afferent activation hypothesis** suggests that cancer and its treatment cause peripheral release of neuroactive molecules that may activate vagal-afferent nerves, resulting in decreased somatic motor output and sustained changes in regions of the brain associated with fatigue.[13,24] Cytokine production in the hypothalamus is especially significant in light of the effect of the HPA axis on fatigue.

The theory behind the **HPA disruption hypothesis** is that tumor-related or treatment-related dysregulation of HPA function might lead to endocrine changes that cause or contribute to fatigue.[13,24] Fatigue has been linked to reduced HPA-axis function and hypocortisolemia in patients with cancer or chronic fatigue syndrome. Reduced levels of cortisol, a stress hormone, may allow for increased levels of proinflammatory cytokines.

The **serotonin dysregulation hypothesis** posits that increases in brain serotonin induced by cancer or its treatment leads to modifications of HPA-axis function and to reductions in a person's ability to perform physical activities.[24] Exercise studies in both animals and humans have shown increased concentrations of serotonin at the point of fatigue and diminished capacity to perform.[38]

According to the **growth factor hypothesis**, elevated levels of vascular endothelial growth factor (VEGF), an angiogenic cytokine that stimulates the formation of new blood vessels necessary for tumor growth and metastasis, may be associated with treatment-induced fatigue.[39]

The **circadian-rhythm modulation hypothesis** focuses on secretion rhythms of the stress hormone cortisol and on rest-activity patterns. Elevated transforming growth factor-α levels have been associated with fatigue,[40] flattened circadian rhythms, and loss of appetite in patients with metastatic colorectal cancer. Alterations in rest – activity cycles, which produce the sleep disruptions commonly seen in patients with cancer – have been correlated with fatigue.

Risk factors beyond the neuroendocrine immune system have been proposed as mechanisms underlying the complex phenomenon of CRF. The **anemia hypothesis** is suggested by a body of literature demonstrating a correlation between anemia management and fatigue reduction. Anemia is known to result in hypoxia, which may compromise organ functioning and lead to fatigue.[41] According to the **adenosine triphosphate hypothesis**, cancer and its treatment may disrupt the metabolism of adenosine triphosphate, a major source of energy for skeletal-muscle contraction.[13,24] The resulting buildup of metabolic byproducts in the neuromuscular joints and skeletal muscle may reduce the patient's physical abilities, a phenomenon known as "peripheral fatigue." It is not known whether peripheral fatigue is a part of CRF.

Current research has promoted a better understanding of how CRF fluctuates according to various triggers and critical moderating factors, which should ultimately advance efforts to develop methods of mechanism-driven symptom intervention and prevention. Chronic fatigue syndrome might possibly be used as a surrogate for studying and understanding CRF, and further investigation into potential shared mechanisms and interventions is thus warranted.

Fatigue assessment: methodological considerations

Efforts to identify effective approaches to treat and manage CRF must be based upon assessments made with validated measurement tools. These tools are also essential in conducting translational mechanism studies and epidemiological studies with fatigue as a primary outcome.

Measuring cancer-related fatigue

CRF is subjectively experienced by individuals and may be accompanied by such symptoms as pain, nausea, and depressed mood. Even though fatigue can cause observable behavioral manifestations and is often associated with objective decrements in performance, fatigue cannot be directly measured by an observer. Subjective patient report (patient-reported outcomes, or PROs) has become the standard method for assessing dimensions of fatigue, such as its severity and interference with daily activities. The US Food and Drug Administration (FDA) encourages investigators to use PRO measures in clinical research for symptom intervention, while emphasizing the importance of utilizing standardized and psychometrically validated assessment tools.[42]

Epidemiological fatigue research

Several approaches for measuring fatigue have been broadly adopted in prevalence studies, but comparisons across studies are limited by the variety of criteria used to define fatigue and grade its severity.[43] For example, in some studies, prevalence is reported as the proportion of patients who have complained of any degree of fatigue (yes or no), whereas in others, prevalence is reported on the basis of complaints of severe fatigue only. The most rigorous approach to identifying fatigue is to apply a strict set of diagnostic criteria to populations of patients with cancer.[44]

Despite the use of various measures of fatigue across studies, several descriptive studies with large databases[3,45,46] have found that the mean fatigue level as measured by, for example, the Brief Fatigue Inventory, the Functional Assessment of Cancer Therapy (FACT), or the fatigue items in the European Organisation for Research and Treatment of Cancer (EORTC) Quality of Life Questionnaire for Cancer Patients (QLQ-C30), was significantly higher for patients with cancer than for healthy individuals.

Comprehensive clinical assessment

The multidimensional nature of fatigue makes it difficult to measure. Although initial efforts to develop a measure of fatigue after World War I were considered impractical, it is now more widely accepted that developing a comprehensive and validated fatigue assessment process is possible. Existing validated fatigue measures typically assess severity first, to determine how bad the situation is for the patient; severity assessment is often followed by an assessment for determining how much the fatigue interferes with daily life. However, assessments of severity and interference must often be integrated, on a patient-by-patient basis, with assessments of other factors, such as quality of fatigue, temporal pattern, history, and expectations associated with a specific disease phase or treatment status. To be clinically meaningful, a fatigue assessment should also include a formal examination of the impact of fatigue on physical function, social function, cognition, mood, and other facets of quality of life.

The assessment process must also give clinical consideration to potential etiologies, eg, cancer treatment, intercurrent systemic disorders such as anemia and infection, sleep disorders, chronic pain, lack of exercise, centrally acting drugs, malnutrition, metabolic disturbance, cachexia, anxiety, and depression,[47] especially to support the identification of treatable causes.

Selecting an assessment tool

Good tools for measuring persistent fatigue should be both practical and psychometrically sound: they should require patients to evaluate only a few aspects of their experience within a reasonable recall period; present aspects for evaluation in easily understood terms; rely on easy-to-use scales and standardized rules for administration and scoring; and be able to detect changes in patient experience. To facilitate cross-cultural validation and comparison, the tool should also be developed to maximize the ease and effectiveness with which it can be translated into other languages. Most important, a good fatigue assessment tool should allow for consistent interpretation of data.

As Hjollund et al. summarized in 2007,[48] between 1975 and 2004 more than 250 fatigue assessment tools were developed for use in patients with either cancer or chronic disease; of these, 150 were used only once. Seventy-one scales specifically designed to measure fatigue were used in 416 studies, and 156 multisymptom scales were used in 670 studies. These tools vary in their construction (coverage, structure), frequency of use, recommended frequency of administration, scoring, and psychometric properties. An earlier review[49] indicated the need for more serious work to be done in the development of new scales and in the further validation of existing tools, including gathering basic data on reliability and on sensitivity to detect changes in severity and prevalence, and studies of severity cut points for clinical use.

An investigator's choice of a standardized method to assess CRF will likely depend on: (1) the user's clinical demands, such as whether quick screening or comprehensive assessment is more important and what medical services and reimbursement are available; (2) the method's psychometric properties (ie, its standardization, reliability, and validity); and (3) its research utility. Quick and easy measures used for screening purposes provide basic information, such as whether fatigue is present or absent and, if present, its intensity, severity, and/or impact. These measures may indicate whether more comprehensive clinical examination is needed and, when used in research or clinical trials, can provide enough data to track changes in fatigue both over time and in response to treatment. Multidimensional measures allow the examination of various facets of fatigue in the mental-cognitive, physical, and emotional domains, which is valuable given that the experiences of patients with CRF are subjective and that the impact of fatigue on everyday life varies from patient to patient.

No single instrument assessing either CRF or other forms of chronic fatigue has attained broad appeal, either in clinical practice or in research. Although the FDA[42] has encouraged investigators to use PRO measures in their research, the agency has emphasized that no gold standard for choosing a particular instrument yet exists. Many of the tools currently available were developed for use in specific patient populations, such as those affected by CRF, chronic fatigue syndrome, or fatigue related to neurological or systemic disorders; some tools have "crossed over" to be used in additional patient populations, whereas others have not. These instruments are all based on patient self-report, but the type of response collected varies. The tools may use, for example, verbal descriptor scales (where patients select a category to describe their fatigue, such as "none," "mild," "moderate," "severe"), visual analogue scales (where patients mark their fatigue severity along a line), or numerical rating scales (where patients choose a number to rate their fatigue severity) with verbal anchors at both ends (such as "no fatigue" and "fatigue as bad as you can imagine").

Although no consensus on the dimensional structure of fatigue has been reached,[50] the currently available fatigue scales may be summarized as falling into three categories: (1) single-item scales or parts of larger instruments; (2) unidimensional scales; and (3) multidimensional scales.

Single-item and subscale measures

At their briefest, PRO assessment tools can measure fatigue with a single item or a multisymptom or quality-of-life subscale. Clinicians commonly use the numeric rating scale as an empirical tool, and several instruments of this type have been standardized and validated. The single-item score given for "fatigue at its worst" in the Brief Fatigue Inventory[3] asks patients to rate their level of worst fatigue/tiredness during the previous 24 hours on a 0–10 scale anchored by "not present" and "as bad as you can imagine." This item can be used as a rapid screening tool or a continuous-monitoring variable in clinical practice.[11] Kirsh et al.[51] used the level of response on a single item from the Zung Self-Rating Depression Scale as a quick screening method for CRF. A single fatigue item assessing presence, severity, and distress is presented in the Memorial Symptom Assessment Scale (MSAS).[52] The 13-item fatigue subscale of the FACT[53] rates CRF on a 0–4 scale with a recall period of the previous seven days. Similarly, a fatigue subscale consisting of three items covering the prior week is a part of the EORTC QLQ-C30.[54]

Unidimensional measures

Whether CRF is unidimensional or multidimensional has not been definitively resolved. Lai et al.[55] conducted exploratory factor analysis using a theory-driven bifactor model and 72-item fatigue item bank populated with data from a sample of 555 patients with cancer. The items included physical, mental, social, and other fatigue experiences. The authors concluded that CRF is sufficiently unidimensional for measurement approaches that require or assume unidimensionality. Single-item, single-dimension measures for CRF include the widely used NCCN patient-reported fatigue intensity rating,[10] which has a 0–10 numeric scale, and the National Cancer Institute's Common Terminology Criteria for Adverse Events (version 3.0),[56] which uses a 5-point Likert scale rated by medical staff. Some unidimensional measures for CRF have multiple items, including the BFI[3] and the Fatigue Severity Scale.[57] Although having responses for all items from every patient is ideal, some instruments with good reliability can, through the use of arithmetic adjustments, generate usable results when a small percentage of responses are missing.

Multidimensional measures

Some argue that although the psychometric accuracy of unidimensional measures may be satisfactory, they fall short of assessing the full spectrum of CRF.[1] Unlike unidimensional measures, multidimensional measures typically distinguish physical from mental fatigue and measure responses in dimensions relating to affect and activity. The relatively short and simple Multidimensional Fatigue Inventory (MFI-20)[58] is a commonly used measure of fatigue. Like unidimensional scales, the MFI-20's General Fatigue subscale can serve as a global index of fatigue severity.

One drawback of using multidimensional scales is that some are too long for very ill patients to complete. Many of these measures also depend upon original phrases or idiomatic expressions that can make them difficult to translate into other languages or cultural settings.

Measures of cancer-related fatigue as a syndrome

Standardizing the criteria for characterizing CRF would facilitate cross-country cooperation among medical care providers, reimbursement systems, and researchers studying prevalence and other aspects of CRF. Some would say that using the word "fatigue" alone is misleading and that the use of syndrome-based criteria is a more accurate way of characterizing the collection of diverse phenomena experienced as fatigue. "Malaise and fatigue" is listed under "Symptoms, signs, and ill-defined conditions" (780 General symptoms) in the *International Classification of Diseases, Ninth Edition, Clinical Modification* (ICD-9-CM). The proposed ICD-10 has been shown to have good internal consistency for all items.[44] Establishing the merits of a criterion-based syndrome approach versus a severity-spectrum approach remains an area worthy of active research, considering that implementing a diagnostic criterion-based method requires trained clinicians to conduct structured patient interviews.

Applying the knowledge gained from fatigue assessment

Fatigue assessment promotes quality assurance in the treatment of cancer by expanding attention and resources along the spectrum of services provided to address this common and debilitating symptom. As an outcome measure, CRF can be an important component of drug trials and clinical practice. A reduction in CRF could represent a reduction in treatment toxicity, improved palliation for advanced disease, patient satisfaction with medical care, or better functional and health status for cancer survivors, and may result in a lower cost of care. In contrast, inadequate assessment can be a significant barrier to good fatigue management in the clinic.

Interpreting clinically significant functional impairment

Several critical research questions must be answered to obtain an accurate interpretation of CRF data. For example, is there a clinically meaningful distinction between the way cancer patients and healthy individuals experience fatigue? Can we define a point at which CRF becomes functionally disabling?

One way to begin answering these questions is to examine the meaning of symptom severity by defining levels at which symptoms interfere with physical and affective functioning. In early research on pain, functional impairment or interference increased in a stair-step manner as pain increased.[59,60] This research has been used as a basis for defining critical pain management pathways, quality assurance, and symptom epidemiology.[61] Using the same methodology with numeric Likert-type fatigue scales, Cleeland and Wang[11] observed that functional interference increased as fatigue worsened. The boundary between mild-moderate and severe fatigue may be a clinically meaningful indicator for determining whether an intervention for fatigue is effective. Although the severity of fatigue may be the most informative indicator of the need for intervention, the frequency and duration of fatigue episodes as well as the degree of increase in severity scores may lead to a diagnosis of CRF and suggest a clinical threshold for intervention.

Studies of CRF interventions should be carefully planned to avoid common pitfalls. Investigators of studies involving interventions for CRF should be encouraged to fully examine the history and natural pattern of fatigue in each specific cohort of patients before introducing an intervention. Lack of a non-cancer comparison group or control group reduces the meaningfulness and interpretability of fatigue severity data. Fatigue studies that use cross-sectional designs do not allow symptom interactions to be observed over time, and the results of such studies may be weakened by recall bias. In contrast, well-designed longitudinal fatigue studies and appropriate statistical-analysis methods improve the understanding of the nature of fatigue over the course and treatment of chronic diseases.[14,43]

Interpreting the effect of response shift on fatigue ratings

Fatigue research that tracks changes in self-report over time has the potential to introduce response shift, which raises methodological concerns. Response shift occurs when patients judge their level of fatigue differently after having experiences that alter their own internal standards, values, or conceptualizations. Response shift may lead to an underreporting of fatigue as patients adapt to a greater "normal" level of fatigue after therapy. Visser[62] reported that response shift occurred in a group of patients receiving radiotherapy who retrospectively minimized their pretreatment fatigue severity compared with their current levels of fatigue.

The patient's illness perception, coping skills, and mood may have important and long-lasting effects on his or her eventual adaptation to chronic fatigue – whether the adaptation is acceptable or a maladjustment – and are important effects to note when interpreting fatigue studies. A response shift in fatigue scores might reflect a change in the respondent's internal standards ("recalibration," in psychometric terms), rather than a change in or redefinition of the value of the response ("reconceptualization"). A meta-analysis of 19 studies[63] reported the largest effect size (ES) of response shift for fatigue (mean ES, 0.32), followed by global quality of life, physical role limitation, psychological well-being, and pain. Studies designed with integrated measures of both accumulated dose of cancer therapy and the change in internal standards can explicitly measure response-shift effects and take them into account in evaluating treatments or interventions.

Interpreting the relationship of fatigue to other symptoms

Severe cancer-related symptoms, such as fatigue, pain, and sleep disturbance, rarely occur as solitary symptoms when patients are undergoing active therapy or have advanced disease. It is believed that the greater the number of symptoms and the greater the perceived disability, the more likely that psychological, behavioral, or social factors will be identified by clinicians as contributors to illness. Cluster analyses of multiple cancer-related symptoms have demonstrated the phenomenon of closely related sickness symptoms,[64] raising a serious question as to the independence of CRF and its measurement. The careful measuring of the development of multiple symptoms in a descriptive study, or of symptom reduction as a response to symptom-directed interventions, may help to characterize the interactions between individual symptoms, if any. That this is a complicated issue was shown by Morrow et al.,[65] who demonstrated a positive response to an antidepressant (a selective serotonin reuptake inhibitor) for mood without a corresponding improvement in fatigue severity.

CRF, as well as other sickness symptoms, may appear in cancer patients undergoing chemotherapy and suffering from "chemobrain" (see Chapter 6); however, current evidence confirms no such association. Future longitudinal study is needed to address the issue.

Interventions for cancer-related fatigue

No gold-standard intervention for CRF exists, even though much attention has been directed toward developing and testing both pharmacological and nonpharmacological treatments for fatigue. As a result, first-line therapy for CRF often calls for the identification and management of factors associated with CRF – anemia, hypothyroidism, pain, distress, sleep disturbance, malnutrition, and other comorbidities – rather than the fatigue itself.[10]

In this section we review the literature on the relative merits of both pharmacological and behavioral interventions. Several systematic reviews and meta-analyses, described below, have analyzed preliminary evidence of the efficacy of some of the most-reported interventions.

Pharmacological treatments

Psychostimulants

Methylphenidate, a central nervous system stimulant similar to amphetamine, was used to treat CRF in two randomized placebo-controlled trials; the meta-analysis that included these studies[66] revealed that treatment with methylphenidate for a mean of five weeks significantly reduced fatigue (overall z score, 2.40; $P = 0.02$). The data support prescribing 10–20 mg daily, although the response and potential minor side effects of the drug should be considered.

Modafinil, another central nervous system stimulant, has been approved by the FDA for narcolepsy. The usual dose of modafinil is 100–200 mg in the morning, with another dose at noon or shortly thereafter; the maximum dosage is 400 mg/day. Fava et al.[67] reported that modafinil is a well-tolerated and potentially effective augmenting agent for patients with fatigue and sleepiness who are partial responders to selective serotonin reuptake inhibitors. In a phase III placebo-controlled trial,[68] modafinil seemed useful for improving severe fatigue during chemotherapy; it had a significant beneficial effect on sleepiness but no effect on depression.

Antidepressants

Although it is not known whether fatigue and depression share pathophysiological characteristics, efforts have been made to treat fatigue with antidepressants in depressed cancer patients. Morrow et al.,[65] reporting the results of a double-blind, randomized, placebo-controlled study of cancer patients with fatigue who were undergoing chemotherapy, noted that paroxetine produced a significant reduction in depressive symptoms but no significant change in levels of fatigue. A meta-analysis of two randomized trials[66] found no benefit of fatigue reduction from paroxetine (overall z score, 1.06; $P = 0.29$).

Studies of other classes of antidepressants in patients undergoing various modes of cancer therapy are necessary to determine whether fatigue can be treated effectively in those circumstances. Patients with sleep difficulties and depression may also benefit from antidepressants such as nortriptyline and amitriptyline because of the sedative qualities of those drugs. Bupropion may benefit patients with CRF because it has the pharmacological properties of a stimulant.[69]

Corticosteroids

Results from four randomized placebo-controlled trials[66] indicated that a mean of 8 weeks of progestational steroid therapy (three studies used megestrol acetate and one used medroxyprogesterone acetate) did not reduce fatigue in a group of patients receiving palliative care without chemotherapy (overall z score, 1.06; $P = 0.29$). Because steroids consistently had no effect in the clinical studies, and because of concerns about adverse effects with long term use, further investigation of steroids for the treatment of persistent CRF is not warranted.

Nonpharmacological interventions

Psychological and activity-based intervention

Interest has been growing in the role of cognitive factors (eg, tendency to perceive catastrophe) and behavioral factors (eg, physical activity) in exacerbating and prolonging fatigue. In a meta-analysis, Schmitz et al.[70] suggested that exercise is an effective way to manage CRF, although the ES was small, both during treatment (weighted mean ES, 0.13; 95% confidence interval [95% CI], −0.06 to 0.33) and after treatment (weighted mean ES, 0.16; 95% CI, −0.23 to 0.54). In another summary of 12 randomized controlled clinical trials, Mustian et al.[71] commented that exercise is safe for and well-tolerated by cancer survivors. Many clinical trials have reported the effect of aerobic or resistance exercise interventions for women receiving adjuvant therapy for breast cancer. The Cochrane collaboration[72] published a meta-analysis of nine trials involving 452 women on exercise study, concluding that exercise results in improved physical fitness and thus in improved capacity for performing activities of daily life for this cohort of patients. However, the difference in improvement in patient-reported fatigue between the intervention and control groups was statistically nonsignificant.

In a recent systematic review and meta-analysis of the literature up to 2005, Jacobsen et al.[73] reported limited scientific evidence of the efficacy of nonpharmacological therapy for CRF in adults. Specifically, the meta-analysis found a small effect size (ES, 0.09; 95% CI, 0.02–0.16) overall in 30 randomized controlled trials of nonpharmacological interventions; the effect sizes in 18 studies with psychological interventions were larger, but 12 studies with activity-based interventions showed no significant benefit. The psychosocial interventions included support-group therapy and individual psychotherapy, both of which provided education, coping strategy programs, tailored behavioral interventions, and professionally or self-administered stress-management training. The activity-based interventions were home-based and supervised exercise programs. In a meta-analytical review, Luebbert et al.[74] found that relaxation interventions had no effect on a patient's vigor, fatigue, or confusion during cancer treatment.

The methodological quality of the psychological and activity-based CRF intervention studies analyzed above was often considered less adequate on the basis of the studies' random selection of patients, the level of participant adherence to the intervention, and whether outcomes were assessed by blind personnel. Evidence was compiled primarily from patients with nonmetastatic breast cancer in active treatment, which may limit the generalizability of the results. None of these trials used a consistent baseline fatigue level as a criterion for eligibility, and 92% of the psychological trials lacked a control condition. An adoption of better reporting standards, such as the Consolidated Standard of Reporting Trials (CONSORT),[75,76] and a more careful study design would improve the methodological quality and documentation of this type of study and thus provide more accurate data on the efficacy of psychosocial therapy for CRF. Overall, there is an encouraging trend toward further serious investigation into behavioral interventions for CRF, which should reduce the occurrence of inconclusive results.

Complementary alternative therapy

Although few well-designed randomized clinical trials have tested herbal treatments, massage therapy, and acupuncture for CRF, there is much interest in these complementary alternative therapies. In subjects with unexplained chronic fatigue of unknown etiology lasting for at least six months, the percentage of users who found a treatment helpful was greatest for coenzyme Q10, dehydroepiandrosterone (DHEA), and ginseng, whereas yoga appeared to be most effective for subjects who did not have unclear thinking associated with their fatigue.[77] Acupuncture has not been thoroughly studied in patients with CRF.

Ginseng, a widely used tonic agent, is challenging to investigate in blind randomized trials,[78] partly because its potent smell and aftertaste make it difficult to mask. Also, it is easily acquired at health food stores and patients may not think of it as medication. A recent trial of American ginseng[79,80] indicated that patients receiving larger doses showed improvements in overall energy levels and in overall mental, physical, spiritual, and emotional well-being. Many patients use herbal and supplemental preparations to deal with CRF, but patients should be cautious in their use of herbal treatments because of possible profound drug interactions.

Conclusion

CRF is the most common complaint of patients with cancer. It is frequently the most distressing symptom because it interferes with multiple aspects of daily life. Debilitating fatigue may result from cancer or its treatment, especially in patients with advanced disease and those undergoing active treatment, and it may persist in some survivors who have otherwise been cured of their cancer. Although the awareness and study of this symptom have grown tremendously in recent years, assessment and management of CRF have not been priorities in routine medical practice and much about the mechanisms underlying the development of CRF is still unknown.[11]

Compared with the leaps in progress made in understanding and managing cancer pain, nausea, and vomiting since the 1980s, only baby steps have been taken in advancing our understanding of CRF. National standards for clinical practice now exist for pain management, and initial barriers to optimal pain management, including inadequate assessment, patient reluctance to report pain, and poor staff knowledge and negative attitudes about pain control, have become outmoded. The same is becoming true for CRF relief. A 2003 NIH State-of-the-Science Statement[81] called for additional research on pain, depression, and fatigue – alone and in combination – in adequately funded prospective studies. This has stimulated a tremendous growth in clinical investigations of the effectiveness of interventions for CRF, even while basic research on CRF remains limited. Creating a more mature scientific literature in the field, including epidemiological studies, creation and validation of measurement tools for CRF screening and use in clinical trials, and reports on effective therapies, is critical to improving fatigue management.

Measuring fatigue in a reliable and valid manner that examines widely accepted dimensions is essential for advancing fatigue research and clinical management. No one tool has been firmly recommended as a gold standard for measuring CRF. Individual circumstance, good clinical practice, and research goals will likely dictate the choice of appropriate tool from among the existing subscales, unidimensional tools, and multidimensional tools.

Education about CRF should be made available to all patients and their caregivers. Having accurate and age-appropriate information about conditions like CRF often alleviates the stress and anxiety that poor communication can provoke.

Finally, there is great need for well-designed clinical trials to evaluate both pharmacological and non-pharmacological methods for treating CRF. Our ability to treat the root causes of CRF will require a good understanding of its underlying pathophysiological mechanisms, about which no widely accepted consensus exists. The development of a mechanism-based method of fatigue classification might lead the way to future physiological-behavioral fatigue research and treatment. It may also lead to the development of drugs that target distinct mechanisms, new guidelines for experimental designs, more reliable and valid diagnostic tools, and therapies that provide patients with greater symptom control.

References

1. Prue G, Rankin J, Allen J, Gracey J, Cramp F. Cancer-related fatigue: a critical appraisal. *Eur J Cancer* **42**(7):846–863, 2006.
2. Cleeland CS, Mendoza TR, Wang XS, et al. Assessing symptom distress in cancer patients: the M. D. Anderson Symptom Inventory. *Cancer* **89**(7):1634–1646, 2000.
3. Mendoza TR, Wang XS, Cleeland CS, et al. The rapid assessment of fatigue severity in cancer patients: use of the Brief Fatigue Inventory. *Cancer* **85**(5):1186–1196, 1999.
4. Wang XS, Giralt SA, Mendoza TR, et al. Clinical factors associated with cancer-related fatigue in patients being treated for leukemia and non-Hodgkin's lymphoma. *J Clin Oncol* **20**:1319–1328, 2002.
5. Bower JE, Ganz PA, Desmond KA, Rowland JH, Meyerowitz BE, Belin TR. Fatigue in breast cancer survivors: occurrence, correlates, and impact on quality of life. *J Clin Oncol* **18**(4):743–753, 2000.
6. Servaes P, Gielissen MF, Verhagen S, Bleijenberg G. The course of severe fatigue in disease-free breast cancer patients: a longitudinal study. *Psychooncology* **16**(9):787–795, 2007.
7. Vogelzang NJ, Breitbart W, Cella D, et al. Patient, caregiver, and oncologist perceptions of cancer-related fatigue: results of a tripart assessment survey. The Fatigue Coalition. *Semin Hematol* **34**(3 Suppl 2):4–12, 1997.
8. Gibson F, Garnett M, Richardson A, Edwards J, Sepion B. Heavy to carry: a survey of parents' and healthcare professionals' perceptions of cancer-related fatigue in children and young people. *Cancer Nurs* **28**(1):27–35, 2005.
9. Meeske KA, Siegel SE, Globe DR, Mack WJ, Bernstein L. Prevalence and correlates of fatigue in long-term survivors of childhood leukemia. *J Clin Oncol* **23**(24):5501–5510, 2005.
10. Mock V, Atkinson A, Barsevick AM, et al. Cancer-related fatigue. Clinical practice guidelines in oncology. *J Natl Compr Canc Netw* **5**(10):1054–1078, 2007.
11. Cleeland CS, Wang XS. Measuring and understanding fatigue. *Oncology* **13**(11A):91–97, 1999.
12. Olson K. A new way of thinking about fatigue: a reconceptualization. *Oncol Nurs Forum* **34**(1):93–99, 2007.
13. Wang XS. Pathophysiology of cancer-related fatigue. *Clin J Oncol Nurs* **12**(5 Suppl):11–20, 2008.
14. Wang XS, Fairclough DL, Liao Z, et al. Longitudinal study of the relationship between chemoradiation therapy for non-small-cell lung cancer and patient symptoms. *J Clin Oncol* **24**(27):4485–4491, 2006.
15. Hickok JT, Morrow GR, Roscoe JA, Mustian K, Okunieff P. Occurrence, severity, and longitudinal course of twelve common symptoms in 1129 consecutive patients during radiotherapy for cancer. *J Pain Symptom Manage* **30**(5):433–442, 2005.
16. Knobel H, Loge JH, Nordøy T, et al. High level of fatigue in lymphoma patients treated with high dose therapy. *J Pain Symptom Manage* **19**(6):446–456, 2000.
17. Jacobsen PB, Hann DM, Azzarello LM, Horton J, Balducci L, Lyman GH. Fatigue in women receiving adjuvant chemotherapy for breast cancer: characteristics, course, and correlates. *J Pain Symptom Manage* **18**(4):233–242, 1999.
18. Wang XS, Shi Q, Williams LA, et al. Serum interleukin-6 predicts the development of multiple symptoms at nadir of allogeneic hematopoietic stem cell transplantation. *Cancer* **113**(8):2102–2109, 2008.
19. Anderson KO, Giralt SA, Mendoza TR, et al. Symptom burden in patients undergoing autologous stem-cell transplantation. *Bone Marrow Transplant* **39**(12): 759–766, 2007.
20. Rubin GJ, Hotopf M. Systematic review and meta-analysis of interventions for postoperative fatigue. *Br J Surg* **89**(8):971–984, 2002.
21. Jones TH, Wadler S, Hupart KH. Endocrine-mediated mechanisms of fatigue during treatment with interferon-alpha. *Semin Oncol* **25**(1 Suppl 1):54–63, 1998.
22. Stone P, Hardy J, Huddart R, A'Hern R, Richards M. Fatigue in patients with prostate cancer receiving hormone therapy. *Eur J Cancer* **36**(9):1134–1141, 2000.

23. Chaudhuri A, Behan PO. Fatigue and basal ganglia. *J Neurol Sci* **179**(S 1-2):34–42, 2000.

24. Ryan JL, Carroll JK, Ryan EP, Mustian KM, Fiscella K, Morrow GR. Mechanisms of cancer-related fatigue. *Oncologist* **12**(Suppl 1):22–34, 2007.

25. Dantzer R, Kelley KW. Twenty years of research on cytokine-induced sickness behavior. *Brain Behav Immun* **21**(2):153–160, 2007.

26. Cleeland CS, Bennett GJ, Dantzer R, et al. Are the symptoms of cancer and cancer treatment due to a shared biologic mechanism? *Cancer* **97**(11):2919–2925, 2003.

27. Kurzrock R. The role of cytokines in cancer-related fatigue. *Cancer* **92**(6 Suppl):1684–1688, 2001.

28. Lee BN, Dantzer R, Langley KE, et al. A cytokine-based neuroimmunologic mechanism of cancer-related symptoms. *Neuroimmunomodulation* **11**(5):279–292, 2004.

29. Collado-Hidalgo A, Bower JE, Ganz PA, Cole SW, Irwin MR. Inflammatory biomarkers for persistent fatigue in breast cancer survivors. *Clin Cancer Res* **12**(9):2759–2766, 2006.

30. Bower JE, Ganz PA, Aziz N, Fahey JL. Fatigue and proinflammatory cytokine activity in breast cancer survivors. *Psychosom Med* **64**(4):604–611, 2002.

31. Schubert C, Hong S, Natarajan L, Mills PJ, Dimsdale JE. The association between fatigue and inflammatory marker levels in cancer patients: a quantitative review. *Brain Behav Immun* **21**(4):413–427, 2007.

32. Monk JP, Phillips G, Waite R, et al. Assessment of tumor necrosis factor alpha blockade as an intervention to improve tolerability of dose-intensive chemotherapy in cancer patients. *J Clin Oncol* **24**(12):1852–1859, 2006.

33. Wang XS, Shi Q, Mao L, Cleeland CS, Liao Z. Association between inflammatory cytokines and the development of multiple symptoms in patients with non-small cell lung cancer undergoing chemoradiation therapy [abstract]. American Society of Clinical Oncology 44th Annual Meeting, Chicago IL, May 30–June 3, 2008. *J Clin Oncol* **26**(15 Suppl), 2008. Abstract 9638.

34. Payne JK, Piper B, Rabinowitz I, Zimmerman B. Biomarkers, fatigue, sleep, and depressive symptoms in women with breast cancer: a pilot study. *Oncol Nurs Forum* **33**(4):775–783, 2006.

35. Raison CL, Capuron L, Miller AH. Cytokines sing the blues: inflammation and the pathogenesis of depression. *Trends Immunol* **27**(1):24–31, 2006.

36. Dantzer R, Capuron L, Irwin MR, et al. Identification and treatment of symptoms associated with inflammation in medically ill patients. *Psychoneuroendocrinology* **33**(1):18–29, 2008.

37. Miller AH, Ancoli-Israel S, Bower JE, Capuron L, Irwin MR. Neuroendocrine-immune mechanisms of behavioral comorbidities in patients with cancer. *J Clin Oncol* **26**(6):971–982, 2008.

38. Davis JM, Bailey SP. Possible mechanisms of central nervous system fatigue during exercise. *Med Sci Sports Exerc* **29**(1):45–57, 1997.

39. Mills PJ, Parker BA, Dimsdale JE, Sadler GR, Ancoli-Israel S. The relationship between fatigue, quality of life and inflammation during anthracycline-based chemotherapy in breast cancer. *Biol Psychol* **69**(1):85–96, 2005.

40. Rich T, Innominato PF, Boerner J, et al. Elevated serum cytokines correlated with altered behavior, serum cortisol rhythm, and dampened 24-hour rest-activity patterns in patients with metastatic colorectal cancer. *Clin Cancer Res* **11**(5):1757–1764, 2005.

41. Hurter B, Bush NJ. Cancer-related anemia: clinical review and management update. *Clin J Oncol Nurs* **11**(3):349–359, 2007.

42. US Food and Drug Administration, Center for Drug Evaluation and Research, Center for Biologics Evaluation and Research, Center for Devices and Radiological Health. Guidance for industry. Patient-reported outcome measures: use in medical product development to support labeling claims. Available from: URL: http://www.fda.gov/downloads/Drugs/GuidanceComplianceRegulatoryInformation/Guidances/UCM071975.pdf. Accessed Dec 18, 2009.

43. Lawrence DP, Kupelnick B, Miller K, Devine D, Lau J. Evidence report on the occurrence, assessment, and treatment of fatigue in cancer patients. *J Natl Cancer Inst Monogr* **32**:40–50, 2004.

44. van Belle S, Paridaens R, Evers G, et al. Comparison of proposed diagnostic criteria with FACT-F and VAS for cancer-related fatigue: proposal for use as a screening tool. *Support Care Cancer* **13**(4):246–254, 2005.

45. Cella D, Lai JS, Chang CH, Peterman A, Slavin M. Fatigue in cancer patients compared with fatigue in the general United States population. *Cancer* **94**(2):528–538, 2002.

46. Hjermstad MJ, Fayers PM, Bjordal K, Kaasa S. Health-related quality of life in the general Norwegian population assessed by the European Organization for Research and Treatment of Cancer Core Quality-of-Life Questionnaire: the QLQ=C30 (+3). *J Clin Oncol* **16**(3):1188–1196, 1998.

47. Portenoy RK, Itri LM. Cancer-related fatigue: guidelines for evaluation and management. *Oncologist* **4**(1):1–10, 1999.

48. Hjollund NH, Andersen JH, Bech P. Assessment of fatigue in chronic disease: a bibliographic study of

fatigue measurement scales. *Health Qual Life Outcomes* **5**:12–16, 2007.

49. Dittner AJ, Wessely SC, Brown RG. The assessment of fatigue: a practical guide for clinicians and researchers. *J Psychosom Res* **56**(2):157–170, 2004.
50. Jacobsen PB. Assessment of fatigue in cancer patients. *J Natl Cancer Inst Monogr* **32**:93–97, 2004.
51. Kirsh KL, Passik S, Holtsclaw E, Donaghy K, Theobald D. I get tired for no reason: a single item screening for cancer-related fatigue. *J Pain Symptom Manage* **22**(5):931–937, 2001.
52. Portenoy RK, Thaler HT, Kornblith AB, et al. The Memorial Symptom Assessment Scale: an instrument for the evaluation of symptom prevalence, characteristics and distress. *Eur J Cancer* **30A**(9):1326–1336, 1994.
53. Yellen SB, Cella DF, Webster K, Blendowski C, Kaplan E. Measuring fatigue and other anemia-related symptoms with the Functional Assessment of Cancer Therapy (FACT) measurement system. *J Pain Symptom Manage* **13**(2):63–74, 1997.
54. Aaronson NK, Ahmedzai S, Bergman B, et al. The European Organization for Research and Treatment of Cancer QLQ-C30: a quality-of-life instrument for use in international clinical trials in oncology. *J Natl Cancer Inst* **85**(5):365–376, 1993.
55. Lai JS, Crane PK, Cella D. Factor analysis techniques for assessing sufficient unidimensionality of cancer related fatigue. *Qual Life Res* **15**(7):1179–1190, 2006.
56. Basch E, Iasonos A, McDonough T, et al. Patient versus clinician symptom reporting using the National Cancer Institute Common Terminology Criteria for Adverse Events: results of a questionnaire-based study. *Lancet Oncol* **7**(11): 903–909, 2006.
57. Krupp LB, LaRocca NG, Muir-Nash J, Steinberg AD. The fatigue severity scale. Application to patients with multiple sclerosis and systemic lupus erythematosus. *Arch Neurol* **46**(10):1121–1123, 1989.
58. Smets EMA, Garssen B, Bonke B, De Haes JCJM. The Multidimensional Fatigue Inventory (MFI): psychometric qualities of an instrument to assess fatigue. *J Psychosom Res* **39**(3):315–325, 1995.
59. Serlin RC, Mendoza TR, Nakamura Y, Edwards KR, Cleeland CS. When is cancer pain mild, moderate or severe? Grading pain severity by its interference with function. *Pain* **61**(2):277–284, 1995.
60. Cleeland CS, Ryan KM. Pain assessment: global use of the Brief Pain Inventory. *Ann Acad Med Singapore* **23**(2):129–138, 1994.
61. Cleeland CS, Gonin R, Hatfield AK, et al. Pain and its treatment in outpatients with metastatic cancer. *N Engl J Med* **330**(9):592–596, 1994.
62. Visser MR, Smets EM, Sprangers MA, de Haes HJ. How response shift may affect the measurement of change in fatigue. *J Pain Symptom Manage* **20**(1):12–18, 2000.
63. Schwartz CE, Bode R, Repucci N, Becker J, Sprangers MA, Fayers PM. The clinical significance of adaptation to changing health: a meta-analysis of response shift. *Qual Life Res* **15**(9):1533–1550, 2006.
64. Cleeland CS. Symptom burden: multiple symptoms and their impact as patient-reported outcomes. *J Natl Cancer Inst Monogr* **37**:16–21, 2007.
65. Morrow GR, Hickok JT, Roscoe JA, et al. Differential effects of paroxetine on fatigue and depression: a randomized, double-blind trial from the University of Rochester Cancer Center Community Clinical Oncology Program. *J Clin Oncol* **21**(24):4635–4641, 2003.
66. Minton O, Richardson A, Sharpe M, Hotopf M, Stone P. A systematic review and meta-analysis of the pharmacological treatment of cancer-related fatigue. *J Natl Cancer Inst* **100**(16):1155–1166, 2008.
67. Fava M, Thase ME, DeBattista C. A multicenter, placebo-controlled study of modafinil augmentation in partial responders to selective serotonin reuptake inhibitors with persistent fatigue and sleepiness. *J Clin Psychiatry* **66**(1):85–93, 2005.
68. Morrow GR, Jean-Peirre P, Roscoe JA, et al. A phase III randomized, placebo-controlled, double-blind trial of a eugeroic agent in 642 cancer patients reporting fatigue during chemotherapy: A URCC CCOP Study [abstract]. American Society of Clinical Oncology 44th Annual Meeting, Chicago IL, May 30–June 3, 2008. *J Clin Oncol* **26**(15 Suppl), 2008. Abstract 9512.
69. Moss EL, Simpson JS, Pelletier G, Forsyth P. An open-label study of the effects of bupropion SR on fatigue, depression and quality of life of mixed-site cancer patients and their partners. *Psychooncology* **15**(3):259–267, 2006.
70. Schmitz KH, Holtzman J, Courneya KS, Mâsse LC, Duval S, Kane R. Controlled physical activity trials in cancer survivors: a systematic review and meta-analysis. *Cancer Epidemiol Biomarkers Prev* **14**(7):1588–1595, 2005.
71. Mustian KM, Morrow GR, Carroll JK, Figueroa-Moseley CD, Jean-Pierre P, Williams GC. Integrative nonpharmacologic behavioral interventions for the management of cancer-related fatigue. *Oncologist* **12**(Suppl 1):52–67, 2007.
72. Markes M, Brockow T, Resch KL. Exercise for women receiving adjuvant therapy for breast cancer. *Cochrane Database Syst Rev***4**:CD005001, 2006.
73. Jacobsen PB, Donovan KA, Vadaparampil ST, Small BJ. Systematic review and meta-analysis of psychological and activity-based interventions for

cancer-related fatigue. *Health Psychol* **26**(6):660–667, 2007.

74. Luebbert K, Dahme B, Hasenbring M. The effectiveness of relaxation training in reducing treatment-related symptoms and improving emotional adjustment in acute non-surgical cancer treatment: a meta-analytical review. *Psychooncology* **10**(6):490–502, 2001.

75. Moher D, Jones A, Lepage L. Use of the CONSORT statement and quality of reports of randomized trials: a comparative before-and-after evaluation. *JAMA* **285**(15):1992–1995, 2001.

76. Moher D, Schulz KF, Altman D. The CONSORT statement: revised recommendations for improving the quality of reports of parallel-group randomized trials. *JAMA* **285**(15):1987–1991, 2001.

77. Bentler SE, Hartz AJ, Kuhn EM. Prospective observational study of treatments for unexplained chronic fatigue. *J Clin Psychiatry* **66**(5):625–632, 2005.

78. Elam JL, Carpenter JS, Shu XO, Boyapati S, Friedmann-Gilchrist J. Methodological issues in the investigation of ginseng as an intervention for fatigue. *Clin Nurse Spec* **20**(4):183–189, 2006.

79. Ginseng may relieve cancer treatment fatigue. *Mayo Clin Health Lett* **25**(12):4, 2007.

80. Barton DL, Soori GS, Bauer B, et al. A pilot, multi-dose, placebo-controlled evaluation of American ginseng (*Panax quinquefolius*) to improve cancer-related fatigue: NCCTG trial N03CA. [abstract]. American Society of Clinical Oncology 43rd Annual Meeting, Chicago IL, June 1–5, 2007. *J Clin Oncol* **25**(18 Suppl), 2007. Abstract 9001.

81. Patrick DL, Ferketich SL, Frame PS, et al. National Institutes of Health State-of-the-Science Conference statement: symptom management in cancer: pain, depression, and fatigue, July 15–17, 2002. *J Natl Cancer Inst* **95**(15):1110–1117, 2003.

Section 2 Chapter 11

Cancer Symptom Mechanisms and Models: Clinical and Basic Science

Developing translational animal models of cancer-related fatigue

Mary W. Meagher

Behavioral symptoms, including fatigue, depression, sleep disturbance, and cognitive alterations, are prevalent among patients with cancer[1–4] and may be induced by both cancer and its treatment. Fatigue is the most prevalent and distressing of these behavioral symptoms.[3,5] Cancer-related fatigue (CRF) and associated behavioral disturbances cause profound functional impairments that can persist for years after treatment ends. Nevertheless, the pathogenic mechanisms that mediate CRF remain poorly understood, and current therapies are only partially effective in reducing symptom burden. Progress has been seriously hindered by the lack of appropriate animal models.

Recent evidence suggests that CRF may be conceptualized as a "sickness behavior" that is mediated in part by the central effects of inflammatory cytokines.[4,6–10] Sickness behaviors reflect the activity of a central perceptual-affective-motivational system that reorganizes behavior to promote survival.[11–13] However, under conditions of chronic activation these inflammatory signals are maladaptive and may contribute to the development of persistent fatigue and associated behavioral disturbances in patients with cancer.[1] The constructs of fatigue and sickness contain multiple psychological components that appear to be mediated by distinct molecular, cellular, and neural systems. Advancing our understanding of the neural basis of CRF will require the development of translational measures that parse fatigue and sickness into their specific psychological components using well-validated animal models. Although other biological mechanisms are likely to contribute to the development of CRF (see Chapter 10), the cytokine hypothesis will be used to illustrate how animal models can help researchers evaluate potential mechanisms.

This chapter will consider how animal models can contribute to translational research on CRF, beginning with a review of the traditional criteria used to evaluate the validity of animal models. The conceptual basis and process of developing animal models of fatigue induced by cancer and its treatment are discussed, with particular attention given to the importance of developing translational measures of specific dimensions of CRF that can be objectively assessed in both cancer patients and animal models. Recent animal research investigating the mechanisms mediating the behavioral effects of cancer and its treatment is highlighted, followed by a presentation of a translational framework for investigating the psychological components of fatigue and associated sickness behaviors.

Animal models and traditional validation criteria

Animal models are experimental preparations designed to emulate specific features of a human condition, including the symptoms induced by cancer and its treatment. A fundamental assumption is made regarding cross-species homology, which allows for the extension of behavioral and biological findings in animals to humans. Thus, an ideal animal model should be similar to the human condition in terms of etiology, biology, symptomatology, and treatment. Animal models provide a more efficient and ethical approach for preclinical studies of the biological substrates of symptoms, such as fatigue. The advantages of animal models include easily studied behaviors and biological substrates, readily controlled environments, and the availability of transgenic techniques. Animal models can be used to increase our understanding of the etiology and mechanisms mediating cancer symptoms and to facilitate the development of treatments designed to prevent or reverse these symptoms. The following paragraphs review the traditional criteria that are typically used to evaluate the validity of animal models.[14–16]

Animal models involve both independent and dependent variables. The induction of cancer and the administration of cancer treatments are the primary

Cancer Symptom Science: Measurement, Mechanisms, and Management, eds. Charles S. Cleeland, Michael J. Fisch, and Adrian J. Dunn. Published by Cambridge University Press.

independent variables, whereas the behavioral and biological measures of cancer-related fatigue are the dependent variables. It is necessary to establish the reliability, or reproducibility, of these variables. This requires the ability to precisely manipulate the independent variables to reproduce the same level of biobehavioral disturbance within and across laboratories. Although reliability is necessary, it is not sufficient for validating a model. The criteria used to validate the model will depend on its purported purpose – for example, elucidating the underlying mechanisms of CRF, facilitating the development of effective treatments, and fostering translation research – and include face, etiological, predictive, pharmacological, and construct validity.

"Face validity" refers to the similarity between a particular behavioral change observed in the animal model and the parallel symptom in the human condition.[16] For example, animals undergoing chemotherapy treatment would be expected to exhibit less spontaneous locomotor activity because cancer patients undergoing chemotherapy report reduced activity during treatment. Although face validity can provide a useful starting point for identifying analogous behaviors that may be mediated by similar neural substrates, it is essential to move beyond it to fully validate the model.

"Etiological validity" refers to the similarity of the inducing conditions between the animal model and human condition. The selection of the inducing conditions involves a hypothesis about the etiology of the human condition that may or may not be correct. For example, a researcher may decide to study the effects of chemotherapy on sickness behavior in animals without cancer. The decision to use healthy animals necessarily assumes the hypothesis that chemotherapy alone causes the behavior disturbance. However, it is possible that chemotherapy affects behavior differentially in healthy versus diseased animals. Although investigating chemotherapy-induced fatigue in an otherwise healthy animal provides an efficient strategy that will yield useful information, it would not be expected to approximate the combined disease and treatment factors that lead to fatigue in patients with cancer. Moreover, cancer treatment typically involves the administration of multiple chemotherapy agents that are often combined with irradiation. Thus, to more fully address the issue of etiological validity, it is important to study the fatigue induced by cancer alone and in combination with the standard treatment regimen for that form of cancer.

A two-pronged approach is recommended to efficiently develop etiologically valid and predictive models. Initial studies should characterize the effects of therapeutically relevant cancer treatments in healthy animals to identify dosing regimens that induce fatigue-like behaviors and to establish the construct validity (see below) of the dependent measures. Ideally, the same route of administration and number of treatment cycles used when treating patients should be used to model treatment conditions in animals. Because the effects of treatment are often lagged, it will be important to longitudinally assess both the short-term and long-term effects of cancer and its treatment.[17,18] The etiological validity of the data derived from these treatment-related fatigue models can be further tested in relevant cancer models. Although discussion of rodent models of cancer[19–21] is beyond the scope of this review, care should be taken to select a model that allows temporal control over tumor emergence to enable large cohorts of mice to be tested in behavioral tasks simultaneously, thereby minimizing experimental variance. Moreover, selecting immunocompetent cancer models (eg, spontaneous, syngeneic, or chemically induced) over immunodeficient xenograft models will enable investigation of the role of inflammatory mediators in the development of cancer-related fatigue.

Studying the combined effects of cancer and its treatment in animals may better approximate the pathogenesis of fatigue in patients with cancer; however, clinical studies suggest that these factors alone do not fully explain individual differences in the severity and duration of cancer symptoms.[3,7] Therefore, a multifactorial approach is needed to examine how cancer and treatment interact with genetic, developmental, and environmental vulnerability factors, such as cytokine gene polymorphisms, age, obesity, chronic medical conditions, and environmental stressors. For example, studies in patients with breast cancer suggest that chronic inflammation and associated symptoms of fatigue during treatment are linked to gene polymorphisms of the cytokines interleukin (IL)-1β, IL-6, and IL-6 receptor (*IL1B*, *IL6*, and *IL6R*, respectively). To experimentally investigate the role of particular cytokines in CRF in genetically modified mice, the production of a specific cytokine can be suppressed by the targeted deletion of its gene. For instance, if IL-6 knockout mice exposed to chemotherapy show reduced fatigue-like behaviors compared with controls, this would provide strong evidence that IL-6 is necessary to the induction of CRF. Identifying the genetic factors that determine individual vulnerability to CRF will allow for the identification of genomic markers for risk and the development of novel immunomodulatory treatments to prevent CRF in these individuals.

"Pharmacological validity" refers to the sensitivity of the animal model to drugs with demonstrated therapeutic efficacy in humans.[15,22] For example, clinical studies suggest that stimulant drugs such as modafinil and methylphenidate reduce fatigue in patients with cancer.[23–25] Other evidence suggests that antidepressants may be pharmacologically active in reducing associated fatigue-like behaviors[26,27] and proinflammatory cytokine activity.[28,29] Thus, demonstrating that stimulants and antidepressants are effective in reducing specific fatigue-like behaviors in animals would support the pharmacological validity of the model.

"Predictive validity" refers to the degree to which the biobehavioral test can predict a criterion of interest measured some time in the future. At the most general level, an animal model of CRF is useful to the extent to which it predicts criteria relevant to fatigue in patients with cancer. For example, does the animal model identify underlying neurobiological mechanisms associated with fatigue in patients with cancer? Similarly, does pharmacological data obtained from the animal model predict the efficacy of new or current agents in patients with cancer? Translational neuroimaging techniques can provide critical cross-validation data to determine the clinical relevance of neural mechanisms implicated in animal models, as well as the efficacy of new agents in altering neural correlates of chemotherapy-induced fatigue. However, to make accurate predictions from animal models to patients with cancer, equal attention must be given to establishing the construct validity (see below) of the particular behavioral tests that are used to assess specific dimensions of CRF. This is essential to ensure that the beneficial effects of potential treatments identified in animal models will result in similar improvements in patients with cancer.

"Construct validity" refers to whether the animal model measures the theoretical and behavioral variables that are considered central to human condition.[16,30] Establishing the construct validity of an animal model is essential because it is the overarching concept that subsumes all other forms of validity. Moreover, evaluating the construct validity of an animal model is essential when less is known about the etiology of a clinical condition and when current drugs have limited therapeutic efficacy for a particular condition. The goal of construct validation is to link the theoretical and conceptual domain to observable variables that can be operationalized. In this case a multifactorial approach is used, wherein multiple behavioral and biological dependent measures provide evidence of convergent and discriminant validity to facilitate progress.[31]

"Convergent validity" refers to the degree to which theoretically related concepts are interrelated.

"Discriminant validity" refers to the degree to which theoretically unrelated concepts are, in fact, not interrelated. To establish that an animal model has construct validity, it is essential to demonstrate both convergence and discrimination. However, this can only be accomplished when emphasis is placed on comparing specific dimensions of fatigue that characterize more than one clinical disorder (eg, inflammation-related sickness, multiple sclerosis, Parkinson's disease, chronic fatigue syndrome).

One could argue that the construct validity of an animal model of chemotherapy-induced fatigue is supported when an array of strong and clear-cut behaviors that are induced by the chemotherapy agent are homologous to the symptoms observed in cancer patients. Although the similarity of the behavior changes alone suggests that the model has strong face validity, a number of other theoretically important issues must be addressed regarding chemotherapy as an inducing condition in models of cancer symptoms. First, biological factors thought to contribute to the etiology of fatigue in patients with cancer should be evaluated to determine whether there is homology between the inducing physiological conditions. For example, clinical studies indicate that chemotherapy-induced fatigue is correlated with increases in circulating inflammatory cytokine levels.[6,9,32] Second, to provide evidence of the construct validity of an animal model, one could investigate whether there is a dose-dependent relationship between the emergence of chemotherapy-induced fatigue behaviors and inflammatory cytokine expression. Third, to further determine whether inflammatory cytokine expression mediates chemotherapy-induced fatigue, one could examine whether fatigue-like behavior is attenuated after administration of selective cytokine antagonist drugs.

As noted above, the etiology of cancer symptom burden is complex and presumably involves the interaction of genetic, developmental, biological, and environmental factors, as well as prior health status and stage of disease. In this regard, it is unlikely that administration of chemotherapy alone in healthy mice will model CRF in its entirety. Even so, this more circumscribed approach is an important first step that is likely to yield useful information regarding the mechanisms of chemotherapy-induced fatigue-like behavior that can be further investigated in cancer-bearing animals.

Moving beyond traditional validation criteria

In addition to considering the traditional criteria used to validate animal models, it is important to consider the scope and conceptual basis of the model.[16,33] With respect to scope, one approach is to develop an animal model that mimics every symptom of fatigue induced by a specific cancer and its treatment. The validity of the model would then be determined by its ability to induce a wide range of behavioral disturbances that are homologous to the range of symptoms reported by patients with cancer. This approach is limited because it depends largely on face validity, which is particularly problematic for modeling CRF symptoms in patients that are subjectively defined and assessed using self-report measures. Moreover, there is little agreement on how to define and measure CRF in clinical settings. Although provisional criteria for a clinical syndrome have been proposed,[3] the specific criteria used may change and new subcategories may emerge with additional research (Table 11.1). Given these limitations, animal researchers have moved away from the concept of modeling every feature of the human condition.[33]

An alternative approach is to focus the animal model on a few observable behavioral symptoms that have been identified in patients with cancer and that can be linked to psychological constructs typically assessed through self-report. The development of homologous measures in animals and humans that tap into the same underlying neural mechanisms is more likely to yield cross-species validity and translation. Because fewer endpoints are assessed, this strategy is more efficient for experimental investigations of the underlying neurobiological mechanisms mediating the behavioral symptoms. Although the development of homologous behavioral measures of CRF in animal and patient experimental studies (eg, functional magnetic resonance imaging, or fMRI) will

Table 11.1. *International Statistical Classification of Diseases and Related Health Problems*, 10th Revision (ICD-10) draft criteria for cancer-related fatigue (CRF)

Patient reports significant fatigue that results in clinically significant distress and/or impairment in social, occupational, or other important areas of functioning. These symptoms are attributed to cancer or its treatment rather than to a psychological disorder. Fatigue (item 1) must be present nearly every day during a two-week period along with six or more of the following symptoms:
(1) Significant fatigue, reduced energy, or greater need for rest, disproportionate to recent activity level
(2) Decreased motivation or interest to engage in usual activities
(3) Difficulty completing daily tasks
(4) Struggle to overcome inactivity
(5) Excessive malaise lasting several hours after exertion
(6) Generalized weakness or limb heaviness
(7) Decreased concentration or attention
(8) Insomnia or hypersomnia
(9) Unrefreshing or nonrestorative sleep

Adapted from Cella et al.[3]

foster translation, it may not be practical to include these measures as endpoints in clinical trials. Nevertheless, clinical trials can enhance translation by including behaviorally anchored self-report measures that assess the same underlying constructs measured in experimental studies of animals and humans.

The development of animal experimental tests of CRF will require modeling the underlying psychological constructs that are affected by cancer and its treatment. The measurement of these psychological processes requires operational definitions of the specific behaviors linked to each hypothetical construct. Ideally, this approach involves robust translational measures with construct validity across the animal model and patient cancer syndrome.[33] For example, studies in cancer patients could be used to develop behaviorally anchored operational definitions of the underlying psychological constructs and to establish the constructs' relevance to the cancer syndrome. An important first step would be to translate the largely subjective language contained in the *International Statistical Classification of Diseases and Related Health Problems*, 10th Revision (ICD-10) draft criteria for CRF into core observable behaviors that can be objectively measured in patients and animal models (Table 11.2). In turn, animal studies of homologous psychological constructs and behaviors could be used to evaluate the similarity to the human cancer syndrome. This approach explicitly acknowledges that the modeling process is central to the experimental study of cancer symptoms in both patients and experimental animals. One advantage of this strategy is that validation studies of the psychological constructs and homology can be conducted in healthy humans and animals, as well as in experimental studies of cancer patients and cancer-bearing animals. Another advantage is that it builds upon well-characterized theoretical constructs in the fields of psychology and neuroscience.

Assessing genetic differences in susceptibility to CRF will require the measurement of endophenotypes.[57] Endophenotypes are behavioral and biological markers reflecting genetic factors that predispose an individual to a disorder. They are intermediate phenotypes between genotype and phenotype that provide a marker of genetic risk that can facilitate the identification of susceptibility genes that are evident prior to overt pathology. For example, deficits in sensory gating revealed by impaired pre-pulse inhibition of startle are evident in individuals with schizophrenia

Table 11.2. Translation of ICD-10 draft criteria for cancer-related fatigue into objective behavioral and physiological measures

Core ICD-10 CRF subjective criteria	Translational objective measures
Fatigue, reduced energy, and reduced activity disproportionate with recent activity and exertion	Reduced locomotor activity using a photobeam activity system[34]
	Reduced spontaneous activity using a running wheel[35]
	Delayed recovery of spontaneous and motivated behavior after forced exercise or swim stress[36,37]
Decreased motivation or interest in usual activities	Loss of sucrose preference[38]
	Altered taste reactivity[39]
	Decreased social behavior[40,41]
	Decreased sexual behavior[42]
	Decreased break point on the progressive ratio test[43]
	Reduced lever pressing for preferred food on the concurrent lever press/free chow feeding procedure[44]
Difficulty completing daily tasks and overcoming inactivity	Reduced nest building[45]
	Reduced burrowing behavior[46]
	Increased brain activation using awake magnetic resonance imaging in rats after an effortful task or forced activity[47]
Generalized weakness or limb heaviness	Wire hang[48]
	Forelimb grip strength using a strain gauge[49]
Insomnia or hypersomnia, unrefreshing or nonrestorative sleep	Circadian alterations in sleep/activity/temperature/endocrine cycles[50]
	Electroencephalographic analysis of sleep architecture[51]
Heightened emotional reactivity (eg, sadness, frustration, or irritability)	Heightened acoustic startle and conditioned potentiation startle[52]
	Heightened contextual fear conditioning[53]
	Increased immobility on the forced-swim test[38]
	Elevated plus-maze test for anxiety-like behaviors[48]
Cognitive dysfunction	Novel object recognition task[53]
	Morris water maze task/medial temporal lobe dependent[54]
	Delayed-nonmatching-to-sample task/frontal-executive dependent[54]
	Set-shifting and reversal learning tasks[55]
	Interval timing with gaps and distracters[56]

as well as unaffected relatives.[58] An example applicable to CRF is provided by a model of depression in which mice were selectively bred for extremes in stress reactivity to study clinically relevant endophenotypes – namely, disturbances in the rhythmicity of locomotor behavior, diurnal corticosterone rhythms, and sleep.[59] Because sleep disorders are associated with fatigue in patients with cancer,[4,60–62] these mice may be useful for investigating whether vulnerability to disturbances in sleep–activity cycles and diurnal rhythms may provide useful translational measures.[63]

Translational measures of CRF are needed to bridge the gap between animal and human research and to facilitate bidirectional flow of information. To accomplish this goal, objective measures should be designed to assess homologous psychological and biological CRF constructs in both experimental animals and humans. One strategy is to design animal measures that are more human-like by using tests that are analogous to the clinical criteria. For example, the draft ICD-10 criteria for CRF could be used to select or design relevant animal behavioral tests (Table 11.2). An alternative strategy is to design human tests that are more animal-like. Thus, rather than using self-report measures of fatigue to assess decreases in activity and sleep disturbance, automated measures of activity/rest cycles commonly used in rodents could be used to assess fatigue in humans.

For example, actigraphy can be used to objectively measure fatigue-related alterations in activity/rest cycles. Actigraphy provides a noninvasive method for continuous monitoring of human activity/rest cycles using a wrist-worn accelerometer along with ecological momentary assessment of self-reported fatigue.[64,65] For more detailed laboratory analyses of motor activity, Young et al.[66] have developed a human activity monitoring system that is analogous to rodent motor activity monitoring systems. Similar to rodent measures, human motor and exploratory activity is monitored in a small novel room. This method is more sensitive and allows for multivariate assessment of locomotor activity in humans, which may be used to elucidate underlying neural substrates.[66] Using this reverse-translational approach, other measures of sickness behavior in animals can be adapted to assess fatigue-like behaviors in patients with cancer. Although the language used to describe human symptoms tends to be more subjective than the concrete operational definitions used to describe sickness behaviors in animals, a common language can be developed by focusing on the underlying psychological components of sickness behavior.

Parsing the psychological components of cancer-related fatigue

What are the psychological components of cancer-related fatigue and associated sickness behaviors? Cancer and its treatment can influence behavior by altering emotional, motivational, and effort-related processes. It can also influence behavior by altering one of many forms of learning and memory, including explicit and implicit knowledge produced by associative conditioning and cognitive processes. In addition, it can alter behavior by dysregulating circadian rhythms related to sleep/wake cycles. These psychological components provide foundational constructs that can be used to systematically characterize the behavioral syndrome induced by cancer and its treatment in both cancer patients and animal models.

To effectively study the psychological components of sickness across human and animal models, it is important to recognize that the perceptual, emotional, motivational, learning/memory, and circadian components can exist objectively apart from conscious awareness of them. For example, emotions, motives, and knowledge can be either explicit or implicit. Why is it important to examine implicit components of fatigue-related sickness? One reason is that fatigued cancer patients may respond to internal and external stimuli without explicit awareness of either the stimuli or the basis of their reactions. At times they may not have conscious access to what is guiding their behavior. For example, evidence suggests that the amygdala plays a critical role in both conditioned and unconditioned implicit emotional processes that are independent of conscious awareness, whereas the medial temporal lobe memory system is necessary for explicit processes.[67–70] Thus, self-report measures that assume awareness are likely to provide an incomplete characterization of cancer-related sickness behaviors.

A second reason is that measures of implicit components of sickness may lead to the development of translational measures of CRF. As noted above, the methods used to assess CRF in humans are based almost entirely on self-report and in some cases the constructs assessed may not map directly onto the behavioral measures that are likely to involve both implicit and explicit processes. A third advantage of dissociating implicit from explicit processes is that the core neural and psychological processes that mediate fatigue might be more amenable to objective measurement in experiments where brain systems are manipulated.

The construct of CRF contains multiple components that are likely to be mediated by distinct molecular, cellular, and neural systems. Advances in understanding the neural basis of cancer-related behavioral disturbances will require the development of translational measures that parse fatigue and associated behavioral disturbances into its specific psychological components. Cancer and its treatment may induce neuroimmune and neurodegenerative changes that affect any or all of these psychological processes, and a change in just one component may be sufficient to change behavior. To develop selective treatments designed to prevent or reverse fatigue, we need to understand the underlying neurobiological mechanisms. However, the role of specific molecular, cellular, or neural systems in the pathogenesis of CRF cannot be understood without precisely linking the changes to higher-level changes in these psychological processes.

The similarities between CRF and cytokine-induced sickness behavior are remarkable.[1,71] Both conditions induce reductions in motivated behavior, behavioral activation, effort-related processes, and social behavior, as well as disturbances in mood, sleep, and cognition. A growing body of evidence has established a link between cytokines and fatigue. For example, fatigue develops in humans treated for viral infections and cancer with interferon-α.[72,73] Consistent with these findings, fatigue is prevalent in medical conditions that induce chronic inflammation, such as cancer, multiple sclerosis, rheumatoid arthritis, and heart disease.[7,74–76] However, it is important to recognize that sickness behavior is a short-term adaptive response to immune challenge that resolves once the pathogen is cleared. In contrast, the behavioral disturbance induced by cancer and its treatment represents a maladaptive response, which appears to be mediated in part by an imbalance between proinflammatory and anti-inflammatory mechanisms resulting in chronic activation of the innate immune response and inflammation.[77]

Although most early animal studies of chemotherapy agents focused on nausea, vomiting, and conditioned taste aversions, with the development of more effective antinausea drugs attention is now focused on fatigue. To model the reduction in activity associated with fatigue, animal researchers have assessed the effects of chemotherapy on spontaneous locomotor activity and running-wheel activity. For example, Malik et al.[34] have shown that cisplatin (6 mg/kg administered intraperitoneally) reduced spontaneous nocturnal activity in rats at 24 hours and that this effect lasted for up to eight days. Interestingly, two drugs that were effective in altering indices of nausea and vomiting had no effect on the cisplatin-induced reduction in locomotor activity, suggesting that the effects on locomotor activity were not secondary to nausea.[78] However, dexamethasone administration was effective in ameliorating both nausea and reduced activity. The latter finding suggests that dexamethasone may have its effects by targeting a common inflammatory mechanism that contributes to both sickness behaviors. Wood et al.,[35] investigating the chemotherapy agent etoposide (VP-16), observed increased sickness behaviors in mice and increased IL-6 production by macrophages. VP-16 decreased food intake, body weight, voluntary running-wheel activity, and hemoglobin levels, while increasing p38 mitogen-activated protein kinase (MAPK)-dependent IL-6 production. Using model cell systems, p38 MAPK inhibition blocked chemotherapy-induced inflammatory cytokine production without decreasing drug-induced cytotoxicity.[79] Although *in vivo* studies are needed to confirm this finding, these results suggest that inhibition of inflammatory cytokine production does not reduce the therapeutic efficacy of chemotherapy drugs.

Recent research suggests that cancer alone causes an increase in inflammatory cytokine expression and depressive-like behavior in rats.[38] Mammary tumor-bearing rats exhibited increased floating time and number of floating bouts in the Porsolt forced-swim test, a reduction in sucrose preference, and increased marble burying. However, they showed normal plus-maze and open-field activity, social interaction, food intake, body weight, and body temperature. These results suggest that tumors alone induce depressive-like behaviors, but only mild sickness behaviors relative to those observed in mice administered lipopolysaccharide (LPS). In the periphery, mammary tumor tissue expression of IL-1ß was increased along with plasma IL-1ß and IL-10. In the CNS, tumors increased cytokine expression for IL-1ß, IL-6, TNF-α, and IL-10 in the hippocampus but not in the hypothalamus. Consistent with the lower levels of sickness behaviors, cytokine levels were much lower than those observed after LPS challenge. Tumor-bearing rats also showed blunted corticosterone responses to stress, suggesting that stress might amplify the adverse effects of tumor-induced cytokines on depressive-like behaviors. Other work from this group suggests that social isolation stress increases the mammary gland gene expression and tumor burden.[80–82]

Framework for investigating the psychological components of CRF

This section provides an overview of the psychological components and behavioral tests that may be used to characterize animal models of CRF. Similar to other latent constructs that are subjectively defined (eg, pain, nausea), the construct of fatigue can be indirectly assessed in animals via converging behavioral measures that are used as proxies of the construct. In accordance with ICD-10 draft criteria, the components discussed below focus on measures of fatigue-like behavior and associated changes in emotion, motivation, effort, learning/memory, and sleep/wake cycles.

Fatigue-like behavior

Several investigators have used behavioral measures of spontaneous and forced activity to assess fatigue in animals. One approach is to compare obligatory home-cage activities that are essential for survival, such as eating and drinking, to spontaneous behaviors that are not essential, such as running-wheel activity[35,63] or burrowing.[46,83] Manipulations that induce mild sickness can selectively suppress nonessential spontaneous behaviors without altering general activity.[46,63]

To assess whether fatigue is disproportionate to recent physical activity, behavioral recovery can be assessed after forced exercise.[36,84–86] For example, subsequent to an immune challenge, recovery of spontaneous running-wheel activity has been assessed after forced activity on a motorized treadmill.[36] Mice are acclimated to the running wheels prior to the treadmill session to obtain a stable baseline. During the 20-minute treadmill session, the speed and grade of the treadmill are gradually increased to 22 m/min at a grade of −14% (downhill) or +14% (uphill). The mice run for 150 minutes, motivated by occasional gentle prodding. An advantage of this model is that it allows comparison of the effects of uphill running, which requires more energy but produces little muscle damage and inflammation, with downhill running, which induces significant muscle damage, inflammation, and delayed-onset soreness. Fatigue is defined as a decrease in spontaneous running-wheel activity over the next seven days. In addition, mice can be tested again on the treadmill at 36 m/min and 8% grade either 48 or 72 hours after their initial uphill/downhill run. In this case, fatigue is defined as the time when mice stop running despite gentle prodding for one minute.

Other studies have examined fatigue-like behavior after a forced-swim stress.[37,84,87] After immune challenge, mice are forced to swim individually in a glass jar containing room-temperature water for 10-minute sessions administered weekly.[37] After an initial period of activity the mice become immobile during the swim test. Fatigue is defined as an increased period of immobility during the swim test, as well as delayed recovery of grooming and rearing behavior and hyperalgesia on the tail immersion test after the swim stressor.

Emotional and motivational processes

Cancer and its treatment can alter behavior by disrupting affective (emotional) or motivation processes. Neurobiological studies of sickness and reward behaviors have identified components of emotional and motivational processes mediated by distinct neural circuits.

Affect

Is the effect of the cancer treatment on behavior due to a change in emotional and hedonic responses? If so, which form of affect? For example, healthy mice normally exhibit a sucrose preference when they are given a choice between 2% sucrose water and regular tap water, whereas sick mice lose their preference for the sweeter solution.[88] Similarly, chemotherapy may decrease sucrose preference and it may do so by altering affect or motivation.

Hedonic "liking" and "disliking" reactions include affective facial expressions elicited by the hedonic impact of tastes. One of the best methods to assess hedonic activity is the taste reactivity test developed by Grill and Norgren[39] and later used by Berridge et al.[67,89,90] These authors' research indicates that sucrose elicits positive facial expressions (liking) such as tongue protrusions, whereas bitter quinine elicits negative facial expressions (disliking) such as gaping and chin rubbing. These affective expressions are homologous in humans and rodents, suggesting that the same neural circuits may be involved. Thus, studies of chemotherapy-induced changes in hedonic liking/disliking in rodents may provide insights into the hedonic circuits involved in humans. Conversely, studies of facial electromyography and neuroimaging studies could evaluate whether cancer treatment has a similar hedonic impact in patients with cancer. Previous research indicates that a distributed neural circuit involved in liking includes opioid neural transmission onto γ-aminobutyric acid (GABA)ergic neurons in the nucleus accumbens along with mesolimbic outputs to the ventral pallidum and associated structures. However, dopamine neural transmission is not involved in generating liking, but rather is implicated in incentive motivation or "wanting" (instrumental performance and consumption of rewards). Thus, it is possible that cancer and its treatment may alter liking and conditioned taste aversion through this distinct neural system without necessarily altering motivation and dopamine neural transmission, or vice versa.

Motivation

Alternatively, cancer and its treatment may alter behavior due to a change in motivation. Despite the popular view that sickness behavior reflects the physical debilitation and weakness caused by disease, evidence suggests that it reflects a highly organized motivational state. Motivations are central states that organize perception and behavior toward a goal. When an individual is sick, behavior is reorganized to facilitate recuperation from disease to enhance survival. Neal Miller was the first to show that sickness behavior is a motivational state that reorganizes other behavioral priorities.[91,92] He showed that in some circumstances behavior is suppressed during sickness, but under other circumstances behavior can be increased. For example, rats injected with endotoxin show a decrease in effortful lever pressing to receive a water reward, even though they continue to drink when given free access to a cup of water in the test chamber. This suggests that the sick rats were no longer motivated to work for water, but they were still thirsty. The same general pattern of results was obtained using either food reward or rewarding brain stimulation. In contrast, when rats were subjected to forced exercise on a rotating wheel that could be stopped temporarily by lever pressing, the endotoxin-treated rats showed an increase in lever pressing. This indicates that the sick rats were motivated to work for periods of rest. Thus, sickness can flexibly increase or decrease behavior depending on the consequences of the response. We propose that this motivational account may be useful in conceptualizing CRF and in developing translational behavioral tasks.

Several behavioral tasks that have been used to assess the motivational component of sickness may also be used to assess the motivational dimension of CRF. For example, the progressive-ratio test provides a measure of incentive motivation. The progressive-ratio test was originally developed to examine the reinforcing effects of sweetened milk in rats.[93] The schedule begins with one response requirement for the initial presentation of the reinforcer (the sweetened milk), after which the response requirement for each subsequent presentation of the reinforcer is increased. The primary outcome variable of the progressive-ratio test is the "break point," defined as the final ratio completed, which provides a measure of the maximum effort that an animal will expend to receive the reinforcer.[94] Thus, the progressive-ratio test provides a measure of the motivation to obtain the reward, rather than the amount of intake of a palatable substance. Importantly, the results can be used to determine whether differences in fatigue or differential satiation explain differences between groups. Thus, if cancer treatment induces satiation, treated mice would be expected to stop responding after a consistent number of rewards, independent of the response requirement. In contrast, if cancer treatment induces fatigue, treated subjects would stop responding after a fixed number of responses, independent of the response requirement.

Previous studies have demonstrated that the progressive-ratio test is sensitive to the motivational effects of IL-1ß in mice,[43,95] with IL-1ß causing a dose-dependent decrease in the break point. Importantly, Larson observed greater effects in mice maintained on *ad libitum* chow than in food-restricted mice. Although the anorexic and anhedonic effects of cytokines can be difficult to dissociate, Merali et al.[95] have shown that antidepressants can be used to discriminate these effects. Specifically, chronic pretreatment with fluoxetine selectively attenuated the anhedonic effects of IL-1ß on the progressive-ratio test without altering the anorexic effects on free chow consumption.[96] For example, if inflammation and its downstream effects contribute to CRF, the progressive-ratio test may provide a useful technique to measure changes in incentive motivation induced by cancer and its treatment.

There are several translational advantages to using the progressive-ratio test. First, progressive ratio methodologies have been used in a number of human laboratory studies evaluating the reinforcing effects of stimulants.[97] For example, D-amphetamine and methylphenidate maintain increased break points relative to placebo levels in humans.[98] Thus, parallel human laboratory studies could examine whether cancer therapies decrease break points in humans. Second, human laboratory studies using the progressive-ratio test have demonstrated predictive validity for clinical findings regarding drug abuse and dependence, suggesting that the test may have predictive validity for the motivational deficits induced by cancer therapies. Third, the progressive-ratio test provides a method for comparing the motivational effects of various cancer therapies because the test provides a single outcome (break point) that can be compared across drugs without relying on response rates.[99,100]

Changes in progressive-ratio break points are thought to reflect changes in effort-related decision making. The organism makes a cost/benefit analysis about whether to continue responding, based in part on the work-related response costs and the reinforcer's benefits. Therefore, one must be careful when interpreting the effects of a particular cancer treatment. A treatment may alter the progressive-ratio break point by altering several psychological processes, such as reward value or liking, the exertion of effort, or decision making processes. Thus, the progressive-ratio test should be conducted in conjunction with the sucrose preference and taste-reactivity test to determine whether the treatment was differentially altering liking, and in conjunction with other tests of effort-related choice behavior and cognition.

An experimental strategy to further analyze group differences on the progressive-ratio test has been developed by P. Balsam (personal communication, 2010). One possible explanation for group differences on this task is that extinction might occur sooner in animals receiving chemotherapy compared with controls. This hypothesis can be evaluated in a follow-up experiment by examining whether treated animals extinguish more rapidly than controls after training on a variable interval schedule of reinforcement (VI 20 seconds). Another possibility is that chemotherapy-treated animals might not tolerate delays in reward as well as control animals because the delay increases from one reinforcer to the next on the progressive-ratio schedule. This possibility can be evaluated by requiring the mouse to make a single response during a delay period that increases after each reward. In this case, the delay period would double after each reward until it exceeded the length of the delays experienced by the animal during the original progressive-ratio test.

To further evaluate the effects of cancer therapies on effort-related choice behavior, a modified version of the concurrent lever pressing/chow feeding procedure may be used.[44] In this test, the animal has the choice to work either for a preferred food (eg, condensed milk) by lever pressing on a fixed-ratio schedule, or to consume less-preferred lab chow that is concurrently available.[44] Under normal circumstances, animals will most often work to obtain the preferred food by lever pressing, rather than consume the nonpreferred chow. However, administration of low doses of dopamine antagonists or depletions of accumbens dopamine causes an abrupt shift in behavior that is characterized by reduced lever pressing for the preferred food accompanied by increased consumption of the nonpreferred chow.[44,101] It is expected that therapies that induce fatigue in patients with cancer will cause animals to reallocate their response choices based on response costs and to select low-effort response options for obtaining rewards.

Learning and memory

Is cancer-related fatigue due, in part, to a change in learning and memory? If so, which form of learning has been altered (eg, Pavlovian S-S or S-R associations, instrumental response outcome relationships, cognitive expectancics, or working memory)? Cancer treatment may induce fatigue by altering one or all of these forms of learning and memory, and a change in just one form of learning may lead to a change in fatigue-like behavior. Neuropsychological studies of patients with cancer have identified impairments in working memory tasks dependent on medial temporal lobe function and in executive functions dependent on frontal lobe function, but these are somewhat tentative conclusions because of a lack of adequate controls, small sample sizes, and other methodological limitations. To resolve these issues, behavioral tests developed in animals can be used to determine how different forms of learning and memory and associated brain circuits are adversely affected by cancer and its treatment.

Fear conditioning. Previous studies have shown that chemotherapy alters hippocampal-dependent memory assessed by the contextual fear conditioning task.[53,102] In this test, rats are placed in a chamber where they receive a foot shock. When they are re-exposed to the test context the next day, they show a conditioned fear response of "freezing." Mice treated with therapeutically relevant doses of 5-fluorouracil and methotrexate for several weeks prior to context conditioning show enhanced freezing when re-exposed to the context,[53] suggesting that therapeutic doses of chemotherapy enhance learning. In contrast, rats receiving high-dose methotrexate (250 mg/kg) after foot shock show decreased contextual fear conditioning compared with control rats when tested one month later, suggesting that high doses disrupt memory consolidation. Although contextual fear conditioning is altered by chemotherapy, there is reason to believe that treated mice may show normal amygdala-dependent learning assessed by the auditory-cued fear conditioning task. After LPS treatment, the mice still exhibit conditioned freezing in response to a tone that was previously paired with electric shocks, but impaired contextual fear conditioning.[103] While this paradigm can be used to test the effects of cancer therapies on both amygdala and hippocampal-dependent memory systems, other tasks are needed to fully characterize the impact on learning and memory.

Morris water maze. The Morris water maze task also has been used to assess the effects of cancer therapies on hippocampal-dependent memory.[54,102] In this task, the animal is placed into a large circular tank filled with water made opaque by the addition of white paint. An escape platform located within the tank is submerged just below the surface of the water. Because the animal cannot see the platform directly, it must learn and remember the location of the escape platform using spatial cues surrounding the tank. Performance on this task is hippocampal-dependent and is impaired by administration of chemotherapy agents and other toxins.

Executive function. Several behavioral tasks that tap into frontal-lobe function, including the delayed-nonmatching-to-sample, set-shifting, and reversal-learning tasks, can be used to assess executive function. These are tasks that assess cognitive flexibility and that are sensitive to frontal lobe lesions. For example, rats treated with therapeutically relevant doses of 5-fluorouracil and methotrexate for several weeks prior to testing show deficits on spatial and nonspatial versions of the delayed-nonmatching-to-sample test.[54] For mice, a delayed-nonmatching-to-sample T-maze task, conditional associative learning operant task, and set-shifting task can be used to assess prefrontal executive function.[55,104,105] For example, in set-shifting and reversal learning tasks, mice are placed in test chambers where they are given multiple computer-controlled trials. Each trial involves the presentation of two response levers and illumination of a cue light over one of the two levers. In the set-shifting task, the mice must be flexible enough to learn a series of rules regarding cues that predict reward. At first the mouse must learn to press the lever under the illuminated cue light to receive food. Once this is learned, then the rule change or "set-shift" occurs. Now the mice must press only the left lever to receive food. In the reversal-learning task, the mice must initially learn to press only the left lever for food (irrespective of the position of the cue light). Once learned, the "reversal" (rule change) occurs, and now the mice must press only the right lever to receive food. Because patients with cancer exhibit deficits on similar executive tasks, deficits are likely to be observed in mouse models of cancer. However, other components of executive function (eg, attention) may be disrupted in cancer-related fatigue, which will require additional behavioral testing to resolve.

One limitation to the behavioral tests commonly used to parse cognitive function is that they differ on several dimensions (P. Balsam, personal communication, 2010). For example, an investigator may examine learning using fear conditioning, memory using the Morris water maze, and executive function using reversal learning. When a manipulation alters performance on one test but not the others, the results are interpreted as evidence of a selective effect on one cognitive process. However, it is important to recognize that these behavioral tests vary on dimensions other than the cognitive process they are designed to assess. They differ in the response requirements of the task; the use of contextual versus discrete conditioned stimuli; the use of aversive versus appetitive stimuli; and the duration of training required. The diverse nature of these testing procedures will complicate interpretation of behavioral changes induced by cancer and its treatment. To address this limitation, behavioral tasks that involve similar testing procedures should be used to measure specific cognitive processes (P. Balsam, personal communication, 2010). Balsam and colleagues have developed a strategy to assess distinct cognitive functions using behavioral tasks that are variations of a basic timing task in which mice press a lever to earn a reward.[106] Using this approach, one can assess long-term memory,[107] working memory (P. Balsam, personal communication, 2010),[106] attention,[56] and decision making[108] processes under similar test conditions.

Activity/sleep cycles

Research using objective measures of sleep quality (actigraphy) indicates that sleep disturbances induced by cancer and chemotherapy are associated with fatigue and depression in patients with cancer.[64] Although polysomnography is considered the ideal measure of sleep stage, it is labor intensive and expensive and requires patients to spend several nights in a sleep laboratory. In contrast, actigraphy provides a more efficient, cost effective, and unobtrusive approach and has been shown to correlate well with both the use of sleep logs and polysomnography.[109] Likewise, a simple approach to investigating changes in circadian activity in mice is to measure changes in 24-hour spontaneous running-wheel activity along with circadian changes in gross body activity and core body temperature. The term "circadian rhythm" refers to the normal 24-hour cycles of behavioral and physiological processes. Investigating CRF-related disturbances in circadian rhythms in animals may help elucidate the underlying mechanisms of fatigue. It is possible that CRF may be largely driven by disruption of circadian regulation of sleep, endocrine, and neural systems. Alternatively, circadian alterations may be consequences of CRF or an independent condition that shares some overlapping mechanisms. The prevalence and co-occurrence of CRF and circadian alterations highlight the importance of developing animal models to investigate possible shared mechanisms, with the goal of developing treatments to improve both conditions.[63]

Assessment of sensory and motor function

Before intensive behavioral testing can be conducted it is necessary to evaluate whether sensory and motor functions are intact after cancer treatment.[48,110] For example, odor and taste discrimination tests should be conducted to assess potential changes induced by cancer treatments that could alter performance on affect and motivation tests.[111] Behavioral tasks should not be performed until odor and taste discrimination have recovered. Likewise, the use of appetitively motivated tasks (eg, progressive-ratio) to assess persistent fatigue-like behavior should be delayed until mice have regained their appetite after chemotherapy and radiation treatments. Neuropathic pain should be evaluated using the von Frey test prior to aversively motivated (eg, fear conditioning) and motor activity tests. Under most circumstances, testing can be delayed until animals recover normal function, typically within seven days.[112] Because intact motor function is essential for all performance-based measures, it is necessary to evaluate whether cancer treatment has induced neurological changes that could complicate interpretation of the data. In addition to evaluating clinical signs of neurological impairment (eg, alterations in grooming, posture, gait, righting responses, grid hang, vocalization to tail pinch), the open-field test can be used to quantitatively assess general locomotor activity and the rotarod test can be used to assess coordination and balance.[63,113] Again, animals should not be behaviorally tested for persistent fatigue-like behavior unless motor function has recovered after acute treatment. If motor impairment persists, then behavioral tasks that require less physical effort and are less influenced by motor deficits should be selected.[106]

Neuroimaging fatigue

Animal research has played a critical role in elucidating the psychological components and neurobiological substrates of sickness. Recent imaging studies in humans suggest that similar brain circuits mediate sickness in humans.[114–116] Peripheral inflammation induced by typhoid vaccination is associated with significant increases in IL-6 and self-reported fatigue, confusion, and impaired concentration. Performance of a demanding cognitive task during the inflammatory challenge resulted in increased activation of brain regions that receive afferent interoceptive fibers from the vagus nerve. Moreover, performance-related changes in interoceptive brain regions predicted individual differences in inflammation-induced fatigue and confusion. Increased prefrontal cortical activation was associated with the maintenance of cognitive task performance during inflammation-induced fatigue.

Likewise, translational neuroimaging studies are needed to elucidate the neural mechanisms involved in cancer-related fatigue. To date, neuroimaging studies of fatigue have not been conducted in patients with cancer or animal models of cancer. However, studies of fatigue in multiple sclerosis and other patient populations suggest that fatigue is linked to alterations in basal ganglia and frontal cortical function.[117,118] There is also evidence that the performance of fatiguing cognitive tasks, but not simple tasks, is associated with increased and more diffuse cerebral activation patterns in patients with chronic fatigue or traumatic head injury.[119,120] This increased level of activation is thought to reflect a compensatory strategy in the face of mental fatigue. Changes in performance suggestive of fatigue in patients with multiple sclerosis are associated with increased activation in the basal ganglia and frontal areas (including superior, medial, middle and inferior regions), parietal regions, thalamus, and the occipital lobes.[118] This pattern of activation is consistent with the central-fatigue model,[121] which proposes that nonmotor functions of the basal ganglia contribute to fatigue. Immune, neuroendocrine, and cytokine insults that alter basal ganglia function and motivation may induce alterations in this neural circuit.

Recent studies investigating the effects of peripheral inflammation postvaccination indicate that circulating cytokines modulate the activity of a brain network that represents internal bodily states.[115,116] Consistent with animal studies, circulating cytokines appear to act on autonomic vagal afferents to reorganize motivated behavior during inflammation. In addition, inflammation-induced fatigue and psychomotor slowing were associated with alterations in substantia nigra and insula activation.[114] Furthermore, inflammation-induced deterioration in mood was linked to enhanced activity within the subgenual anterior cingulate cortex (sACC) during an emotional-face task.[116] Other studies suggest that the sACC is implicated in depression after exposure to the exogenous cytokine interferon, which can alter cerebral blood flow.[122] Thus, inflammation-induced alterations in basal ganglia and thalamic pathways may act to suppress prefrontal cortical activity, which may provide a common central mechanism mediating fatigue in cancer and other conditions.

These human imaging findings are consistent with findings from a recent animal study that immune activation decreases neural activation in brain regions linked with positively motivated behavior while it increases neural activity in brain regions associated with stress.[123] Stone and colleagues proposed that neural activation of these two brain regions may be opponently organized and that a shift toward the stress regions contributes to the loss of positively motivated behaviors in sickness behavior and depressive illness. Similarly, cancer and its treatment may bias the activation of brain regions associated with stress, resulting in a decrease in positively motivated behaviors and an increase in fatigue, depression, and cognitive dysfunction.

Conclusions

Translational measures of cancer-related fatigue are needed to bridge the gap between clinical and animal research to facilitate the bidirectional flow of information. Animal models of CRF will play a critical role in elucidating the mechanisms of CRF and will lay the foundation for new treatments designed to prevent or ameliorate treatment-related symptoms. The construct of CRF contains multiple components that are likely to be mediated by distinct molecular, cellular, and neural systems. Therefore, advances in understanding the neural basis of CRF will require the development of behavioral measures in well-validated animal models that parse fatigue and associated behavioral disturbances into their specific components.

Animal models of CRF are also needed to determine whether genetic factors predict risk for CRF and to test the effectiveness of new and existing drugs designed to prevent and control CRF. High-throughput animal models will be especially important to speed the translation of research findings into treatments that can be used in the clinic. A major bottleneck in drug discovery for symptom-directed therapy is limited *in vivo* testing of candidate drugs in neurobehavioral paradigms in normal or genetically modified mice. Efficient animal models of CRF can be designed to remove this bottleneck, to elucidate gene function and to predict the potential efficacy of cancer therapies and symptom burden in humans. This will allow rapid and accurate evaluation of the neurobehavioral symptom-burden profile of new and current drugs and treatments designed to ameliorate their adverse effects. This approach will not only accelerate the process of drug discovery, it will allow for comparisons with nonpharmacological therapeutic strategies, including nutritional and behavioral interventions.

References

1. Bower JE. Cancer-related fatigue: links with inflammation in cancer patients and survivors. *Brain Behav Immun* **21**(7):863–871, 2007.
2. Bower JE. Behavioral symptoms in patients with breast cancer and survivors. *J Clin Oncol* **26**(5): 768–777, 2008.
3. Cella D, Davis K, Breitbart W, Curt G. Cancer-related fatigue: prevalence of proposed diagnostic criteria in a United States sample of cancer survivors. *J Clin Oncol* **19**(14):3385–3391, 2001.

4. Wang XS, Shi Q, Williams LA, et al. Serum interleukin-6 predicts the development of multiple symptoms at nadir of allogeneic hematopoietic stem cell transplantation. *Cancer* **113**(8):2102–2109, 2008.

5. Lawrence DP, Kupelnick B, Miller K, Devine D, Lau J. Evidence report on the occurrence, assessment, and treatment of fatigue in cancer patients. *J Natl Cancer Inst Monogr(32)*:40–50, 2004.

6. Bower JE, Ganz PA, Aziz N, Fahey JL. Fatigue and proinflammatory cytokine activity in breast cancer survivors. *Psychosom Med* **64**(4):604–611, 2002.

7. Bower JE, Ganz PA, Aziz N, Olmstead R, Irwin MR, Cole SW. Inflammatory responses to psychological stress in fatigued breast cancer survivors: relationship to glucocorticoids. *Brain Behav Immun* **21**(3):251–258, 2007.

8. Cleeland CS, Bennett GJ, Dantzer R, et al. Are the symptoms of cancer and cancer treatment due to a shared biologic mechanism? *Cancer* **97**(11):2919–2925, 2003.

9. Collado-Hidalgo A, Bower JE, Ganz PA, Cole SW, Irwin MR. Inflammatory biomarkers for persistent fatigue in breast cancer survivors. *Clin Cancer Res* **12**(9):2759–2766, 2006.

10. Lee BN, Dantzer R, Langley KE, et al. A cytokine-based neuroimmunologic mechanism of cancer-related symptoms. *Neuroimmunomodulation* **11**(5):279–292, 2004.

11. Dantzer R. Cytokine-induced sickness behavior: where do we stand? *Brain Behav Immun* **15**(1):7–24, 2001.

12. Dantzer R, Kelley KW. Twenty years of research on cytokine-induced sickness behavior. *Brain Behav Immun* **21**(2):153–160, 2007.

13. Larson SJ, Dunn AJ. Behavioral effects of cytokines. *Brain Behav Immun* **15**(4):371–387, 2001.

14. McKinney WT, Jr., Bunney WE, Jr. Animal model of depression. I. Review of evidence: implications for research. *Arch Gen Psychiatry* **21**(2):240–248, 1969.

15. Willner P. The validity of animal models of depression. *Psychopharmacology (Berl)* **83**(1):1–16, 1984.

16. Geyer MA, Markou A. Animal models of psychiatric disorders. In: Bloom FE, Kupfer DJ, eds. *Psychopharmacology: the Fourth Generation of Progress*. New York: Raven Press, 1995:787–798.

17. Dietrich J, Han R, Yang Y, Mayer-Pröschel M, Noble M. CNS progenitor cells and oligodendrocytes are targets of chemotherapeutic agents in vitro and in vivo. *J Biol* **5**(7):22.1–22.23, 2006.

18. Han R, Yang YM, Dietrich J, Luebke A, Mayer-Pröschel M, Noble M. Systemic 5-fluorouracil treatment causes a syndrome of delayed myelin destruction in the central nervous system. *J Biol* 7(4):12.1–12.22, 2008.

19. Anisimov VN, Ukraintseva SV, Yashin AI. Cancer in rodents: does it tell us about cancer in humans? *Nat Rev Cancer* **5**(10):807–819, 2005.

20. Gutmann DH, Hunter-Schaedle K, Shannon KM. Harnessing preclinical mouse models to inform human clinical cancer trials. *J Clin Invest* **116**(4):847–852, 2006.

21. Sharpless NE, DePinho RA. The mighty mouse: genetically engineered mouse models in cancer drug development. *Nat Rev Drug Discov* **5**(9):741–754, 2006.

22. McKinney WT. Animal models of depression: an overview. *Psychiatr Dev* **2**(2):77–96, 1984.

23. Sarhill N, Walsh D, Nelson KA, Homsi J, Legrand S, Davis MP. Methylphenidate for fatigue in advanced cancer: a prospective open-label pilot study. *Am J Hosp Palliat Care* **18**(3):187–192, 2001.

24. Sugawara Y, Akechi T, Shima Y, et al. Efficacy of methylphenidate for fatigue in advanced cancer patients: a preliminary study. *Palliat Med* **16**(3):261–263, 2002.

25. Escalante CP. Treatment of cancer-related fatigue: an update. *Support Care Cancer* **11**(2):79–83, 2003.

26. Cullum JL, Wojciechowski AE, Pelletier G, Simpson JS. Bupropion sustained release treatment reduces fatigue in cancer patients. *Can J Psychiatry* **49**(2):139–144, 2004.

27. Moss EL, Simpson JS, Pelletier G, Forsyth P. An open-label study of the effects of bupropion SR on fatigue, depression and quality of life of mixed-site cancer patients and their partners. *Psychooncology* **15**(3):259–267, 2006.

28. Kubera M, Holan V, Mathison R, Maes M. The effect of repeated amitriptyline and desipramine administration on cytokine release in C57BL/6 mice. *Psychoneuroendocrinology* **25**(8):785–797, 2000.

29. Kubera M, Maes M, Kenis G, Kim YK, Lason W. Effects of serotonin and serotonergic agonists and antagonists on the production of tumor necrosis factor alpha and interleukin-6. *Psychiatry Res* **134**(3):251–258, 2005.

30. Cronbach LJ, Meehl PE. Construct validity in psychological tests. *Psychol Bull* **52**(4):281–302, 1955.

31. Campbell DT, Fiske DW. Convergent and discriminant validation by the multitrait-multimethod matrix. *Psychol Bull* **56**(2):81–105, 1959.

32. Mills PJ, Parker BA, Dimsdale JE, Sadler GR, Ancoli-Israel S. The relationship between fatigue, quality of life and inflammation during anthracycline-based chemotherapy in breast cancer. *Biol Psychol* **69**(1):85–96, 2005.

33. Markou A, Chiamulera C, Geyer MA, Tricklebank M, Steckler T. Removing obstacles in neuroscience drug discovery: the future path for animal models. *Neuropsychopharmacology* **34**(1):74–89, 2009.
34. Malik NM, Moore GB, Smith G, Liu YL, Sanger GJ, Andrews PL. Behavioural and hypothalamic molecular effects of the anti-cancer agent cisplatin in the rat: a model of chemotherapy-related malaise? *Pharmacol Biochem Behav* **83**(1):9–20, 2006.
35. Wood LJ, Nail LM, Perrin NA, Elsea CR, Fischer A, Druker BJ. The cancer chemotherapy drug etoposide (VP-16) induces proinflammatory cytokine production and sickness behavior-like symptoms in a mouse model of cancer chemotherapy-related symptoms. *Biol Res Nurs* **8**(2):157–169, 2006.
36. Carmichael MD, Davis JM, Murphy EA, et al. Recovery of running performance following muscle-damaging exercise: relationship to brain IL-1beta. *Brain Behav Immun* **19**(5):445–452, 2005.
37. Sachdeva AK, Kuhad A, Tiwari V, Chopra K. Epigallocatechin gallate ameliorates chronic fatigue syndrome in mice: behavioral and biochemical evidence. *Behav Brain Res* **205**(2):414–420, 2009.
38. Pyter LM, Pineros V, Galang JA, McClintock MK, Prendergast BJ. Peripheral tumors induce depressive-like behaviors and cytokine production and alter hypothalamic-pituitary-adrenal axis regulation. *Proc Natl Acad Sci U S A* **106**(22):9069–9074, 2009.
39. Grill HJ, Norgren R. The taste reactivity test. I. Mimetic responses to gustatory stimuli in neurologically normal rats. *Brain Res* **143**(2):263–279, 1978.
40. Bluthé RM, Michaud B, Poli V, Dantzer R. Role of IL-6 in cytokine-induced sickness behavior: a study with IL-6 deficient mice. *Physiol Behav* **70**(3–4):367–373, 2000.
41. Moy SS, Nadler JJ, Young NB, et al. Mouse behavioral tasks relevant to autism: phenotypes of 10 inbred strains. *Behav Brain Res* **176**(1):4–20, 2007.
42. Avitsur R, Cohen E, Yirmiya R. Effects of interleukin-1 on sexual attractivity in a model of sickness behavior. *Physiol Behav* **63**(1):25–30, 1997.
43. Larson SJ, Romanoff RL, Dunn AJ, Glowa JR. Effects of interleukin-1beta on food-maintained behavior in the mouse. *Brain Behav Immun* **16**(4):398–410, 2002.
44. Salamone JD, Steinpreis RE, McCullough LD, Smith P, Grebel D, Mahan K. Haloperidol and nucleus accumbens dopamine depletion suppress lever pressing for food but increase free food consumption in a novel food choice procedure. *Psychopharmacology (Berl)* **104**(4):515–521, 1991.
45. Deacon RMJ. Assessing nest building in mice. *Nat Protoc* **1**(3):1117–1119, 2006.
46. Deacon RMJ. Burrowing: a sensitive behavioural assay, tested in five species of laboratory rodents. *Behav Brain Res* **200**(1):128–133, 2009.
47. Ferris CF, Stolberg T. Imaging the immediate non-genomic effects of stress hormone on brain activity. *Psychoneuroendocrinology* **35**(1):5–14, 2010.
48. Crawley JN. Behavioral phenotyping of transgenic and knockout mice: experimental design and evaluation of general health, sensory functions, motor abilities, and specific behavioral tests. *Brain Res* **835**(1):18–26, 1999.
49. Nevins ME, Nash SA, Beardsley PM. Quantitative grip strength assessment as a means of evaluating muscle relaxation in mice. *Psychopharmacology (Berl)* **110**(1–2):92–96, 1993.
50. Taylor AN, Rahman SU, Tio DL, et al. Lasting neuroendocrine-immune effects of traumatic brain injury in rats. *J Neurotrauma* **23**(12):1802–1813, 2006.
51. Olivadoti MD, Opp MR. Effects of i.c.v. administration of interleukin-1 on sleep and body temperature of interleukin-6-deficient mice. *Neuroscience* **153**(1):338–348, 2008.
52. Lockey AJ, Kavaliers M, Ossenkopp KP. Lipopolysaccharide produces dose-dependent reductions of the acoustic startle response without impairing prepulse inhibition in male rats. *Brain Behav Immun* **23**(1):101–107, 2009.
53. Gandal MJ, Ehrlichman RS, Rudnick ND, Siegel SJ. A novel electrophysiological model of chemotherapy-induced cognitive impairments in mice. *Neuroscience* **157**(1):95–104, 2008.
54. Winocur G, Vardy J, Binns MA, Kerr L, Tannock I. The effects of the anti-cancer drugs, methotrexate and 5-fluorouracil, on cognitive function in mice. *Pharmacol Biochem Behav* **85**(1):66–75, 2006.
55. Brigman JL, Rothblat LA. Stimulus specific deficit on visual reversal learning after lesions of medial prefrontal cortex in the mouse. *Behav Brain Res* **187**(2):405–410, 2008.
56. Buhusi CV, Meck WH. Interval timing with gaps and distracters: evaluation of the ambiguity, switch, and time-sharing hypotheses. *J Exp Psychol Anim Behav Process* **32**(3):329–338, 2006.
57. Gould TD, Gottesman II. Psychiatric endophenotypes and the development of valid animal models. *Genes Brain Behav* **5**(2):113–119, 2006.
58. Cadenhead KS, Swerdlow NR, Braff DL. Relative risk of prepulse inhibition deficits in schizophrenia patients and their siblings [abstract]. Society of Biological Psychiatry 56th Annual Meeting, New Orleans LA, May 3–5, 2001. *Biol Psychiatry* **49**(8 Suppl 1):126S, 2001. Abstract 439.
59. Touma C, Fenzl T, Ruschel J, et al. Rhythmicity in mice selected for extremes in stress reactivity:

behavioural, endocrine and sleep changes resembling endophenotypes of major depression. *PLoS One***4**(1):e4325, 2009.

60. Kirkova J, Walsh D. Cancer symptom clusters – a dynamic construct. *Support Care Cancer* **15**(9):1011–1013, 2007.

61. Roscoe JA, Morrow GR, Hickok JT, et al. Temporal interrelationships among fatigue, circadian rhythm and depression in breast cancer patients undergoing chemotherapy treatment. *Support Care Cancer* **10**(4):329–336, 2002.

62. Mulrooney DA, Ness KK, Neglia JP, et al. Fatigue and sleep disturbance in adult survivors of childhood cancer: a report from the childhood cancer survivor study (CCSS). *Sleep* **31**(2):271–281, 2008.

63. Ray M, Rogers LQ, Trammell RA, Toth LA. Fatigue and sleep during cancer and chemotherapy: translational rodent models. *Comp Med* **58**(3): 234–245, 2008.

64. Beck SL, Berger AM, Barsevick AM, Wong B, Stewart KA, Dudley WN. Sleep quality after initial chemotherapy for breast cancer. *Support Care Cancer: e-pub ahead of print*, 2009.

65. Berger AM, Wielgus K, Hertzog M, Fischer P, Farr L. Patterns of circadian activity rhythms and their relationships with fatigue and anxiety/depression in women treated with breast cancer adjuvant chemotherapy. *Support Care Cancer: e-pub ahead of print*, 2009.

66. Young JW, Minassian A, Paulus MP, Geyer MA, Perry W. A reverse-translational approach to bipolar disorder: rodent and human studies in the Behavioral Pattern Monitor. *Neurosci Biobehav Rev* **31**(6):882–896, 2007.

67. Berridge KC, Robinson TE. Parsing reward. *Trends Neurosci* **26**(9):507–513, 2003.

68. LeDoux JE. *The Emotional Brain: the Mysterious Underpinnings of Emotional Life*. New York: Simon & Schuster, 1996.

69. Phelps EA. Emotion and cognition: insights from studies of the human amygdala. *Annu Rev Psychol* **57**:27–53, 2006.

70. Phelps EA, LeDoux JE. Contributions of the amygdala to emotion processing: from animal models to human behavior. *Neuron* **48**(2):175–187, 2005.

71. Miller AH, Ancoli-Israel S, Bower JE, Capuron L, Irwin MR. Neuroendocrine-immune mechanisms of behavioral comorbidities in patients with cancer. *J Clin Oncol* **26**(6):971–982, 2008.

72. Majer M, Welberg LA, Capuron L, Pagnoni G, Raison CL, Miller AH. IFN-alpha-induced motor slowing is associated with increased depression and fatigue in patients with chronic hepatitis C. *Brain Behav Immun* **22**(6):870–880, 2008.

73. Miller AH. Norman Cousins Lecture. Mechanisms of cytokine-induced behavioral changes: psychoneuroimmunology at the translational interface. *Brain Behav Immun* **23**(2):149–158, 2009.

74. Kos D, Kerckhofs E, Nagels G, D'hooghe MB, Ilsbroukx S. Origin of fatigue in multiple sclerosis: review of the literature. *Neurorehabil Neural Repair* **22**(1):91–100, 2008.

75. Levy MR. Cancer fatigue: a neurobiological review for psychiatrists. *Psychosomatics* **49**(4):283–291, 2008.

76. Leocani L, Colombo B, Comi G. Physiopathology of fatigue in multiple sclerosis. *Neurol Sci***29**(Suppl 2):S241–S243, 2008.

77. Serhan CN, Brain SD, Buckley CD, et al. Resolution of inflammation: state of the art, definitions and terms. *FASEB J* **21**(2):325–332, 2007.

78. Malik NM, Liu YL, Cole N, Sanger GJ, Andrews PL. Differential effects of dexamethasone, ondansetron and a tachykinin NK1 receptor antagonist (GR205171) on cisplatin-induced changes in behaviour, food intake, pica and gastric function in rats. *Eur J Pharmacol* **555**(2–3):164–173, 2007.

79. Elsea CR, Roberts DA, Druker BJ, Wood LJ. Inhibition of p38 MAPK suppresses inflammatory cytokine induction by etoposide, 5-fluorouracil, and doxorubicin without affecting tumoricidal activity. *PLoS One***3**(6):e2355, 2008.

80. Hermes GL, Delgado B, Tretiakova M, et al. Social isolation dysregulates endocrine and behavioral stress while increasing malignant burden of spontaneous mammary tumors. *Proc Natl Acad Sci U S A* **106**(52):22393–22398, 2009.

81. Hermes GL, McClintock MK. Isolation and the timing of mammary gland development, gonadarche, and ovarian senescence: implications for mammary tumor burden. *Dev Psychobiol* **50**(4):353–360, 2008.

82. Williams JB, Pang D, Delgado B, et al. A model of gene-environment interaction reveals altered mammary gland gene expression and increased tumor growth following social isolation. *Cancer Prev Res (Phila Pa)* **2**(10):850–861, 2009.

83. Deacon RMJ. Burrowing in rodents: a sensitive method for detecting behavioral dysfunction. *Nat Protoc* **1**(1):118–121, 2006.

84. Burne TH, Johnston AN, McGrath JJ, Mackay-Sim A. Swimming behaviour and post-swimming activity in Vitamin D receptor knockout mice. *Brain Res Bull* **69**(1):74–78, 2006.

85. Carmichael MD, Davis JM, Murphy EA, et al. Role of brain macrophages on IL-1beta and fatigue following eccentric exercise-induced muscle damage. *Brain Behav Immun* **24**(4): 564–568, 2010.

86. Davis JM, Murphy EA, Carmichael MD, et al. Curcumin effects on inflammation and performance recovery following eccentric exercise-induced muscle damage. *Am J Physiol Regul Integr Comp Physiol* **292**(6):R2168–R2173, 2007.

87. Sachdeva AK, Kuhad A, Tiwari V, Arora V, Chopra K. Protective effect of epigallocatechin gallate in murine water-immersion stress model of chronic fatigue syndrome. *Basic Clin Pharmacol Toxicol: e-pub ahead of print*, 2010.

88. Meagher MW, Johnson RR, Young EE, et al. Interleukin-6 as a mechanism for the adverse effects of social stress on acute Theiler's virus infection. *Brain Behav Immun* **21**(8):1083–1095, 2007.

89. Berridge KC. The debate over dopamine's role in reward: the case for incentive salience. *Psychopharmacology (Berl)* **191**(3):391–431, 2007.

90. Berridge KC, Robinson TE. What is the role of dopamine in reward: hedonic impact, reward learning, or incentive salience? *Brain Res Brain Res Rev* **28**(3):309–369, 1998.

91. Holmes JE, Miller NE. Effects of bacterial endotoxin on water intake, food intake, and body temperature in the albino rat. *J Exp Med* **118**:649–658, 1963.

92. Miller NE. Some psychophysiological studies of the motivation and of the behavioral effects of illness. *Bull British Psychol Soc* **17**:1–20, 1964.

93. Hodos W. Progressive ratio as a measure of reward strength. *Science* **134**:943–944, 1961.

94. Richardson NR, Roberts DC. Progressive ratio schedules in drug self-administration studies in rats: a method to evaluate reinforcing efficacy. *J Neurosci Methods* **66**(1):1–11, 1996.

95. Merali Z, Brennan K, Brau P, Anisman H. Dissociating anorexia and anhedonia elicited by interleukin-1beta: antidepressant and gender effects on responding for "free chow" and "earned" sucrose intake. *Psychopharmacology (Berl)* **165**(4):413–418, 2003.

96. Barr AM, Phillips AG. Withdrawal following repeated exposure to d-amphetamine decreases responding for a sucrose solution as measured by a progressive ratio schedule of reinforcement. *Psychopharmacology (Berl)* **141**(1):99–106, 1999.

97. Stoops WW. Reinforcing effects of stimulants in humans: sensitivity of progressive-ratio schedules. *Exp Clin Psychopharmacol* **16**(6):503–512, 2008.

98. Stoops WW, Glaser PE, Fillmore MT, Rush CR. Reinforcing, subject-rated, performance and physiological effects of methylphenidate and d-amphetamine in stimulant abusing humans. *J Psychopharmacol* **18**(4):534–543, 2004.

99. Comer SD, Ashworth JB, Foltin RW, Johanson CE, Zacny JP, Walsh SL. The role of human drug self-administration procedures in the development of medications. *Drug Alcohol Depend* **96**(1–2):1–15, 2008.

100. Stafford D, LeSage MG, Glowa JR. Progressive-ratio schedules of drug delivery in the analysis of drug self-administration: a review. *Psychopharmacology (Berl)* **139**(3):169–184, 1998.

101. Salamone JD, Correa M. Dopamine/adenosine interactions involved in effort-related aspects of food motivation. *Appetite* **53**(3):422–425, 2009.

102. Seigers R, Schagen SB, Coppens CM, et al. Methotrexate decreases hippocampal cell proliferation and induces memory deficits in rats. *Behav Brain Res* **201**(2):279–284, 2009.

103. Pugh CR, Kumagawa K, Fleshner M, Watkins LR, Maier SF, Rudy JW. Selective effects of peripheral lipopolysaccharide administration on contextual and auditory-cue fear conditioning. *Brain Behav Immun* **12**(3):212–229, 1998.

104. Bach ME, Simpson EH, Kahn L, Marshall JJ, Kandel ER, Kellendonk C. Transient and selective overexpression of D2 receptors in the striatum causes persistent deficits in conditional associative learning. *Proc Natl Acad Sci U S A* **105**(41):16027–16032, 2008.

105. Kellendonk C, Simpson EH, Polan HJ, et al. Transient and selective overexpression of dopamine D2 receptors in the striatum causes persistent abnormalities in prefrontal cortex functioning. *Neuron* **49**(4):603–615, 2006.

106. Ward RD, Kellendonk C, Simpson EH, et al. Impaired timing precision produced by striatal D2 receptor overexpression is mediated by cognitive and motivational deficits. *Behav Neurosci* **123**(4):720–730, 2009.

107. Drew MR, Simpson EH, Kellendonk C, et al. Transient overexpression of striatal D2 receptors impairs operant motivation and interval timing. *J Neurosci* **27**(29):7731–7739, 2007.

108. Davison M, McCarthy D. The interaction of stimulus and reinforcer control in complex temporal discrimination. *J Exp Anal Behav* **48**(1):97–116, 1987.

109. Jean-Louis G, Kripke DF, Cole RJ, Assmus JD, Langer RD. Sleep detection with an accelerometer actigraph: comparisons with polysomnography. *Physiol Behav* **72**(1–2):21–28, 2001.

110. Karl T, Pabst R, von Hörsten S. Behavioral phenotyping of mice in pharmacological and toxicological research. *Exp Toxicol Pathol* **55**(1):69–83, 2003.

111. Smith DR, Burruss DR, Johnson AW. An assessment of olfaction and responses to novelty in three strains of mice. *Behav Brain Res* **201**(1):22–28, 2009.

112. Garcia JM, Cata JP, Dougherty PM, Smith RG. Ghrelin prevents cisplatin-induced mechanical hyperalgesia and cachexia. *Endocrinology* **149**(2):455–460, 2008.

113. Sieve AN, Steelman AJ, Young CR, et al. Chronic restraint stress during early Theiler's virus infection exacerbates the subsequent demyelinating disease in SJL mice. *J Neuroimmunol* **155**(1–2):103–118, 2004.

114. Brydon L, Harrison NA, Walker C, Steptoe A, Critchley HD. Peripheral inflammation is associated with altered substantia nigra activity and psychomotor slowing in humans. *Biol Psychiatry* **63**(11):1022–1029, 2008.

115. Harrison NA, Brydon L, Walker C, et al. Neural origins of human sickness in interoceptive responses to inflammation. *Biol Psychiatry* **66**(5):415–422, 2009.

116. Harrison NA, Brydon L, Walker C, Gray MA, Steptoe A, Critchley HD. Inflammation causes mood changes through alterations in subgenual cingulate activity and mesolimbic connectivity. *Biol Psychiatry* **66**(5): 407–414, 2009.

117. Filippi M, Rocca MA, Colombo B, et al. Functional magnetic resonance imaging correlates of fatigue in multiple sclerosis. *Neuroimage* **15**(3):559–567, 2002.

118. DeLuca J, Genova HM, Hillary FG, Wylie G. Neural correlates of cognitive fatigue in multiple sclerosis using functional MRI. *J Neurol Sci* **270**(1–2):28–39, 2008.

119. Lange G, Steffener J, Cook DB, et al. Objective evidence of cognitive complaints in chronic fatigue syndrome: a BOLD fMRI study of verbal working memory. *Neuroimage* **26**(2):513–524, 2005.

120. Cook DB, O'Connor PJ, Lange G, Steffener J. Functional neuroimaging correlates of mental fatigue induced by cognition among chronic fatigue syndrome patients and controls. *Neuroimage* **36**(1):108–122, 2007.

121. Chaudhuri A, Behan PO. Fatigue and basal ganglia. *J Neurol Sci* **179**(S 1–2):34–42, 2000.

122. Rocca MA, Agosta F, Colombo B, et al. fMRI changes in relapsing-remitting multiple sclerosis patients complaining of fatigue after IFNbeta-1a injection. *Hum Brain Mapp* **28**(5):373–382, 2007.

123. Stone EA, Lehmann ML, Lin Y, Quartermain D. Depressive behavior in mice due to immune stimulation is accompanied by reduced neural activity in brain regions involved in positively motivated behavior. *Biol Psychiatry* **60**(8):803–811, 2006.

Section 2 Chapter 12

Cancer Symptom Mechanisms and Models: Clinical and Basic Science

Cancer anorexia/weight loss syndrome: clinical science

Nisha Lassi and Aminah Jatoi

Cancer-related anorexia/weight-loss syndrome, commonly experienced by patients with advanced incurable cancer, is characterized by general weight loss and muscle wasting, loss of appetite, overall decline in quality of life, and shortened survival.[1] Most patients with advanced cancer develop this syndrome at some point during the course of their disease.

The approach to managing patients with cancer anorexia/weight-loss syndrome has improved dramatically over the past 50 years. A 1955 article[2] described efforts to force-feed a cohort of 64 "terminal cancer patients" with various advanced malignancies, including cancer of the cervix, colon, stomach, pancreas, and breast. Study participants were subjected to nasogastric tube feedings. The investigators described how "many who were bedfast in the hospital were temporarily restored to family living without special care." Even so, the investigators were not able to determine whether the patients' length of life was extended or shortened, further noting that "tumors that were palpable or visible seemed to increase in size..." Today, force-feeding patients with advanced, incurable cancer is viewed as ineffective and is almost obsolete. Despite progress in the management of cancer-related anorexia/weight-loss syndrome, however, many aspects of this syndrome continue to be vexing from a clinical and research perspective.

This chapter outlines areas of progress and ongoing challenge. We address: (1) the clinical significance of cancer anorexia/weight-loss syndrome; (2) the current thinking on its pathophysiology; (3) current treatment approaches; and (4) recent inconsistencies between translational and clinical research, all of which underscore the need for avid, continued clinical investigation.

The clinical significance of cancer anorexia/weight-loss syndrome

The ramifications of anorexia and weight loss for patients with cancer are profound. First, the sign of weight loss clearly predicts a poor prognosis. In a landmark study, Dewys et al.[3] examined 3047 patients with cancer who had participated in a dozen different Eastern Cooperative Oncology Group (ECOG) chemotherapy trials and found that a weight reduction of as little as 6% in the preceding two months predicted significantly shortened survival. This prognostic effect remained even after the investigators adjusted for factors such as performance status score and extent of tumor burden. Chemotherapy response rates were also lower in a limited set of patients, as observed in a subgroup analysis. Thus, weight loss is a strong predictor of poor outcomes in patients with cancer.

The prognostic significance of cancer anorexia/weight-loss syndrome is not limited to weight loss. Anorexia, or loss of appetite, is also prognostic of poor outcomes. In a study of 115 patients with lung and colorectal cancer conducted by the North Central Cancer Treatment Group,[4] the patients contending with anorexia did not live as long as the patients who had maintained their appetites.

Strong justification for incorporating the study of anorexia/weight-loss syndrome into a comprehensive cancer-care research agenda is provided by one particular aspect of the syndrome: it bothers patients. At the end of life, patients with cancer consistently describe anorexia as one of their five most troubling symptoms.[5] This rating is also reported by children with cancer[6] and even by patients who are not receiving active cancer treatment, indicating that anorexia can occur as a result of the cancer itself and not just from the administration of chemotherapy. Although the data on weight loss are not as clear-cut, patients with cancer who have lost weight appear to suffer from a functional decline, which may well have a negative impact on quality of life. In an ECOG study, Finkelstein et al.[7] observed that decrease in Functional Living Index-Cancer scores, which correlated with poor performance status (P = 0.0002), also correlated with a greater than 5% weight loss (P = 0.004). Such observations suggest that weight

Cancer Symptom Science: Measurement, Mechanisms, and Management, eds. Charles S. Cleeland, Michael J. Fisch, and Adrian J. Dunn.
Published by Cambridge University Press.

loss has far-reaching ramifications that extend even to overall quality of life for the patient with cancer.

The pathophysiology of the cancer anorexia/weight-loss syndrome

If we probe further into this syndrome, what clinical observations become apparent? The approach of the investigators who tested forced feeding in the 1950s[2] notwithstanding, this syndrome does not resemble starvation. It is true that cancer patients can starve and that they can benefit from caloric supplementation under specific circumstances. These circumstances are relatively uncommon, however, and primarily reflect a situation where the cancer is potentially curable and the patient is suffering from severe malnutrition or is at risk for developing severe malnutrition – for example, a preoperative patient who is being considered for a potentially curative cancer resection and who has lost more than 10% of his or her premorbid weight.[8] This relatively rare patient is likely to benefit from nutrition support in the perioperative setting.

Whereas most weight-losing patients with advanced, incurable cancer may appear to be starving, in actuality they are not. Three clinically evident distinctions set these patients apart from the starving patient. First, body composition studies show that the clinical findings observed in patients with cancer anorexia/weight-loss syndrome contrast with clinical findings observed in patients experiencing starvation: patients with cancer anorexia/weight-loss syndrome waste lean tissue. Cohn et al.[9] utilized a variety of body-composition measurement techniques, such as prompt gamma neutron activation, total body potassium, and total body water as measured by tritiated water, in an effort to better understand what occurs at the tissue level in weight-losing patients with cancer. These investigators concluded, "The loss of body weight by patients with solid tumors [consists] primarily of the loss of muscle mass and body fat… It is the skeletal muscle which is predominantly lost." With starvation, the exact opposite occurs: lean tissue is preserved. Instead, patients preferentially waste fat. These seminal observations were derived from Keys et al.[10] in the setting of semistarvation among men who were conscientious war objectors and participated in a Minnesota experiment on starvation. Body-composition studies showed that these young men preserved their lean tissue and squandered fat. Thus, from a qualitative standpoint, the changes that occur in patients with cancer who suffer from anorexia/weight-loss syndrome appear to be in direct contradistinction to the changes that occur in an individual who is starving.

Second, many of the studies evaluating resting energy expenditure have shown it to increase in patients with cancer. Our group took these observations one step further in a study of patients with non-metastatic, potentially curable non-small cell lung cancer.[11] Utilizing a case-control study design, we compared the resting energy expenditure of 18 patients with nonmetastatic non-small cell lung cancer and 18 healthy individuals matched for age (± 5 years), gender, and body mass index (± 3 kg/m^2). Of note, only four of the patients with cancer had experienced weight loss. Resting energy expenditure measurements were adjusted for lean mass as measured by dual x-ray absorptiometry, potassium-40 measurements, and total body water as measured by tritiated water. Adjusting resting energy expenditure results demonstrated an increase in resting energy expenditure to mean values as high as 724 kJ/day for the patients with cancer, based on a body cell mass adjustment (potassium-40). These results suggest that even when the cancer has not metastasized extensively, metabolic changes, including alterations in resting energy expenditure, are occurring.

Third, as suggested above, cancer patients with anorexia/weight-loss syndrome eat less. The noxious symptom of anorexia leads to decreased caloric intake. Hutton et al.[12] looked at dietary patterns of 151 patients with cancer who were evaluated approximately 8 months before death. Although there were wide variations in daily caloric intake among these patients with cancer, weight-losing patients were definitely consuming fewer calories. Admittedly, this observation may seem too obvious to report. However, the sobering fact is that weight-losing cancer patients, amid growing caloric needs, are providing a physiological response – namely, anorexia – that dooms them to failure; hence, they eat less. Again, this observation is very much at odds with what occurs during starvation, where hunger drives starving individuals to eat more.

The juxtaposition of these discordant nutritional responses – poor appetite accompanied by poor oral intake, a wearing down of lean tissue, and an unexpected revving up of the metabolic rate – conspires to create a dangerous situation for the patient with cancer. As caloric needs increase (sometimes inexplicably), anorexia nonetheless sets in and patients eat less. At the same time, lean tissue, a body compartment that plays a critical role in sustaining life, is sacrificed to meet the body's growing energy needs. Thus, the epidemiological data that describe the negative prognostic effect of weight loss becomes easier to understand in view of this odd constellation of unexpected and seemingly illogical pathophysiological events.

Current palliative approaches

Given that caloric repletion does not have a major favorable impact on patients with cancer anorexia/weight-loss syndrome and can even be detrimental, what is an appropriate standard of care for patients with incurable cancer who experience weight loss and loss of appetite? Is it acceptable to consider pharmacological interventions? The pathophysiology of cancer anorexia/weight-loss syndrome as described above indicates that pharmacological appetite-stimulation treatment can be justified under certain circumstances.

First, the patient must have a malignancy that likely will not respond to anticancer therapy. Anecdotal reports indicate that patients do gain weight and improve their appetites with successful antineoplastic treatment, and clinical studies suggest the same. Second, the patient must not have other comorbidities, such as severe dysphagia, bowel obstruction, or pain with eating, that are physically causing the poor oral intake. When a patient is physically unable to eat, appetite stimulants will play a negligible role at best and may actually increase the patient's frustration. Third, the cancer patient and his or her family must be well educated about the cancer anorexia/weight-loss syndrome, so that the patient can make an informed decision about opting for an appetite stimulant. Although appetite stimulants may improve appetite and weight, they do not improve survival or global quality of life.[13] It is therefore important for patients to be thoroughly educated and realistic about the benefits as well as the side effects of appetite stimulants.

Two classes of drugs – corticosteroids and progestational agents – have proven effective in palliating anorexia in patients with cancer. Both groups of agents have been tested in numerous randomized, double-blinded, placebo-controlled trials. For example, Moertel et al.[14] studied patients with gastrointestinal cancer who were approaching the end of life and demonstrated that 2–4 mg/day of the corticosteroid dexamethasone assuaged anorexia on a short-term basis. It is not exactly clear how dexamethasone or corticosteroids work, but it is thought that they somehow exert central nervous system effects on appetite stimulation. Other studies have confirmed the original observations from Moertel et al.[15,16]

Patients and health care providers should be aware that corticosteroid therapy produces long-term effects that make this intervention less than optimal for the cancer patient, who might require several months of such treatment. Corticosteroid side effects include muscle weakness, gastritis and other irritation of the gastrointestinal tract, increased risk for bone fractures, and increased risk for infections. Thus, although corticosteroids can be used for appetite stimulation in patients with cancer, they should be restricted to short-term administration only.

Progestational agents are a second option for appetite stimulation. Megestrol acetate is perhaps the best studied and its efficacy as an appetite stimulant has been proven by means of multiple placebo-controlled, double-blinded, randomized trials. The first-published of these studies, conducted by the North Central Cancer Treatment Group, focused on 133 patients with advanced cancer who were experiencing appetite loss, weight loss, or both.[17] These patients were randomly assigned to megestrol acetate 800 mg/day or to placebo. Seventy percent of the patients treated with megestrol acetate reported an improved appetite, but fewer than half of the placebo-exposed patients reported similar favorable effects. Other investigations, including a recent meta-analysis,[18] have underscored the role of megestrol acetate as a palliative intervention for cancer patients suffering from anorexia.

From a practical standpoint, megestrol acetate can be prescribed at doses between 480 and 800 mg/day to induce appetite stimulation, although doses as low as 160 mg/day can also be effective.[19] In a phase III, dose-finding trial of 342 patients with cancer randomly assigned to receive megestrol acetate at oral doses of 160, 480, 800, or 1280 mg/day,[19] a positive dose–response effect occurred but no increase in benefit was observed beyond the 800 mg dose. Side effects of megestrol acetate, which include blood clots, impotence, vaginal bleeding, and adrenal insufficiency upon abrupt withdrawal, occur in fewer than 10% of patients. Nonetheless, any side effects should be carefully noted and discussed with patients.

Finally, one comparative study provides guidance on when to prescribe corticosteroids and when to prescribe megestrol acetate.[20] This three-arm clinical trial included 475 patients who were randomly assigned to either megestrol acetate 800 mg/day, dexamethasone 0.75 mg four times a day, or an androgen that did not perform as well and will not be discussed. Megestrol acetate and dexamethasone performed comparably as appetite stimulants. However, dexamethasone produced more notable short-term side effects that resulted in higher rates of drug discontinuation. Patients treated with megestrol acetate exhibited a trend toward higher rates of blood-clot formation. Thus, if a patient has a history of blood clots, megestrol acetate should be avoided; in this case, corticosteroids such as dexamethasone may be preferable. If a patient is likely to use an appetite stimulant long-term, megestrol acetate would be the better choice.

Despite the widespread use of corticosteroids and megestrol acetate, the mechanisms that explain how these agents work remain unknown. Some authors have suggested that these agents act directly on the inflammatory cytokine environment, but other studies have not been conclusive in this regard.

Unifying translational and clinical observations: a need for further clinical research

The past several years of research have provided major advances in our understanding of the pathophysiology of cancer anorexia/weight-loss syndrome. Recently, there has been a greater focus on the hormonal milieu of patients with cancer and its impact on alterations in appetite,[21] along with heightened attention to myostatin, nuclear factor kappa B, and the dystrophin–glycoprotein complex.[22] The remainder of this review focuses on three purported mediators of cancer anorexia/weight-loss syndrome that are being tested in clinical settings: the proteolysis-inducing factor, tumor necrosis factor (TNF)-α, and the ubiquitin-proteasome pathway.

The proteolysis-inducing factor

In 1996, Todorov et al.[23] provided evidence of a newly characterized mediator of weight loss in cancer patients. The investigators isolated a 24-kilodalton proteoglycan (herein referred to as the proteolysis-inducing factor) derived from a MAC16 tumor, and concluded that this isolate mediated cachexia, a general wasting of tissue and loss of appetite that accompanies chronic disease, in both mice and humans. Indeed, the data suggesting that the proteolysis-inducing factor is a true mediator of anorexia/weight-loss syndrome appeared compelling. Mice given the proteolysis-inducing factor lost more weight than mice given vehicle; further, administering an antibody to the proteolysis-inducing factor prior to administering the proteolysis-inducing factor seemed to prevent such weight loss.

The human data from this 1996 publication were even more compelling.[23] Sixteen healthy individuals, 17 patients who had lost weight as a result of trauma or sepsis, and 25 patients with cancer participated in this portion of the study. Assays of urine from all participants found proteolysis-inducing factor in only the weight-losing cancer patients; in contrast, patients with cancer who had lost less than 1.3 kg of weight per month did not have detectable levels of the proteolysis-inducing factor. Similarly, patients who were losing weight from noncancer causes did not have this mediator in their urine. These results suggested that in a clinical setting the proteolysis-inducing factor is highly sensitive and specific for cancer-associated weight loss.

Since this early work, numerous other studies, primarily from the same group and primarily derived in a laboratory setting, have focused on the proteolysis-inducing factor. In general, however, the clinical relevance of this mediator has not been fully validated. Deans et al.[24] recently evaluated proteolysis core peptide expression in tumor and benign tissue from patients with esophageal or gastric cancer and from benign esophageal or gastric tissue from healthy volunteers. Forty-six biopsies from the former group and 11 biopsies from the latter group were studied. Relying upon baseline and prospectively gathered clinical data, the investigators drew several conclusions. First, expression of the proteolysis core peptide was greater in patients with cancer regardless of whether the sampled tissue was benign or malignant. Second, in patients with cancer, expression of the proteolysis core peptide did not correlate with the extent of weight loss or prognosis. The investigators concluded that "post-translational modification of proteolysis-inducing factor may be a key step in determining the biological role of proteolysis-inducing factor in the patient with advanced cancer and cachexia."

Similarly, our group evaluated proteolysis-inducing factor in a cohort of 41 patients with metastatic gastric or esophageal cancer.[25] All patients received the same cancer treatment and participated in the same prospective follow-up. Proteolysis-inducing factor was found in the urine of 23 patients (56%) at the time of study entry; however, there was no correlation between the presence of proteolysis-inducing factor and weight loss, nor between its presence and patient-reported anorexia. Importantly, the presence of proteolysis-inducing factor did not predict tumor response or patient survival. Thus, the clinical relevance of proteolysis-inducing factor requires further clinical investigation.

A series of additional studies, some of which were clinical, have demonstrated the need for further research on the proteolysis-inducing factor to better understand its role. Early preclinical work suggested that inhibition of the proteolysis-inducing factor attenuated weight loss in tumor-bearing animals. Smith et al.[26] utilized an *in vitro* murine myotube model as a surrogate for skeletal muscle and observed that at a concentration of 50 μmol/L, eicosapentaenoic acid (an omega-3 fatty acid) abrogated protein degradation induced by proteolysis-inducing factor. However, when such provocative, mechanism-based preclinical data led to the testing of eicosapentaenoic acid in a clinical setting, results were disappointing. At least four large comparative trials of eicosapentaenoic acid conducted in more than 1000 patients yielded negative results with respect to showing clinical benefits of eicosapentaenoic acid,[27–30] even though previous studies seemed to show that this agent worked by means of inhibiting proteolysis-inducing factor, and even though other mechanisms of action besides inhibition of proteolysis-inducing factor had been invoked to support these trials. These negative trials cast doubt on the role of eicosapentaenoic acid in this setting.

In summary, the above studies have been inconsistent in showing the clinical correlative significance of proteolysis-inducing factor. Although the early work from 1996[23] pointed to this mediator as being highly sensitive and specific for cancer-associated weight loss, some of the subsequent clinical data[27–30] have not validated these results. More clinically relevant research on this purported mediator is needed.

Tumor necrosis factor-α

TNF-α is one of several inflammatory cytokines implicated in mediating cancer anorexia/weight-loss syndrome. This cytokine has likely received the greatest degree of research focus. Not all studies have consistently reported that TNF-α is a mediator of this syndrome. For example, our group found that among 118 cancer patients with anorexia and/or weight loss, 54% had undetectable serum levels of TNF-α.[31]

However, other data do provide strong evidence to implicate this cytokine as a mediator of cancer anorexia/weight-loss syndrome. Implantation of Lewis lung carcinoma into gene knockout mice that are TNF-α deficient results in rates of protein degradation that are much lower than the rates seen in tumor-bearing wild-type mice.[32] In addition, TNF-α in combination with interferon-γ downregulates myosin heavy chains,[33] an observation that might shed light on how muscle wasting occurs in this syndrome. Further, nuclear factor kappa B, which has been implicated in muscle wasting, is upregulated by TNF-α.[34]

Earlier animal data are even more compelling. Torelli et al.[35] examined changes in eating habits and weight in tumor-bearing rodents. Testing a dimeric, pegylated 55-kilodalton TNF receptor construct that, in effect, served as a TNF-α inhibitor, these investigators observed that the eight mice receiving the inhibitor ate more and gained more weight over a one-week period than the mice receiving vehicle. These findings suggest that the inflammatory cytokine TNF-α plays a role in mediating the cancer anorexia/weight-loss syndrome.

Are there clinical data to suggest that TNF-α inhibition can result in reversal of the cancer-associated weight loss syndrome? On the basis of very preliminary data, several agents are thought to mediate cancer anorexia/weight-loss syndrome, and some of these agents are thought to work by means of inhibition of TNF-α. At least five pilot studies in patients with cancer suggest that thalidomide, a TNF-α inhibitor, may be effective in the treatment of cancer-associated weight loss.[36–40] For example, Gordon et al.[40] studied 50 patients with advanced pancreatic cancer and observed preliminary evidence of weight gain in thalidomide-treated patients, but not in placebo-exposed patients. Melatonin is yet another drug that at least preliminarily appears to play a potential role in treating cancer anorexia/weight-loss syndrome. This agent is also thought to inhibit TNF-α.[41,42] Lissoni et al.[41] studied melatonin in 100 patients with metastatic cancer and observed that an oral dose of melatonin 20 mg/day seemed to stabilize weight, whereas patients who received standard supportive care experienced continued weight loss. Taken together, such findings suggest that TNF-α might be a mediator of this syndrome and might also serve as a therapeutic target for palliation.

However, not all clinical data have consistently indicated that TNF-α inhibition palliates cancer-associated anorexia and weight loss. Our group recently completed a study that looked at the agent etanercept, a dimeric soluble recombinant form of the extracellular domain of the p75 TNF receptor.[43] Etanercept has been used successfully in the treatment of rheumatoid arthritis, ankylosing spondylitis, and psoriatic arthritis at dosages of 25 mg administered subcutaneously twice a week. As a highly specific inhibitor of TNF-α, etanercept provided an excellent opportunity to test whether TNF-α is truly a clinically relevant mediator of cancer anorexia/weight-loss syndrome. We conducted a randomized, double-blind, placebo-controlled trial with 63 patients who had various tumor types and the overarching features of weight loss and/or anorexia in the setting of an incurable cancer.[43] Etanercept was administered to patients in the intervention arm subcutaneously at a dose of 25 mg twice a week. No patient in either the intervention or control group gained more than 10% of his or her baseline body weight. Moreover, when we examined lesser degrees of weight gain or overall appetite improvement, we found no evidence of improvement in appetite or weight in the patients who received etanercept.

How might these negative findings be explained? Apart from the possibility that TNF-α might not be a mediator of cancer anorexia/weight-loss syndrome after all, several alternate explanations merit consideration. First, it is possible that a higher dose of etanercept might have resulted in a better clinical outcome. The dose used in our trial was derived from studies that demonstrated efficacy in other disease settings, such as rheumatoid arthritis. If tissue concentrations of TNF-α in the setting of cancer are in fact higher, a higher dose of etanercept might be needed to counter the higher concentrations of TNF-α. Second, studies have suggested that inflammatory cytokines often act in concert. Thus, if one cytokine is inhibited, there is a possibility that redundant mechanisms might kick in and compensate for diminished concentrations of that cytokine. Further clinical study of the role of inflammatory cytokines in cancer anorexia/weight-loss syndrome is indicated.

The ubiquitin–proteasome pathway

The ubiquitin-proteasome pathway is well known to allow for senescent, damaged, and other proteins to be effectively degraded and cleared away in the body. This pathway has also been implicated in cancer anorexia/weight-loss syndrome. In a seminal animal model study, Baracos et al.[44] observed that the ubiquitin-proteasome system accounts for 80% of muscle wasting in cancer. Other investigators demonstrated a link that implicates TNF-α as a direct mediator of this pathway.[32] Overall, a burgeoning group of studies focused on this pathway have suggested that the ubiquitin-proteasome system might serve as an effective target for palliating some aspects of cancer anorexia/weight-loss syndrome. A review of such studies was recently published.[45]

Despite the growing interest in the ubiquitin-proteasome pathway, few studies have attempted to understand its role in cancer-associated weight loss from a clinical vantage point. Bossola et al[46] evaluated this pathway in patients with gastric cancer. Careful examination of muscle biopsies revealed no direct correlations between weight loss and ubiquitin-related overexpression of mRNA in muscle.

Similarly, our group recently evaluated bortezomib as a potential palliative agent for cancer anorexia/weight-loss syndrome in patients with metastatic pancreatic cancer.[47] Bortezomib is a dipeptide boronic acid analogue and a reversible proteasome inhibitor. This study was undertaken as part of a subgroup analysis that included two previously conducted treatment trials, one of which included single-agent bortezomib and the other of which included octreotide, an agent that is thought to have negligible antineoplastic activity in patients with metastatic pancreatic cancer. None of the 88 patients evaluated manifested a tumor response either with bortezomib 1.5 or 1.3 mg/m^2 administered intravenously on days 1, 4, 8, and 11 of a 21-day cycle, or with octreotide 200 or 500 μg administered subcutaneously three times a day. Adverse events with bortezomib, which were sometimes severe, included abdominal pain, fatigue, nausea, thrombosis, and thrombocytopenia. Comparing mean change in weight from baseline through three cycles of chemotherapy, we observed no statistically significant differences between groups to suggest that bortezomib exerted favorable effects on weight. Quality-of-life data were available only for bortezomib patients and, at first glance, suggested stability over time. However, notable dropout rates over time invite caution in interpreting such stability as favorable. We believe that a more realistic interpretation of these data is that bortezomib did not provide a favorable impact on appetite.

Again the question arises, how might these negative findings be explained? Once more, the issue of dose might partly explain these results. The dosages used in this study were based on dosing that is most commonly utilized in antineoplastic trials; a reduced, less-toxic dosage might have resulted in better outcomes from the standpoint of anorexia and weight loss. Even so, to our knowledge no reports have ever demonstrated that weight loss predicts a poor outcome in patients with pancreatic cancer. It may well be that the aggressive nature of pancreatic cancer carries tremendous morbidity that may not be easily reversed by a therapy that primarily targets the reversal of weight loss. In short, further clinical research is needed to better understand whether proteasome inhibition can have a positive impact on patients with cancer anorexia/weight-loss syndrome.

Conclusions

Anorexia/weight-loss syndrome continues to be a source of major morbidity and mortality for patients with advanced cancer. In contrast to 50 years ago, we now understand that this syndrome does not represent classic starvation, that forced feeding is not an appropriate treatment approach, and that pharmacological therapy to palliate some aspects of this syndrome can be justified. Further clinical research into the roles of proteolysis-inducing factor, TNF-α, and the proteasome promises to provide better palliative options in the future.

References

1. Giordano KF, Jatoi A. The cancer anorexia/weight loss syndrome: therapeutic challenges. *Curr Oncol Rep* 7(4):271–276, 2005.
2. Pareira MD, Conrad EJ, Hicks W, Elman R. Clinical response and changes in nitrogen balance, body weight, plasma proteins, and hemoglobin following tube feeding in cancer cachexia. *Cancer* **8**(4):803–808, 1955.
3. Dewys WD, Begg C, Lavin PT, et al. Prognostic effect of weight loss prior to chemotherapy in cancer patients. Eastern Cooperative Oncology Group. *Am J Med* **69**(4):491–497, 1980.
4. Loprinzi CL, Laurie JA, Wieand HS, et al. Prospective evaluation of prognostic variables from patient-completed questionnaires. North Central Cancer Treatment Group. *J Clin Oncol* **12**(3):601–607, 1994.
5. Walsh D, Rybicki L. Symptom clustering in advanced cancer. *Support Care Cancer* **14**(8):831–836, 2006.
6. Wolfe J, Grier HE, Klar N, et al. Symptoms and suffering at the end of life in children with cancer. *N Engl J Med* **342**(5):326–333, 2000.
7. Finkelstein DM, Cassileth BR, Bonomi PD, Ruckdeschel JC, Ezdinli EZ, Wolter JM. A pilot study of the Functional Living Index-Cancer (FLIC) Scale for the assessment of quality of life for metastatic lung cancer patients. An Eastern Cooperative Oncology Group study. *Am J Clin Oncol* **11**(6):630–633, 1988.
8. The Veterans Affairs Total Parenteral Nutrition Cooperative Study Group. Perioperative total parenteral nutrition in surgical patients. *N Engl J Med* **325**(8):525–532, 1991.
9. Cohn SH, Gartenhaus W, Sawitsky A, et al. Compartmental body composition of cancer patients by measurement of total body nitrogen, potassium, and water. *Metabolism* **30**(3):222–229, 1981.
10. Keys A. The residues of malnutrition and starvation. *Science* **112**(2909):371–373, 1950.
11. Jatoi A, Daly BD, Hughes VA, Dallal GE, Kehayias J, Roubenoff R. Do patients with nonmetastatic non-small cell lung cancer demonstrate altered resting energy expenditure? *Ann Thorac Surg* **72**(2):348–351, 2001.
12. Hutton JL, Martin L, Field CJ, et al. Dietary patterns in patients with advanced cancer: implications for anorexia-cachexia therapy. *Am J Clin Nutr* **84**(5):1163–1170, 2006.
13. Jatoi A. Pharmacologic therapy for the cancer anorexia/weight loss syndrome: A data-driven, practical approach. *J Support Oncol* **4**(10):499–502, 2006.
14. Moertel CG, Schutt AJ, Reitemeier RJ, Hahn RG. Corticosteroid therapy of preterminal gastrointestinal cancer. *Cancer* **33**(6):1607–1609, 1974.
15. Bruera E, Roca E, Cedaro L, Carraro S, Chacon R. Action of oral methylprednisolone in terminal cancer patients: a prospective randomized double-blind study. *Cancer Treat Rep* **69**(7–8):751–754, 1985.
16. Popiela T, Lucchi R, Giongo F. Methylprednisolone as palliative therapy for female terminal cancer patients. The Methylprednisolone Female Preterminal Cancer Study Group. *Eur J Cancer Clin Oncol* **25**(12):1823–1829, 1989.
17. Loprinzi CL, Ellison NM, Schaid DJ, et al. Controlled trial of megestrol acetate for the treatment of cancer anorexia and cachexia. *J Natl Cancer Inst* **82**(13):1127–1132, 1990.
18. Berenstein EG, Ortiz Z. Megestrol acetate for the treatment of anorexia-cachexia syndrome. *Cochrane Database Syst Rev* **2**:CD004310, 2005.
19. Loprinzi CL, Michalak JC, Schaid DJ, et al. Phase III evaluation of four doses of megestrol acetate as therapy for patients with cancer anorexia and/or cachexia. *J Clin Oncol* **11**(4):762–767, 1993.
20. Loprinzi CL, Kugler JW, Sloan JA, et al. Randomized comparison of megestrol acetate versus dexamethasone versus fluoxymesterone for the treatment of cancer anorexia/cachexia. *J Clin Oncol* **17**(10):3299–3306, 1999.

21. Davis MP, Dreicer R, Walsh D, Lagman R, LeGrand SB. Appetite and cancer-associated anorexia: a review. *J Clin Oncol* **22**(8):1510–1517, 2004.

22. Acharyya S, Guttridge DC. Cancer cachexia signaling pathways continue to emerge yet much still points to the proteasome. *Clin Cancer Res* **13**(5):1356–1361, 2007.

23. Todorov P, Cariuk P, McDevitt T, Coles B, Fearon K, Tisdale M. Characterization of a cancer cachectic factor. *Nature* **379**(6567):739–742, 1996.

24. Deans DA, Wigmore SJ, Gilmour H, Tisdale MJ, Fearon KC, Ross JA. Expression of the proteolysis-inducing factor core peptide mRNA is upregulated in both tumour and adjacent normal tissue in gastro-oesophageal malignancy. *Br J Cancer* **94**(5):731–736, 2006.

25. Jatoi A, Foster N, Wieland B, et al. The proteolysis-inducing factor: in search of its clinical relevance in patients with metastatic gastric/esophageal cancer. *Dis Esophagus* **19**(4):241–247, 2006.

26. Smith HJ, Mukerji P, Tisdale MJ. Attenuation of proteasome-induced proteolysis in skeletal muscle by β-hydroxy-β-methylbutyrate in cancer-induced muscle loss. *Cancer Res* **65**(1):277–283, 2005.

27. Bruera E, Strasser F, Palmer JL, et al. Effect of fish oil on appetite and other symptoms in patients with advanced cancer and anorexia/cachexia: a double-blind, placebo-controlled study. *J Clin Oncol* **21**(1):129–134, 2003.

28. Jatoi A, Rowland K, Loprinzi CL, et al. An eicosapentaenoic acid supplement versus megestrol acetate versus both for patients with cancer-associated wasting: a North Central Cancer Treatment Group and National Cancer Institute of Canada collaborative effort. *J Clin Oncol* **22**(12):2469–2476, 2004.

29. Fearon KC, von Meyenfeldt MF, Moses AG, et al. Effect of a protein and energy dense N-3 fatty acid enriched oral supplement on loss of weight and lean tissue in cancer cachexia: a randomised double blind trial. *Gut* **52**(10):1479–1486, 2003.

30. Fearon KC, Barber MD, Moses AG, et al. Double-blind, placebo-controlled, randomized study of eicosapentaenoic acid diester in patients with cancer cachexia. *J Clin Oncol* **24**(21):3401–3407, 2006.

31. Jatoi A, Egner J, Loprinzi CL, et al. Investigating the utility of serum cytokine measurements in a multi-institutional cancer anorexia/weight loss trial. *Support Care Cancer* **12**(9):640–644, 2004.

32. Llovera M, García-Martínez C, López-Soriano J, et al. Role of TNF receptor 1 in protein turnover during cancer cachexia using gene knockout mice. *Mol Cell Endocrinol* **142**(1–2):183–189, 1998.

33. Acharyya S, Ladner KJ, Nelsen LL, et al. Cancer cachexia is regulated by selective targeting of skeletal muscle gene products. *J Clin Invest* **114**(3):370–378, 2004.

34. Langen RC, Van Der Velden JL, Schols AM, Kelders MC, Wouters EF, Janssen-Heininger YM. Tumor necrosis factor-alpha inhibits myogenic differentiation through MyoD protein destabilization. *FASEB J* **18**(2):227–237, 2004.

35. Torelli GF, Meguid MM, Moldawer LL, et al. Use of recombinant human soluble TNF receptor in anorectic tumor-bearing rats. *Am J Physiol* **277**(3 Pt 2):R850–R855, 1999.

36. Mahmoud FA, Walsh D, Davis M, Legrand S, Lagman R, Mekhail T. A dose titration study of thalidomide in cancer anorexia [abstract]. *American Society of Clinical Oncology 39th Annual Meeting*, Chicago IL. Proc Am Soc Clin Oncol 2003;22.

37. Boasberg P, O'Day S, Weisberg M, Deck G, Frost J, Ye W. Thalidomide-induced cessation of weight loss and improved sleep in advanced cancer patients with cachexia [abstract]. *American Society of Clinical Oncology 36th Annual Meeting*, New Orleans LA. Proc Am Soc Clin Oncol 2000;19.

38. Khan ZH, Simpson EJ, Cole AT, et al. Oesophageal cancer and cachexia: the effect of short-term treatment with thalidomide on weight loss and lean body mass. *Aliment Pharmacol Ther* **17**(5):677–682, 2003.

39. Bruera E, Neumann CM, Pituskin E, Calder K, Ball G, Hanson J. Thalidomide in patients with cachexia due to terminal cancer: preliminary report. *Ann Oncol* **10**(7):857–859, 1999.

40. Gordon JN, Trebble TM, Ellis RD, Duncan HD, Johns T, Goggin PM. Thalidomide in the treatment of cancer cachexia: a randomised placebo controlled trial. *Gut* **54**(4):540–545, 2005.

41. Lissoni P, Paolorossi F, Tancini G, et al. Is there a role for melatonin in the treatment of neoplastic cachexia? *Eur J Cancer* **32A**(8):1340–1343, 1996.

42. Lissoni P, Paolorossi F, Ardizzoia A, et al. A randomized study of chemotherapy with cisplatin plus etoposide versus chemoendocrine therapy with cisplatin, etoposide and the pineal hormone melatonin as a first-line treatment of advanced non-small cell lung cancer patients in a poor clinical state. *J Pineal Res* **23**(1):15–19, 1997.

43. Jatoi A, Dakhil SR, Nguyen PL, et al. A placebo-controlled double blind trial of etanercept for the cancer anorexia/weight loss syndrome: results from N00C1 from the North Central Cancer Treatment Group. *Cancer* **110**(6):1396–1403, 2007.

44. Baracos VE, DeVivo C, Hoyle DH, Goldberg AL. Activation of the ATP-ubiquitin-proteasome pathway in skeletal muscle of cachectic rats bearing a hepatoma. *Am J Physiol* **268**(5 Pt 1):E996–1006, 1995.

45. Camps C, Iranzo V, Bremnes RM, Sirera R. Anorexia-Cachexia syndrome in cancer: implications of the

ubiquitin-proteasome pathway. *Support Care Cancer* **14**(12):1173–1183, 2006.

46. Bossola M, Muscaritoli M, Costelli P, et al. Increased muscle proteasome activity correlates with disease severity in gastric cancer patients. *Ann Surg* **237**(3):384–389, 2003.

47. Jatoi A, Alberts SR, Foster N, et al. Is bortezomib, a proteasome inhibitor, effective in treating cancer-associated weight loss? Preliminary results from the North Central Cancer Treatment Group. *Support Care Cancer* **13**(6):381–386, 2005.

Section 2 Chapter 13

Cancer Symptom Mechanisms and Models: Clinical and Basic Science

Appetite loss/cachexia: basic science

Tristin D. Brisbois Clarkson, Wendy V. Wismer, and Vickie E. Baracos

Involuntary weight loss is one of the hallmarks of advanced cancer. Healthy adults are generally highly resistant to attempts to lose body fat, which stores a remarkably constant amount of energy overall. Normally, highly precise controls work to ensure that energy expenditure and energy intake are matched (energy homeostasis), so that there is neither net loss nor net gain of body energy stores. In the patient with advanced cancer, however, a failure to maintain food intake relative to energy expenditure results in a failure to maintain energy homeostasis and is a primary contributor to involuntary weight loss. Reported levels of food intake in weight-losing patients with cancer are often lower than the basal metabolic rate of the same or similar patient populations.[1]

A full understanding of this weight loss is intimately linked to an understanding of the factors coordinating the balance between food intake and energy expenditure. Body weight is controlled by centers in the brain, notably the hypothalamus. Specific hypothalamic nuclei integrate cognitive, visual, taste, and olfactory sensory inputs, as well as peripheral signals indicating the status of physiological reserves of energy and protein in the whole body, the activity of the gastrointestinal tract, and nutrient intake. Three main elements of the appetite regulatory systems are considered here: the hypothalamic control of appetite, the reward pathway, and the sensory inputs that support food intake.

Central regulation of appetite

Food intake is controlled by highly complex processes that reside in the hypothalamus. A group of neuropeptides, systemically generated hormones, and paracrine factors play a critical role in the control of food intake and energy expenditure (Table 13.1). The list of mediators exerting orexigenic and anorexigenic actions in the brain to regulate energy balance has expanded considerably in recent years and has been the subject of many reviews.[2–7] Neuropeptide Y (NPY), Agouti-related protein (AgRP), melanin-concentrating hormone, ghrelin, and the orexins act to stimulate feeding behavior, whereas melanocortin (α- and γ-melanocyte-stimulating hormone), cocaine- and amphetamine-regulated transcript, thyrotropin-releasing hormone, corticotropin-releasing hormone, and urocortin have an inhibitory action. Among the key systemic hormones modulating energy homeostasis are insulin,[8] leptin,[9,10] corticosteroids,[11,12] ghrelin,[13–15] peptide YY, cholecystokinin, and glucagon-like peptide-1. Whereas leptin, insulin, and glucagon-like peptide-1 inhibit feeding, corticosteroids and ghrelin can stimulate feeding. Proinflammatory cytokines, such as interleukin-1β and tumor necrosis factor-α, have been noted to act as central players in appetite inhibition during disease and injury, and it is suggested that these mediators serve to initiate both appetite loss and coordinated mobilization of body energy and protein reserves.[16,17]

Although these many inputs are known to contribute to the regulation of energy balance, it is not fully clear which signals and which brain regions are the most critical. Experiments involving lesions in parts of the brain, especially the hypothalamus, or the injection, overexpression, or genetic ablation of chemical messengers and/or their receptors in the brain, have been used to clarify the participation of individual factors. The integration of the multiple participants in physiological regulation of energy balance is less well understood. The current epidemic of obesity is one motivation for intense research activity in appetite control; however, as a category, syndromes of anorexia (such as cancer anorexia) have not been well investigated.

The primary neurons in the arcuate nucleus of the hypothalamus may be divided into two major categories: (1) neurons that stimulate appetite through secretion of NPY and AgRP; and (2) neurons that depress appetite through secretion of proopiomelanocortin

Cancer Symptom Science: Measurement, Mechanisms, and Management, eds. Charles S. Cleeland, Michael J. Fisch, and Adrian J. Dunn.

Table 13.1. Signaling molecules in appetite regulation: abbreviations and actions

Abbreviation	Molecule name	Effect on feeding
2AG	2-Arachidonylglycerol (endocannabinoid)	+
5-HT	Serotonin	–
AgRP	Agouti-related protein	+
α-MSH	α-melanocyte-stimulating hormone	–
Amylin	Gut peptide	–
Anandamide	*N*-arachidonylethanolamine (endocannabinoid)	+
CART	Cocaine- and amphetamine-regulated transcript	–
CCK	Cholecystokinin	–
Cort	Corticosterone, cortisol (species-dependent)	+
CRF = CRH	Corticotropin-releasing factor	–
DA	Dopamine	+
Gal	Galanin	+
Ghrelin	Natural ligand of GHS-R	+
GHS-R	Growth hormone secretagogue receptor	+
GIP	Gastrin inhibitory peptide	–
GLP-1, GLP-2	Glucagon-like peptide-1 and -2	–
IL-1β	Interleukin-1β proinflammatory cytokine	–
Insulin	Natural ligand of insulin receptor	–
Leptin	Adipocyte-secreted hormone	–
MC4-R	Melanocortin-4 receptor	–
MCH	Melanin-concentrating hormone	+
Norepinephrine	Noradrenaline	+
NPY	Neuropeptide Y	+
OEA	Oleoylethanolamide	–
OX	Orexin A and B	+
POMC	Proopiomelanocortin	–
PYY	Peptide YY–Y2 receptor ligand	–
TNF-α	Tumor necrosis factor proinflammatory cytokine	–
TRH	Thyrotropin-releasing hormone	–
UCN 1, 2, 3	Urocortins 1, 2, 3	–
UCP 1, 2, 3	Uncoupling proteins 1, 2, 3	–
Y1R, Y5R	NPY-1 and NPY-5 receptors	+
Y2R	NPY-2 receptors	–

(POMC). A feeling of hunger can be induced through several mechanisms. Activation of the NPY/AgRP-releasing neurons will increase appetite, as will inhibition of the POMC-releasing neurons. Conversely, inhibition of the NPY/AgRP-secreting cells will dampen appetite, as will activation of the POMC-producing neurons. Overall, these controls appear to be shifted in cancer anorexia, resulting in decreased NPY production and response. NPY and Y(1) receptor immunohistochemistry revealed reduced NPY staining in paraventricular and arcuate nuclei of tumor-bearing and pair-fed rats.[18] Y(1) receptor immunostaining was also reduced in the arcuate nucleus and paraventricular nuclei of tumor-bearing rats, while pair-fed rats exhibited elevated Y(1) R in the paraventricular nuclei. NPY concentrations were decreased in paraventricular nuclei, ventromedial nuclei, and lateral hypothalamic areas in tumor-bearing rats compared with pair-fed controls, and these changes were reversed by tumor resection.[19] These results implicate dysfunction of NPY controls in experimental cancer anorexia and suggest downregulation of Y(1) receptors as well as possible problems in NPY translation.

Stimulation of the hypothalamic melanocortin-4 receptor (MC4-R) produces relative anorexia and increased metabolic rate, even in a relatively starved state. It has been demonstrated that cachexia induced by administration of lipopolysaccharide or interleukin-1β and by tumor growth is blocked by MC4-R blockade.[20,21] MC4-R knockout mice or mice administered the MC4-R antagonist, AgRP, resist tumor-induced loss of lean body mass.[22] The recent advent of nontoxic, orally active, small-molecule MC4-R antagonists that pass the blood–brain barrier has raised the possibility of direct intervention at this level.[23]

Corticosteroids have long been recognized as potent stimuli to food intake.[11,12] The use of synthetic glucocorticoids, such as dexamethasone, to achieve acute increases in food intake is common in the care of patients with advanced cancer who are affected by the most profound anorexia; however, the use of these agents is limited by their ability to directly and markedly favor insulin resistance and visceral fat deposition. They may also act secondarily to suppress inflammatory cytokine production.

Hormones released directly from the digestive system are important regulators, and some of these may have applications in cancer anorexia therapy. Ghrelin, a peptide hormone released by the empty stomach, stimulates appetite by activation of NPY/AgRP-releasing neurons. Ghrelin secretion abruptly stops after food intake. Early evidence suggests that exogenously administered ghrelin or ghrelin-mimetic small molecules may override cancer anorexia in animal models.[24,25]

The neurobiology of appetite in cancer anorexia has been the subject of very little research, and the research that has been conducted remains quite heterogeneous with respect to the animal models used. This paucity of evidence is the principal limitation in the development of therapeutic approaches.

Reward and food intake

Human beings derive pleasure from food properties, particularly the qualities of sweetness and fattiness. A preference for foods with these properties promotes consumption of foods with high energy density, and this is generally understood to have had adaptive value over the course of human evolution. The intrinsic sensory attractiveness of food is mediated by brain pathways referred to as reward pathways. Thus, in addition to the hypothalamic control of appetite, reward systems are also involved in food intake regulation.

Reward pathways promote various types of pleasure and involve particular neurochemical transmitters, including dopamine, endogenous opioids, and cannabinoids, together with their specific receptors. Reward is defined as both *wanting* (motivational) and *liking* (hedonic).[26] *Wanting* is the incentive motivational value of a stimulus, ie, the drive to obtain the reward, whereas *liking* is purely hedonic, ie, the pleasure that is obtained from the reward. The reward pathway is thought to have the capacity to override the homeostatic system for appetite control, generating net energy storage in response to exposure to high-energy-density foods.[26,27] The combination of an environment saturated with high-energy-density foods and the genetic susceptibility of some individuals to food-reward stimuli is an important current theme of obesity research. Conversely, the status of the reward pathway in cancer anorexia is largely unknown, although it has been suggested that stimulating the reward pathway through pleasant and varying visual, textural, gustatory, and olfactory food stimuli or through exogenous agents such as cannabinoids may prove to be effective treatments for cancer anorexia.[28]

The reward system involves several brain regions – the ventral tegmental area, nucleus accumbens, ventral pallidum, and medial prefrontal cortex.[29] These areas of the brain are linked together and to the medial forebrain bundle by synaptically interconnected neurons to form the circuit.[30] Stimulation of the circuit induces pleasure in humans,[29] resulting in increased dopamine levels in the nucleus accumbens.[31] Two types of dopamine receptors (D1-like and D2-like) are involved in mediating the action of rewards.[32]

Both the endogenous opioid and cannabinoid systems are involved in reward. The endogenous opioid system consists of three types of opioid receptors (μ, δ, κ), with the μ-opioid receptor primarily involved in food reward,[30] and several endogenous opioids such as β-endorphin, enkephalin, and dynorphin. Opioid receptors are concentrated in brain areas involved in food intake and reward (eg, the hypothalamus and ventral tegmental area). The endogenous opioid system is directly connected to the dopamine brain reward axis and is more involved in the hedonic aspects of rewards.[27,33] It is of note that chronic stimulation with morphine results in a downregulation of G-coupled proteins involved in reward systems, such as cannabinoid receptors[34]; in cancer patients chronically treated with opioid analgesics, the reward pathway may have a lowered responsiveness as a consequence. We speculate that this is potentially a highly important limitation to reward-based ingestive behavior, but it remains to be tested.

The endocannabinoid system consists of endogenous cannabinoid receptors (CB1, CB2) and their endogenous agonists, such as anandamide. CB1 is found in the hypothalamus, ventral tegmental area, and nucleus accumbens. Cannabinoids increase appetite through activation of the CB1 receptors, which causes increases in NPY.[35] How cannabinoids interact with the reward pathway is not completely understood, although they have been shown to increase dopamine levels in various reward-related areas.[29] Thus, stimulation of the CB1 receptors with either endogenous or exogenous agonists (eg, Δ-9-tetrahydrocannabinol, THC) increases extracellular dopamine levels in the brain, causing a rewarding effect.[36] This increase in dopamine levels can be mitigated with CB1 antagonists (eg, SR141716).[37]

Sensory features, such as sight, texture, taste, and smell, determine the reward value of food.[38] The evaluation of the pleasantness of food takes place in the orbitofrontal cortex (the secondary gustatory cortex).[39] The orbitofrontal cortex is mediated by dopamine levels in the striatum; thus, stimulation of the orbitofrontal cortex increases the desire for food.[40] Overall, the ventral striatum is the interface between taste perception (brainstem visceral taste nuclei and gustatory cortex) and reward-related behavior.[41] Because the taste and smell of food heavily influence the rewarding aspects of eating (ie, the motivation to eat and the liking of food), it seems important that the taste and smell changes commonly experienced by patients with cancer may undermine the pleasure incentives of food. These chemosensory alterations have been noted to decrease the pleasure of eating.[42,43]

Enhanced sensory cues, food variety, or exogenous agents, such as cannabinoids, that activate the reward pathway may be useful approaches to restore the rewarding aspects of food. One way to increase dopamine levels is to consume a variety of foods. The orbitofrontal cortex is responsible for rating the pleasure aspects of food and is involved with sensory-specific satiety. When a food is eaten to satiety, even if it is palatable, it becomes unappealing.[38] In other words, repeated exposure to the same food causes dopamine signals to adapt, resulting in a tolerance to the natural reward similar to the tolerance effect of drugs.[31] Replacing the food item with a different palatable food reinstates reward (ie, increases dopamine levels in the nucleus accumbens) and the pleasure of eating, which may increase overall food intake.[38] Thus, increasing food variety, such as changing the flavor, texture, or even appearance of foods, may increase overall food intake and food enjoyment. Sensory enhancement interventions to promote food intake, such as flavor amplification, have been tried in elderly individuals with some success.[44,45]

Stimulating the reward pathway with exogenous cannabinoids is also a plausible approach. Cannabinoids increase the motivation to eat and increase sensitivity to the sensory properties of foods, creating a preference for highly palatable foods even when satiated.[46,47] In animals, cannabinoids increased the pleasantness of sucrose solutions and decreased the aversiveness of bitter solutions.[48] Cannabinoids have been shown to increase food intake in healthy[49–51] and AIDS[52] populations, but their effectiveness in cancer anorexia is limited and controversial.[53–56]

Chemosensory perception of foods

The chemosensory perception of food determines its reward value,[38] the motivation to eat, and the liking of the food. Although all five senses are used in the evaluation of foods, gustation and olfaction collectively result in the perception of food flavor, a defining attribute of "overall unitary perception."[57] Thus chemosensation (combined gustatory and olfactory function) is the usual measure of potential food appreciation. Alterations of these senses decrease food appreciation and reward and interfere with the motivation and continuation of feeding, thus negatively affecting the appetitive systems outlined above.

Knowledge of gustatory and olfactory perception has progressed tremendously in the past decade with advances in genetics, molecular biology, electrophysiology, and brain imaging.[58] Jones et al.[58] present a complex taste-processing model describing more than 40 connections among 20 brain regions, and the complexity of olfactory processing (recognition and discrimination) was recently reviewed by Hatt.[59] The anatomy, neurobiology, and functional measurement of gustation and olfaction are detailed in the second edition of the *Handbook of Olfaction and Gustation*.[60]

Our appreciation of the effect of aging and disease states on olfactory and gustatory processing is also advancing. Declines in both olfactory and gustatory acuity are associated with normal aging.[61] Although the impact on food selection and preference and subsequent nutrient intake is not clear,[61] the simple strategy of flavor enhancement of nutrient-dense foods and the subsequent increase in their consumption has shown physiological benefits and improved nutritional parameters when offered to hospitalized patients with clinical manifestations of malnutrition.[44,62]

Taste and smell alterations are a commonly cited problem in patients with cancer,[63–65] although the specific nature and prevalence of these alterations are unclear.[66] Variously, 15%–100% of patients with cancer are reported to experience taste alterations during the course of their illness.[43,63,67]

The effect of cancer itself (ie, prior to therapy) has received limited attention. Normal taste sensitivity in patients with cancer has been observed using threshold testing and perceived taste intensities.[68] However, self-assessed changes in taste prior to therapy have been reported by patients with advanced-stage cancer of the oropharynx.[69] Pretreatment assessments of chemosensory perception are limited, and a comprehensive approach would be beneficial.

There has been a substantial focus in the literature on chemotherapy and radiation as possible causes of chemosensory alterations. As both gustatory and olfactory cells are regularly replaced throughout the lifespan (every 10 and 30 days, respectively[66]) and chemotherapy and radiotherapy affect the body's cellular regenerative abilities, it is not surprising that chemosensory perception is in some way altered during or after cancer therapy. The impact of radiotherapy on taste function was reviewed by Ruo Redda and Allis.[70] Taste impairment (reduced, altered, or lost) occurs a few weeks after radiotherapy begins and persists for six months to one year. Radiation dose, fraction size, volume of irradiated tissue, and technique affect the extent of damage to the oral mucosa and taste buds. In particular, loss of both bitter and salty taste perception was noted. Taste impairment clusters with other radiation-induced symptoms (xerostomia, dysphagia, mucositis), which may also affect sensation and hedonic aspects.[70] For example, thickened saliva may prevent tastants from being diluted and reaching receptors.[69,71]

The effects of chemotherapy on chemosensory perception appear to be less extensively studied than the effects of radiation. Because a variety of drugs pass into saliva and can be tasted or smelled when they reach the appropriate receptors,[66] chemotherapeutic agents may be responsible for a variety of unpleasant tastes and smells during treatment. Some drugs are known to generate a bitter background taste and cisplatin therapy results in a persistent metallic taste,[66] either of which would alter the perceived taste of food. Chemotherapy has been associated with higher recognition thresholds for bitter taste, higher detection thresholds, and taste recognition errors.[72,73] Berteretche et al.[72] suggested that chemotherapy decreases the regeneration of taste cells, resulting in decreased taste sensitivity overall, and that the postchemotherapy synchronous regeneration of many taste cells and their mapping to nerve fibers may alter taste coding.

It should be noted that there are important questions relating to the reliability and validity of the various techniques used to profile taste loss, and that some of the methods may not accurately describe the dysfunction. This may be one reason that attempts to define the exact nature of the chemosensory alterations have been inconclusive. Recognition thresholds of the basic tastes have been most frequently measured as an indicator of functional competence, and both increased and decreased thresholds, as well as no difference in control participants, have been mentioned. Attempts to define the olfactory capabilities of patients with cancer are more recent, and these, too, have yielded inconsistent results. Factors contributing to this variability in perception likely include the variety of chemosensory measurement techniques used (eg, whole-mouth threshold testing is a better choice than the once-standard three-drop stimulus technique), the multiplicity of tumor types and their treatments, and the assessment of perception at a variety of points in time relative to treatment. Further, unrecorded or unrecognized factors that contribute to chemosensory alterations (eg, history of smoking, drugs used in treatment of comorbid conditions) may also account for variation within a study population.

The utility of threshold measurements is debated in the field of sensory science. There is great appeal in using physical intensity units to describe psychophysical perception because this gives the researcher the feel of objectivity, yet variability within a population and in individual perception diminishes the "absolutivity" of measured thresholds, and in any case thresholds may best be described by ranges rather than a single concentration.[74] Bartoshuk[75] suggests that the perceived intensity of a taste is a more useful measure of taste function than a recognition threshold, as the ability to identify a taste at its lowest concentration does not predict or relate to perception of a tastant at high concentrations. Thus, although our clinically evaluative techniques are improving in their reliability and validity and may serve to describe the chemosensory abilities of cancer populations relative to other populations or controls, they may not provide insight into "the lived experience" of distorted chemosensory perception.

The most relevant evaluations of real-life chemosensory perception that affects food selection are those made by the patients themselves. Self-assessment allows for enhanced description and appreciation of the type and severity of the chemosensory alteration and can provide insight into the effect of chemosensory changes on food intake and food enjoyment. A variety of chemosensory self-assessment tools and their application are reported in the literature. Huldij et al.[42] presented 108 cancer patients (30 females with endometrial or cervical cancer, 52 males with bladder or prostate cancer, 28 patients with lymphoma) with a questionnaire evaluating their appreciation of the four basic tastes and 31 food items. Bitter taste was increasingly disliked after seven weeks of cancer therapy, whereas no significant change occurred in appreciation of the other tastes. The participants demonstrated various patterns of food appreciation over time and relative to tumor type.

Hutton et al.[43] used a tool previously validated in patients with AIDS-related cachexia to score chemosensory complaints in patients with advanced cancer. A unique feature of this tool is that participants can rate their sense of both taste and smell as being reduced, the same, or heightened relative to the onset of their disease. This aspect allowed these authors to observe that chemosensory complaints were often of heightened or distorted acuity.[43] In particular, increased olfactory sensitivity and enhanced salt perception were mentioned by participants. Few instances of abnormally acute olfactory function (hyperosmia) are documented in the literature (eg, pregnancy, migraine onset, multiple-chemical intolerance).[76] Altered chemosensory perception in patients with advanced cancer is thus very different from the changes observed with aging and other illnesses (eg, Alzheimer's disease, liver diseases) in which chemosensory sensitivity is reduced.[77]

Chemotherapy-induced alterations in taste and smell can cause food preference changes and food aversions, which are likely to produce a decrease in food intake and loss of food enjoyment. A heightened sensitivity to odors in patients undergoing chemotherapy has been observed to result in nausea and vomiting when food odors are introduced, which in turn results in lack of appetite and conditioned taste aversions.[66] Some researchers suggest that taste aversions can be particularly detrimental if the food or beverage is a favorite or makes an important nutrient contribution to the patient's diet,[75,78] whereas Mattes et al.[79] conclude that posttherapy food aversions are of limited clinical significance. Skolin et al.[73] noted that pediatric patients receiving chemotherapy and their parents both indicated that altered taste perception was the cause of reduced food intake.

Hutton et al.[43] demonstrated that patients with advanced cancer who experienced a greater number and severity of chemosensory complaints had nutrient intakes reduced by nearly 900 kcal/day compared with similar patients lacking chemosensory alterations. Although a clear causal link will be difficult to establish, it seems likely that altered sensation is an important contributor to altered food intake in patients with cancer.

Conclusions

Food intake regulation is a complex process involving various systems of the hypothalamus and reward centers, as well as sensory inputs. These systems work synergistically, enabling healthy individuals to maintain energy balance by sustaining an appropriate level of food intake. Any alteration of these systems or their interactions can cause weight loss or weight gain. In cancer, the mobilization of fat and muscle, combined with a disproportion of anorexic to orexigenic signals, paints a complicated picture of energy homeostasis, one that has yet to be fully understood. Further, the aberrant chemosensations experienced by most patients with cancer hinder the motivation and incentive to eat by dampening food-related reward. Together, the multitude of food-intake-related problems in cancer is complex and difficult to treat, and thus a multidimensional approach is required to effectively halt or reverse cancer-induced anorexia. Research and palliation of chemosensory alterations in cancer is scant, regardless of their impact on food enjoyment, reward, and quality of life. Future research should aim to integrate appetite, reward, and sensory systems in the investigation and palliation of cancer-induced anorexia.

References

1. Hutton JL, Martin L, Field CJ, et al. Dietary patterns in patients with advanced cancer: implications for anorexia-cachexia therapy. *Am J Clin Nutr* **84**(5):1163–1170, 2006.
2. Cone RD. The central melanocortin system and energy homeostasis. *Trends Endocrinol Metab* **10**(6):211–216, 1999.
3. Elmquist JK. Anatomic basis of leptin action in the hypothalamus. *Front Horm Res* **26**:21–41, 2000.
4. Schwartz MW, Woods SC, Porte D, Jr., Seeley RJ, Baskin DG. Central nervous system control of food intake. *Nature* **404**(6778):661–671, 2000.
5. Sleeman MW, Anderson KD, Lambert PD, Yancopoulos GD, Wiegand SJ. The ciliary neurotrophic factor and its receptor, CNTFR alpha. *Pharm Acta Helv* **74**(2–3):265–272, 2000.
6. Williams G, Harrold JA, Cutler DJ. The hypothalamus and the regulation of energy homeostasis: lifting the lid on a black box. *Proc Nutr Soc* **59**(3):385–396, 2000.
7. Woods SC, Schwartz MW, Baskin DG, Seeley RJ. Food intake and the regulation of body weight. *Annu Rev Psychol* **51**:255–277, 2000.
8. Schwartz MW, Figlewicz DP, Baskin DG, Woods SC, Porte D, Jr. Insulin in the brain: a hormonal regulator of energy balance. *Endocr Rev* **13**(3):387–414, 1992.
9. Ahima RS, Flier JS. Leptin. *Annu Rev Physiol* **62**:413–437, 2000.
10. Friedman JM, Halaas JL. Leptin and the regulation of body weight in mammals. *Nature* **395**(6704):763–770, 1998.
11. Cabanac M, Richard D. The nature of the ponderostat: Hervey's hypothesis revived. *Appetite* **26**(1):45–54, 1996.
12. Dallman MF, Akana SF, Strack AM, Hanson ES, Sebastian RJ. The neural network that regulates energy balance is responsive to glucocorticoids and insulin and also regulates HPA axis responsivity at a site proximal to CRF neurons. *Ann N Y Acad Sci* **771**:730–742, 1995.
13. Kojima M, Hosoda H, Date Y, Nakazato M, Matsuo H, Kangawa K. Ghrelin is a growth-hormone-releasing acylated peptide from stomach. *Nature* **402**(6762): 656–660, 1999.
14. Nakazato M, Murakami N, Date Y, et al. A role for ghrelin in the central regulation of feeding. *Nature* **409**(6817):194–198, 2001.
15. Tschöp M, Smiley DL, Heiman ML. Ghrelin induces adiposity in rodents. *Nature* **407**(6806):908–913, 2000.
16. Turrin NP, Ilyin SE, Gayle DA, et al. Interleukin-1beta system in anorectic catabolic tumor-bearing rats. *Curr Opin Clin Nutr Metab Care* **7**(4):419–426, 2004.
17. Tracey KJ, Morgello S, Koplin B, et al. Metabolic effects of cachectin/tumor necrosis factor are modified by site of production: cachectin/tumor necrosis factor-secreting tumor in skeletal muscle induces chronic cachexia, while implantation in brain induces predominantly acute anorexia. *J Clin Invest* **86**(6): 2014–2024, 1990.
18. Chance WT, Xiao C, Dayal R, Sheriff S. Alteration of NPY and Y1 receptor in dorsomedial and ventromedial areas of hypothalamus in anorectic tumor-bearing rats. *Peptides* **28**(2):295–301, 2007.
19. Ramos EJ, Suzuki S, Meguid MM, et al. Changes in hypothalamic neuropeptide Y and monoaminergic system in tumor-bearing rats: pre- and post-tumor resection and at death. *Surgery* **136**(2):270–276, 2004.
20. Marks DL, Ling N, Cone RD. Role of the central melanocortin system in cachexia. *Cancer Res* **61**(4):1432–1438, 2001.
21. Marks DL, Butler AA, Turner R, Brookhart G, Cone RD. Differential role of melanocortin receptor subtypes in cachexia. *Endocrinology* **144**(4):1513–1523, 2003.
22. Whitaker KW, Reyes TM. Central blockade of melanocortin receptors attenuates the metabolic and locomotor responses to peripheral interleukin-1beta administration. *Neuropharmacology* **54**(3):509–520, 2008.
23. Chen C, Jiang W, Tucci F, et al. Discovery of 1-[2-[(1S)-(3-dimethylaminopropionyl)amino-2-methylpropyl]-4-methylphenyl] -4-[(2R)-methyl-3-(4-chlorophenyl)-propionyl]piperazine as an orally active antagonist of the melanocortin-4 receptor for the potential treatment of cachexia. *J Med Chem* **50**(22): 5249–5252, 2007.
24. Wang W, Andersson M, Iresjö BM, Lönnroth C, Lundholm K. Effects of ghrelin on anorexia in tumor-bearing mice with eicosanoid-related cachexia. *Int J Oncol* **28**(6):1393–1400, 2006.
25. DeBoer MD, Zhu XX, Levasseur P, et al. Ghrelin treatment causes increased food intake and retention of lean body mass in a rat model of cancer cachexia. *Endocrinology* **148**(6):3004–3012, 2007.

26. Kelley AE, Baldo BA, Pratt WE. A proposed hypothalamic-thalamic-striatal axis for the integration of energy balance, arousal, and food reward. *J Comp Neurol* **493**(1):72–85, 2005.

27. Berridge KC. Motivation concepts in behavioral neuroscience. *Physiol Behav* **81**(2):179–209, 2004.

28. Brisbois TD, Hutton JL, Baracos VE, Wismer WV. Taste and smell abnormalities as an independent cause of failure of food intake in patients with advanced cancer – an argument for the application of sensory science. *J Palliat Care* **22**(2):111–114, 2006.

29. Gardner EL. Addictive potential of cannabinoids: the underlying neurobiology. *Chem Phys Lipids* **121**(1–2): 267–290, 2002.

30. Cota D, Tschöp MH, Horvath TL, Levine AS. Cannabinoids, opioids and eating behavior: the molecular face of hedonism? *Brain Res Rev* **51**(1):85–107, 2006.

31. Spanagel R, Weiss F. The dopamine hypothesis of reward: past and current status. *Trends Neurosci* **22**(11):521–527, 1999.

32. Epstein LH, Leddy JJ. Food reinforcement. *Appetite* **46**(1):22–25, 2006.

33. van den Bos R, de Ridder D. Evolved to satisfy our immediate needs: self-control and the rewarding properties of food. *Appetite* **47**(1):24–29, 2006.

34. Manzanares J, Corchero J, Romero J, Fernández-Ruiz JJ, Ramos JA, Fuentes JA. Pharmacological and biochemical interactions between opioids and cannabinoids. *Trends Pharmacol Sci* **20**(7):287–294, 1999.

35. Kirkham TC. Endocannabinoids in the regulation of appetite and body weight. *Behav Pharmacol* **16**(5–6): 297–313, 2005.

36. Lupica CR, Riegel AC, Hoffman AF. Marijuana and cannabinoid regulation of brain reward circuits. *Br J Pharmacol* **143**(2):227–234, 2004.

37. Tanda G, Pontieri FE, Di Chiara G. Cannabinoid and heroin activation of mesolimbic dopamine transmission by a common mu1 opioid receptor mechanism. *Science* **276**(5321):2048–2050, 1997.

38. Rolls ET. Taste, olfactory, and food texture processing in the brain, and the control of food intake. *Physiol Behav* **85**(1):45–56, 2005.

39. Cooper SJ. Endocannabinoids and food consumption: comparisons with benzodiazepine and opioid palatability-dependent appetite. *Eur J Pharmacol* **500**(1–3):37–49, 2004.

40. Wang GJ, Volkow ND, Telang F, et al. Exposure to appetitive food stimuli markedly activates the human brain. *Neuroimage* **21**(4):1790–1797, 2004.

41. Kelley AE, Bakshi VP, Haber SN, Steininger TL, Will MJ, Zhang M. Opioid modulation of taste hedonics within the ventral striatum. *Physiol Behav* **76**(3):365–377, 2002.

42. Huldij A, Giesbers A, Klein Poelhuis EH, Hart AA, Hulshof KF, Bruning PF. Alterations in taste appreciation in cancer patients during treatment. *Cancer Nurs* **9**(1):38–42, 1986.

43. Hutton JL, Baracos VE, Wismer WV. Chemosensory dysfunction is a primary factor in the evolution of declining nutritional status and quality of life in patients with advanced cancer. *J Pain Symptom Manage* **33**(2):156–165, 2007.

44. Schiffman SS. Intensification of sensory properties of foods for the elderly. *J Nutr* **130**(4S Suppl):927S–930S, 2000.

45. Schiffman SS. Taste and smell losses in normal aging and disease. *JAMA* **278**(16):1357–1362, 1997.

46. Williams CM, Rogers PJ, Kirkham TC. Hyperphagia in pre-fed rats following oral delta9-THC. *Physiol Behav* **65**(2):343–346, 1998.

47. Fride E, Bregman T, Kirkham TC. Endocannabinoids and food intake: newborn suckling and appetite regulation in adulthood. *Exp Biol Med (Maywood)* **230**(4):225–234, 2005.

48. Jarrett MM, Limebeer CL, Parker LA. Effect of Delta9-tetrahydrocannabinol on sucrose palatability as measured by the taste reactivity test. *Physiol Behav* **86**(4):475–479, 2005.

49. Mattes RD, Engelman K, Shaw LM, Elsohly MA. Cannabinoids and appetite stimulation. *Pharmacol Biochem Behav* **49**(1):187–195, 1994.

50. Foltin RW, Fischman MW, Byrne MF. Effects of smoked marijuana on food intake and body weight of humans living in a residential laboratory. *Appetite* **11**(1):1–14, 1988.

51. Greenberg I, Kuehnle J, Mendelson JH, Bernstein JG. Effects of marihuana use on body weight and caloric intake in humans. *Psychopharmacology (Berl)* **49**(1): 79–84, 1976.

52. Beal JE, Olson R, Laubenstein L, et al. Dronabinol as a treatment for anorexia associated with weight loss in patients with AIDS. *J Pain Symptom Manage* **10**(2):89–97, 1995.

53. Nelson K, Walsh D, Deeter P, Sheehan F. A phase II study of delta-9-tetrahydrocannabinol for appetite stimulation in cancer-associated anorexia. *J Palliat Care* **10**(1):14–18, 1994.

54. Jatoi A, Windschitl HE, Loprinzi CL, et al. Dronabinol versus megestrol acetate versus combination therapy for cancer-associated anorexia: a North Central Cancer Treatment Group study. *J Clin Oncol* **20**(2): 567–573, 2002.

55. Strasser F, Luftner D, Possinger K, et al. Comparison of orally administered cannabis extract and delta-9-tetrahydrocannabinol in treating patients with cancer-related anorexia-cachexia syndrome: a multicenter, phase III, randomized, double-blind, placebo-controlled clinical trial from the Cannabis-In-Cachexia-Study-Group. *J Clin Oncol* **24**(21):3394–3400, 2006.
56. Regelson W, Butler JR, Schulz J. Delta-9-tetrahydrocannabinol as an effective antidepressant and appetite-stimulating agent in advanced cancer patients. In: Braude MC, Szara SI, National Institute on Drug Abuse, eds. *Pharmacology of marihuana: a monograph of the National Institute on Drug Abuse.* New York: Raven Press, 1976:163–173.
57. Small DM, Prescott J. Odor/taste integration and the perception of flavor. *Exp Brain Res* **166**(3–4):345–357, 2005.
58. Jones LM, Fontanini A, Katz DB. Gustatory processing: a dynamic systems approach. *Curr Opin Neurobiol* **16**(4):420–428, 2006.
59. Hatt H. Molecular and cellular basis of human olfaction. *Chem Biodivers* **1**(12):1857–1869, 2004.
60. Doty RL. *Handbook of Olfaction and Gustation*, 2nd ed. New York: Marcel Dekker, 2003.
61. Rolls BJ. Do chemosensory changes influence food intake in the elderly? *Physiol Behav* **66**(2):193–197, 1999.
62. Schiffman SS. Sensory enhancement of foods for the elderly with monosodium glutamate and flavors. *Food Rev Int* **14**(2–3):321–333, 1998.
63. Ravasco P. Aspects of taste and compliance in patients with cancer. *Eur J Oncol Nurs* **9**(Suppl 2):S84–S91, 2005.
64. Sherry VW. Taste alterations among patients with cancer. *Clin J Oncol Nurs* **6**(2):73–77, 2002.
65. Grant M, Kravits K. Symptoms and their impact on nutrition. *Semin Oncol Nurs* **16**(2):113–121, 2000.
66. Comeau TB, Epstein JB, Migas C. Taste and smell dysfunction in patients receiving chemotherapy: a review of current knowledge. *Support Care Cancer* **9**(8):575–580, 2001.
67. Dewys WD, Begg C, Lavin PT, et al. Prognostic effect of weight loss prior to chemotherapy in cancer patients. Eastern Cooperative Oncology Group. *Am J Med* **69**(4):491–497, 1980.
68. Trant AS, Serin J, Douglass HO. Is taste related to anorexia in cancer patients? *Am J Clin Nutr* **36**(1):45–58, 1982.
69. Logemann JA, Smith CH, Pauloski BR, et al. Effects of xerostomia on perception and performance of swallow function. *Head Neck* **23**(4):317–321, 2001.
70. Ruo Redda MG, Allis S. Radiotherapy-induced taste impairment. *Cancer Treat Rev* **32**(7):541–547, 2006.
71. Wickham RS, Rehwaldt M, Kefer C, et al. Taste changes experienced by patients receiving chemotherapy. *Oncol Nurs Forum* **26**(4):697–706, 1999.
72. Berteretche MV, Dalix AM, d'Ornano AM, Bellisle F, Khayat D, Faurion A. Decreased taste sensitivity in cancer patients under chemotherapy. *Support Care Cancer* **12**(8):571–576, 2004.
73. Skolin I, Wahlin YB, Broman DA, Koivisto Hursti UK, Vikström Larsson M, Hernell O. Altered food intake and taste perception in children with cancer after start of chemotherapy: perspectives of children, parents and nurses. *Support Care Cancer* **14**(4):369–378, 2006.
74. Lawless HT, Heymann H. *Sensory Evaluation of Food: Principles and Practices.* New York: Chapman & Hall, 1998.
75. Bartoshuk LM. Chemosensory alterations and cancer therapies. *NCI Monogr* **9**:179–184, 1990.
76. Miller CS. Multiple chemical intolerance, 2nd ed. In: Doty RL, ed. *Handbook of Olfaction and Gustation.* New York: Marcel Dekker, 2003:871–908. Neurological disease and therapy; vol. 32.
77. Mattes RD. Nutritional implications of taste and smell. In: Doty RL, ed. *Handbook of Olfaction and Gustation*, 2nd ed. New York: Marcel Dekker, 2003:1446–1481. Neurological disease and therapy; vol. 32.
78. Karlin D. Anorexia and taste abnormalities in cancer patients. *Med Times* **111**(1):71–78, 1983.
79. Mattes RD, Curran WJ, Jr., Powlis W, Whittington R. A descriptive study of learned food aversions in radiotherapy patients. *Physiol Behav* **50**(6):1103–1109, 1991.

Section 2 Chapter 14

Cancer Symptom Mechanisms and Models: Clinical and Basic Science

Sleep and its disorders: clinical science

Lianqi Liu and Sonia Ancoli-Israel

Sleep disturbances are common in patients with cancer[1] yet are often neglected.[2] Most of the sleep studies conducted in patients with cancer have been related almost exclusively to insomnia; other kinds of sleep disturbances – for example, sleep-disordered breathing[3] and periodic limb movement[4] – have rarely been studied in relation to cancer. Systematic research into other sleep disorders commonly seen in the general population, such as circadian-rhythm disturbances and restless legs syndrome, is rare in patients with cancer.

To understand the relationship between sleep disorders and cancer, one must first have a general understanding of the various sleep disorders. The sleep disorders most common in patients with cancer are insomnias, sleep-related breathing disorders, sleep-related movement disorders, and circadian-rhythm sleep disorders. In this chapter we present a brief introduction of several of these relatively common sleep problems, followed by discussion of the prevalence, possible reasons, and treatment of sleep disturbance in cancer and a consideration of future research and treatment directions.

Common sleep disorders

Insomnia

Insomnia is defined as difficulty with sleep initiation or maintenance that (1) occurs despite adequate time and opportunity for sleep, and (2) results in some form of daytime impairment, such as clinically significant distress, fatigue, or impairment in social, occupational, or other important areas of functioning. Insomnia can be divided into two types of complaints, depending upon the duration of the sleep difficulty. Acute (short-term, transient) insomnia has a short duration, typically lasting a few days to a few weeks, and generally improves without intervention or with short-term therapy. Chronic insomnia lasts at least one month, is usually comorbid with other conditions, and has a serious impact on daily functioning. These daytime dysfunctions include fatigue, difficulty with memory and concentration, decreased vigilance, increased functional impairment, decreased quality of life, increased risk of future psychiatric disorders, and increased health care costs.[5]

Sleep-related breathing disorders

Sleep-disordered breathing is a condition characterized by repeated episodes of breathing cessation during sleep that last 10 seconds or longer. These interruptions in breathing can be complete (apneas) or partial (hypopneas). The Respiratory Disturbance Index, also called the Apnea-Hypopnea Index, is the number of breathing interruptions per hour of sleep and represents a measure of severity of sleep-disordered breathing. A Respiratory Disturbance Index or Apnea-Hypopnea Index of 10 or higher is generally considered clinically relevant and pathological.

Apneas can be obstructive, central, or mixed. Obstructive apneas are caused by an anatomical collapse (obstruction) of the upper airway. Persons with obstructive sleep apnea cannot breathe despite efforts to do so, which frequently results in choking and panting sounds and loud snoring (often reported by frustrated bed partners). In contrast, central apneas result from failure of the brain to appropriately regulate the breathing process at the central nervous system level. People with central apneas do not even attempt to breathe, but simply stop breathing until the apneic event is over. Mixed apneas are a combination of central and obstructive apnea, beginning with a central component and ending with an obstructive component. The apneic events can occur in any stage of sleep, but tend to occur primarily in stage 1, 2, or rapid-eye-movement (REM) sleep and tend to be longer and more severe in REM sleep. The supine position during sleep can aggravate the apnea (positional apnea), most likely due to gravity pulling the

Cancer Symptom Science: Measurement, Mechanisms, and Management, eds. Charles S. Cleeland, Michael J. Fisch, and Adrian J. Dunn.

tongue back toward the anterior oropharynx, thus hindering the flow of air.

Each apneic episode disrupts and fragments sleep. It is important to note that more often than not, people with sleep-disordered breathing do not remember waking up during the night, most likely because the arousals are very brief. Hypoxia, excessive daytime sleepiness, and impaired cognitive and memory functioning are additional consequences of both the sleep fragmentation and the hypoxia associated with sleep-disordered breathing. People with this condition are at greater risk for hypertension and cardiovascular disease.

Sleep-related movement disorders

Periodic limb movements in sleep (PLMS) and restless legs syndrome are the two most common types of sleep-related movement disorders in adults. PLMS is a condition characterized by involuntary jerking or kicking of the limbs, most often the legs, during sleep. The movements are repetitive, typically occurring in clustered episodes that last between 0.5 and 5.0 seconds, repeating every 20–40 seconds. PLMS are often associated with arousals. The Periodic Limb Movements in Sleep Index is a measure of the number of jerks per hour of sleep, each causing an arousal, and represents a measure of the severity of the condition. A Periodic Limb Movements in Sleep Index of 5 or more is considered clinically significant. The presence of PLMS can be confirmed only with an overnight sleep study.

In addition to causing complaints of insomnia at night, PLMS can so thoroughly disrupt sleep that it produces fatigue and sleepiness during the day (eg, excessive daytime sleepiness). As is true for sleep-disordered breathing, the awakenings associated with PLMS are often not remembered. Therefore, people with PLMS are frequently unaware of their poor sleep quality. Some may also suffer from other sleep disturbances, such as sleep-disordered breathing and REM sleep behavior disorder.

Restless legs syndrome is characterized by unpleasant creeping-crawling and sometimes painful sensations in the legs that are associated with uncontrollable leg movements during a resting, but awake, state. The symptoms disturb the person's ability to go to sleep or return to sleep after an awakening, thus significantly affecting sleep quality and quantity. Many people with restless legs syndrome also suffer from PLMS, making their sleep even worse. A diagnosis of restless legs syndrome is based on a history of difficulty keeping the legs still in quiet, relaxed situations.

Circadian-rhythm sleep disorders

Circadian rhythms are important biological regulators in all mammals. Hormone secretion, body temperature, and sleep–wake cycles are examples of the many physiological systems that fluctuate routinely within 24-hour intervals. Studies have shown that in humans, the sleep–wake cycle is regulated by the combined effect of (1) an endogenous pacemaker situated in neurons of the suprachiasmatic nucleus in the central nervous system, and (2) various exogenous and environmental stimuli (zeitgebers), such as amount of light exposure, food intake, and time spent awake.

Delayed sleep-phase syndrome and advanced sleep-phase syndrome are the two most common circadian-rhythm sleep disorders. Delayed sleep-phase syndrome is characterized by very late habitual sleep–wake times, whereas advanced sleep-phase syndrome is characterized by very early habitual sleep–wake times. The delay and advance are typically greater than two hours relative to conventional or socially acceptable bed times and arising times. People affected by delayed sleep-phase syndrome complain of difficulty falling asleep and difficulty waking up at a socially acceptable time, often preferring to sleep from 1:00 AM or 2:00 AM until the late morning hours. Those affected by advanced sleep-phase syndrome complain of sleepiness in the late afternoon or early evening and awakening too early in the morning ("in the middle of the night"). Delayed sleep-phase syndrome is most common in adolescents, whereas advanced sleep-phase syndrome is most common in older adults; however, each condition can be found in all age groups.

Sleep disturbance in cancer

Prevalence

Sleep disturbances are reported among 30%–75% of patients with newly diagnosed or recently treated cancer,[1] a rate that is about two times that of the general population.[6] In a 1979 study, Derogatis et al.[7] found that the most frequent psychotropic medications prescribed for patients with cancer were hypnotics, accounting for 48% of all prescriptions. In the same study, physicians reported that of the 814 prescriptions for hypnotics, 85% were prescribed for sleep, compared with 14% for medical procedures, 1% for nausea and vomiting, 1% for psychological distress,

0% for pain, and 0% for "other." The same results were replicated 10 years later by Stiefel et al.,[8] who reported that 44% of approximately 400 prescriptions written in the clinic for more than 200 consecutive patients with cancer were for hypnotic medications. The patient sample in this particular study encompassed a broad range of cancer diagnoses and disease severities, with the time since diagnosis ranging from 1 to 204 months (mean = 23 months). The large number of prescriptions for hypnotics in these studies indicates that sleeping difficulties are a major problem for patients with cancer.

Surveys have suggested that cancer patients' complaints range from difficulty falling asleep to difficulty staying asleep, with frequent and prolonged nighttime awakenings. Patients reported these complaints both before treatment[9] and during treatment.[10] Anderson et al.,[11] in a comparison of 354 patients with cancer, 72 patients with depression, and 290 nonpatient volunteers, found that 62% of the patients with cancer reported moderate to severe sleep disturbance, whereas only 30% of the volunteers and 53% of the depressed patients reported the same complaint. Studies investigating sleep disturbances among patients with advanced cancer are relatively few; however, one recent study found that 30% of 123 patients with advanced cancer reported sleeping fewer than five hours per night, suggesting significant sleep problems.

Other prevalence studies have relied on surveys of larger samples. Engstrom et al.[10] administered an extensive sleep-specific telephone survey to 150 patients with lung or breast cancer in various stages of a variety of treatments. Of those interviewed, 44% reported a sleep problem in the previous month, but only 17% had communicated the problem to their doctors. In the second phase of the survey, a group of 20 patients with cancer was interviewed, 45% of whom reported a sleep problem in the previous month; half of these rated the sleep problem as moderate, severe, or intolerable. The most frequent type of sleep complaint was awakening during the night, reported by more than 90% of the patients. Approximately 85% complained of sleeping fewer hours than normal, 75% complained of difficulty getting back to sleep, and 39% reported napping at unusual times, such as midmorning and midafternoon.

In a large survey conducted by Davidson et al.[12] among 982 patients with various types of cancer and at different treatment phases, 31% of patients reported insomnia, 28% reported excessive sleepiness, and 41% complained of restless legs. The data also suggested that the prevalence of sleep problems varied among patients according to their cancer type. Patients with lung cancer had the highest or second-highest prevalence of sleep problems in general, whereas patients with breast cancer had a high prevalence of insomnia and fatigue. In another survey,[13] the degree of insomnia was as high in patients with cancer as it was in patients with depression. Savard et al.[4] studied the prevalence of insomnia in 300 women with breast cancer and found that 19% met the diagnostic criteria for insomnia; of these, 95% experienced chronic insomnia. In addition, the investigators found that the onset of insomnia followed the breast cancer diagnosis in 33% of the cases, and that 58% of the patients reported that cancer either caused or aggravated their sleep problems.

The above data help to identify the types of sleep complaints experienced by patients with cancer and suggest that sleep difficulties, particularly insomnia, are a major problem for these patients.

Objective sleep measures

Polysomnography

The gold standard for recording sleep is polysomnography, in which overnight sleep measurements record brain waves, eye movement, muscle tension, and, often, respiration, heart rate, and leg movements. Although not invasive, polysomnography involves the use of electrodes and wire leads and can thus be cumbersome, particularly for patients with cancer who are already fatigued or in pain. Therefore, only a few studies have used polysomnography to study sleep in cancer.

Silberfarb et al.[14] compared polysomnography recordings from patients with lung cancer, patients with breast cancer, otherwise healthy patients with insomnia, and normal volunteers and found that, as expected, the patients with insomnia had the shortest total sleep time of all the groups, followed by the lung cancer patients. Although the patients with lung cancer spent more time in bed than did the patients with breast cancer or the normal controls, they did not sleep more: they had lower sleep efficiency (the percentage of time in bed actually spent asleep) and longer sleep-onset latency (time to fall asleep), and they spent more time awake during the night than the patients with breast cancer or the normal sleepers.

In the same study, none of the patients with cancer were found to have sleep-disordered breathing, but there was a higher preponderance of PLMS in the cancer patients than in controls or insomnia patients. Data from our own studies showed that 36% of women with breast cancer had PLMS.[15] Because PLMS is treatable, these data suggest that it would be important to explore PLMS as a cause of sleep disturbance in patients with cancer.

Savard et al.[16,17] performed polysomnographies in a randomized study of the efficacy of cognitive-behavioral therapy for insomnia in survivors of breast cancer. Hot flashes were found to be associated with sleep disturbances in the patients complaining of insomnia; nights with hot flashes were significantly worse than nights without hot flashes, with increased wake time, lower percentage of stage-2 sleep, and longer REM latency. Because there was no control group in this study, however, it is difficult to determine whether the sleep problems were secondary to hot flashes or to other aspects of breast cancer.

Actigraphy

Because polysomnography can be cumbersome to record, many researchers have turned to actigraphy to study sleep–wake patterns.[18] Actigraphs are small devices, about the size of a large watch and worn on the wrist of the nondominant hand, that record movement via motion-sensitive accelerometers.[18] Special algorithms have been developed to estimate sleep and wake time from the movement, and studies correlating actigraphy and EEG readings suggest high reliability.

Miaskowski and Lee[19] recorded wrist actigraphy over a 48-hour period in 24 patients at various points during radiation therapy for bone metastases. As radiation therapy progressed, subjective sleep complaints increased in concert with the objective actigraphy measurements. Sleep efficiency declined, with frequent urination, rather than pain intensity, reported as the main cause of awakening in the night. The results of a recent pilot study by Payne et al.[20] showed that, compared with healthy controls, patients with breast cancer had significantly shorter total sleep time as estimated from actigraphy.

We conducted a sleep study of 82 women before and during chemotherapy for breast cancer.[21] We collected both objective data (actigraphic sleep measures) and subjective data (patient reports of sleep quality). Subjects reported having sleep difficulties before beginning chemotherapy; at the baseline assessment, the women were asleep on average for 77% of the night (mean = 6.1 hours) and awake for 23% of the night (mean = 1.9 hours). The sleep was intermittent, with a mean duration of 32.4 minutes; bouts of wakefulness lasted 6.3 minutes, on average. During chemotherapy, the percentage of time spent asleep at night dropped from 77% to 74%.

Results from this study also suggested that the disturbed sleep was correlated with fatigue, depressive symptoms, and functional outcome.[21] The causal relationship between sleep and these factors could not be determined from the study data. However, pretreatment sleep disturbance predicted more fatigue, more depressive symptoms, and worse quality of life throughout the chemotherapy.[22]

These data suggest that sleep disturbances in cancer patients may be a result of factors other than chemotherapy, such as the cancer itself or cancer-related symptoms.

Possible reasons for sleep disturbance in cancer

General factors

There are multiple factors related to sleep disruption in patients with cancer. Using Speilman's three-factor model,[23] Savard and Morin[2] summarized insomnia-related factors in cancer into three categories: (1) predisposing factors that increase the individual's general vulnerability to develop insomnia, such as hyperarousability, being female, aging, and a personal or familial history of insomnia; (2) precipitating factors that trigger the onset of sleep disturbances, such as the cancer itself, cancer-related emotional impact and functional loss, and cancer-related treatments, pain, and delirium; and (3) perpetuating factors that contribute to the maintenance of sleep disturbance over time, such as maladaptive sleep behaviors and faulty beliefs and attitudes about sleep. Some of these are discussed below.

Disease-related precipitating factors

Most of the studies on sleep problems in cancer have been conducted in women with breast cancer. The population of women with breast cancer is possibly more prone to insomnia than other cancer populations for various reasons, including disruption of sleep due to increased frequency and severity of the hot flashes associated with sudden menopause secondary to the breast cancer treatment. Other possible factors include depression in response to the breast cancer diagnosis, along with increased anxiety and fatigue levels. In a study of the clinical characteristics, prevalence of, and risk factors for insomnia in 300 patients with breast cancer, Savard et al.[4] found that factors associated with high risk of insomnia included being on sick leave, being unemployed, being a widow, having had a lumpectomy, being on chemotherapy, and having less severe cancer at diagnosis.

Anxiety, depression, confusion, and poor performance status have been reported to be associated with sleep disturbance in patients with advanced cancer. In the large survey of 982 patients with different types of cancer, Davidson et al.[12] found that insomnia-related risk factors included fatigue, age, restless legs, use of sedatives or hypnotic drugs, low or variable mood, unpleasant dreams or dreaming more than usual, various concerns, and recent cancer surgery.

Radiation and chemotherapy are both known to produce sleep disturbances. However, as mentioned above, some studies have shown that sleep disturbances already exist before the start of treatment, lending credence to the thought that poor sleep can be caused by the cancer itself. Cimprich[9] administered self-report items relating to sleep quality, fatigue and distress to patients with breast cancer who had not yet undergone treatment. Insomnia was correlated with high levels of distress and was the most frequent symptom, with 88% of the sample reporting difficulty sleeping. Subjective reports of distress and anxiety were correlated with insomnia, and even before treatment had begun, self-ratings of fatigue and sleep difficulty were high. In patients whose self-ratings of anxiety (as well as anger) were low, levels of insomnia and fatigue were still high. This contrasts with the general notion that disturbed sleep prior to treatment is attributable simply to the increased anxiety and stress accompanying the recent diagnosis of a life-threatening illness.

Physiological and psychological precipitating factors

Pain and psychiatric disorders (eg, depression and anxiety) have also been reported as possible causes of poor sleep and fatigue in cancer,[24] as these factors may work together to induce sleep difficulties. Engstrom et al.[10] posit that pain may be the cause of nocturnal awakenings, but that the return to sleep is prevented by psychological distress. Lewin and Dahl[25] point out that in various medical conditions, the management of pain interrelates with sleep quality in many ways. They theorize that because sleep allows for recovery and repair of tissue and may offer a temporary cessation of the psychological awareness of pain, poor sleep can lead to difficulty managing pain. In this way, a cycle of pain and poor sleep may become self-perpetuating. However, surprisingly few studies support the notion that pain leads to disrupted sleep. Silberfarb et al.[14] compared 32 cancer patients (15 with breast cancer, 17 with lung cancer), 32 age-matched and sex-matched normal volunteers, and 32 patients with insomnia, and found that only the patients with breast cancer complained of pain before bedtime; even so, their sleep quality was not significantly affected. The poor sleep quality of the patients with insomnia or lung cancer was not associated with reports of pain.

Cancer pain is often treated with opioids, a common side effect of which is sedation, yet the relationship between opioid use and sleep has not been well studied. Limited polysomnography data show that opioids decrease REM sleep and slow-wave sleep,[26] suggesting that, rather than improving sleep via their sedative effect, opioids may contribute to the sleep disturbances experienced by cancer patients with chronic pain. In addition, the most serious adverse effect of opioids is respiratory depression, which may exacerbate hypoxemia in individuals with sleep-disordered breathing, leading to more interrupted sleep.

The relationship between sleep disturbance and depressive symptoms in cancer also is not well described. It is known that insomnia is often comorbid with depression, that sleep disturbance is a risk factor for depressive symptoms, and that the amount of insomnia in patients with cancer and patients with depression is equally as high, yet studies have shown that depression and sleep disturbances exist before the start of any cancer treatment.[9,21] This suggests that sleep problems may be independent of these psychological and physiological factors.

It is unknown whether the disruptions in sleep are partially secondary to or cormorbid with pain or secondary to the medications used to counteract the pain, anxiety, or depression. Additional, well-controlled research studies are needed to tease out the answers to these questions.

Biological rhythms

There is growing interest in examining the biological rhythms of patients with cancer. Although circadian rhythms and sleep have been widely studied in healthy individuals and in patients with other illnesses, little is known about the links between these domains in cancer.[27] However, evidence from cancer patients is beginning to show a strong correlation between sleep disturbances and interrupted circadian rhythms. Studies in animals and humans suggest that cancer itself may result from disturbed biological rhythms.[28] The disruptions in biological rhythmicity are relevant to cancer, to the mitotic properties of cancerous cells themselves, to the treatments of cancer and the time of day they are administered, and possibly to the cancer patient's quality of life.

Actigraphy, described above, is a convenient and effective instrument to measure circadian activity rhythms. Mormont et al.[29] used actigraphy to study the circadian rhythms of the rest–activity cycle and of serum cortisol, leukocyte, and neutrophil levels in patients with metastatic colorectal cancer for three consecutive days prior to beginning chronomodulated chemotherapy. Patients with marked activity rhythms (ie, more activity when out of bed than when in bed) had a fivefold higher survival rate at their two-year follow-up than did the patients with less-synchronized rhythms. Patients with marked activity rhythms also had better quality of life and reported significantly less fatigue. Circadian rhythms in activity and in white blood cells were jointly prognostic of response. The authors concluded that the rest–activity cycle can be used to determine prognosis for cancer patients' survival and tumor response.

Our laboratory also used actigraphy to measure circadian activity rhythms and sleep–wake patterns in patients with breast cancer. The circadian rhythms were robust at baseline but desynchronized during the chemotherapy. This desynchronization was correlated with fatigue, low daytime light exposure, and decreased quality of life.[30,31]

Circadian rhythms can influence tissues and cells as well as sleep–wake activity. Certain tumor types appear to undergo mitosis (cell division) at specific times of day. In some cases, tumor-cell mitosis appears to fall out of phase with the patient's rhythms. In other words, there are indications that the tumor as well as the host (ie, the patient) shows signs of abnormal circadian rhythmicity as the disease progresses. This rhythmicity can be used to develop new therapeutic methods, such as chronotherapy.

Chronotherapy involves choosing the timing of administration of a drug to minimize its side effects and maximize therapeutic effects. This approach is possible because both the toxicity and the antitumor activity of cancer drugs are time dependent. Chronotherapy has been extensively studied in cancer by Levi and colleagues,[32] who have shown that it is more effective and has lower toxicity and fewer side effects than regular treatment. Other benefits include improved quality of life and fewer days of hospitalization.[33]

Inflammatory markers

Inflammation is now recognized as a critical component of tumor progression. Secreted by inflammatory leukocytes and some nonleukocytic cells, cytokines are nonantibody polypeptides that act as intercellular mediators. Cytokines are induced not only by infectious agents, but also by cancer cells. Elevated levels of cytokines have been found in the blood, ascites, pleural effusions, and urine of patients with cancer. Recent data suggest that elevated cytokine levels in cancer patients are correlated with circadian parameters.[34] Because cytokines are generally elevated in patients with cancer, they may also play a role in cancer-related sleep disturbance. Clinical and animal studies suggest that cancer-related symptom clusters, such as sleep disturbance, circadian rhythm patterns, pain, fatigue, cognitive dysfunction, and affective symptoms, may share common cytokine-based neuroimmunological mechanisms.[35]

Some inflammatory cytokines, such as interferon (IFN)-α, interleukin (IL)-2, and tumor necrosis factor (TNF)-α, are used in the treatment of patients with particular cancers. Systemic administration of cytokines often leads to development of a condition known as systemic inflammatory response syndrome, which includes lethargy, weakness, malaise, listlessness, inability to concentrate, fatigue, anorexia, fever, and sleep changes.[35] Kelley et al.[36] collectively termed these nonspecific changes "sickness behavior." Sickness behavior is a protective reaction of the central nervous system to the organism itself. Peripherally produced cytokines may affect the central nervous system through transport mechanisms that permit their passage into brain tissue through the blood–brain barrier and by vagal nerve stimulation. They affect skin and core body temperatures through the release of the fever-regulating hormone prostaglandin E2 and by stimulating the synthesis and release of corticotropin-releasing factor in the hypothalamus, which then affects sleep–wake states.[36,37]

The daytime sleepiness and longer sleep times seen in some patients with cancer may be an exaggeration of the physical effects of IL-1 and TNF-α that promote non-REM sleep.[37] In patients with metastatic cancer, significant correlations have been reported between elevated serum cytokines, serum cortisol rhythm and 24-hour rest–activity rhythm, and tumor-related symptoms.[34] This suggests a possible role for cytokines in mediating an array of signals through the hypothalamic-pituitary-adrenal axis or the circadian axis,[34] which consequently affects the sleep–wake cycle and results in sleep disturbances.

Some cytokines have been reported to be directly correlated to sleep disturbances. Excessive daytime sleepiness is associated with elevated plasma cytokines, and sleep deprivation is known to cause elevation of proinflammatory cytokine levels, including IL-6. On the other hand, a good night's sleep, or a daytime nap after one night's sleep loss, can decrease the secretion of IL-6.[38]

Data from our laboratory showed that inflammatory markers such as vascular endothelial growth factor (VEGF) and soluble intercellular adhesion molecule-1 (sICAM-1) were significantly elevated during chemotherapy in patients with breast cancer,[39] and that elevated VEGF levels were associated with poorer sleep during treatment.[40] Using a different approach, Savard et al[41] investigated the relationship between insomnia and the immune system in breast cancer. Preliminary results suggested that immediately after successful treatment of insomnia with cognitive-behavioral therapy, the women had increased levels of IFN-γ secretion activity; at follow-up, they showed increased levels of various immune variables. These results suggest that insomnia and immune regulation are related and that amelioration of insomnia symptoms might boost the immune system.

Sleep disturbances may be a direct result of the cytokines' effect on the brain or a secondary effect of other cytokine-induced sickness behavior, such as fatigue, fever, and disrupted circadian rhythms. Cytokines have been studied widely in patients with cancer, but further research is needed. Additional studies will help us to understand the mechanisms of sleep disturbance and other cancer-related symptoms, and may possibly lead to new treatments for these complaints.

Treatment of sleep disturbance in cancer

Pharmacotherapy

Pharmacological interventions are the most common treatment for sleep disturbances, in both the general population and in patients with cancer. Nonetheless, there is a paucity of studies related to pharmacological interventions for cancer patients. Two recent reviews concluded that there is not sufficient evidence to recommend specific pharmacological interventions for sleep disturbances in cancer patients.[6,42] A recent NIH State-of-the-Science Conference on Insomnia[43] concluded that the newer, shorter-acting benzodiazepine receptor agonists are efficacious in the management of insomnia and that the frequency and severity of associated adverse effects are much lower than those seen with the older, longer-acting benzodiazepines. However, they also concluded that all antidepressants, antihistamines (H1 receptor antagonists), and antipsychotics have potentially significant adverse effects, raising concerns about the risk–benefit ratio. Thus, their use in the treatment of chronic insomnia cannot be recommended. Clinicians need to evaluate the relative effectiveness and side-effect profiles of pharmacological agents, and researchers need to be challenged to evaluate the impact of pharmacological treatment on sleep disturbances among cancer patients.[6]

Nonpharmacotherapy

Many nonpharmacological interventions, such as cognitive-behavioral therapy, have been developed and tested in otherwise healthy people with sleep disturbances. These treatments target the perpetuating factors associated with insomnia. Numerous randomized controlled clinical trials in insomnia among general populations have shown that cognitive-behavioral therapy for insomnia is at least as effective, and may be more effective, than pharmacological treatment.[44] The NIH State-of-the-Science Conference on Insomnia[43] concluded that cognitive-behavioral therapy is as effective as prescription medications for brief treatment of chronic insomnia and that there are indications that the beneficial effects of cognitive-behavioral therapy, in contrast to the effects produced by medications, may last well beyond termination of treatment.

Available data indicate that a potential benefit may exist for selected nonpharmacological interventions and suggest that these interventions should be considered for future clinical trials of sleep disturbance in cancer patients. Two published studies examined the effect of cognitive-behavioral therapy on insomnia in patients with cancer. Quesnel et al.[45] used group cognitive-behavioral therapy in patients with breast cancer and found significant improvements in sleep efficiency, total sleep time, mood, and cognitive aspects of quality of life. Savard et al.[17] conducted a randomized wait-list controlled study of the effects of cognitive-behavioral therapy on insomnia in women with breast cancer. Results suggested that cognitive-behavioral therapy was effective in decreasing sleep complaints and levels of depression and anxiety, and increasing quality of life. Therapeutic effects were maintained at follow-up.

Combination therapies

The combination of pharmacological and nonpharmacological therapies has been studied in noncancer populations,[46] with better short-term improvement found with a combinatorial approach than with each therapy alone. As reviewed by Theobald,[47] treating insomnia in cancer patients with a combination of pharmacological and nonpharmacological modalities may have a positive impact not only on the insomnia itself, but also on related symptoms, including pain, fatigue, and psychological distress. Whereas cognitive-behavioral therapy alone produces better long-term gains than pharmacological interventions alone,[46] it is not often used as an adjunct to pharmacological therapies in clinical practice, as few practitioners are trained in the techniques.[48] Nonetheless, most cognitive-behavioral therapy strategies can easily and effectively be integrated into the cancer-care routine.[2]

Conclusion and future directions

Sleep disturbances are common in patients with cancer, and the causes are multifactorial. More descriptive studies are needed to determine baseline levels of sleep and sleep disturbances in cancer patients. Sleep disturbance may share common cytokine-based neuroimmunological mechanisms with other symptoms, such as pain, fatigue, depression, disturbed circadian rhythms, and cognitive dysfunction. Because of the possible role of cytokines in producing sleep disturbances in patients with cancer, much more needs to be learned about the basic neuroscience of how cytokines act on their receptors in the central nervous system, and on how the intracellular signaling pathways activated by cytokines interact with receptors. Further animal and clinical trials are needed to clarify the cellular and molecular mechanisms of those symptoms, particularly the roles of cytokines.

Pharmacological treatments are the most common interventions for sleep disturbances in cancer patients, yet combined cognitive-behavioral therapy and pharmacotherapy may be more advantageous due to the rapid effect of pharmacological therapy and durability of cognitive-behavioral modification. Nonpharmacological treatments and combined therapeutic methods need to be developed and tested in patients with cancer. The long-term goal of research on sleep disturbance in cancer should be to illuminate approaches that might improve patients' quality of life during treatment and even improve the treatment itself.

References

1. Ancoli-Israel S, Moore P, Jones V. The relationship between fatigue and sleep in cancer patients: a review. *Eur J Cancer Care (Engl)* **10**(4):245–255, 2001.
2. Savard J, Morin CM. Insomnia in the context of cancer: a review of a neglected problem. *J Clin Oncol* **19**(3):895–908, 2001.
3. Nesse W, Hoekema A, Stegenga B, van der Hoeven JH, de Bont LG, Roodenburg JL. Prevalence of obstructive sleep apnoea following head and neck cancer treatment: a cross-sectional study. *Oral Oncol* **42**(1): 108–114, 2006.
4. Savard J, Simard S, Blanchet J, Ivers H, Morin CM. Prevalence, clinical characteristics, and risk factors for insomnia in the context of breast cancer. *Sleep* **24**(5): 583–590, 2001.
5. Ancoli-Israel S. The impact and prevalence of chronic insomnia and other sleep disturbances associated with chronic illness. *Am J Manag Care* **12**(8 Suppl): S221–S229, 2006.
6. Berger AM, Parker KP, Young-McCaughan S, et al. Sleep wake disturbances in people with cancer and their caregivers: state of the science. *Oncol Nurs Forum* **32**(6):E98–126, 2005.
7. Derogatis LR, Feldstein M, Morrow G, et al. A survey of psychotropic drug prescriptions in an oncology population. *Cancer* **44**:1919–1929, 1979.
8. Stiefel FC, Kornblith AB, Holland JC. Changes in the prescription patterns of psychotropic drugs over a 10-year period. *Cancer* **65**:1048–1053, 1990.
9. Cimprich B. Pretreatment symptom distress in women newly diagnosed with breast cancer. *Cancer Nurs* **22**:185–194, 1999.
10. Engstrom CA, Strohl RA, Rose L, Lewandowski L, Stefanek ME. Sleep alterations in cancer patients. *Cancer Nurs* **22**:143–148, 1999.
11. Anderson KO, Getto CJ, Mendoza TR, et al. Fatigue and sleep disturbance in patients with cancer, patients with clinical depression, and community-dwelling adults. *J Pain Symptom Manage* **25**(4):307–318, 2003.

12. Davidson JR, MacLean AW, Brundage MD, Schulze K. Sleep disturbance in cancer patients. *Soc Sci Med* **54**(9):1309–1321, 2002.
13. Holland JC, Plumb M. A comparative study of depressive symptoms in patients with advanced cancer. *Proc Am Assoc Cancer Res* **18**:201, 1977.
14. Silberfarb PM, Hauri PJ, Oxman TE, Schnurr PP. Assessment of sleep in patients with lung cancer and breast cancer. *J Clin Oncol* **11**(5):997–1004, 1993.
15. Ancoli-Israel S. Sleep and fatigue in cancer patients. In: Kryger MH, Roth T, Dement WC, eds. *Principles and Practice of Sleep Medicine*. Philadelphia: W.B. Saunders, 2005:1218–1224.
16. Savard J, Davidson JR, Ivers H, et al. The association between nocturnal hot flashes and sleep in breast cancer survivors. *J Pain Symptom Manage* **27**(6): 513–522, 2004.
17. Savard J, Simard S, Ivers H, Morin CM. Randomized study on the efficacy of cognitive-behavioral therapy for insomnia secondary to breast cancer, part I: sleep and psychological effects. *J Clin Oncol* **23**(25): 6083–6096, 2005.
18. Ancoli-Israel S, Cole R, Alessi CA, Chambers M, Moorcroft WH, Pollak C. The role of actigraphy in the study of sleep and circadian rhythms. *Sleep* **26**(3): 342–392, 2003.
19. Miaskowski C, Lee KA. Pain, fatigue and sleep disturbances in oncology outpatients receiving radiation therapy for bone metastasis: a pilot study. *J Pain Symptom Manage* **17**(5):320–332, 1999.
20. Payne JK, Piper B, Rabinowitz I, Zimmerman B. Biomarkers, fatigue, sleep, and depressive symptoms in women with breast cancer: a pilot study. *Oncol Nurs Forum* **33**(4):775–783, 2006.
21. Ancoli-Israel S, Liu L, Marler M, et al. Fatigue, sleep and circadian rhythms prior to chemotherapy for breast cancer. *Support Care Cancer* **14**(3):201–209, 2006.
22. Liu L, Fiorentino L, Natarajan L, et al. Pre-treatment symptom cluster in breast cancer patients is associated with worse sleep, fatigue and depression during chemotherapy. *Psychooncology:* e-pub ahead of print, 2008.
23. Speilman AJ, Glovinsky PB. Case studies in insomnia. In: Hauri PJ, ed. *The Varied Nature of Insomnia*. New York: Plenum Press, 1991:1–15.
24. Hu D, Silberfarb PM. Management of sleep problems in cancer patients. *Oncology* **5**:23–27, 1991.
25. Lewin DS, Dahl RE. Importance of sleep in the management of pediatric pain. *J Dev Behav Pediatr* **20**(4):244–252, 1999.
26. Dimsdale JE, Norman D, DeJardin D, Wallace MS. The effect of opioids on sleep architecture. *J Clin Sleep Med* **3**(1):33–36, 2007.
27. Lee K, Cho M, Miaskowski C, Dodd M. Impaired sleep and rhythms in persons with cancer. *Sleep Med Rev* **8**(3):199–212, 2004.
28. Moser M, Schaumberger K, Schernhammer E, Stevens RG. Cancer and rhythm. *Cancer Causes Control* **17**(4):483–487, 2006.
29. Mormont MC, Waterhouse J, Bleuzen P, et al. Marked 24-h rest/activity rhythms are associated with better quality of life, better response and longer survival in patients with metastatic colorectal cancer and good performance status. *Clin Cancer Res* **6**:3038–3045, 2000.
30. Liu L, Marler M, Parker BA, et al. The relationship between fatigue and light exposure during chemotherapy. *Support Care Cancer* **13**(12):1010–1017, 2005.
31. Mercadante S, Girelli D, Casuccio A. Sleep disorders in advanced cancer patients: prevalence and factors associated. *Support Care Cancer* **12**(5):355–359, 2004.
32. Lévi F. Chronotherapeutics: the relevance of timing in cancer therapy. *Cancer Causes Control* **17**(4):611–621, 2006.
33. Wood PA, Hrushesky WJM. Circadian rhythms and cancer chemotherapy. *Crit Rev Eukaryot Gene Expr* **6**:299–343, 1996.
34. Rich T, Innominato PF, Boerner J, et al. Elevated serum cytokines correlated with altered behavior, serum cortisol rhythm, and dampened 24-hour rest-activity patterns in patients with metastatic colorectal cancer. *Clin Cancer Res* **11**(5):1757–1764, 2005.
35. Lee BN, Dantzer R, Langley KE, et al. A cytokine-based neuroimmunologic mechanism of cancer-related symptoms. *Neuroimmunomodulation* **11**(5):279–292, 2004.
36. Kelley KW, Bluthé RM, Dantzer R, et al. Cytokine-induced sickness behavior. *Brain Behav Immun* **17**:S112–S118, 2003.
37. Vena C, Parker K, Cunningham M, Clark J, McMillan S. Sleep-wake disturbances in people with cancer part I: an overview of sleep, sleep regulation, and effects of disease and treatment. *Oncol Nurs Forum* **31**(4):735–746, 2004.
38. Vgontzas AN, Pejovic S, Zoumakis E, et al. Daytime napping after a night of sleep loss decreases sleepiness, improves performance, and causes beneficial changes in cortisol and interleukin-6 secretion. *Am J Physiol Endocrinol Metab* **292**(1):E253–E261, 2007.
39. Mills PJ, Parker BA, Jones V, et al. The effects of standard anthracycline-based chemotherapy on soluble ICAM-1 and vascular endothelial growth factor levels in breast cancer. *Clin Cancer Res* **10**(15):4998–5003, 2004.

40. Mills PJ, Parker BA, Dimsdale JE, Sadler GR, Ancoli-Israel S. The relationship between fatigue, quality of life and inflammation during anthracycline-based chemotherapy in breast cancer. *Biol Psychol* **69**(1):85–96, 2005.

41. Savard J, Simard S, Ivers H, Morin CM. Randomized study on the efficacy of cognitive-behavioral therapy for insomnia secondary to breast cancer, part II: immunologic effects. *J Clin Oncol* **23**(25):6097–6106, 2005.

42. Clark J, Cunningham M, McMillan S, Vena C, Parker K. Sleep-wake disturbances in people with cancer part II: evaluating the evidence for clinical decision making. *Oncol Nurs Forum* **31**(4):747–771, 2004.

43. National Institutes of Health. National Institutes of Health State of the Science Conference statement on manifestations and management of chronic insomnia in adults, June 13–15, 2005. *Sleep* **28**(9):1049–1058, 2005.

44. Bastien CH, Morin CM, Ouellet MC, Blais FC, Bouchard S. Cognitive-behavioral therapy for insomnia: comparison of individual therapy, group therapy, and telephone consultations. *J Consult Clin Psychol* **72**(4):653–659, 2004.

45. Quesnel C, Savard J, Simard S, Ivers H, Morin CM. Efficacy of cognitive-behavioral therapy for insomnia in women treated for nonmetastatic breast cancer. *J Consult Clin Psychol* **71**(1):189–200, 2003.

46. Morin CM, Colecchi C, Stone J, Sood R, Brink D. Behavioral and pharmacological therapies for late life insomnia. *JAMA* **281**(11):991–999, 1999.

47. Theobald DE. Cancer pain, fatigue, distress, and insomnia in cancer patients. *Clin Cornerstone* **6**(Suppl 1D):S15–S21, 2004.

48. Cohrs S, Rodenbeck A, Guan Z, et al. Sleep-promoting properties of quetiapine in healthy subjects. *Psychopharmacology (Berl)* **174**(3):421–429, 2004.

Section 2 Chapter 15

Cancer Symptom Mechanisms and Models: Clinical and Basic Science

Sleep and its disorders: basic science

Mark R. Opp and Luca Imeri

Sleep is a fundamental biological process that is as important to survival as are eating and breathing. We now know that adequate sleep is essential for physical and mental health. Yet, the precise functions of sleep – what sleep does for the brain and body – remain elusive. The relationship among cancer, sleep disruption, and sleep disorders is discussed in Chapter 14. The focus of this chapter is basic sleep mechanisms that can lead to cancer-related sleep disturbances, particularly those mechanisms that may be susceptible to perturbation during pathology.

Sleep consists of two major *phases*, rapid-eye-movement (REM) sleep and non-REM (NREM) sleep. In human sleep research and in sleep-disorders medicine, the NREM sleep phase is further subdivided into three stages that may generally be considered to parallel a continuum of sleep depth: stage N1 is the light sleep that follows wakefulness; during stage N2, two electroencephalogram (EEG) features, spindles and K-complexes, are typically found; stage N3 is referred to as slow-wave sleep and is characterized by a preponderance of high-amplitude, low-frequency EEG components. Preclinical sleep researchers generally find it sufficient to define only the two sleep phases, REM sleep and NREM sleep, in laboratory research animals.

Healthy sleep consists of cycles of orderly transitions from wakefulness to NREM sleep to REM sleep. Healthy human adults during the course of a night's sleep will have four to six NREM–REM cycles of about 80–110 minutes duration, whereas rodents will have many NREM–REM cycles, each lasting about 8–10 minutes.

Variations in arousal state are associated with well-defined variations in multiple physiological parameters. Irrespective of whether subjects of sleep studies are humans or animals, the physiological parameters most often recorded include the EEG and one or more of the following: muscle tone (electromyogram), eye movements (electrooculogram), respiration, body movements, and body or brain temperature. Human sleep studies employ multiple surface electrodes to record the EEG, whereas preclinical studies of laboratory animals generally employ surgically implanted electrodes. For most preclinical studies using laboratory animals, recording the EEG and either the electromyogram or body movements provides sufficient information to determine phases of sleep or wakefulness.

Sleep–wake regulatory mechanisms

Systems involved in the regulation of sleep–wake behavior are diffusely distributed throughout the brain. The neurons in the neuroanatomic regions involved in the regulation of sleep contain multiple neurotransmitters. In addition to neurotransmitters, various peptides and hormones act on receptors contained on neurons in brain regions involved in controlling the arousal state. Because the regulation of sleep–wake behavior is complex, a comprehensive review of regulatory mechanisms for sleep–wake behavior is beyond the scope of this chapter. The interested reader is referred to several recent reviews,[1,2] from which much of the following discussion was derived.

In this section, we provide a very brief overview of some of the neuroanatomic regions and neurotransmitter systems involved in regulating sleep–wake behavior. We highlight systems that, as we shall see, are affected by immunomodulators.

Wakefulness

Brainstem aminergic neurons

Wakefulness is directly promoted by noradrenergic neurons of the locus coeruleus and serotonergic neurons of the dorsal raphe nucleus and other midline raphe nuclei. The firing rate of these aminergic neurons is maximal during wakefulness, decreases during NREM sleep, and almost ceases during REM sleep.

Cancer Symptom Science: Measurement, Mechanisms, and Management, eds. Charles S. Cleeland, Michael J. Fisch, and Adrian J. Dunn. Published by Cambridge University Press.

The release of noradrenaline and serotonin (5-hydroxytryptamine [5-HT]) parallels changes in neuronal discharge. Noradrenergic and serotonergic neurons, known because of their pattern of activity as REM-off neurons, project diffusely to the entire central nervous system (CNS) and, in particular, to the cerebral cortex, hippocampus, thalamus, and hypothalamus/basal forebrain. Brainstem aminergic neurons inhibit cholinergic and cholinoceptive neurons in the brainstem that are involved in REM sleep generation. In the basal forebrain, cholinergic neurons are excited by noradrenaline and inhibited by serotonin. As described below, gamma-aminobutyric acid (GABA)ergic neurons in both the locus coeruleus and dorsal raphe nucleus may also inhibit aminergic neurons.

Although experimental and clinical observations show that serotonin directly promotes wakefulness, it also appears to be necessary for the sleep that follows wakefulness. Experimental depletion of brain serotonin has been shown to induce insomnia, and sleep researchers now believe that serotonin may stimulate the synthesis and/or release of yet unidentified sleep factor(s). Serotonin may be necessary for NREM sleep, due to its action in the hypothalamic preoptic area/basal forebrain.

Observations of the effects of serotonergic activation in rats support this dual role for serotonin in sleep regulation. Activity of the serotonergic system may be increased by administering 5-hydroxytryptophan, the direct serotonin precursor. Administration of 5-hydroxytryptophan into rats or mice first enhances wakefulness and then, after a delay, increases NREM sleep.

Experimental and clinical observations suggest that dopamine promotes wakefulness. Dopamine is synthesized primarily by neurons in the substantia nigra and in the ventral tegmental area. Although the firing rate of dopaminergic neurons is generally similar across the various phases of the sleep–wake cycle, dopaminergic neurons active during wakefulness have recently been described in the ventral part of the periaqueductal gray. These neurons could account for the wake-promoting effects of dopamine. Even more recently, dopaminergic REM-active neurons have been described in the ventral tegmental area.

Histamine and hypocretin (also known as orexin) promote wakefulness. Histaminergic neurons in the tuberomammillary nucleus diffusely project to essentially all of the CNS. Histaminergic neurons discharge during wakefulness and are silent during REM sleep. Drugs acting as histamine antagonists (antihistamines) decrease vigilance and increase sleepiness and time spent asleep. Hypocretinergic neurons in the posterior hypothalamus are essential for the maintenance of wakefulness. Loss of hypocretin or mutations of the hypocretin receptor result in symptoms of narcolepsy in animals; similarly, hypocretin neurons appear degenerated in postmortem brain tissue from humans who suffered from narcolepsy.

Brainstem cholinergic nuclei

Brainstem cholinergic neurons involved in arousal-state regulation are localized within the laterodorsal and peduncolopontine tegmental nuclei. In addition to neurons that are active during REM sleep, the laterodorsal and peduncolopontine tegmental nuclei also contain neurons that are active during both wakefulness and REM sleep. These neurons are known as REM-on neurons. They project primarily to the hypothalamus and to both the relay nuclei and the intralaminar and midline nuclei of the thalamus. During wakefulness and REM sleep, elevated acetylcholine release depolarizes thalamic neurons, thus sustaining cortical desynchronization and activation. When acetylcholine release is reduced during NREM sleep, the firing pattern of thalamic neurons changes: bursts of spikes alternate with periods of hyperpolarization. Such a pattern of thalamic activity sustains cortical synchronization. As further described below, laterodorsal and peduncolopontine tegmental nuclei also contain GABAergic neurons, which can inhibit aminergic neurons in the locus coeruleus and dorsal raphe nucleus during REM sleep.

NREM sleep

Systems involved in the promotion of NREM sleep include neurons in the lower brainstem and upper forebrain that inhibit wake-generating neurons. The nucleus of the solitary tract and the anterior hypothalamus-preoptic region contain neurons that discharge at higher rates during NREM sleep. Lesions of the nucleus of the solitary tract reduce NREM sleep, whereas electrical stimulation of this region induces NREM sleep. These neurons project to the forebrain, where they are able to stimulate other systems involved in the promotion of sleep. Lesions of the preoptic area result in insomnia, whereas stimulation of this area elicits sleep. Many of the preoptic-area neurons discharge at higher rates during NREM sleep than during wakefulness. The adjacent basal forebrain also contains neurons that discharge at higher rates during NREM sleep than during wakefulness. Because the preoptic area and basal forebrain also contain neurons that are more active during wakefulness, these brain regions contribute to the regulation of sleep–wake behavior in a complex manner.

Sleep-active neurons in the basal forebrain commonly contain the inhibitory neurotransmitter GABA, although the basal forebrain also contains cholinergic neurons. Sleep-active GABAergic neurons of the basal forebrain are inhibited by noradrenaline released from neurons in the locus coeruleus. Some GABAergic neurons from the basal forebrain project to the cortex and directly promote EEG slow-wave activity, whereas other GABAergic neurons may inhibit cholinergic wake-active neurons within the basal forebrain. Still other GABAergic neurons project to the hypocretinergic, histaminergic, and noradrenergic neurons of the arousal-promoting systems and inhibit their activity.

REM sleep

REM sleep is characterized by cortical activation and peripheral inhibition, an observation leading Jouvet to refer to this phase of sleep as "paradoxical sleep." During REM sleep, the brainstem cholinergic system is active and the cerebral cortex is activated. At the same time, peripheral inhibition manifests as loss of muscle tone. Certain neurons in the pontine tegmentum inhibit postural muscle tone, while other neurons in the lower medullary reticular formation that project to the spinal cord also participate in the motor inhibition characteristic of REM sleep.

Cholinergic neurons within the brainstem laterodorsal and peduncolopontine tegmental nuclei are active during REM sleep (REM-on neurons), whereas their firing rate is very low during wakefulness and NREM sleep. REM-on neurons project mainly to the pontine reticular formation and, in particular, to the oral part of the pontine reticular nucleus, where cholinoceptive neurons activated by acetylcholine are located. Cholinoceptive neurons (which, in part, release glutamate), project back to cholinergic neurons (facilitating their discharge) and project caudally and rostrally to the brain structures responsible for the phasic and tonic events that characterize REM sleep. The physiological increase in acetylcholine release that occurs in the pontine reticular formation during REM sleep can be experimentally mimicked by the local administration into these areas of drugs that activate cholinergic receptors (cholinomimetic drugs). Administration of cholinomimetics into the pontine reticular formation induces REM sleep-like states, whereas administration of cholinergic antagonists inhibits REM sleep. Lesions of the cholinergic neurons in the laterodorsal or peduncolopontine tegmentum nuclei inhibit REM sleep. It has been recently proposed that within the pontine reticular formation, the sublaterodorsal nucleus (also known as the peri-LC-alpha nucleus) may be particularly important for REM sleep generation.

The laterodorsal and peduncolopontine tegmental nuclei also contain GABAergic neurons that inhibit noradrenergic (arousal-promoting) neurons in the locus coeruleus, which must be silent for REM sleep to be manifest. Glycine, another inhibitory neurotransmitter that is contained in neurons of the brainstem and spinal cord, inhibits motor neurons and thus plays a role in the muscle atonia characteristic of REM sleep.

Immunomodulators and sleep regulation

The brain was once considered an immune-privileged site because of its protection by the blood–brain barrier. We now know that many immunomodulatory systems – ligands, receptors, endogenous receptor antagonists, and binding proteins – are present in the normal, healthy brain. Among the immunomodulators implicated in normal physiology in the absence of pathology are members of a class of molecules referred to as cytokines. Cytokines in the brain act on numerous systems to contribute to the regulation of sleep during health and are likely involved in alterations in sleep under pathological conditions.

Historical perspective

Current knowledge of the role played by immunomodulators in sleep regulation grew out of the ancient notion that sleep is regulated by humoral mechanisms (sleep factors). The concept that "vapors" were responsible for sleep induction was prevalent in ancient times and persisted for thousands of years. Renewed interest in "fatigue substances" during the latter part of the nineteenth century led Ishimori in Japan[3] and Legendre and Piéron in France[4] in the early twentieth century to experiment with cerebrospinal fluid extracted from sleep-deprived dogs. The cerebrospinal fluid from the sleep-deprived dogs was injected into rested recipient dogs, inducing a deep sleep that resembled a narcosis. Speaking of these studies, Ishimori wrote, "That the cerebral matter of sleep-deprived animals contains a potent hypnogenic substance which cannot be detected in the brain of normally sleeping animals leads to clarify the cause of induction of our normal sleep A special substance… is gradually produced [during waking]… and induces the so-called state of drowsiness, and finally causes natural sleep."

The work of Ishimori and Legendre and Piéron was largely ignored for many years. Studies conducted in the 1960s by John Pappenheimer at Harvard rekindled interest in humoral factors and sleep, and these studies have had the greatest impact on our current understanding of interactions between sleep and the immune system.[5] Pappenheimer et al. demonstrated that cerebrospinal fluid extracted from sleep-deprived goats induced sleep when injected into rats. It took 15 years for this unknown substance, termed Factor S by Pappenheimer, to be extracted, purified, characterized, and ultimately identified as muramyl peptide. Muramyl peptide was already known to induce the synthesis and secretion of a substance termed lymphocyte-activating factor/endogenous pyrogen, now known as the proinflammatory cytokine interleukin (IL)-1. This link – muramyl peptide (Factor S) inducing the synthesis of IL-1 – provided the impetus for researchers to attempt to discover whether IL-1 possessed sleep-inducing properties. Abstracts and papers published in 1983 and 1984 demonstrated that IL-1 injected intracerebroventricularly into rabbits and rats increased the amount of time spent in NREM sleep, suppressed REM sleep, and altered EEG properties.[6–8]

Cytokines and sleep

Since the early 1980s, numerous cytokines, chemokines (small cytokines that activate and mobilize immune cells throughout the body), and growth factors have been studied with respect to sleep–wake behavior. However, most of our knowledge about the role of cytokines in the regulation and modulation of sleep has been derived from studies of three cytokines: IL-1β (hereafter referred to as IL-1), tumor necrosis factor (TNF)–α (hereafter referred to as TNF), and IL-6. Data derived from electrophysiological, biochemical, and molecular genetic studies indicate a role for IL-1 and TNF in the regulation of spontaneously occurring, physiological NREM sleep, whereas it is likely that IL-6 is a modulator of NREM sleep during chronic pathology. Evidence indicating a role for IL-1, TNF, and IL-6 in the regulation and modulation of sleep–wake behavior has been extensively reviewed.[9–11]

Although electrophysiology studies demonstrate direct, receptor-mediated effects of IL-1 and TNF on neurons in brain regions implicated in the regulation of sleep, most studies on the role of cytokines as regulators of sleep have used biochemical or molecular genetic approaches. Central or peripheral administration of IL-1 or TNF into laboratory animals increases the amount of time spent in NREM sleep. Doses of IL-1 or TNF that are effective in increasing NREM sleep in laboratory studies generally reduce REM sleep. Diurnal changes in IL-1 and TNF mRNA and protein within the laboratory rodent brain parallel the diurnal changes in sleep–wake behavior. Similarly, IL-1–like activity detected in the cerebrospinal fluid of cats is in phase with sleep–wake activity, and human plasma concentrations of IL-1 peak at sleep onset.[11] Mice whose IL-1 or TNF signaling receptors have been genetically ablated spend less time in NREM sleep than do genetically intact control animals.

Substances or manipulations that increase endogenous IL-1 or TNF increase NREM sleep. For example, IL-1 and TNF increase during the course of prolonged wakefulness (sleep deprivation) or in response to mild elevations of ambient temperature; conversely, increases in NREM sleep induced by sleep deprivation or ambient temperature are blocked when IL-1 or TNF receptors are antagonized.

Recent clinical and preclinical studies suggest that IL-6 may be a modulator of sleep during some pathologies characterized by excessive daytime sleepiness, such as insomnia, narcolepsy, sleep apnea, and obesity.[12–15] Although IL-6 does not alter the sleep of laboratory rabbits, when species-specific IL-6 is administered into laboratory rats there are periods during which NREM sleep increases. In contrast to IL-1 or TNF, intracerebroventricular administration of IL-6 does not alter REM sleep in rats. Unlike antagonism of the IL-1 or TNF systems, targeting the rat IL-6 system with monoclonal or polyclonal IL-6 antibodies does not alter any aspect of rat sleep.[16] In addition to studies in rats, experiments using IL-6-deficient (knockout) mice indicate that the rhythms of body temperature and NREM and REM sleep are normal in IL-6 knockout mice and that the amount of time spent in NREM sleep does not differ between the IL-6 knockout mice and C57BL/6J control mice.[17] Collectively, these human, rat, and mouse data suggest that IL-6 may not be involved in the regulation of physiological sleep, but may modulate sleep under conditions in which IL-6 is elevated.

IL-1, TNF, and IL-6, the three cytokines studied most extensively with respect to sleep–wake behavior, are proinflammatory cytokines. Anti-inflammatory cytokines are so called because their actions antagonize many of the effects of proinflammatory cytokines, often by direct inhibition of protein synthesis via interference with signal transduction or transcription. Therefore, it stands to reason that proinflammatory cytokines and anti-inflammatory cytokines would have opposite effects on sleep–wake behavior. This appears to be the case: administration of two anti-inflammatory cytokines, IL-4 and IL-10, into laboratory rats and rabbits reduced the amount of time these animals spent in NREM sleep.[18–20] In addition, mice lacking a functional IL-10 gene spent more time in NREM sleep during the dark period of the light–dark cycle than did genetically intact mice.[21] The increase in the amount of time mice lacking IL-10 spent in NREM sleep during the dark period was presumably due to the fact that IL-10 normally inhibits the synthesis of IL-1.

Other endogenous systems serve to antagonize cytokine actions before they become deleterious to the host. For example, stimuli that increase the production of IL-1 also increase the production of IL-1 receptor antagonist (IL-1RA). IL-1RA binds to the IL-1 type I receptor with approximately the same affinity as IL-1 itself does, thus limiting the effects of IL-1. When administered into laboratory rabbits, IL-1RA transiently reduces NREM sleep.[22] The hypothalamic-pituitary-adrenocortical (HPA) axis, via actions of glucocorticoids, inhibits the synthesis of multiple cytokines in the brain. Components of the HPA axis, such as corticotropin-releasing hormone (CRH),[23] increase wakefulness and reduce spontaneous NREM sleep when administered into laboratory animals. In addition, CRH antagonizes the effects of IL-1 on sleep and temperature regulation.

Rat strains that differ in production of CRH exhibit different responses to IL-1 administration. For example, Fischer 344 rats, which hypersecrete CRH, respond to IL-1 with a CRH surge that is larger than that observed in Lewis rats, which are deficient in CRH production. Lewis rats respond to IL-1 with rapid increases in NREM sleep, whereas Fischer 344 rats respond to the same dose of IL-1 with enhanced wakefulness, after which NREM sleep increases. These differences in response to IL-1 are attributed to differences in CRH secretion, as pretreatment of Fischer 344 rats with the CRH receptor antagonist α-hCRH blocks the IL-1-induced wakefulness normally observed in this rat strain.[23]

Because the HPA axis provides negative feedback inhibition for cytokine synthesis in the brain via actions of corticosteroids, cytokine mRNA and protein in the rodent brain are out of phase with HPA axis activity. That is, when HPA axis activity is high, cytokine mRNA and protein in rodent brain are low. Accordingly, modulating HPA axis activity affects cytokine mRNA and protein in the rodent brain.[24,25] This relationship between HPA axis activity and cytokine mRNA and protein in the rodent brain is of functional consequence to the regulation of physiological sleep. When HPA axis activity in rats is reduced by intracerebroventricular administration of a CRH receptor antagonist prior to the dark period – the time when HPA axis activity would normally be at its highest and when laboratory rodents are most awake – there are increases in NREM sleep and IL-1 mRNA in the brain. Pretreating rats intracerebroventricularly with antibodies directed against IL-1 blocks this increase in NREM sleep after HPA-axis antagonism.[23]

Interactions among immunomodulators and sleep-regulatory mechanisms

As briefly reviewed above, several cytokines are involved in the regulation of sleep. The brain cytokine network is complex, with cytokines exerting effects on each other and on various neuroendocrine, peptide, and neurotransmitter systems. We focus in this section on IL-1 because most studies of the mechanisms mediating cytokine effects on sleep (and specifically those studies investigating a direct action of cytokines on neurons and their neurotransmitters) have been performed using IL-1. Cytokine effects on REM sleep have received little attention; thus, we will focus on interactions relevant to NREM sleep regulation only.

Mechanisms by which IL-1 affects NREM sleep have been investigated at length.[11] Evidence gathered since the mid-1990s shows that IL-1 interactions with the serotonergic system (at the level of both serotonergic cell bodies and serotonergic axon terminals) are essential for the NREM sleep responses to IL-1 to be fully manifest. IL-1 interactions with the GABAergic and cholinergic systems, as they pertain to sleep regulation, have also been investigated.

In addition to direct actions on neurons, it has been proposed that IL-1-induced enhancement of NREM sleep may be mediated by actions on

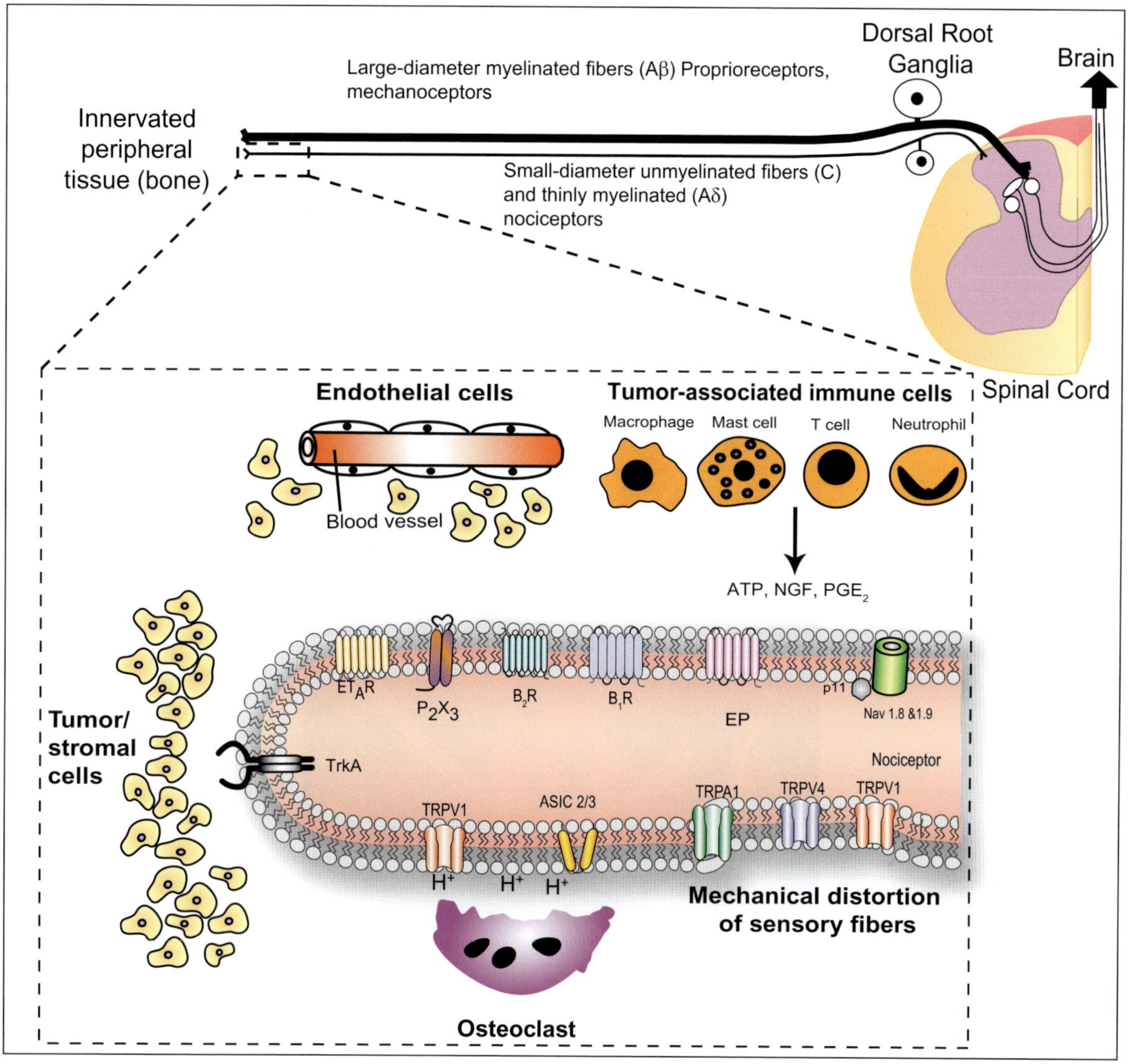

Figure 5.1. Primary afferent sensory nerve fibers involved in generating the cancer pain. Primary afferent neurons innervating the body have their cell bodies in the dorsal root ganglia (DRG) and transmit sensory information from the periphery to the spinal cord and brain. Myelinated A fibers (Aβ) containing large-diameter cell bodies, which project centrally to the dorsal column nuclei and deep spinal cord, are involved in detecting nonnoxious sensations including light touch, vibration, and proprioception. Unmyelinated C fibers and thinly myelinated Aδ fibers contain small-diameter cell bodies which project centrally to the superficial spinal cord. These fibers are involved in detecting multiple noxious stimuli (chemical, thermal, and mechanical). Box: Nociceptors use several different types of receptors to detect and transmit signals about noxious stimuli produced by cancer cells (yellow), tumor-associated immune cells (orange), or other aspects of the tumor microenvironment. Multiple factors may contribute to the pain associated with cancer. The transient receptor potential vanilloid receptor-1 (TRPV1) and acid-sensing ion channels (ASICs) detect extracellular protons produced by tumor-induced tissue damage or abnormal osteoclast-mediated bone resorption. Several mechanosensitive ion channels may be involved in detecting high-threshold mechanical stimuli that occur when distal aspects of sensory nerve fiber are distended from mechanical pressure due to the growing tumor or as a result of destabilization or fracture of bone. Tumor cells and associated inflammatory (immune) cells produce a variety of chemical mediators, including prostaglandins (PGE2), nerve growth factor (NGF), endothelins, bradykinin, and extracellular ATP. Several of these proinflammatory mediators have receptors on peripheral terminals and can directly activate or sensitize nociceptors. NGF, together with its cognate receptor trkA, may serve as a master regulator of bone cancer pain by modulating the sensitivity of or increasing the expression of several receptors and ion channels contributing to increased excitability of nociceptors in the vicinity of the tumor.

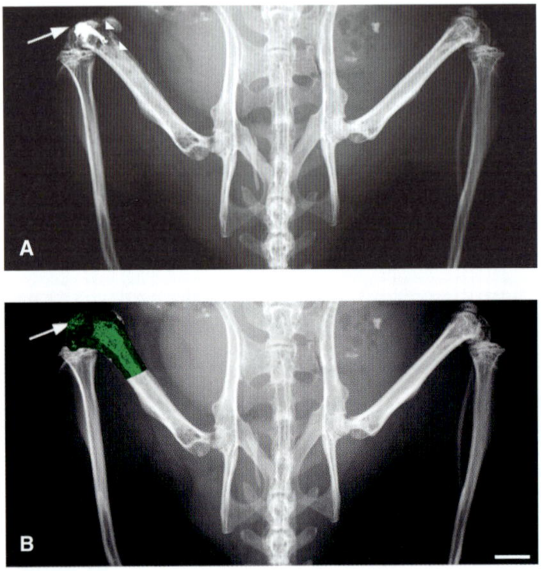

Figure 5.2. Development of a murine bone-cancer pain model. A. Low power anterior-posterior radiograph of mouse pelvis and hind limbs after a unilatereal injection of sarcoma cells into the distal part of the femur and closure of the injection site with an amalgam plug (arrow), which prevents the tumor cells from growing outside the bone. Extensive bone destruction occurs as tumor progression continues, characterized by multifocal radiolucencies and complete loss of trabecular bone regions as compared with contralateral hind limb (arrowheads). B. Tumor burden may be visualized and quantified using sarcoma cancer cells genetically manipulated to express enhanced green fluorescent protein (GFP), as in shown in the overlapping confocal immunofluorescence picture. By day 14 postinjection, GFP-expressing tumor cells (green) had completely filled the intramedullary space. Scale bar 3 mm.

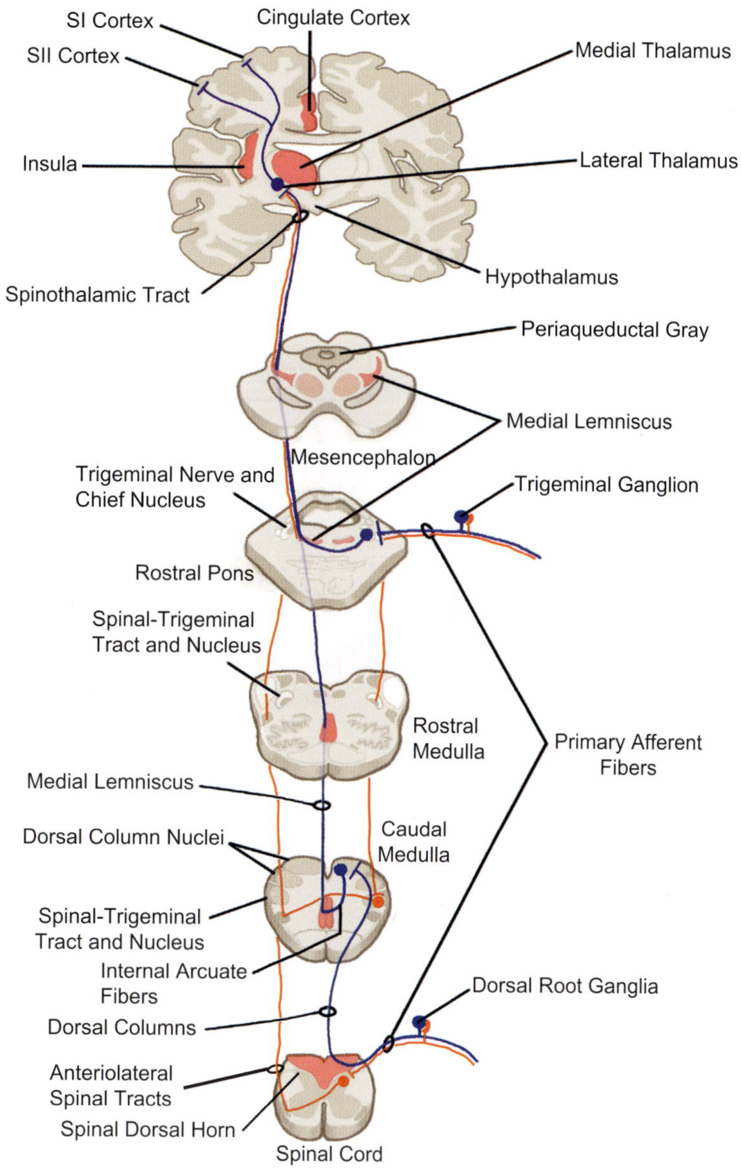

Figure 5.3. The central nociceptive pathways. Primary afferent fibers enter the neuraxis via spinal nerves with cell bodies in the dorsal root ganglia, or via the trigeminal nerve with cell bodies in the trigeminal ganglion. In anteriolateral spinal nociceptive pathway (gray lines), primary afferents from the dorsal root ganglia form synapses on the secondary-order neurons in spinal dorsal horn. The secondary-order axons then cross the midline in the anterior white commissure and gather into the anteriolateral spinal columns. Primary afferent fibers from trigeminal ganglia descend in the spinal-trigeminal tract and form synapses on the secondary-order neurons in the spinal-trigeminal nucleus. The secondary-order axons from spinal-trigeminal nucleus cross the midline to join in the anteriolateral tract. The axons in anteriolateral tract send collaterals to the reticular formation, midbrain, and hypothalamus while ascending and finally terminating in the lateral or medial thalamus. The third-order neurons in thalamus project to various cortical areas. In the dorsal column-medial lemniscal sensory pathway (medial lemniscus: black line), primary afferents from dorsal root ganglia ascend in the dorsal spinal columns and form synapses on the secondary-order neurons in the dorsal column nuclei. The axons from the secondary-order neurons cross the midline in the internal arcuate fibers and gather to form the medial lemniscus. The primary afferents from trigeminal ganglia enter and synapse in the chief (main) sensory trigeminal nucleus, and axons from the secondary-order neurons cross the midline and join in the medial lemniscus. The secondary-order axons then ascend and terminate in the lateral thalamus. Finally, the third-order neurons in thalamus project to cortical areas.

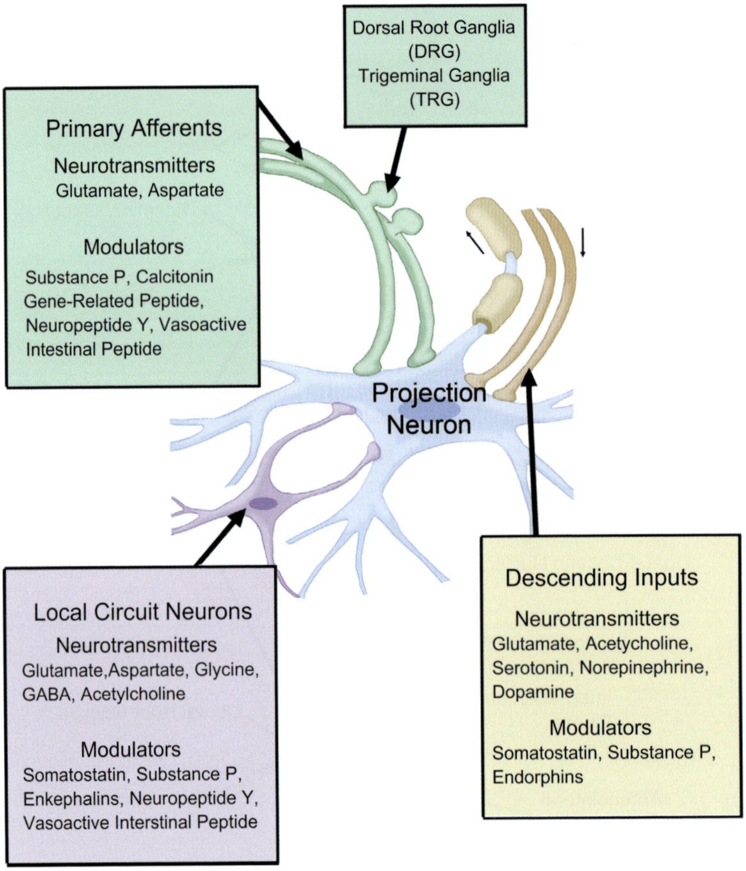

Figure 5.4. Neurotransmission in the spinal dorsal horn. This schematic summarizes the neurochemical pathways involved in somatosensory neurotransmission in the dorsal horn. Intrinsic sources of each transmitter are indicated by the labeled boxes.

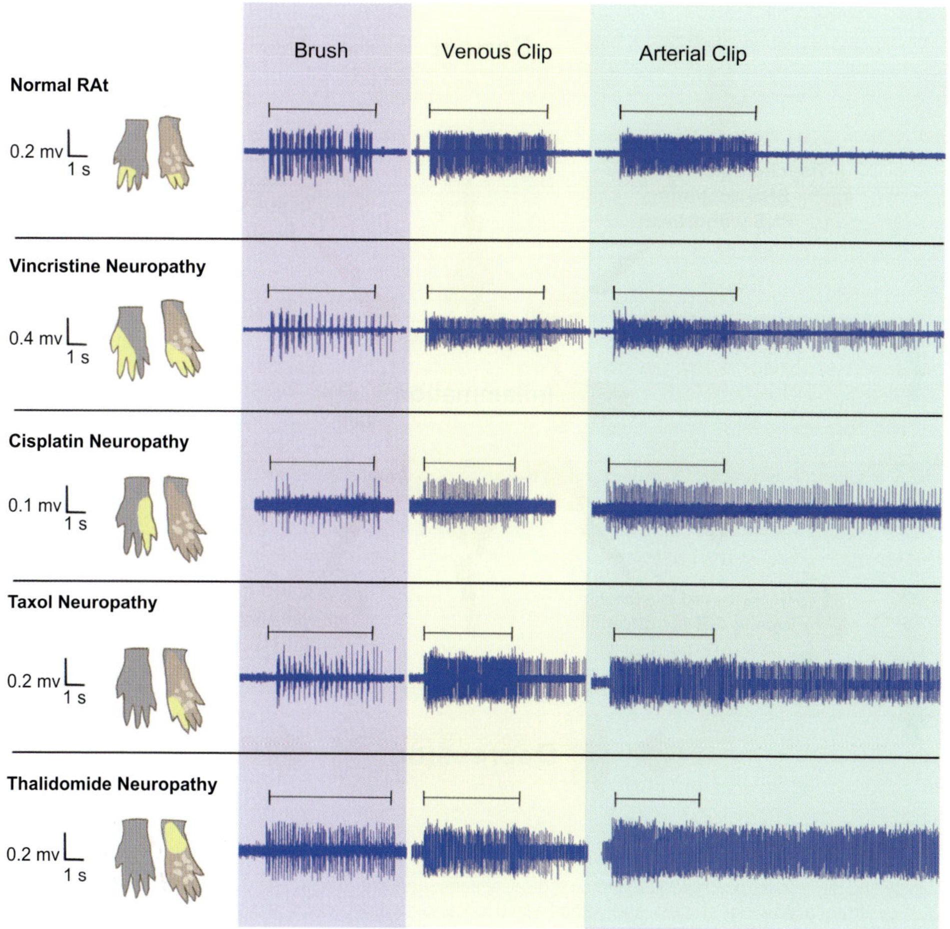

Figure 5.5. Analogue recordings of neuronal activity from the spinal cord. Hyperalgesic rats that had been treated for three to five days with vincristine or cisplatin exhibited excess neuronal afterdischarge in response to cutaneous stimuli. The times of each stimulus application are indicted by the lines over each trace, and the receptive field locations are shown in the drawings at the left.

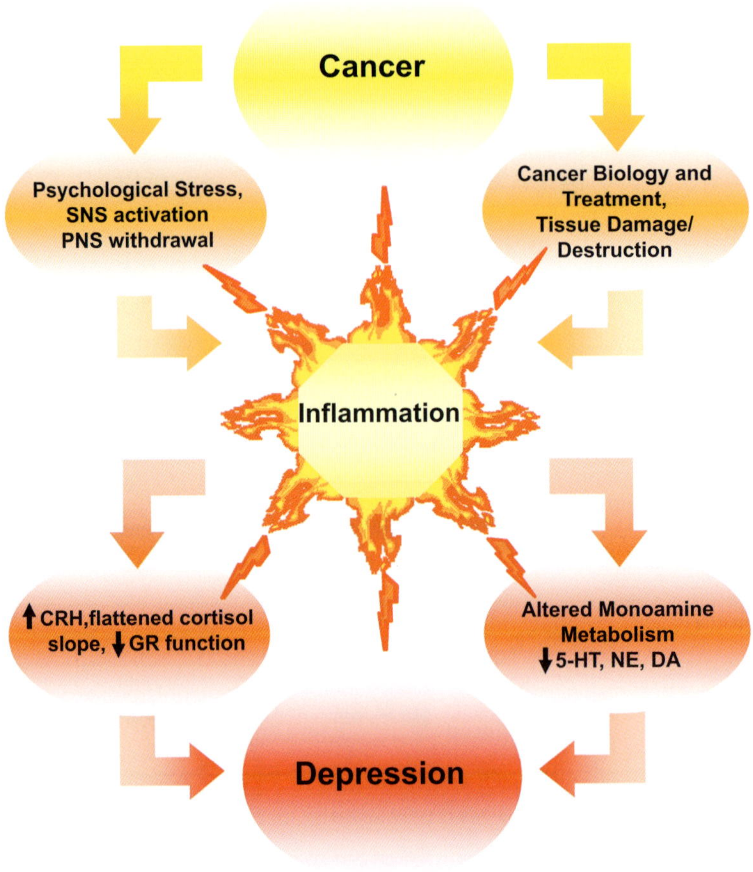

Figure 8.1. Cancer and depression: psychological and biological influences on inflammation and the brain. Receiving a cancer diagnosis frequently causes significant psychological stress, and being treated for cancer is associated with tissue damage and destruction. Together, these processes are potent activators of the innate immune response and inflammation. In the context of psychological stress, sympathetic nervous system (SNS) pathways can activate inflammatory responses, whereas parasympathetic nervous system (PNS) responses can inhibit inflammation. Stress can also sensitize the immune system to the activation of inflammatory pathways by cancer and its treatment. In turn, activation of innate immune responses and inflammation can alter neuroendocrine function by increasing corticotropin-releasing hormone (CRH), flattening the diurnal cortisol curve and disrupting glucocorticoid receptor (GR) function, all of which have been associated with the development of depression. Activation of inflammation and innate immune cytokines can also disrupt monoamine metabolism, leading to reductions in serotonin (5-hydroxytryptophan [5-HT]), norepinephrine (NE), and dopamine (DA). Reduced availability of these neurotransmitters is believed to play an important role in mood regulation.

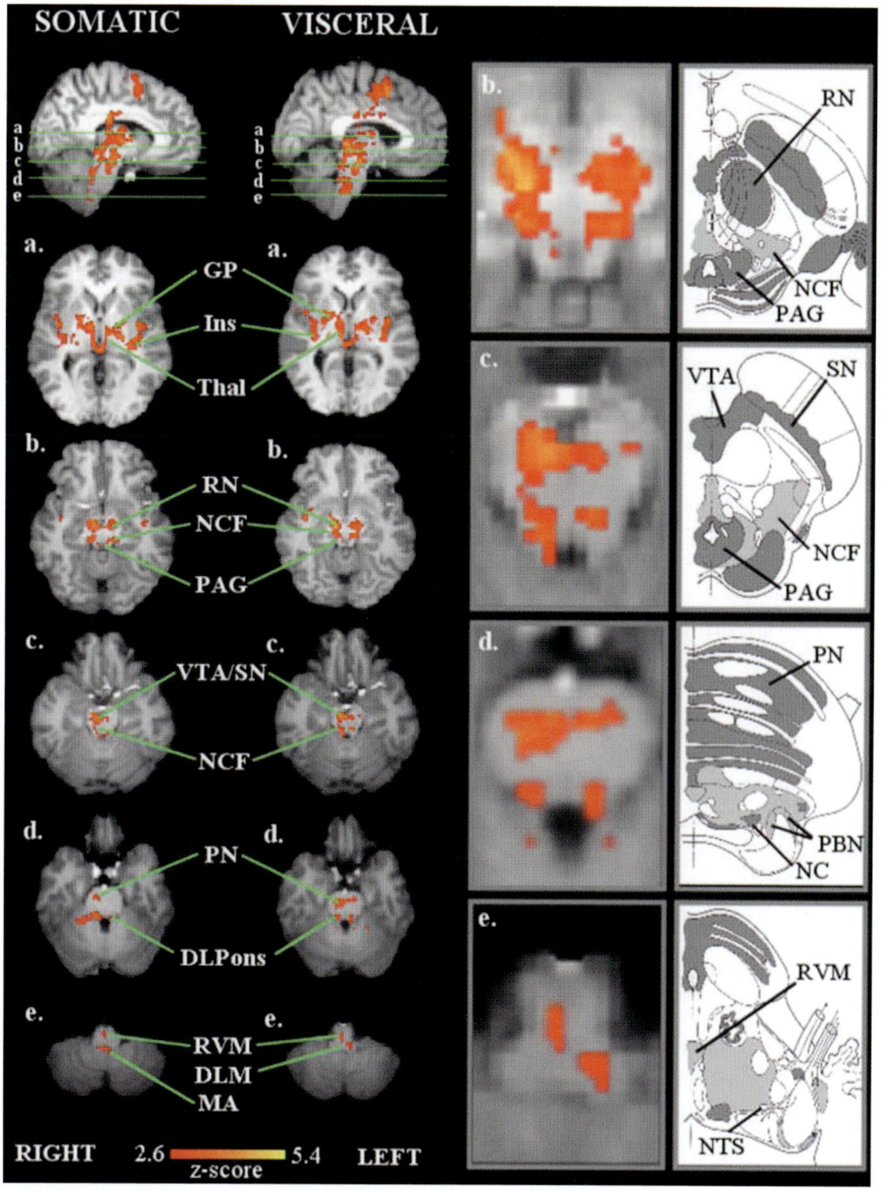

Figure 18.2. Differences and similarities in group activation maps for somatic and visceral pain. The sagittal slices show columns of activation within the brainstem in each group. Axial slices (a–e) correspond to the plane indicated in the sagittal slice. Regions commonly activated in whole-brain pain-imaging studies are significantly activated: thalamus (Thal) and posterior insula (Ins) bilaterally. Activation was also seen in the globus pallidus (GP) bilaterally in both groups. Significantly, activated brainstem nuclei included the red nucleus (RN), nucleus cuneiformis (NCF), periaqueductal gray (PAG), ventral tegmental area (VTA, which extended laterally into the substantia nigra [SN]), and the dorsolateral pons (DLPons) bilaterally. Bilateral activation of the pontine nuclei (PN) occurred in the visceral group but was limited to the right side in the somatic group. Activation in the region of the rostral ventromedial medulla (RVM) was also seen in both groups. In the visceral group alone, a region of activation occurred in the left dorsolateral medulla (DLM). The axial slices in the visceral group have been magnified and juxtaposed to drawings at the same anatomical location. Modified from Duvernoy (1995) with permission.

Source: Reprinted from the Journal of Neuroscience, vol. 25, Dunckley P, Wise RG, Fairhurst M, et al. A comparison of visceral and somatic pain processing in the human brainstem using functional magnetic resonance imaging, Pages 7333–7341, Copyright 2005, with permission from the Society for Neuroscience.

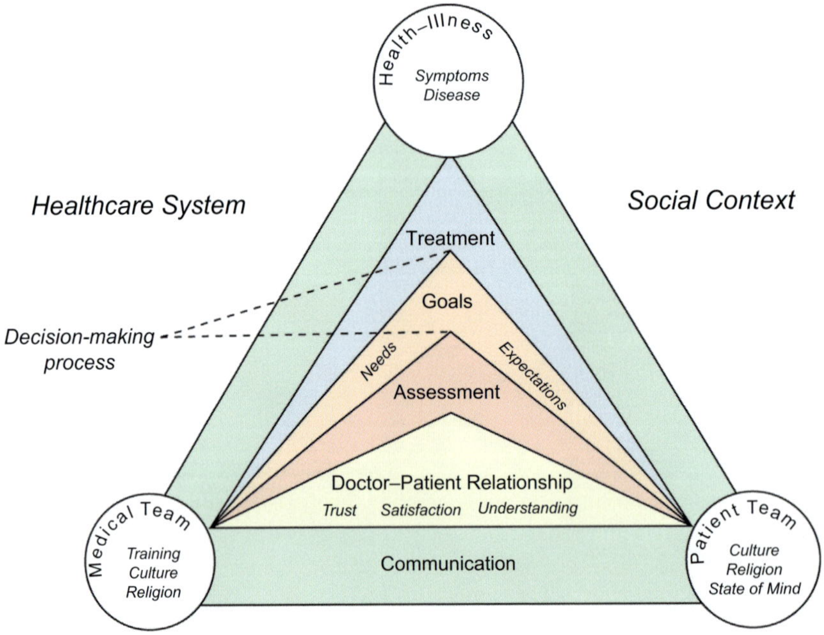

Figure 21.2. The Lee-Epner-Walsh Doctor-Patient-Health Model.

(1) growth-hormone-releasing hormone (GHRH), (2) prostaglandins, such as PGD_2, (3) adenosine, and (4) nitric oxide. A comprehensive review of the role played by these substances in sleep regulation and in mediating IL-1 effects on sleep is beyond the scope of this chapter; see Obal et al.[26] for an in-depth discussion. Briefly: (1) IL-1 stimulates the production of GHRH, PGD_2, nitric oxide and adenosine; (2) GHRH, PGD_2, and adenosine enhance NREM sleep; and (3) antagonism of these same substances decreases NREM sleep and IL-1-induced NREM sleep enhancement. GHRH is a secretagogue for growth hormone, most of which is released during NREM sleep. GHRH promotes NREM sleep in laboratory animals and humans; conversely, experimental suppression of GHRH reduces NREM sleep. Mice and rats with deficiencies in the GHRH system spend less time in NREM sleep.

Adenosine has received considerable attention with respect to the regulation of sleep–wake behavior. Adenosine plays a critical role in brain metabolism. Adenosine levels in the brain progressively increase during prolonged wakefulness. Adenosine enhances the activity of GABAergic neurons in the preoptic area and basal forebrain that promote NREM sleep, as discussed above. On the other hand, adenosine inhibits aminergic neurons that sustain wakefulness and cholinergic neurons involved in cortical activation. Caffeine and other methylxanthines stimulate wakefulness and vigilance because they antagonize adenosine binding to its receptors.

IL-1 interactions with the serotonergic and other brain aminergic systems

As mentioned previously, serotonin is now thought to promote wakefulness and to induce subsequent NREM sleep by stimulating the synthesis or release of sleep factor(s).[27] The manner by which IL-1 affects the serotonergic system suggests that these interactions have a role in regulating NREM sleep. IL-1 actions on the serotonergic system may be mediated by two distinct neuroanatomic regions: (1) the dorsal raphe nucleus, in which IL-1 inhibits cell bodies of the wake-promoting serotonergic system; and (2) the hypothalamic preoptic area/basal forebrain (a brain region where serotonin is essential for the promotion of NREM sleep), in which IL-1 increases the release of serotonin from axon terminals.

IL-1 increases NREM sleep when microinjected into the dorsal raphe nucleus and inhibits firing rates of serotonergic neurons in that region.[28] Because serotonergic neurons in the dorsal raphe nucleus are wake-active, their inhibition could contribute to the NREM sleep enhancement induced by IL-1. Recent data suggest that IL-1-induced inhibition of DRN serotonergic neurons could be caused by the IL-1-induced enhancement of GABAergic inhibitory postsynaptic potentials.[29] This IL-1 action could be interpreted as a potentiation of physiological GABAergic inhibition that is crucial in shaping the state-dependent discharge of serotonergic neurons in the dorsal raphe nucleus. Data showing that IL-1 potentiates GABAergic inhibition are in agreement with evidence reviewed in the next section.

In the hypothalamic preoptic area/basal forebrain, IL-1 stimulates the release of serotonin from axon terminals. Serotonin is essential for IL-1 effects on NREM sleep to be fully manifest; depletion of brain serotonin by para-chlorophenylalanine (PCPA, which inhibits tryptophan hydroxylase, a rate-limiting enzyme in serotonin formation from tryptophan)[30] or blockade of 5-HT_2 receptors[31] impairs IL-1-induced enhancement of NREM sleep. The hypothalamic preoptic area/basal forebrain is the only brain area in which increasing serotonergic activity by local administration of the direct serotonin precursor 5-hydroxytryptophan restores physiological sleep in cats made insomniac by PCPA. In the preoptic area/basal forebrain, serotonin may be essential for NREM sleep because it hyperpolarizes and inhibits cholinergic neurons responsible for cortical activation. Moreover, serotonergic activation promotes IL-1 mRNA expression in the hypothalamus at times during which serotonergic activation (after the first phase of increased wakefulness) enhances NREM sleep. IL-1 mRNA and protein are under potent inhibitory control by the HPA axis, whose activity is stimulated by the activation of the serotonergic system.[32]

In summary, in addition to other mechanisms, IL-1 may promote NREM sleep through two opposite, yet complementary actions at two levels of the serotonergic system: inhibition of serotonergic cell bodies in the brainstem, and the selective stimulation of serotonin release from axon terminals in one specific brain region crucial for NREM sleep, the hypothalamic preoptic area/basal forebrain.

IL-1 activates brain aminergic systems other than the serotonergic system, including the the noradrenergic, histaminergic, and dopaminergic systems.[33] Activation of these systems is thought to mediate some IL-1 effects on various CNS processes; in relation to sleep, these brain aminergic systems promote wakefulness, as reviewed above. Accordingly, it is likely that IL-1-induced increases in NREM sleep occur not because of brain aminergic activation, but in spite of it. It could be further hypothesized that brain aminergic activation induced by IL-1 could counteract IL-1 behavioral effects, contributing to the return to homeostasis. Within the conceptual framework of this hypothesis, IL-1-induced activation of brain aminergic systems could play the same functional role as IL-1-induced activation of the HPA axis.

IL-1 interactions with the GABAergic and cholinergic systems

Data demonstrate that IL-1 increases the activity of the GABAergic system and inhibits activity of the cholinergic system. IL-1 enhances GABA inhibitory effects at multiple levels. Presynaptically, IL-1 increases GABA release in slice preparations from the preoptic and anterior hypothalamic areas of the brain and in brain explants. IL-1 increases cytosolic Ca^{2+} in a subset of hypothalamic neurons, the majority of which are GABAergic. Postsynaptically, IL-1 increases Cl^- uptake in synaptosomes derived from mouse cortex by acting on $GABA_A$ receptors. As previously stated, IL-1 also enhances GABAergic inhibitory postsynaptic potentials in hippocampal neurons and in serotonergic neurons of the dorsal raphe nucleus.[34] In rat-cultured hippocampal neurons and in *Xenopus* oocytes expressing GABA receptors, IL-1 increases recruitment of $GABA_A$ receptors to the cell surface. In the *Xenopus* oocyte model this $GABA_A$ receptor recruitment is due to the IL-1-induced stimulation of an IL-1 receptor, type I (IL-1RI)-dependent phosphatidylinositol 3-kinase/Akt pathway. Moreover, in voltage-clamped oocytes IL-1 induces a delayed potentiation of the GABA-elicited Cl^- current, an effect suppressed by IL-1RA.[35] It has also been suggested that the inhibitory effects of IL-1 on supraoptic neurons are mediated by activation of local GABAergic interneurons.[36] Collectively, these data indicate that IL-1 could enhance GABAergic-induced hyperpolarization and inhibition. Because GABAergic neurons play a crucial role in inhibiting the neuronal systems promoting wakefulness and cortical activation, IL-1-induced enhancement of GABA effects could account, at least in part, for the reduction in wakefulness induced by this cytokine.

IL-1 inhibits acetylcholine release *in vivo* in the hippocampus[37] and inhibits acetylcholine synthesis *in vitro* in cultured pituitary cells.[38] IL-1 also increases acetylcholine degradation by increasing acetylcholinesterase activity and mRNA expression in both neuron–glia co-cultures and *in vivo* in the rat cortex.[39] Recent data suggest that IL-1 inhibits the firing rate of physiologically and pharmacologically identified cholinergic neurons in the laterodorsal and pedunculopontine tegmental nuclei.[40] Because the cholinergic system plays a role in regulating REM sleep, as well as in thalamic and cortical desynchronization, IL-1-induced inhibition of the cholinergic system could, at least in part, account for the reduction in REM sleep observed after IL-1 administration in laboratory animals.

In addition to increasing the duration of NREM sleep, IL-1 also increases the amplitude of the EEG in the slow frequency band, so-called delta waves. EEG delta waves are considered a reliable index of sleep depth; they also represent a measure of sleep drive and, as such, their amplitude is reduced during night sleep from the first to the last NREM sleep episode.[41] IL-1 actions on the cholinergic system could also contribute to enhancement of delta waves.

Conclusions

Compelling evidence suggests that cytokines, notably IL-1 and TNF, are involved in the regulation of normal physiological sleep in the absence of pathology. It is therefore likely that alterations in sleep through the course of an immune challenge result from alterations in cytokine networks in the brain. Actions of cytokines may directly alter sleep–wake behavior, as briefly reviewed in this chapter. Alterations in cytokine profiles may also indirectly alter sleep–wake behavior due to the actions of these immunomodulators on various neurotransmitter, peptide, and hormone systems.

Much of the knowledge of mechanisms by which cytokines contribute to the regulation of sleep in health and disruptions to sleep during immune challenge has been derived from acute studies in which cytokines have been administered to laboratory animals or human volunteers. These acute manipulations result in responses that are useful for dissecting the mechanisms and pathways by which these systems function. However, such acute studies do not adequately reflect the clinical conditions encountered during prolonged illness.

As reviewed in Chapter 14, sleep disturbances are reported twice as often by patients with cancer as by the general population. The factors contributing to sleep disturbances in patients with cancer are myriad, and much additional clinical and preclinical research is necessary to further our understanding of the etiology of sleep disturbances in these patients. Such information may lead to new treatment modalities for sleep disturbances in the cancer patient population. Given the importance of sleep to physical and mental health, improving the quality of nighttime sleep for patients with cancer may result in improved quality of daytime life.

References

1. Jones BE. From waking to sleeping: neuronal and chemical substrates. *Trends Pharmacol Sci* **26**(11): 578–586, 2005.
2. Pace-Schott EF, Hobson JA. The neurobiology of sleep: genetics, cellular physiology and subcortical networks. *Nature Rev Neurosci* **3**(8):591–605, 2002.
3. Ishimori K. True cause of sleep: a hypnogenic substance as evidenced in the brain of sleep-deprived animals. *Tokyo Igakkai Zasshi* **23**:429–459, 1909.
4. Legendre R, Piéron H. Le problème des facteurs du sommeil: résultats d'injections vasculaires et intracérébrales de liquides insomniques. *C R Seances Soc Biol Fil* **68**:1077–1079, 1910.
5. Krueger JM, Karnovsky ML. Sleep as a neuroimmune phenomenon: a brief historical perspective. *Adv Neuroimmunol* **5**:5–12, 1995.
6. Krueger JM, Dinarello CA, Chedid L. Promotion of slow-wave sleep (SWS) by a purified interleukin-1 (IL-1) preparation [abstract]. *Fed Proc* **42**:356, 1983.
7. Krueger JM, Walter J, Dinarello CA, Wolff SM, Chedid L. Sleep-promoting effects of endogenous pyrogen (interleukin-1). *Am J Physiol* **246**:R994–R999, 1984.
8. Tobler I, Borbély AA, Schwyzer M, Fontana A. Interleukin-1 derived from astrocytes enhances slow wave activity in sleep EEG of the rat. *Eur J Pharmacol* **104**:191–192, 1984.
9. Krueger JM, Obal FJ, Fang J, Kubota T, Taishi P. The role of cytokines in physiological sleep regulation. *Ann N Y Acad Sci* **933**:211–221, 2001.
10. Opp MR, Toth LA. Neural-immune interactions in the regulation of sleep. *Front Biosci* **8**:d768–d779, 2003.
11. Opp MR. Cytokines and sleep. *Sleep Med Rev* **9**(5):355–364, 2005.
12. Alberti A, Sarchielli P, Gallinella E, et al. Plasma cytokine levels in patients with obstructive sleep apnea syndrome: a preliminary study. *J Sleep Res* **12**(4):305–311, 2003.
13. Okun ML, Giese S, Lin L, Einen M, Mignot E, Coussons-Read ME. Exploring the cytokine and endocrine involvement in narcolepsy. *Brain Behav Immun* **18**(4):326–332, 2004.
14. Burgos I, Richter L, Klein T, et al. Increased nocturnal interleukin-6 excretion in patients with primary insomnia: a pilot study. *Brain Behav Immun* **20**:246–253, 2006.
15. Vgontzas AN, Papanicolaou DA, Bixler EO, Chrousos GP. Elevation of plasma cytokines in disorders of excessive daytime sleepiness: role of sleep disturbance and obesity. *J Clin Endocrinol Metab* **82**:1313–1316, 1997.
16. Hogan D, Morrow JD, Smith EM, Opp MR. Interleukin-6 alters sleep of rats. *J Neuroimmunol* **137**(1–2):59–66, 2003.
17. Morrow JD, Opp MR. Sleep-wake behavior and responses of interleukin-6-deficient mice to sleep deprivation. *Brain Behav Immun* **19**(1):28–39, 2005.
18. Opp MR, Smith EM, Hughes TK, Jr. IL-10 (cytokine synthesis inhibitory factor) acts in the central nervous system of rats to reduce sleep. *J Neuroimmunol* **60**:165–168, 1995.
19. Kushikata T, Fang J, Wang Y, Krueger JM. Interleukin-4 inhibits spontaneous sleep in rabbits. *Am J Physiol* **275**:R1185–R1191, 1998.
20. Kushikata T, Fang J, Krueger JM. Interleukin-10 inhibits spontaneous sleep in rabbits. *J Interferon Cytokine Res* **19**:1025–1030, 1999.
21. Toth LA, Opp MR. Cytokine- and microbially-induced sleep responses of interleukin-10 deficient mice. *Am J Physiol* **280**:R1806–R1814, 2001.
22. Opp MR, Krueger JM. Interleukin 1-receptor antagonist blocks interleukin 1-induced sleep and fever. *Am J Physiol* **260**:R453–R457, 1991.
23. Chang FC, Opp MR. Corticotropin-releasing hormone (CRH) as a regulator of waking. *Neurosci Biobehav Rev* **25**(5):445–453, 2001.
24. Goujon E, Parnet P, Layé S, Combe C, Dantzer R. Adrenalectomy enhances pro-inflammatory cytokines gene expression, in the spleen, pituitary and brain of mice in response to lipopolysaccharide. *Mol Brain Res* **36**:53–62, 1996.
25. Mustafa M, Mustafa A, Nyberg F, Mangat H, Elhassan A, Adem R. Hypophysectomy enhances interleukin-1b, tumor necrosis factor-a, and interleukin-10 mRNA expression in the rat brain. *J Interferon Cytokine Res* **19**(6):583–587, 1999.
26. Obal F, Jr., Alt J, Taishi P, Gardi J, Krueger JM. Sleep in mice with nonfunctional growth hormone-releasing hormone receptors. *Am J Physiol Regul Integr Comp Physiol* **284**(1):R131–R139, 2003.

27. Jouvet M. Sleep and serotonin: an unfinished story. *Neuropsychopharmacology* **21**:24s–27s, 1999.

28. Brambilla D, Franciosi S, Opp MR, Imeri L. Interleukin-1 inhibits firing of serotonergic neurons in the dorsal raphe nucleus and enhances GABAergic inhibitory post-synaptic potentials. *Eur J Neurosci* **26**(7):1862–1869, 2007.

29. Brambilla D, Opp MR, Imeri L. Interleukin-1 enhances GABAergic inhibitory post-synaptic potentials in dorsal raphe serotonergic neurons [abstract]. *Sleep* **28**(Abstract Supplement):A1, 2 005.

30. Imeri L, Bianchi S, Mancia M. Muramyl dipeptide and IL-1 effects on sleep and brain temperature after inhibition of serotonin synthesis. *Am J Physiol Regul Integr Comp Physiol* **273**(5):R1663–R1668, 1997.

31. Imeri L, Mancia M, Opp MR. Blockade of 5-HT_2 receptors alters interleukin-1-induced changes in rat sleep. *Neuroscience* **92**:745–749, 1999.

32. Gemma C, Imeri L, Opp MR. Serotonergic activation stimulates the pituitary-adrenal axis and alters interleukin-1 mRNA expression in rat brain. *Psychoneuroendocrinology* **28**(7):875–884, 2003.

33. Imeri L, De Simoni MG. Immune alterations in neurotransmission. In: Lydic R, Baghdoyan HA, eds. *Handbook of Behavioral State Control: Cellular and Molecular Mechanisms.* Boca Raton: CRC Press, 1999:659–674.

34. Brambilla D, Chapman D, Greene R. Adenosine mediation of presynaptic feedback inhibition of glutamate release. *Neuron* **46**(2):275–283, 2005.

35. Serantes R, Arnalich F, Figueroa M, et al. Interleukin-1beta enhances GABAA receptor cell-surface expression by a phosphatidylinositol 3-kinase/Akt pathway: relevance to sepsis-associated encephalopathy. *J Biol Chem* **281**(21):14632–14643, 2006.

36. Li Z, Inenaga K, Yamashita H. GABAergic inputs modulate effects of interleukin-1b on supraoptic neurones in vitro. *Neuroreport* **5**:181–183, 1993.

37. Rada P, Mark GP, Vitek MP, et al. Interleukin-1b decreases acetylcholine measured by microdialysis in the hippocampus of freely moving rats. *Brain Res* **550**:287–290, 1991.

38. Carmeliet P, Van Damme J, Denef C. Interleukin-1 beta inhibits acetylcholine synthesis in the pituitary corticotropic cell line AtT20. *Brain Res* **491**(1):199–203, 1989.

39. Li Y, Liu L, Kang J, Sheng JG, Mrak RE, Griffin WST. Neuronal-glial interactions mediated by interleukin-1 enhance neuronal acetylcholinesterase activity and mRNA expression. *J Neurosci* **20**:1–149, 2000.

40. Brambilla D, Franciosi S, Opp MR, Imeri L. Interleukin-1 inhibits firing rate of pharmacologically identified cholinergic neurons of the laterodorsal tegmental nucleus recorded in vitro [abstract]. 18th Congress of the European Sleep Research Society, Innsbruck, Austria, September 12–16, 2006. *J Sleep Res***15**(Suppl 1):235, 2006.

41. Borbély AA. A two process model of sleep regulation. *Hum Neurobiol* **1**:195–204, 1982.

Section 2 Chapter 16

Cancer Symptom Mechanisms and Models: Clinical and Basic Science

Proteins and symptoms

Bang-Ning Lee and James M. Reuben

Multiple and severe symptoms profoundly affect the quality of life of cancer patients and their families, and also are a significant challenge for those who manage patients with cancer. Untreated symptoms can negatively influence the effectiveness of curative treatment by interrupting or terminating therapy. It is likely that the association of co-occurring symptoms reflects a common underlying mechanism.

Some self-reported symptoms have been related to the actions of specific cytokines that appear to produce a constellation of symptoms and behavioral signs when given exogenously to both humans and animals.[1] The notion that proinflammatory cytokines play a pivotal role in the pathophysiology of cancer-related symptoms comes from several convergent lines of experimental and clinical research that are not limited to the study of cancer. Inflammation is now recognized as a critical component of tumor progression because many cancers arise from sites of infection, chronic irritation, and inflammation, and tumor cells co-opt some of the signaling molecules of the innate immune system for invasion, migration, and metastasis.[2]

This chapter considers the role of inflammation in the production of symptoms in cancer and other chronic diseases and examines emerging therapeutic approaches for treating cancer and its symptoms.

Proteins, cytokines, and chemokines

Proteins

Proteins, essential to all living organisms, are large organic compounds characterized by specific sequences of amino acids that are encoded by specific genes. Proteins participate in all cellular functions to ensure cell survival. Some proteins are enzymes that catalyze biochemical reactions. Some have structural or mechanical functions, and others act as membrane receptors that bind signaling molecules. These proteins have effector domains in the cytoplasm that possess enzymatic activity and are involved in cell signaling and signal transduction. Other membrane proteins contain internal channels that allow molecules to enter and exit the cells. Many ion channel proteins specifically select a particular ion. Ligand transport proteins bind particular small biomolecules and transport them to discrete locations in the organism. These proteins have a high binding affinity when their ligand is present in the target tissues in high concentrations, but release the ligand when it is present at low concentrations.

Cytokines

Cytokines are a group of proteineous signaling molecules that, like hormones and neurotransmitters, are used extensively for cell-to-cell communication. Cytokines mediate inflammatory reactions that are essential for survival and can stimulate the acute-phase reaction, stress response, and sickness behaviors mediated by the hypothalamic-pituitary-adrenal (HPA) axis and the sympathetic nervous system.

Proinflammatory cytokines are proteins that are predominantly produced by the immune system. Their cell signaling effects are mediated by three major mitogen-activated protein (MAP) kinase pathways, p38, SAPK/JNK, and ERK.[3] Through phosphorylation, these kinases can induce or suppress apoptosis, cell growth, and cell proliferation. They can activate various transcription factors, including nuclear factor kappa B (NF-κB)[4] and signal transducers and activators of transcription (STAT).[5] Proinflammatory cytokines also potently mediate brain functions. For example, stress hormones can facilitate inflammation by inducing expression of the cytokines interleukin (IL)-1, IL-6, IL-8, IL-18, and tumor necrosis factor (TNF)-α, by producing C-reactive protein, and by activating corticotropin-releasing hormone (CRH). The inflammatory reaction can also preferentially induce the T-helper (Th) type 2 cytokines IL-4, IL-5,

Cancer Symptom Science: Measurement, Mechanisms, and Management, eds. Charles S. Cleeland, Michael J. Fisch, and Adrian J. Dunn.
Published by Cambridge University Press.

and IL-13, and can protect the organism from harmful effects related to the overproduction of the Th1 type proinflammatory cytokines IL-2, interferon (IFN)-γ, and TNF-α.

Chemokines

Chemokines, or chemotactic cytokines, are small cytokines or proteins that are secreted by cells and can induce directed chemotaxis in responsive cells. The chemokines control the migration of many cell types in the body, including tumor cells. Some chemokines are proinflammatory and can be induced during an immune response, whereas others function in a homeostatic manner. Chemokines are divided into four groups, designated CXC, CC, C, and CX_3C, depending upon the spacing of conserved cysteine domains. Each nucleated cell type produces chemokines; they can be expressed either in response to a stimulus or constitutively in a tissue-specific manner.

Symptoms and diseases affected by cytokines and chemokines

The role of cytokines in cancer-related symptoms

Fatigue, gastrointestinal symptoms, cachexia, anorexia, shortness of breath, and psychological distress are but a few of the symptoms that add tremendously to the affliction that patients experience. Common cancer-related symptoms include anorexia, cognitive dysfunction, depression, dyspnea, fatigue, hormonal disturbances, neutropenia, pain, peripheral neuropathy, and sexual dysfunction.[6] Patients with cancer are likely to experience multiple symptoms concurrently, as symptoms tend to occur together in clusters. For example, pain, fatigue, depression, and sleep disturbances often co-occur.[7,8] Further, patients often report at least some of their symptoms as severe. The symptoms experienced by patients with cancer have much in common with the sickness behavior that occurs in animals after the administration of infectious or inflammatory agents or certain proinflammatory cytokines, suggesting that cancer-related symptom clusters may share common cytokine-based neuroimmunological mechanisms.

Cytokines and brain function

Immunotherapy with cytokines is widely used to treat chronic leukemia, renal cell carcinoma, and melanoma. More than 50% of patients receiving cytokine treatment have documented cognitive impairments.[9] IL-2 and TNF-α can produce dose-dependent toxicities, such as decreased attention abilities, verbal memory deficits, motor coordination impairments, and frontal lobe executive dysfunction.[10] Headache, anorexia, stroke-like events (eg, transient amnesia), and demyelination in the brain are other adverse effects of TNF-α. IL-1 and its receptors are found in many areas of the brain, particularly the hippocampus. IL-1 suppresses the influx of calcium into hippocampal neurons, which may explain the preponderance of memory impairments in patients with IL-1-associated toxicity.[10]

Cytokines and fatigue

Changes in serum concentrations of IL-1 receptor antagonist (IL-1RA), TNF-α, IL-6, IL-8, and epidermal growth factor are associated with fatigue and reduced quality of life in patients with myelodysplastic syndrome and acute leukemia before treatment.[11] Interferon-induced proteins are elevated in the blood of patients suffering from chronic fatigue syndrome, which is related to viral infections such as Epstein-Barr virus, human herpes virus-6, and cytomegalovirus.[12] Similarly, fluctuations in peripheral cytokines are associated with cancer-related fatigue.[13] Compared with nonfatigued survivors of breast cancer, fatigued survivors have shown significantly higher serum levels of IL-1RA, TNF-α receptor p75, and neopterin.[14] Cancer-related fatigue may also be associated with anemia, low serum albumin, and abnormal hemoglobin levels.[15] High serum levels of IL-1, IL-6, and TNF-α have been observed in patients with advanced-stage cancer, particularly those with anorexia/cachexia syndrome.[16]

Cytokines and neuropathic pain

The induction of proinflammatory cytokines around nerve endings may play a role in chemotherapy-induced peripheral neuropathy, as cytokines are released from tissues exposed to chemotherapeutic drugs. Coadministration of vincristine and granulocyte-macrophage colony-stimulating factor (GM-CSF) markedly increases the severity and magnitude of treatment-induced pain and neurological impairment.[17,18] Release of the proinflammatory cytokines IFN-γ, TNF-α, and IL-1β is increased by cisplatin[19,20] and taxol.[21,22] Vincristine does not induce release of the same cytokines as taxol and cisplatin but rather upregulates GM-CSF and downregulates TNF-α receptors.[23] Nevertheless, all three chemotherapeutic drugs directly activate the NF-κB signaling pathway. This mechanism provides a link to the generation of pain as it is also activated in response to *N*-methyl-D-aspartate and substance P receptors in neural tissues.[23] These are the key spinal neurotransmitter systems involved in cutaneous hyperalgesia.[24]

The role of cytokines in allogeneic stem cell transplantation

Acute myeloid leukemia is a clonal disorder of hematopoiesis characterized by the accumulation of myeloblasts that are incapable of normal differentiation. Treatment of the disease usually involves intensive chemotherapy to induce remission, followed by allogeneic stem cell transplantation. However, tissue damage caused by the pretransplantation conditioning therapy and alloreactive responses to the allogeneic transplant produce various proinflammatory cytokines, including IL-1β and TNF-α. In a recent study, we observed that patients with acute myeloid leukemia were prone to experience physical symptoms (pain, nausea, and fatigue), affective symptoms (depression, anxiety), and cognitive symptoms (poor problem solving, memory, and attention) during treatment. Because many cancer-related symptoms might be induced by common biological mechanisms, we hypothesized that altered levels of inflammatory cytokines would be associated with the production of symptoms. Understanding this connection is critical to appropriate symptom management.

To test this hypothesis, we conducted a longitudinal study to determine whether a correlation existed between plasma cytokines, cortisol, and the severity of the self-reported symptoms in patients with acute myeloid leukemia undergoing allogeneic stem cell transplantation.[25] Peripheral blood was obtained from 46 patients with acute myeloid leukemia before and after conditioning therapy with IV fludarabine (40 mg/m^2) and busulfan (130 mg/m^2), which was administered before transplantation and at weekly intervals thereafter up to day 60. Plasma levels of cytokines (IL-1β, IL-6, IL-8, IL-10, IL-12, and TNF-α) were measured using a cytometric bead array assay. Self-reported symptoms, rated on a 0–10 scale with 10 as the worst possible score, were assessed using the M. D. Anderson Symptom Inventory (MDASI) instrument in a subset of 13 patients.

The symptoms with an average MDASI score greater than 3 were pain, fatigue, and drowsiness (physical symptoms); distress, feeling sad (affective symptoms); and sleep disturbance. Before conditioning therapy, patients had significantly elevated plasma levels of IL-1β and IL-6 compared with normal controls. Principal component analysis of the cytokine profiles over the posttransplantation evaluation period identified two clusters of cytokines consisting of IL-1β, IL-12, and TNF-α (Cluster 1, which peaked around day 42 posttransplantation) and IL-6, IL-8, and IL-10 (Cluster 2, which peaked around day 10–14 posttransplantation). Moreover, the highest cumulative symptom score coincided with the peak in Cluster 2 cytokines and accounted for much of the variation in symptom severity. Among the 13 patients with MDASI symptoms scores, four developed acute graft-versus-host disease with a time-dependent elevation in Cluster 1 cytokines. These data suggest that IL-6, IL-8, and IL-10 are related to the tissue damage induced by the conditioning regimen and onset of self-reported symptoms, whereas IL-1β, IL-12, and TNF-α are more likely to be associated with alloreactivity and the development of acute graft-versus-host disease.

The role of chemokines in angiogenesis and inflammatory response

Cytokines and chemokines exert both direct and indirect control over angiogenesis. Pathological angiogenesis and physiological angiogenesis are usually associated with an inflammatory-cell infiltrate. Chemokines primarily mediate physiological and pathological leukocyte traffic in homeostasis as well as in inflammation.[26] Like cytokines, they are necessary for immune cell differentiation and form a key part of the linkage between innate and adaptive immunity. Some chemokines and cytokines induced during inflammation promote a milieu for angiogenesis, whereas others are potent inhibitors of angiogenesis.

Many reports suggest that the expression of chemokine receptors in many cancers is not random. CXCR4 and CCR7 are likely to be the most important chemokine receptors in many cancers and their expression correlates with enhanced disease aggressiveness and poor prognosis. For example, Laverdiere and Gorlick[27] revealed an association between CXCR4 expression and metastasis in patients with osteosarcoma. Wang et al.[28] found a correlation between the expression of CCR7 and metastasis in squamous cell carcinoma of the head and neck. Diaz[29] described a syndrome called WHIM (warts, hypogammaglobulinemia, infections, and myelokathesis) that is caused by mutations in CXCR4 leading to defects in signaling.

The role of chemokines in allergy and asthma

Chemokines are potent leukocyte chemoattractants, cellular activating factors, histamine-releasing factors, and regulators of homeostatic immunity, making them particularly important in the pathogenesis of airway inflammation in asthma. The asthmatic response is characterized by elevated production of immunoglobulin E (IgE), cytokines and chemokines, mucus hypersecretion, airway obstruction, eosinophilia, and enhanced airway hyperreactivity to spasmogens. Furthermore, there is a strong correlation between the presence of CD4+ and Th2 cells, eosinophils, and disease severity, suggesting an integral role for these cells in the pathophysiology of asthma. Th2 cells are thought to induce asthma through the secretion of an array of cytokines (IL-4, IL-5, and IL-13) that activate inflammatory and residential effector pathways. In particular, IL-4 and IL-13 are produced at elevated levels in the asthmatic lung and are thought to be major regulators of many of the clinical features of asthma.

The role of cytokines in rheumatoid arthritis

Proinflammatory cytokines such as TNF-α, IL-1, IL-6, GM-CSF, and chemokine IL-8 are abundant in the lesions of patients with rheumatoid arthritis. This phenomenon is compensated for by the increased production of anti-inflammatory cytokines IL-10 and transforming growth factor-β, and of cytokine inhibitors such as IL-1RA and soluble receptors of TNF-α. Further, TNF-α, which is spontaneously produced by rheumatoid joint cell cultures, has been shown to be the dominant regulator of IL-1. The notion that TNF-α is a major player in rheumatoid arthritis has provided the rationale for clinical trials of anti-TNF-α therapy in patients with long-standing rheumatoid arthritis.[30] Several clinical trials using a chimeric anti-TNF-α antibody demonstrated a marked clinical benefit, supporting the hypothesis that TNF-α is of major importance in rheumatoid arthritis.[30]

The role of cytokines in inflammatory bowel disease

Inflammatory bowel disease and its treatment are not yet completely delineated. Both types of inflammatory bowel disease (ulcerative colitis and Crohn's disease) have been investigated for more than half a century. Advances in immunology have recently provided a more complete understanding of the underlying mechanisms of inflammatory bowel disease. The mucosal immune system is the central effector of intestinal inflammation and injury, with cytokines playing a central role in modulating inflammation. Under normal situations, the intestinal mucosa is in a state of homeostatic inflammation, regulated by a balance between proinflammatory cytokines (IFN-γ, IL-1, IL-6, IL-12, and TNF-α) and anti-inflammatory cytokines (IL-4, IL-10, and IL-11). Inflammatory bowel disease is produced by an exaggerated response to bacterial flora within the intestinal mucosa. T lymphocytes, in particular, are key players during the development and maintenance of inflammatory bowel disease, although the cytokine profile in Crohn's disease (mostly Th1 cytokines) differs from that in ulcerative colitis (mainly Th2 cytokines). After the inflammation has been established, the balance between proinflammatory and regulatory cytokines determines the degree of mucosal damage and the form of disease presentation. Biotherapies targeted against leukocyte adhesion, Th1 polarization, T-cell activation, TNF-α, or NF-κB are being evaluated as potential therapies for inflammatory bowel disease.[31]

Transcription factors, proinflammatory cytokines, and symptoms

In general, chronic inflammation predisposes to cancer formation and progression. It is commonly accepted that chemokines contribute to this process. NF-κB, which regulates innate and adaptive immune responses, is constitutively active in various types of cancer, including leukemia, lymphoma, breast cancer, and colorectal cancer.[32] Many different triggers, including bacteria and viruses, can lead to the activation of NF-κB, which, in turn, controls the expression of many inflammatory cytokines, chemokines, immune receptors, and cell-surface adhesion molecules. A schematic illustration of the steps involved in the activation of the NF-κB pathway in inflammatory cells that promote malignant conversion and progression of cancer is shown in Figure 16.1.[33]

Recent studies have shown that NF-κB is activated by various stressful conditions, including physical

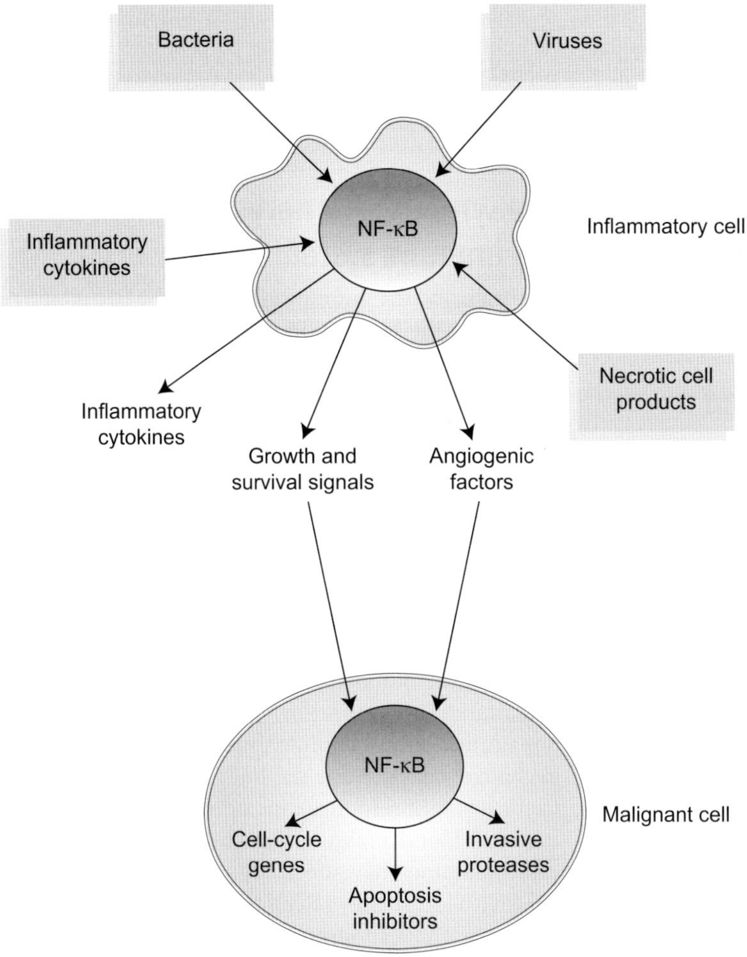

Figure 16.1. NF-κB activation and the interaction between inflammatory and malignant cells can promote malignant conversion and progression.
Source: Reprinted by permission from Macmillan Publishers Ltd: *Nature* 441(7092): 431–436, copyright 2006.[33]

stress, oxidative stress, and exposure to certain chemicals, and that NF-κB can also regulate stress responses. In particular, IL-1β and TNF-α produced by an NF-κB-dependent mechanism can directly activate the NF-κB pathway, thus establishing a positive feedback loop.[34] In addition, NF-κB activates the expression of genes coding for enzymes involved in the pathogenesis of inflammatory processes, including inducible nitric oxide synthetase and inducible cyclooxygenase (COX)-2.[35] COX-2 enables prostaglandin formation (phospholipase A2 initiates the cascade), and the active products of the arachidonate metabolism produced by the cerebral microvasculature have critical roles in initiating the neuronal responses and the neurophysiological outcomes that take place during immunogenic stimuli, including sickness behaviors, fever, and increased activity in the HPA axis.[36] Therefore, activation of NF-κB is a potential link between the expression of inflammatory cytokines and the production of cancer-related symptoms.

Cytokine signaling through the transcription factors

A family of cytoplasmic transcription factors, the STATs, is known to mediate the responsiveness of cells to several cytokines and growth factors. Recent studies have shown that the mechanism of intracellular signaling of inflammatory cytokines such as TNF-α, IFN-γ, and IL-6. STAT1, STAT3, and NF-κB is involved in transmitting inflammatory cytokine signals to the nucleus. NF-κB and STAT1 induce inflammatory mediators from inflammatory cells, especially macrophages, whereas STAT3 has both proinflammatory and anti-inflammatory actions, depending on the cell-specific and stimulus-specific context.[37] NF-κB and STAT3 in tumor cells can promote cell growth and cell survival through the induction of target genes. In contrast, STAT1 is generally believed to be antiproliferative because it promotes apoptosis through the p53 pathway, but it may also promote inflammation-mediated tumor development by enhancing tissue injury and inflammation. Inhibition of NF-κB and STATs offers yet another strategy for treating various malignancies and abrogating associated subjective symptoms.

The neuroendocrine system and peptide hormones

Several peptide hormones are secreted from the pituitary gland and are important for maintaining physiological homeostasis. The anterior pituitary synthesizes and secretes important endocrine hormones that are released from the gland under the influence of hypothalamic hormones. Adrenocorticotrophic hormone, in particular, acts on the adrenal cortex to regulate the secretion of glucocorticoids and growth hormone. The posterior pituitary gland secretes antidiuretic hormone, also called vasopressin, which causes the kidneys to conserve water by concentrating urine and reducing urine volume. Vasopressin also has various functions in the brain and blood vessels. Some neuropeptides act as neurotransmitters in the nervous system in addition to acting as hormones when released into the blood.

It has been shown that neuropeptides are potent stimulators of cytokine production in several cell types, including macrophages, lymphocytes, and mast cells. For example, substance P is capable of stimulating the release of IL-1, IL-6, and TNF-α from human monocytes.[38] When a peptide hormone binds to receptors on the surface of the cell, a second messenger appears in the cytoplasm, triggering intracellular responses. Tachykinins (including substance P), neurokinin A and B, hemokinin-1, and endokinins are a family of neuropeptides that act through three types of transmembrane G-protein-coupled tachykinin receptors. Beside their role as neurotransmitters in the peripheral and central nervous systems, tachykinins and their receptors are expressed in nonneuronal cells, thereby connecting the central nervous system with peripheral organ systems, including the respiratory, cardiovascular, immune, endocrine, gastrointestinal, and genitourinary systems. Tachykinin-receptor-expressing tumors, such as astrocytoma, glioma, neuroblastoma, pancreatic cancer, and melanoma, use tachykinin-induced signaling to promote cancer-cell proliferation and survival and to release cytokines and soluble mediators, thereby contributing to the development of cancer-related symptoms.

The sympathetic nervous system and the immune system

The brain and the immune system are the two adaptive systems in the body and are linked by two pathways. The autonomic nervous system provides communication via direct neural influences, and neuroendocrine humoral outflow via the pituitary. The sympathetic nervous system, a major component of the autonomic nervous system, innervates all lymphoid organs; the catecholamines, the end product of the sympathetic nervous system, modulate several immune parameters. Catecholamines, which are chemical compounds derived from the amino acid tyrosine, are biogenic amines of which 50% bind to plasma proteins and circulate in the bloodstream. The most abundant catecholamines are epinephrine, norepinephrine, and dopamine. Catecholamines cause general physiological changes that prepare the body for physical activity (fight-or-flight response), including increases in heart rate and blood pressure. Similar to glucocorticoids, catecholamines have been regarded as immunosuppressive because they selectively inhibit Th1 functions and favor Th2 responses.

Considerable data suggest that stress, accompanied by increased levels of peripheral catecholamines, inhibits several components of cellular immunity, particularly natural-killer-cell activity, an effect that is mediated mainly by the CRH-directed sympathetic nervous system axis. The potent suppressive effect of catecholamines on natural-killer-cell activity is probably due to the fact that, among the lymphoid cells, natural killer cells possess the greatest amount of beta 2 adrenergic receptor (β_2-AR). In contrast, the effect of catecholamines on macrophage activity appears to be more complex and is not completely understood. Apart from the modulatory effects of norepinephrine acting through adrenergic receptors, it is possible that macrophage activity is affected by substance P secreted locally by peptidergic/sensory nerve fibers or by mast cell-secreted histamine (Figure 16.2).[39] The release of substance P and CRH might trigger the secretion of histamine, which, in turn, mediates acute inflammation, vasodilatation, or neurogenic inflammation through stimulation of H1 histamine receptors. The

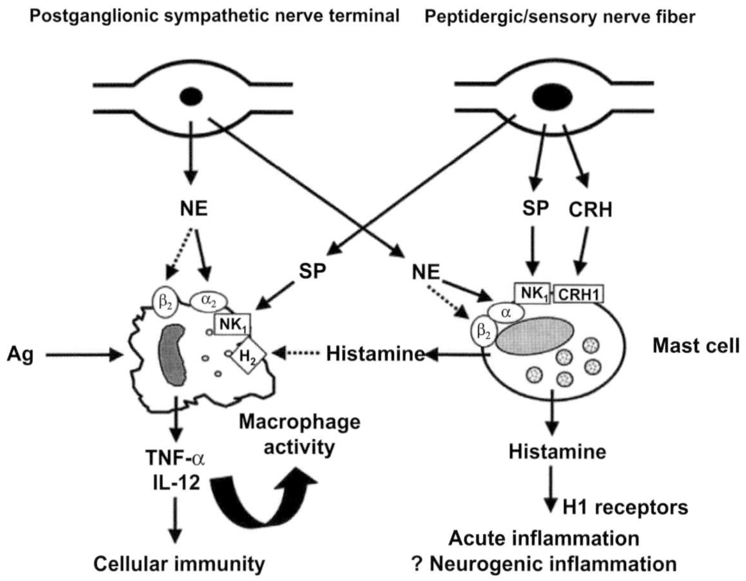

Figure 16.2. The effects of locally released mediators on the secretion of TNF-α and IL-12, and macrophage activity. Ag indicates antigen; α, α2 and β2, adrenoreceptor; CRH, corticotropin-releasing hormone; H1 and H2, histamine receptor; NE, norepinephrine; NK, natural killer cell; SP, substance P.
Source: Reprinted by permission from American Society for Pharmacology and Experimental Therapeutics: *Pharmacol Rev* 52: 595–638, copyright 2000.[39]

anti-inflammatory effect of catecholamines exerted through stimulation of β_2-AR depends on the presence and expression of α-AR on macrophages and mast cells, and other local mediators or cellular factors. Through stimulation of α-AR and β_2-AR, catecholamines stimulate and inhibit the release of histamine from mast cells, whereas histamine, through stimulation of H2 histamine receptors, suppresses the production of TNF-α and IL-12.[40] Catecholamine-mediated suppression of cellular immunity may promulgate the growth of some tumors and the development of cancer-related symptoms.

Building a hypothetical model of an immunoneurological pathway in the development of cancer-related symptoms

It is known that IL-6 is elevated in various types of cancer, including multiple myeloma, chronic lymphocytic leukemia, and malignant melanoma.[41] To study the role of the immunoneuroendocrine network in the development of cancer-related symptoms, we propose a conceptual model (Figure 16.3). The model suggests that IL-6 is a driving force that can trigger many symptoms, particularly fatigue, depression, and sleep disturbances. As illustrated in Figure 16.3, in addition to activating the HPA axis, IL-6 can induce the production of IL-1RA and soluble receptor 1 of TNF-α (sTNF-R1)[42] to block the action of IL-1β and TNF-α, respectively.[43] Further, an increase in IL-6 could augment the activity of the HPA axis and the release by the hypothalamus of growth-hormone-releasing hormone, a somnogenic molecule,[44] and CRH.[45] IL-1β and TNF-α also induce the secretion of growth-hormone-releasing hormone through an NF-κB-independent pathway.

Positive feedback loops are characteristic of nonlinear systems of amplification and are dependent upon a suppressive mechanism. For example, IL-1β induces the production of CRH that, in turn, inhibits IL-1β production. Control of the immunoneurological pathway occurs when cortisol binds to the glucocorticoid receptor and forms a complex that represses transcriptional activity of the transcription factors AP-1 and NF-κB.[46] NF-κB can be found in the cytoplasm of all cell types and is inactivated by the induction of inhibitory proteins known as inhibitors of NF-κB (IκB). IκB prevent the nuclear translocation of NF-κB and the subsequent transcription of inflammatory cytokines IL-1β and TNF-α.[47–49] We believe this model can be used to better understand the development of symptom burden in patients with cancer.

Therapeutic interventions for cancer and its symptoms

Based on current knowledge, therapeutic interventions that target cytokines, chemokines, and their

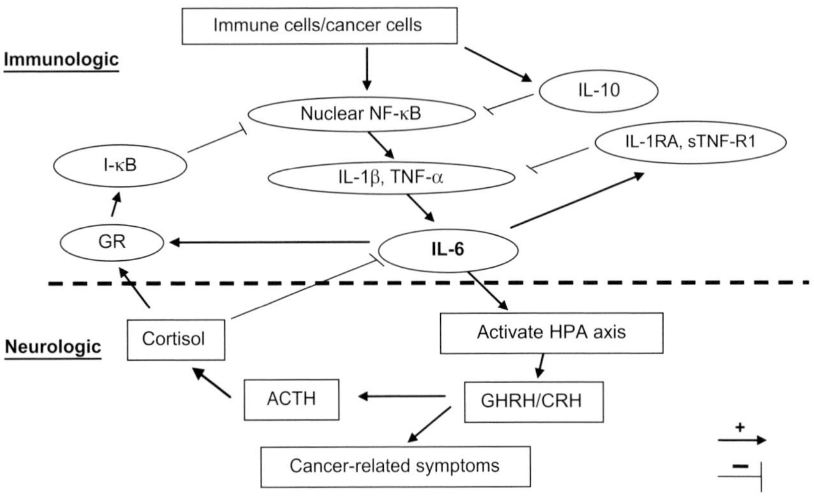

Figure 16.3. The immunoneuroendocrine network in the development of cancer-related symptoms. ACTH indicates adrenocorticotrophic hormone; CRH, corticotropin-releasing hormone; GHRH, growth-hormone-releasing hormone; GR, glucocorticoid receptor; HPA axis, hypothalamic-pituitary-adrenal axis; IκB, inhibitor of NF-κB.

receptors are highly promising candidates for suppressing and possibly protecting the organism from the development of cancer-related symptoms. Future cancer treatment will employ a multidisciplinary approach, incorporating targeted therapies into current standard regimens. Many molecules are currently in the pharmaceutical pipeline and under investigation. These molecules can be categorized according to their mechanisms of action.

Anti-TNF agents

Blocking TNF bioactivity and inhibiting TNF production may be effective anticancer therapies. TNF-α is involved in tumor initiation and progression, in part by inducing the production of angiogenic factors, chemokines, and matrix metalloproteinases. Several clinical studies reported abnormally high levels of circulating TNF in patients with pancreatic,[50] kidney,[51] breast,[52] or prostate cancer.[53] Higher levels of TNF have also been correlated with tumor stage, extent of anorexia-cachexia syndrome, and shorter survival time. However, circulating TNF is not always detectable in patients with cancer and may vary within individual patients over time and the course of their disease.

A few anti-TNF molecules block or inactivate TNF, specifically the soluble TNF receptor fusion protein. These include etanercept (Enbrel®; Amgen Inc., Thousand Oaks, California) and the anti-TNF monoclonal antibody infliximab (Remicade®; Centocor Inc., Horsham, Pennsylvania). Small molecules, such as thalidomide (Thalomid®; Celgene Corp., Summit, New Jersey) and its derivatives, which are structural and functional analogues of thalidomide, represent another promising new class of immunomodulators of various inflammatory, autoimmune, and neoplastic diseases. The anti-angiogenic and T cell costimulatory functions of immunomodulator compounds have led to the investigation of these agents for treatment of multiple myeloma, myelodysplastic syndromes, chronic lymphocytic leukemia, and some solid tumors. In clinical studies, immunomodulators appear to have fewer of the sedative and neurotoxic effects that are often associated with long-term thalidomide dosing.

In general, immunomodulators have effects on inflammatory-cytokine secretion, T cell modulation, angiogenesis, and the expression of adhesion molecules. However, each immunomodulator has a unique potency, which may provide selective applicability for distinct diseases. Lenalidomide, a second-generation immunomodulator, has been used to treat myelodysplastic syndrome and multiple myeloma, with a reported better safety profile than thalidomide and no evidence of teratogenicity. Lenalidomide is clinically active in myelodysplastic syndrome,[54] multiple myeloma,[55] and chronic lymphocytic leukemia.[56] Because of its improved side-effect profile and potent anti-inflammatory and anticancer properties, lenalidomide and other immunomodulators are expected to become important alternatives to thalidomide.

The US Food and Drug Administration (FDA) approved the use of the proteasome inhibitor bortezomib (Velcade®; Millennium Pharmaceuticals Inc, Cambridge, Massachusetts), which acts by blocking

NF-κB activity via inhibiting the degradation of ubiquininated IκB in the proteosome and preventing the translocation of NF-κB to the nucleus. Velcade not only inhibits myeloma cell growth and induces myeloma cell death, but also inhibits the production of growth and survival factors by blocking the production of adhesion molecules on the myeloma cell surface, thereby interfering with the interaction between myeloma and bone marrow cells.[57] Other anti-TNF therapies that inhibit TNF signaling and synthesis include inhibitors of P38 MAP kinase LY2228820 (Eli Lilly and Company, Indianapolis, Indiana), AMG-548 (Amgen Inc., Thousand Oaks, California), BIRB-796 (Boehringer Ingelheim Pharmaceuticals, Inc., Ridgefield, Connecticut), SCIO-469 and SCIO-323 (Scios Inc., Fremont, California), and VX-702 (Vertex Pharmaceuticals, Cambridge, Massachusetts).[58] As P38 MAPK represents a point of convergence for multiple signaling processes that are activated during inflammation, it serves as a potential target for the modulation of cytokine production.

Anti-IL-6 agents

IL-6 is a multifunctional acute-phase protein that is upregulated in many types of cancer.[41] It plays an important role in hematopoiesis, in the proliferation and survival of specific hematological malignancies, and as an autocrine growth factor for some solid tumors. IL-6 is believed to be a causative factor for cancer-related symptoms, including cachexia, flu-like symptoms, and fatigue. Anti-IL-6 therapies could potentially alleviate these symptoms and improve the quality of life for some patients. In fact, monoclonal IL-6 antibody CNTO 328 (Centocor Inc., Malvern, Pennsylvania), a mouse–human chimeric anti-IL-6 antibody, is in phase II development for the potential treatment of multiple myeloma and renal cell carcinoma. CNTO 328 (1) potentiated bortezomib-mediated activation of caspase-8 and caspase-9 and the common downstream effector caspase-3; (2) attenuated bortezomib-mediated induction of anti-apoptotic heat shock protein-70, which correlated with downregulation of phosphorylated STAT-1; and (3) inhibited bortezomib-mediated accumulation of myeloid cell leukemia-1, an effect that was associated with downregulation of phosphorylated STAT-3.[59]

Because murine monoclonal antibodies frequently induce human antimouse antibodies, the clinical use of a murine monoclonal antibody in humans is limited. A humanized anti-IL-6 receptor antibody, tocilizumab, was codeveloped by Chugai Pharmaceuticals Inc., Tokyo, Japan and F. Hoffmann-La Roche, Basel, Switzerland (also known as MRA, R-1569, humanized PM-1, or, in Japan, Actemra™). A clinical trial of tocilizumab was recently approved in Japan for the treatment of Castleman's disease, a rare lymphoproliferative disease associated with high levels of IL-6 production from enlarged lymph nodes.[60,61] This therapy is also in clinical development for rheumatoid arthritis, Crohn's disease, myeloproliferative disorder, and systemic lupus erythematosus.[60,61]

Anti-chemokine therapy

IL-8 is an 8-kilodalton chemokine with endothelial-cell chemotactic and proliferative activity.[62] High IL-8 expression levels render tumor cells highly tumorigenic, angiogenic, and invasive. The expression of IL-8 is associated with angiogenesis in metastatic melanoma[63] and non-small cell lung carcinoma,[64] and with prognosis in head and neck squamous cell carcinoma.[65] A humanized anti-IL-8 antibody, ABX-IL8 (Abgenix, Inc., Fremont, California), was used for treating various inflammatory and malignant diseases.[66] This high-affinity antibody blocks the binding of IL-8 to its receptors and inhibits IL-8-dependent neutrophil activation, migration, and degranulation.[67] A recent report on the development of anti-IL-8 (ABX-IL8) and anti-MUC18 (ABX-MA1; Abgenix) agents suggests that ABX-IL8 and ABX-MA1 could serve as new modalities for the treatment of melanoma either alone, or in combination with conventional chemotherapy or other antitumor agents.[68] The therapeutic value of blocking IL-8 has yet to be realized in cancer patients.

CXCR4 is a chemokine receptor that belongs to the seven transmembrane G protein-coupled receptor family, with SDF-1 (CXCL12) as its endogenous ligand. CXCR4 is involved in several diseases, including HIV infection and rheumatoid arthritis. It is also involved in cancer progression, especially metastasis.[69] In preclinical models, the BKT140 derivative (Biokine Therapeutics Ltd., Rehovot, Israel) significantly reduced pulmonary metastasis of breast cancer[70] and melanoma cells.[71] Blockade of the SDF-1/CXCR4 signaling axis by targeting either the ligand or the receptor was shown to inhibit cancer metastasis.[72] CTCE-9908 (Chemokine Therapeutics Corporation, Vancouver, Canada), an analogue of SDF-1 and antagonist of SDF-1 receptors, did not reveal any significant toxicity when administered to healthy adults[73] and has the potential to become part of a new generation of drugs that act to inhibit the spread and growth of cancer cells from the primary tumor. Another CXCR4 antagonist, AMD3100 (AnorMed Inc, Langley BC, Canada), appears to be a safe and effective agent for the rapid mobilization of CD34+ cells in patients who previously received chemotherapy.[74]

Targeting multiple signaling pathways with kinase inhibitors

Signal transduction in cancer cells involves receptor tyrosine kinases that trigger multiple cytoplasmic kinases, such as serine/threonine kinases. Tumor models have identified several key cellular signaling pathways that work independently, in parallel, or through interconnections to promote cancer development. Three major signaling pathways that have played important roles in tumorigenesis include the phosphatidyl inositol-3-kinase (PI3K)/AKT, protein kinase C family, and mitogen-activated protein kinase (MAPK)/Ras signaling cascades. However, specific or highly selective blocking of one of the kinases involved in these signaling pathways has been associated with limited or sporadic responses in clinical trials. Current understanding of the complexity of signal transduction processes and their roles in cancer suggests that simultaneous inhibition of several key kinases at the level of receptors and/or downstream serine/threonine kinases may improve the therapeutic benefit of the kinase-targeted anticancer agents. Preclinical and clinical studies also point to molecules on vascular endothelial cells and pericytes as being important targets for anticancer therapies. These studies suggest that an optimal anticancer therapy may involve targeting multiple molecules found in both the tumor and supportive vascular tissues.

Conclusions

The paradigm that persistent infection and chronic inflammation contribute via cytokine-mediated and chemokine-mediated dysregulation of immune responses to carcinogenesis is acknowledged in biomedical research. Inflammation is believed to trigger chronic diseases, and the major signaling pathway that controls inflammation-associated gene expression is the very one that activates the transcription factor NF-κB. The activation of the NF-κB, a hallmark of inflammatory responses, is frequently detected in tumors and contributes to the development of cancer-related symptoms.

New therapeutic opportunities for treating cancer are emerging, and the challenge for clinical oncologists and experimental cancer researchers will be to identify the appropriate molecular targets, cancer types, and disease stages for a particular type of therapy. In addition to traditional immune modulatory regimens, complementary therapies exemplified by epigallocatechin gallate from green tea, curcumin from curry, and soya isoflavones have been studied and shown to possess cancer chemopreventive properties. Curcumin has anti-proliferative and pro-apoptotic effects in melanoma cells that are related to the suppression of IκB kinase and NF-κB activity,[75] and the compound has been used in clinical trials as maintenance therapy for ulcerative colitis [76] and for treating inflammatory bowel disease.[77] In addition, curcumin has chemosensitizing properties in prostate, breast, hepatic, and lung tumors.

Finally, combining anti-inflammatory agents with another mode of therapy, such as cytotoxic, cytostatic, or antiangiogenic drugs, may prove to be an effective treatment strategy. Selecting the appropriate patient population for a given approach will involve pinpointing a set of biomarkers to reflect the nature of inflammatory responses in tumor tissues, and to enable selection of patients most likely to benefit from such therapies in terms of disease regression and reduction of symptom burden.

References

1. Lee BN, Dantzer R, Langley KE, et al. A cytokine-based neuroimmunologic mechanism of cancer-related symptoms. *Neuroimmunomodulation* **11**(5):279–292, 2004.

2. Coussens LM, Werb Z. Inflammation and cancer. *Nature* **420**(6917):860–867, 2002.

3. Rivest S, Lacroix S, Vallières L, Nadeau S, Zhang J, Laflamme N. How the blood talks to the brain parenchyma and the paraventricular nucleus of the hypothalamus during systemic inflammatory and infectious stimuli. *Proc Soc Exp Biol Med* **223**(1):22–38, 2000.

4. Craig R, Larkin A, Mingo AM, et al. p38 MAPK and NF-kappa B collaborate to induce interleukin-6 gene expression and release: evidence for a cytoprotective autocrine signaling pathway in a cardiac myocyte model system. *J Biol Chem* **275**(31):23814–23824, 2000.

5. Hierholzer C, Kalff JC, Bednarski B, et al. Rapid and simultaneous activation of Stat3 and production of interleukin 6 in resuscitated hemorrhagic shock. *Arch Orthop Trauma Surg* **119**:332–336, 1999.
6. Oncology Nursing Society. Welcome to CancerSymptoms.org. Available from: URL: www.cancersymptoms.org. Accessed Oct 29, 2008.
7. Cleeland CS. Cancer-related symptoms. *Semin Radiat Oncol* **10**(3):175–190, 2000.
8. Patrick DL, Ferketich SL, Frame PS, et al. National Institutes of Health State-of-the-Science Conference Statement: Symptom Management in Cancer: Pain, Depression, and Fatigue, July 15–17, 2002. *J Natl Cancer Inst Monogr* **32**:9–16, 2004.
9. Meyers CA, Abbruzzese JL. Cognitive functioning in cancer patients: effect of previous treatment. *Neurology* **42**:434–436, 1992.
10. Meyers CA, Valentine AD. Neurological and psychiatric adverse effects of immunological therapy. *CNS Drugs* **3**:56–68, 1995.
11. Valentine AD, Meyers CA. Neurobehavioral effects of interferon therapy. *Curr Psychiatry Rep* **7**:391–395, 2005.
12. Vojdani A, Lapp CW. Interferon-induced proteins are elevated in blood samples of patients with chemically or virally induced chronic fatigue syndrome. *Immunopharmacol Immunotoxicol* **21**:175–202, 1999.
13. Kurzrock R. The role of cytokines in cancer-related fatigue. *Cancer* **92**(6 Suppl):1684–1688, 2001.
14. Bower JE, Ganz PA, Aziz N, Fahey JL. Fatigue and proinflammatory cytokine activity in breast cancer survivors. *Psychosom Med* **64**(4):604–611, 2002.
15. Wang XS, Giralt SA, Mendoza TR, et al. Clinical factors associated with cancer-related fatigue in patients being treated for leukemia and non-Hodgkin's lymphoma. *J Clin Oncol* **20**:1319–1328, 2002.
16. Mantovani G, Macciò A, Lai P, Massa E, Ghiani M, Santona MC. Cytokine involvement in cancer anorexia/cachexia: role of megestrol acetate and medroxyprogesterone acetate on cytokine downregulation and improvement of clinical symptoms. *Crit Rev Oncog* **9**:99–106, 1998.
17. Rowinsky EK, Chaudhry V, Forastiere AA, et al. Phase I and pharmacologic study of paclitaxel and cisplatin with granulocyte colony-stimulating factor: neuromuscular toxicity is dose-limiting. *J Clin Oncol* **11**:2010–2020, 1993.
18. Weintraub M, Adde MA, Venzon DJ, et al. Severe atypical neuropathy associated with administration of hematopoietic colony-stimulating factors and vincristine. *J Clin Oncol* **14**:935–940, 1996.
19. Basu S, Sodhi A. Increased release of interleukin-1 and tumor necrosis factor by interleukin-2-induced lymphokine-activated killer cells in the presence of cisplatin and FK-565. *Immunol Cell Biol* **70**:15–24, 1992.
20. Gan XH, Jewett A, Bonavida B. Activation of human peripheral blood-derived monocytes by cis-diamminedichloroplatinum: enhanced tumoricidal activity and secretion of tumor necrosis factor-alpha. *Nat Immun* **11**:144–155, 1992.
21. O'Brien JM, Jr., Wewers MD, Moore SA, Allen JN. Taxol and colchicine increase LPS-induced pro-IL-1 beta production, but do not increase IL-1 beta secretion: a role for microtubules in the regulation of IL-1 beta production. *J Immunol* **154**(8):4113–4122, 1995.
22. Zaks-Zilberman M, Zaks TZ, Vogel SN. Induction of proinflammatory and chemokine genes by lipopolysaccharide and paclitaxel (Taxol) in murine and human breast cancer cell lines. *Cytokine* **15**(3):156–165, 2001.
23. Ogura K, Ohta S, Ohmori T, et al. Vinca alkaloids induce granulocyte-macrophage colony stimulating factor in human peripheral blood mononuclear cells. *Anticancer Res* **20**:2383–2388, 2000.
24. Dougherty PM, Palecek J, Palecková V, Sorkin LS, Willis WD. The role of NMDA and non-NMDA excitatory amino acid receptors in the excitation of primate spinothalamic tract neurons by mechanical, thermal, chemical, and electrical stimuli. *J Neurosci* **12**:3025–3041, 1992.
25. Lee BN, Andersson B, Cohen MZ, et al. Relationship between plasma cytokine levels and self-reported symptoms in AML patients pre- and post-transplantation with allogeneic peripheral blood stem cells [abstract]. American Society of Hematology 45th Annual Meeting and Exposition, *San Diego CA*, December 6–9, 2003. *Blood* **102**(11):966A, 2003. Abstract 3600.
26. Zlotnik A. Chemokines and cancer. *Int J Cancer* **119**:2026–2029, 2006.
27. Laverdiere C, Gorlick R. CXCR4 expression in osteosarcoma cell lines and tumor samples: evidence for expression by tumor cells. *Clin Cancer Res* **12**(17):5254, 2006.
28. Wang J, Xi L, Gooding W, Godfrey TE, Ferris RL. Chemokine receptors 6 and 7 identify a metastatic expression pattern in squamous cell carcinoma of the head and neck. *Adv Otorhinolaryngol* **62**:121–133, 2005.
29. Diaz GA. CXCR4 mutations in WHIM syndrome: a misguided immune system? *Immunol Rev* **203**:235–243, 2005.
30. Feldmann M. What is the mechanism of action of anti-tumour necrosis factor-alpha antibody in

rheumatoid arthritis? *Int Arch Allergy Immunol* **111**:362–365, 1996.

31. Ardizzone S, Bianchi Porro G. Biologic therapy for inflammatory bowel disease. *Drugs* **65**:2253–2286, 2005.
32. Karin M, Cao Y, Greten FR, Li ZW. NF-kB in cancer: from innocent bystander to major culprit. *Nature Rev Cancer* **2**(4):301–310, 2002.
33. Karin M. Nuclear factor-kappaB in cancer development and progression. *Nature* **441**:431–436, 2006.
34. Yamamoto Y, Gaynor RB. Therapeutic potential of inhibition of the NF-kB pathway in the treatment of inflammation and cancer. *J Clin Invest* **107**(2):134–142, 2001.
35. Surh YJ, Chun KS, Cha HH, et al. Molecular mechanisms underlying chemopreventive activities of anti-inflammatory phytochemicals: down-regulation of COX-2 and iNOS through suppression of NF-kappa B activation. *Mutation Res* **480–481**:243–268, 2001.
36. Rivest S. What is the cellular source of prostaglandins in the brain in response to systemic inflammation? Facts and controversies. *Molec Psychiatry* **4**:500–507, 1999.
37. O'Shea JJ, Murray PJ. Cytokine signaling modules in inflammatory responses. *Immunity* **28**(4):477–487, 2008.
38. Lotz M, Vaughan JH, Carson DA. Effect of neuropeptides on production of inflammatory cytokines by human monocytes. *Science* **241**:1218–1221, 1988.
39. Elenkov IJ, Wilder RL, Chrousos GP, Vizi ES. The sympathetic nerve – an integrative interface between two supersystems: the brain and the immune system. *Pharmacol Rev* **52**:595–638, 2000.
40. Elenkov IJ, Webster E, Papanicolaou DA, Fleisher TA, Chrousos GP, Wilder RL. Histamine potently suppresses human IL-12 and stimulates IL-10 production via H2 receptors. *J Immunol* **161**:2586–2593, 1998.
41. Trikha M, Corringham R, Klein B, Rossi JF. Targeted anti-interleukin-6 monoclonal antibody therapy for cancer: a review of the rationale and clinical evidence. *Clin Cancer Res* **9**:4653–4665, 2003.
42. Tilg H, Trehu E, Atkins MB, Dinarello CA, Mier JW. Interleukin-6 (IL-6) as an anti-inflammatory cytokine: induction of circulating IL-1 receptor antagonist and soluble tumor necrosis factor receptor p55. *Blood* **83**(1):113–118, 1994.
43. Schindler R, Mancilla J, Endres S, Ghorbani R, Clark SC, Dinarello CA. Correlations and interactions in the production of interleukin-6 (IL- 6), IL-1, and tumor necrosis factor (TNF) in human blood mononuclear cells: IL-6 suppresses IL-1 and TNF. *Blood* **75**(1):40–47, 1990.
44. Korth C, Mullington J, Schreiber W, Pollmächer T. Influence of endotoxin on daytime sleep in humans. *Infect Immun* **64**:1110–1115, 1996.
45. Born J, Späth-Schwalbe E, Schwakenhofer H, Kern W, Fehm HL. Influences of corticotropin-releasing hormone, adrenocorticotropin, and cortisol on sleep in normal man. *J Clin Endocrinol Metab* **68**(5):904–911, 1989.
46. Cidlowski JA, Bellingham DL, Powell-Oliver FE, Lubahn DB, Sar M. Novel antipeptide antibodies to the human glucocorticoid receptor: recognition of multiple receptor forms in vitro and distinct localization of cytoplasmic and nuclear receptors. *Mol Endocrinol* **4**:1427–1437, 1990.
47. Auphan N, DiDonato JA, Rosette C, Helmberg A, Karin M. Immunosuppression by glucocorticoids: inhibition of NF-kappaB activity through induction of I kappa B synthesis. *Science* **270**:286–290, 1995.
48. Ramdas J, Harmon J. Glucocorticoid-induced apoptosis and regulation of NF-kappaB activity in human leukemic T cells. *Endocrinology* **139**:3813–3821, 1998.
49. Scheinman R, Cogswell P, Lofquist A, Baldwin A. Role of transcriptional activation of I kappaB in mediation of immunosuppression by glucocorticoids. *Science* **270**:283–286, 1995.
50. Karayiannakis AJ, Syrigos KN, Polychronidis A, Pitiakoudis M, Bounovas A, Simopoulos K. Serum levels of tumor necrosis factor-alpha and nutritional status in pancreatic cancer patients. *Anticancer Res* **21**:1355–1358, 2001.
51. Yoshida N, Ikemoto S, Narita K, et al. Interleukin-6, tumour necrosis factor alpha and interleukin-1beta in patients with renal cell carcinoma. *Br J Cancer* **86**:1396–1400, 2002.
52. Bozcuk H, Uslu G, Samur M, et al. Tumour necrosis factor-alpha, interleukin-6, and fasting serum insulin correlate with clinical outcome in metastatic breast cancer patients treated with chemotherapy. *Cytokine* **27**:58–65, 2004.
53. Michalaki V, Syrigos KN, Charles P, Waxman J. Serum levels of IL-6 and TNF-alpha correlate with clinicopathological features and patient survival in patients with prostate cancer. *Br J Cancer* **90**:2312–2316, 2004.
54. List A, Kurtin S, Roe DJ, et al. Efficacy of lenalidomide in myelodysplastic syndromes. *N Engl J Med* **352**(6):549–557, 2005.
55. Richardson PG, Blood E, Mitsiades CS, et al. A randomized phase 2 study of lenalidomide therapy for patients with relapsed or relapsed and refractory multiple myeloma. *Blood* **108**(10):3458–3464, 2006.

56. Ferrajoli A, Lee BN, Schlette EJ, et al. Lenalidomide induces complete and partial remissions in patients with relapsed and refractory chronic lymphocytic leukemia. *Blood* **111**(11):5291–5297, 2008.

57. Field-Smith A, Morgan GJ, Davies FE. Bortezomib (Velcade®) in the treatment of multiple myeloma. *Ther Clin Risk Manag* **2**(3):271–279, 2006.

58. Dominguez C, Powers DA, Tamayo N. p38 MAP kinase inhibitors: many are made, but few are chosen. *Curr Opin Drug Discov Devel* **8**(4):421–430, 2005.

59. Voorhees PM, Chen Q, Kuhn DJ, et al. Inhibition of interleukin-6 signaling with CNTO 328 enhances the activity of bortezomib in preclinical models of multiple myeloma. *Clin Cancer Res* **13**(21):6469–6478, 2007.

60. Paul-Pletzer K. Tocilizumab: blockade of interleukin-6 signaling pathway as a therapeutic strategy for inflammatory disorders. *Drugs Today (Barc)* **42**: 559–576, 2006.

61. Nishimoto N. Clinical studies in patients with Castleman's disease, Crohn's disease, and rheumatoid arthritis in Japan. *Clin Rev Allergy Immunol* **28**: 221–230, 2005.

62. Baggiolini M, Dewald B, Moser B. Interleukin-8 and related chemotactic cytokines – CXC and CC chemokines. *Adv Immunol* **55**:97–179, 1994.

63. Singh RK, Varney ML, Bucana CD, Johansson SL. Expression of interleukin-8 in primary and metastatic malignant melanoma of the skin. *Melanoma Res* **9**:383–387, 1999.

64. Masuya D, Huang CL, Liu D, et al. The intratumoral expression of vascular endothelial growth factor and interleukin-8 associated with angiogenesis in nonsmall cell lung carcinoma patients. *Cancer* **92**(10):2628–2638, 2001.

65. Eisma RJ, Spiro JD, Kreutzer DL. Role of angiogenic factors: coexpression of interleukin-8 and vascular endothelial growth factor in patients with head and neck squamous carcinoma. *Laryngoscope* **109**(5):687–693, 1999.

66. Huang S, Mills L, Mian B, et al. Fully humanized neutralizing antibodies to interleukin-8 (ABX-IL8) inhibit angiogenesis, tumor growth, and metastasis of human melanoma. *Am J Pathol* **161**:125–134, 2002.

67. Yang XD, Corvalan JR, Wang P, Roy CM, Davis CG. Fully human anti-interleukin-8 monoclonal antibodies: potential therapeutics for the treatment of inflammatory disease states. *J Leukoc Biol* **66**:401–410, 1999.

68. Melnikova VO, Bar-Eli M. Bioimmunotherapy for melanoma using fully human antibodies targeting MCAM/MUC18 and IL-8. *Pigment Cell Res* **19**:395–405, 2006.

69. Harvey JR, Mellor P, Eldaly H, Lennard TW, Kirby JA, Ali S. Inhibition of CXCR4-mediated breast cancer metastasis: a potential role for heparinoids? *Clin Cancer Res* **13**:1562–1570, 2007.

70. Tamamura H, Hori A, Kanzaki N. T140 analogs as CXCR4 antagonists identified as anti-metastatic agents in the treatment of breast cancer. *FEBS Lett* **550**:79–83, 2003.

71. Takenaga M, Tamamura H, Hiramatsu K. A single treatment with microcapsules containing a CXCR4 antagonist suppresses pulmonary metastasis of murine melanoma. *Biochem Biophys Res Commun* **320**:226–232, 2004.

72. Liang Z, Yoon Y, Votaw J, Goodman MM, Williams L, Shim H. Silencing of CXCR4 blocks breast cancer metastasis. *Cancer Res* **65**:967–971, 2005.

73. Kim SY, Lee CH, Midura BV, et al. Inhibition of the CXCR4/CXCL12 chemokine pathway reduces the development of murine pulmonary metastases. *Clin Exp Metastasis* **25**(3):201–211, 2008.

74. Devine SM, Flomenberg N, Vesole DH, et al. Rapid mobilization of CD34+ cells following administration of the CXCR4 antagonist AMD3100 to patients with multiple myeloma and non-Hodgkin's lymphoma. *J Clin Oncol* **22**:1095–1102, 2004.

75. Siwak DR, Shishodia S, Aggarwal BB, Kurzrock R. Curcumin-induced antiproliferative and proapoptotic effects in melanoma cells are associated with suppression of Ikappa B kinase and nuclear factor kappaB activity and are independent of the B-Raf/mitogen-activated/extracellular signal-regulated protein kinase pathway and the Akt pathway. *Cancer* **104**(4):879–890, 2005.

76. Hanai H, Iida T, Takeuchi K, et al. Curcumin maintenance therapy for ulcerative colitis: randomized, multicenter, double-blind, placebo-controlled trial. *Clin Gastroenterol Hepatol* **4**(12):1502–1506, 2006.

77. Holt PR, Katz S, Kirshoff R. Curcumin therapy in inflammatory bowel disease: a pilot study. *Dig Dis Sci* **50**:2191–2193, 2005.

Section 2 Chapter

17

Cancer Symptom Mechanisms and Models: Clinical and Basic Science

Genetic approaches to treating and preventing symptoms in patients with cancer

Qiuling Shi and Charles S. Cleeland

Disease-related and treatment-related symptoms vary among patients with cancer, even when disease severity and treatment modality are comparable. Numerous studies document that age, gender, race/ethnicity, mood states, and other environmental factors can influence the individual's symptom experience. However, the large interindividual variation not explained by such factors suggests that genetic characteristics may contribute to the variability. Genetic variations and the differences in proteins they encode affect individuals' predispositions to symptoms and to other common diseases. As a complex process, development of cancer-related symptoms is influenced by multiple genetic variations, each of which makes a small contribution to the patient's overall symptom susceptibility.

Identifying the associations between cancer-related symptoms and common genetic variations provides several potential benefits. First, investigating the relationship between patients' genetic variations and their predispositions to certain symptoms may reveal the biological mechanisms or pathways governing symptom development. Second, determining the genotypes that are highly correlated to specific symptoms may help clinicians identify patients who have a high risk for symptom burden and who would benefit from preventive therapy. Third, using genotypes to evaluate an individual patient's sensitivity to specific treatments could enable clinicians to manage multiple symptoms by targeting underlying biological mechanisms instead of treating individual symptoms empirically (eg, stimulants for fatigue, opioids for pain). Controlling or even preventing symptoms in such a personalized way would potentially benefit thousands of cancer patients and survivors.

The effects of genes on cancer-related symptoms have been investigated simultaneously in both animals and humans. Knockout and transgenic animal models have been used to explore the functions and variations of target genes affecting the biological pathways involved in symptom development and treatment response. New high-throughput techniques such as proteomics have been used to identify novel pathways and new treatment targets. Whereas research using animal models might reveal symptom-relevant genes, molecular epidemiological studies focused on genetic polymorphisms are able to evaluate individual patients' susceptibility to multiple symptoms and sensitivity to treatment. Described more fully below, linkage analysis has been used to identify candidate genomic regions that may relate to specific phenotypes in family samples, and association analysis is being used to identify a patient's risk for genetic variations that could exacerbate multiple symptoms or affect symptom treatment (Figure 17.1).

In this chapter, we discuss the genetic variations associated with the incidence, development, and management of symptoms in patients with cancer. We propose a new concept, "symptom phenotype," to describe the observable characteristics of an individual patient's multiple symptoms. We also introduce the genotype markers used to identify associations between common genetic variations and cancer-related symptoms, and we summarize three molecular epidemiological approaches to evaluating these associations. Finally, we discuss genetic variations that have been associated with several common cancer-related and treatment-related symptoms – pain, analgesic response, depression, fatigue, sleep disturbance, and cognitive impairment.

Phenotyping and genotyping

Symptom phenotyping

A living organism's phenotype is anything that is part of the observable structure, function, or behavior of that organism, as determined by a combination of its genotype and the environment. Investigators of the molecular mediators of behavior have used the concept of "behavioral phenotype" to describe delayed

Cancer Symptom Science: Measurement, Mechanisms, and Management, eds. Charles S. Cleeland, Michael J. Fisch, and Adrian J. Dunn.

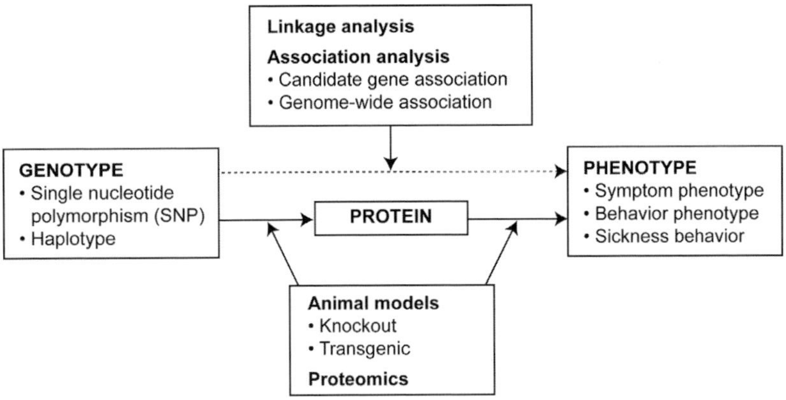

Figure 17.1. Approaches for gene–symptom associations. Knockout and transgenic animal models allow researchers to explore the functions and variations in target genes affecting the biological pathways involved in symptom development and treatment response. Proteomics identify novel proteins that may imply new pathways and novel targets for drug search. Linkage analyses identify candidate genomic regions that may relate to specific phenotypes in family samples, and association studies identify patients' risk for genetic polymorphisms to enhance the prevention and treatment of multiple symptoms.

cognitive development and mental retardation in humans with genetic disorders such as Down syndrome and fragile X syndrome[1], and in animal models of sickness behaviors such as depression, anorexia, hyperalgesia, and impaired cognitive ability.[2] Given the similarities in the occurrence of and molecular mechanisms of symptoms in cancer patients and sickness behaviors in animal models,[3] we propose the concept "symptom phenotype" to describe a cancer patient's co-occurring symptoms that share molecular mechanisms.

In studies of gene–symptom associations, symptoms are commonly assessed and treated individually or classified separately as physical symptoms (eg, pain), cognitive symptoms (eg, impaired memory), or affective symptoms (eg, anxiety and depression). In contrast, symptom phenotype comprises cancer-related symptoms as a whole. Because symptom phenotype is a novel concept, the methods for describing it and applying it are still emerging. One consideration in symptom phenotyping is the need to assess the impact of multiple symptoms (eg, symptom burden) and to interpret the impact in a meaningful way, especially because a patient's phenotype is not known *a priori*. Symptom burden has been successfully measured via instruments that assess patient report of symptoms (patient-reported outcomes, or PROs).[4] In studies that investigate the association between genetic variations and symptoms, PROs are typically continuous or categorical outcomes with cut points. However, because symptom phenotype considers the effect of all symptoms a patient experiences, we propose that cluster analysis be used to assign patients to groups of either high or low overall symptom burden on the basis of their scores of multiple symptoms.

Cluster analysis is a simple, descriptive statistical method that identifies sets of similar individuals with minimal within-group variation and maximum between-group variation. Cluster analysis allows investigators to establish groups and analyze group membership without prior knowledge of classification values or the number of groups required. A number of clustering algorithms, including hierarchical, partitional, density-based, and two-way clustering algorithms, can be used to investigate associations between genetic variations and symptom development.[5] Choosing the appropriate algorithm for applying cluster analysis to assign patients to groups according to their symptom burden is a contentious issue, however, and clear guidelines for conducting and reporting cluster analyses are needed to obtain an accurate and replicable symptom phenotype.

Another consideration for symptom phenotyping is that cancer patients' symptoms usually change over time because of disease progression and/or treatment response. To obtain replicable genetic markers and gene–symptom associations that can be interpreted within specific clinical applications, phenotyping techniques must be able to describe the longitudinal characteristics of symptoms. To date, there is no recommendation for how the longitudinal symptom burden should be described in a gene–symptom association study.

One attempt to address the considerations above (the multiplicity of cancer-related symptoms and the longitudinal nature of disease and treatment) is the group-based trajectory model exemplified in Figure 17.2.[6] The developmental trajectories shown in the figure indicate variations in symptom susceptibility among individual patients that are likely caused by

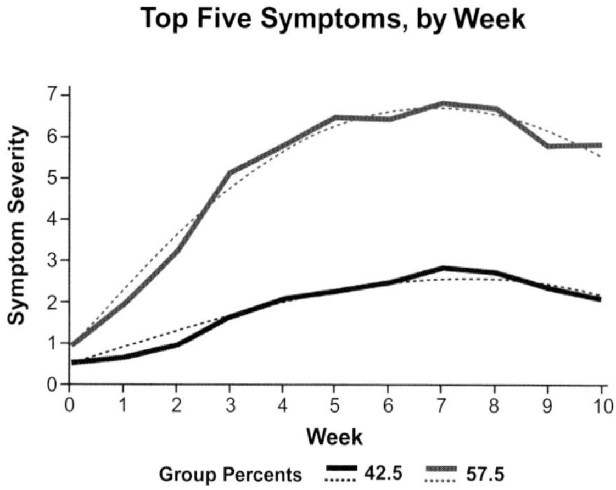

Figure 17.2. Phenotyping longitudinal symptoms. Group-based modeling was used to phenotype multiple longitudinal symptoms in cancer patients undergoing chemotherapy and/or radiotherapy. A total of 182 patients with head and neck cancer or breast cancer were followed for 10 weeks; symptoms were assessed repeatedly on a 0–10 numeric rating scale. At the end of treatment, the five symptoms experienced most frequently were fatigue, pain, disturbed sleep, lack of appetite, and drowsiness. On the basis of the longitudinal measurements of these symptoms, patients with distinct developmental trajectories were divided into two groups. Seventy-eight patients (43%) with no or mild symptom burden over the course of treatment were assigned to one group; the remaining 104 patients (57%), who were asymptomatic at the beginning of treatment but suffered increasing symptom burden as treatment progressed, were assigned to the second group.

patients' genetic backgrounds and environmental interactions. Rather than assuming the existence of specific developmental trajectories before performing statistical analyses, researchers can use group-based modeling to classify patients regardless of whether or not hypothesized trajectories emerge. In addition, group-based modeling of longitudinal PRO data produces phenotypes that are comparable to the known phenotypes of other common diseases, thus enabling researchers to apply established statistical analyses in genetic association studies and to interpret the clinical relevance of these associations.

Genotyping

Humans, even monozygotic twins, are genetically diverse. The Human Genome Projects have identified millions of genetic variations, including single nucleotide polymorphisms (SNPs), copy number variation, epigenetics, and variable number tandem repeats. These genetic variations, especially SNPs, have been used as biological markers to locate genes associated with disease and to predict an individual's susceptibility to environmental factors and response to drugs.

SNPs, which account for about 90% of the variations in DNA sequence, are the genetic markers most frequently used to analyze individual genomic backgrounds for their association with disease phenotypes. An SNP is a variation of a single nucleotide (A, T, C, or G) in the DNA sequence of a gene. SNPs occur normally throughout human DNA, with an approximate frequency of one in every 300 nucleotides. There are approximately 10 million common SNPs in the human genome. The three major types of SNPs include substitution, in which a single nucleotide is replaced; deletion, in which a single nucleotide is removed from the polynucleotide sequence; and insertion, in which a single nucleotide is added.

SNPs occur throughout the genome, in coding regions, noncoding sequences, and intergenic regions. SNPs in the coding region are usually classified as either nonsynonymous or synonymous. In a nonsynonymous SNP, the DNA base change results in an altered polypeptide sequence. A nonsynonymous change may influence the function of the gene product (mRNA or protein) by altering the amino acid sequence of the protein or may produce a nonfunctional protein as a result of premature termination. Because of their impact on protein function, nonsynonymous SNPs have been primary candidate markers in gene–disease association studies. For example, *rs4680*, a nonsynonymous SNP of the catechol-*O*-methyltransferase (COMT) gene, *COMT*, causes the substitution of methionine for valine at position 158, which is associated with a 3-fold to 4-fold reduction in COMT activity and is thus related to increased pain sensitivity.[7] *rs4680* has been associated with pain perception,[8] the efficacy and side effects of morphine,[9] and depression and anxiety[10] in patients with cancer, and as such is considered a candidate genetic marker in symptom research, especially in pain studies.

Synonymous SNPs lead to the same polypeptide sequence and so seldom affect the function of the protein that is produced. Although synonymous SNPs cause few functional changes, some have been associated with disease onset by influencing protein folding and mRNA splicing and stability.[11] For example, *his62his* (*rs4633*) and *leu136leu* (*rs4818*), two diverse synonymous SNPs of the *COMT* gene that alter the mRNA structure and increase or decrease the amounts of protein,[12] are associated with pain sensitivity.[8]

SNPs in noncoding regions are either intronic or intergenic and may affect gene splicing, transcription factor binding, and noncoding RNA sequencing. For example, the SNP *C-889T* (*rs1800587*) in the promoter region of interleukin *(IL)-1α* does not functionally change the IL-1α protein but decreases mRNA expression and serum protein levels by affecting the enzymatic efficiency of the protease that cleaves pre-IL-1α.[13]

Analyzing multiple SNPs in a region of interest provides more information about gene–disease associations than analyzing a single genetic marker. Theoretically, identifying the genetic markers that are related to a particular disease requires information about all genetic variations in an individual's complete DNA sequence. However, the high cost of full-genome sequencing makes this approach unfeasible. Instead, the haplotype, a set of SNPs in the same chromosome that are generally inherited together and can be identified by patterns of genetic variation, is used to identify potential disease-related genetic markers.[14] Genetic variations, mainly SNPs, in one haplotype are statistically linked, implying that a specific SNP can be predicted on the basis of nearby known SNPs and that a few SNPs are enough to identify the haplotypes in a given chromosomal region. Smaller sets of informative SNPs, known as tag SNPs, can represent the genetic variation across a specific region or the entire genome. By eliminating the redundancy in the information provided by the SNPs, tag SNPs enable researchers to investigate genetic markers without having to genotype every SNP in the chromosomal region of interest.

In gene–disease association studies, tag SNPs are usually selected using data from a dense network of SNPs that have been identified in a relatively small panel of subjects. The National Institute of Environmental Health Sciences' Environmental Genome Project – which aims to genotype SNPs in more than 600 environmental response genes in a panel of 95 individuals of diverse ethnicities – is one of the primary data sources for tag SNP selection.[15] With those data, haplotype-block-dependent and haplotype-block-independent approaches can be used to identify tag SNPs. Haplotype-block-dependent approaches require defined haplotype blocks, which allow SNPs that are highly correlated but outside of those blocks to go undetected.[16,17] Also, because haplotype blocks vary among populations, applying haplotype data obtained from one sample set to a different sample set can be difficult.[18] Haplotype-block-independent approaches, which are used more frequently than haplotype-block-dependent approaches, use correlations between SNPs only (ie, linkage disequilibrium properties of the SNPs) to identify the most informative SNPs across a region of interest.[19,20]

A number of software packages for deriving tag SNPs are available online. Each of those packages usually implements one of the approaches proposed here. Researchers can select one or more software packages to obtain the tag SNP set that will most likely fulfill their specific research purposes.

Approaches for studying gene-linked symptoms in humans

A number of innovative techniques have been used to identify the common biological mechanisms of cancer-related symptoms. Advances in molecular technology, such as high-throughput genotyping techniques, now enable the assessment of genetic variations in diverse populations. Genetic markers are integrated with psychological and physiological measurements to assess symptom risk in individuals and groups. The two main approaches used to identify phenotype-associated genes in humans are linkage analysis and association analysis (Figure 17.1).

Linkage analysis

Linkage analysis, which is typically the first step in identifying gene-related diseases, is used to investigate potential associations between phenotypes and related genes' locations on chromosomes. Genetic markers that are located near each other on the same chromosome tend to be inherited together; therefore, if a patient inherits specific genetic markers along with a particular disease, the disease-related genes can likely be found near the genetic markers on the same chromosome. The base 10 logarithm of odds (LOD) score is the primary statistical means of estimating genetic linkage; a score of 3 or greater indicates that two genetic markers are likely to be inherited together.

Although the method primarily focuses on familial inheritance patterns, linkage analysis can also be used to identify the locations of potential candidate genes in common gene–common disease association studies. For example, Yang et al.[21] linked primary erythermalgia, a condition characterized by burning sensation in the extremities along with redness and increased temperature in the skin, to a 5.98 cM genetic region on chromosome 2q. The region contains the *SCN9A* gene encoding the α-subunit of Nav1.7, the voltage-gated sodium channel, which is strongly expressed in nociceptive neurons. Two *SCN9A* gene mutations, *T2573A* and *T2543C*, were found in a number of patients regardless of whether the patients were related, suggesting that *T2573A* and *T2543C* are candidate markers for patients' predisposition to pain.

Association analysis

The primary purpose of association analysis is to identify susceptibility gene markers for preventing and treating common diseases by determining whether a particular DNA polymorphism occurs more frequently in patients with a phenotype of interest than in patients without the phenotype. Association analyses are generally performed in unrelated patients using a case-control or cohort study design. The approach could be hypothesis-driven, as in a candidate gene association study, or hypothesis-free, as in a genome-wide association study.

Candidate gene studies

Hypothesis-driven candidate gene studies investigate genes that may be involved in the biological pathways that regulate disease development and treatment response. Choosing genetic markers hypothesized to modify targeted phenotypes is crucial to performing a successful candidate gene association study. Researchers can select candidate genetic markers from: (1) the pool of previously reported genetic variations involved in a phenotype that may share the same biological pathways with target phenotypes; (2) genes identified by linkage analysis to be located in a particular chromosomal region; (3) genetic variations already known to alter protein activities; or (4) genetic variations with statistically significant association with a symptom phenotype or with high linkage to such a variation in an initial genome-wide association study.

The identification of a disease-related SNP or haplotype is partially dependent on the number of genetic markers tested. Testing a small set of SNPs that focus on known biological pathways may increase the statistical power of the study[22]; however, because most common diseases are consequences of multiple genes, testing such a limited set of SNPs may also reveal weak associations with symptoms or associations that cannot be replicated.[8,23,24] Genotyping tag SNPs in the candidate gene may partially solve this problem because tag SNPs can theoretically represent all variations throughout a gene of interest. When three or more SNPs are involved in the association study, the problem of multiple comparisons should also be considered. Multiple comparison is a statistical concern that occurs when three or more hypotheses are tested simultaneously, which may cause incorrect rejection of the null hypothesis (false positives). The easiest and most common way to control for multiple comparisons is to use the Bonferroni correction, in which the threshold P value, usually 0.05, is divided by the number of SNPs tested: for example, if 100 SNPs are tested, the P value would be set at 0.0005. However, because the Bonferroni correction is a conservative method, a large sample size is required to obtain a statistically significant association when hundreds of genetic markers are involved.

Genome-wide association studies

Unlike a candidate gene association study, which targets small candidate regions, a genome-wide association study (GWAS) examines genetic variations across a given genome to identify associations between specific genes and common diseases. Because the entire genome is analyzed, a GWAS enables investigators to study the genetics of a phenotype without having to formulate hypotheses about potential mechanisms or candidate genes. A well-designed GWAS can identify previously unknown genetic markers that may indicate novel biological pathways underlying gene–disease associations.[25,26] GWASs have already revealed modest gene-disease associations in, for example, autism, type 2 diabetes, prostate cancer, breast cancer, and colorectal cancer.[27]

Because approximately 1 million SNPs are tested simultaneously in a GWAS, multiple comparisons are a much more overwhelming issue in a GWAS than in a traditional epidemiology or candidate gene association study. Using the Bonferroni correction method to avoid false positives, the threshold for claiming "genome-wide" significance is usually around 5×10^{-8}, thus requiring thousands of patients to detect a gene–disease association. In addition, disease-associated SNPs discovered in a GWAS may not directly reveal the underlying biology of the specific phenotype, because these SNPs may be located in yet unknown chromosome regions or may simply be part of a larger block of SNPs that are highly correlated with each other and involve a functional SNP at some distance. Such SNPs should be considered location markers, and SNPs that are involved in the same region should be considered in future candidate–gene association studies to generate useful markers for investigating disease etiology and developing novel drug targets.[28]

Genetic variations associated with cancer-related symptoms

In candidate gene association studies used to evaluate genetic disposition to cancer-related symptoms, genetic markers are selected from the biological pathways related to specific symptoms, including the inflammation, neurotransmission, and drug metabolism and transport pathways. The genetic variations associated with disease-related or treatment-related symptoms in cancer patients in each of these biological pathways are summarized in Table 17.1.

Inflammation

Patients with cancer exhibit many symptoms that are very similar to animal sickness behaviors caused by inflammation in response to an immune challenge. Sickness behaviors can be elicited by the subcutaneous, intravenous, or intraperitoneal systemic administration of proinflammatory cytokines, including IL-1, tumor necrosis factor (TNF)-α, interferon-α, and IL–2.[36] Cytokines may play a mechanistic role in cancer-related symptoms. Bower et al.[37] found that changes in the serum levels of two inflammatory markers, C-reactive protein and IL-1 receptor antagonist (IL-1RA), were positively associated with increases in fatigue in patients undergoing radiotherapy for breast or prostate cancer. In a study of patients with acute myelogenous leukemia or myelodysplastic syndrome, Wang et al.[38] found that the release of systemic inflammatory cytokines (mainly IL-6) was associated with an increase in treatment-related, multiple-symptom burden during the nadir of allogeneic hematopoietic stem cell transplantation. The findings of Bower et al. and Wang et al. suggest that the genetic variations that increase patients' fatigue or inflammatory cytokine levels may be associated with specific cancer-related symptoms.

Interleukin-1

IL-1 participates in activating T cells and induces adhesion molecule expression. IL-1 administration in rats can lead to mechanical allodynia and hyperalgesia[39] and can enhance rats' responsiveness to stressful environmental stimuli.[40] Two polypeptides, IL-1α and IL-1β, and the competitive inhibitor IL-1RA determine the activity of IL-1. *IL-1α*, *IL-1β*, and *IL-1RA* genes are mapped to a closely linked area on chromosome 2q13-q24. The polymorphisms *IL-1α C889T* (*rs1800587*),[41] *IL-1βC3954T* (*rs1143634*),[42] *IL-1βC-511T* (*rs16944*),[43] and an 86-base-pair repeat VNTR (variable number of tandem repeats polymorphism) in the *IL-1RA* gene,[44] have biological relevance in regulating IL-1 production. Although these polymorphisms are not associated with cancer-related symptoms, the *IL-1β-511 TC* and *TT* genotypes were significantly related to higher toxicity in patients receiving 5-fluorouracil plus cisplatin chemotherapy[45]

Table 17.1. Genetic variants associated with disease-related or treatment-related symptoms in patients with cancer

Gene	Polymorphism	Pain phenotype	Sample	Reference
COMT	rs4680	Morphine consumption	Cancer patients	Rakvåg et al.[29]
	Haplotype of SNPs in intron 1	Opioid side effects	Cancer patients	Ross et al.[30]
	Haplotype of 11 SNPs	Morphine consumption	Cancer patients	Rakvåg et al.[9]
OPRM1	rs1799971	Pain perception, morphine consumption	Cancer patients	Klepstad et al.[31]
IL-6	rs1800795	Opioid response	Lung cancer patients	Reyes-Gibby et al.[32]
IL-8	rs4073	Pain severity	Caucasian lung cancer patients	Reyes-Gibby et al.[33]
TNF-α	rs1800629	Pain severity	Lung cancer patients	Reyes-Gibby et al.[32]
ABCB1	rs1045642 rs2032582	Morphine response	Cancer patients	Campa et al.[34], Klepstad et al.[35]

Abbreviations: COMT, catechol-O-methyltransferase; SNPs, single nucleotide polymorphisms; OPRM1, μ-opioid receptor; IL, interleukin; TNF, tumor necrosis factor; ABCB1, adenosine triphosphate-binding cassette family member B1.

and to fatigue in a limited sample size of breast cancer survivors (33 patients and 14 controls).[46] In patients with low back pain, the *IL-1β 3954T* allele was associated with longer pain duration and higher pain intensity, and *IL-1RA 1812A* was associated with multiple pain phenotypes, including more frequent pain occurrence, increased pain duration, and prolonged limitations on daily activity.[47] The 86-base-pair repeat in the *IL-1RA* gene was associated with higher morphine consumption postsurgery in women.[48]

Interleukin-6

IL-6 plays multiple roles in the physiology of nociception and the pathophysiology of pain. Bianchi et al.[49] found that *IL-6* gene knockout mice showed a reduced analgesic response to morphine and a more rapid development of tolerance to the analgesic effect of morphine. High plasma levels of IL-6 have been associated with the development of post-traumatic stress disorders,[50] pain,[38] and depression[51,52] in patients with cancer and in older patients.[53] In animal models, central administration of rat recombinant IL-6 increases non-rapid-eye-movement sleep in rats,[54] and elevated peripheral IL-6 levels have been linked to long-lasting cognitive deficits in older mice.[55] The *C* allele of the *G–174C* (*rs1800795*) SNP in the *IL-6* gene promoter region was found to be associated with significantly lower levels of plasma IL-6 in healthy people.[56] Patients with lung cancer who were homozygous for the *–174C* allele required an opioid dose for pain relief that was 4.7 times higher than the dose required for patients who were heterozygous or homozygous for the *G* allele.[32] In patients treated with interferon-α and ribavirin for hepatitis C, those who were homozygous for the *G* allele had significantly fewer symptoms of depression than patients who were heterozygous for the allele.[57] Patients with juvenile rheumatoid arthritis who were homozygous for the *G* allele reported higher pain severity than patients who were heterozygous for the *G* allele.[58] In patients with sciatica, the *GGGA* haplotype of four SNPs (*A–596G*, *G–572C*, *G–174C*, and *T+15A*) was found to predict duration of back or leg pain.[59]

Tumor necrosis factor-α

TNF-α plays a major role in the inflammatory response after surgery, infection, and trauma. TNF-α expression has been correlated with the development of allodynia or hyperalgesia in neuropathic pain models.[39,60] In mice with inflammatory pain induced by carrageenan injection, TNF-α mRNA was increased at the site of injection.[61] The *A* allele of the *G–308A* (*rs3093544*) polymorphism in the *TNF-α* gene promoter site has been associated with high promoter activity and increased TNF-α expression.[62] This allele has been associated with greater pain severity in Caucasian patients with non-small cell lung cancer.[32] Findings of associations between *TNF-α* polymorphisms and symptoms other than pain have been contradictory. For example, the *GG* genotype of *G–308A* has been associated with a greater risk of developing major depression in older Caucasian patients[63] but not Asian patients.[64]

Interleukin 8

IL-8, a major mediator of the inflammatory response, attracts neutrophils and macrophages, and manifests a wide range of proinflammatory effects.[65] In a study of 23 patients who underwent surgery for lumbar disc herniations with radiculopathy, IL-8 mRNA expression was associated with the development and duration of radicular pain caused by back extension.[66] A common SNP, *T–251A* (*rs4073*), is located in the *IL-8* gene's promoter region; the *A* allele has been associated with increased IL-8 production in lipopolysaccharide-stimulated whole blood[67] and severe pain in Caucasian patients with lung cancer.[33]

Other cytokines

Other cytokine genes, such as the IL-10 (*IL10*), transforming growth factor-β (*TGF-β*), and interferon (*IFN*) genes, have been associated with the development and prognosis of a number of cancers. Well-designed studies with sufficient sample size and consistent symptom phenotypes are warranted to identify the associations between these cytokine genes' polymorphisms and cancer-related symptoms.

Neurotransmission

Symptoms are the consequences of interactions between a stimulus and the neurotransmission system. When a stimulus is encountered, the sensory neuron releases neurotransmitters, which bind to postsynaptic receptors and activate transmission pathways. Several neurotransmitters and receptors, such as serotonin, certain catecholamines, and γ-aminobutyric acid (GABA), contribute to the transmission of sensations within the brain and spinal cord. Genes that modulate expression and activity of these proteins may explain individual differences in perception of symptoms, and thus are potential targets for development of symptom-control treatments.

Catechol-*O*-methyltransferase

Catechol-*O*-methyltransferase (COMT) mediates the inactivation of catecholamine neurotransmitters, including dopamine, adrenaline, and noradrenaline. Reduced COMT enzymatic activity may increase patients' sensitivity to and temporal summation of pain. Diatchenko et al.[8] found that a haplotype of four *COMT* SNPs (*rs6269*, *rs4818*, *rs4680*, and *rs4633*) was strongly associated with variation in the risk for developing myogenous temporomandibular joint disorder, a common musculoskeletal pain condition. This haplotype has also been found to modulate protein expression by altering mRNA secondary structure.[12] Polymorphisms of the *COMT* gene have also been investigated for their possible roles in symptoms other than pain. Babovic et al.[68] found that mice with the homozygous *COMT* deletion had improved spatial learning and working memory, whereas mice with the heterozygous deletion had cognitive impairment. In humans, the *Val158Met* polymorphism has been found to contribute to multiple cognitive impairment phenotypes, including age-related decline in executive cognition,[69] cognitive deterioration in patients with psychosis,[70] cognitive stability and aggregation in patients with first-onset schizophrenia,[71] and cognitive response to antipsychotic medication.[72] However, a meta-analysis revealed that the *COMT Val158/108Met* polymorphism may have little if any association with cognitive function.[73] The *COMT* gene may also be involved in response to antidepressant treatment. The *Val158Met* polymorphism has been associated with increased response to sleep deprivation plus phototherapy,[74] paroxetine,[75,76] and electroconvulsive therapy.[76] Although their roles in cancer-related symptoms have not been thoroughly investigated, *COMT* polymorphisms, especially the *Val158Met* polymorphism, remain potential candidate genetic variations for multiple cancer-related symptoms.

Opioid receptors

Opioid receptors are specific receptors essential to the analgesic action of morphine and similar opioids.[77] The three types of opioid receptors – μ-opioid, δ-opioid, and κ-opioid – are expressed in both central and peripheral nerve systems,[78] as well as in various circulating immune cells.[79] The μ-opioid receptor is the primary binding site for morphine and other opioid analgesics.[80] The most studied SNP in the μ-opioid receptor gene (*OPRM1*), *A118G*, causes an amino acid exchange from asparagine to aspartate at position 40.[81] This nucleotide shift decreases μ-opioid receptor signaling efficacy in the S2 brain region, an important part of the pain matrix that codes for pain intensity[82] (see Chapter 18). Patients with the *G* allele are more sensitive to pain[83] and less responsive to opioid analgesics than are patients who do not have the *G* allele.[84] As a result, cancer patients who are homozygous for the *G* allele require higher doses of morphine to achieve pain control.[31] This finding was repeated in all but one study,[85] which found increased morphine efficacy in patients with the *G* allele who were given intrathecal fentanyl for labor pain, implying that the effects from a specific SNP may vary among opioids, drug administration routes, and pain etiologies. Few studies have investigated the role of opioid receptors in symptoms other than pain. In animal models of depression, κ-opioid receptor antagonists such as norbinaltorphimine have been found to produce antidepressant-like behavioral effects.[86] In patients with cancer, the μ-opioid receptor has also been found to be associated with short-term effects of acute sciatica on mood.[10]

Serotonin transporter

Serotonin transporter (*5-hydroxytryptamine*, *5-HTT*) affects monoamine neurotransmitter-mediated behaviors, including anxiety, depression, and obsessive-compulsive behavior, as well as response to painful stimuli. The protein product of the serotonin transporter gene (*5-HTT*) causes serotonin reuptake from the synaptic cleft, which regulates serotonin transmission.[87] A 20-base-pair to 23-base-pair unit can be repeated 14 or 16 times in the gene's promoter region, *5-HTT* gene-linked polymorphic region (*5-HTTLPR*; *rs25531*), which is referred to as a 44-base-pair insertion/deletion polymorphism.[88] The short (14-repeat) allele of *5-HTTLPR* results in lower transcriptional activity leading to lower neuronal serotonin reuptake[89] and is associated with higher levels of anxiety-related traits,[88] increased susceptibility to depression,[90] and increased analgesic effect of remifentanil.[91] A study of 11 patients with depression and advanced cancer revealed that the short allele was associated with higher levels of depression and anxiety.[92] Another polymorphism in the second intron of the serotonin transporter gene, *STin2*, which usually contains a 16-base-pair to 17-base-pair sequence with 10 or 12 repeats, was associated with joint pain severity in patients without cancer.[93]

Drug transport and metabolism

Drug efficacy is influenced by multiple factors and varies among individuals. Polymorphic proteins involved in transport and metabolism may contribute to the varied individual responses to symptom-control drugs. Current pharmacogenetic studies are primarily focused on opioids and nonsteroidal anti-inflammatory drugs (NSAIDs). A number of genetic polymorphisms of drug transporters, drug metabolizing enzymes, and opioid receptors have been identified as able to alter analgesic efficacy in cancer patients.

Permeability glycoprotein

Permeability glycoprotein (P-gp) mediates the transport of several opioid peptides across biological membranes and causes the efflux of nonpeptide opiates such as morphine[94–96] from the brain across the blood–brain barrier. P-gp is encoded by the adenosine triphosphate-binding cassette family member B1 (*ABCB1*) gene.[97] A common SNP, *C3435T*, is located in exon 26 of the *ABCB1* gene. Patients who are homozygous for the *T* allele demonstrate 2-fold lower P-gp duodenal expression and digoxin plasma concentration than patients with *CC* genotypes.[98] The *C3435T* affects the efficacy of multiple opioids. In patients who took a variety of opioids for pain, daily opioid doses significantly decreased in a gene dose-dependent manner.[99] Campa et al.[34] found that, among cancer patients receiving opioids, patients who were homozygous for *T* allele reported significantly greater pain relief than patients who were homozygous for *C* allele, whereas the pain relief reported by patients who were heterozygous was not significantly different from that of patients who were homozygous. Similarly, Coller et al.[100] found an association between the *T* allele and lower daily methadone dose requirements in opioid-dependent patients. Park et al.[101] found that Korean patients with *1236TT, 2677TT,* and *3435TT* genotypes who underwent spinal anesthesia with intravenous fentanyl were more likely to have side effects, notably early and profound respiration suppression, than patients with *1236CC, 2677GG,* and *3435CC* genotypes. Kim et al.[102] found that the *T/A* allele of the *G2677T/A* polymorphism was a significant risk factor for grade 3 or 4 hematological and gastrointestinal toxicities in ovarian cancer patients undergoing chemotherapy. Qian et al.[103] found that the *129T – 2677A – 3435C* haplotype was associated with mood disorder in Japanese patients.

Cytochrome P450 enzymes

Cytochrome P450 (CYP) enzymes are phase I enzymes that account for 75% of drug metabolism in humans.[104] Polymorphisms in CYP isoforms may contribute to variations in analgesic efficacy and side effects, generally in a drug-specific manner.[105,106] For example, the polymorphic CYP2D6 enzyme controls the *O*-demethylation of codeine to morphine and thus the rate of morphine production. To date, more than 100 allelic variants of *CYP2D6* have been discovered. Based on those polymorphisms, patients with distinct enzymatic activities are classified into one of four groups: poor metabolizers, who have complete enzymatic deficiency; intermediate metabolizers, who have decreased enzymatic activity; extensive metabolizers, who have normal enzymatic activity; and ultrarapid metabolizers, who have increased enzymatic activity.[107] In poor metabolizers, codeine is an ineffective analgesic because it is not activated into morphine.[108] In addition, in the initial 48 hours after surgery for gastric cancer, patients who were homozygous for *CYP2D6*10* consumed significantly higher amounts of tramadol than patients without *CYP2D6*10*.[109] Genetic polymorphisms in other P450 enzymes are also reported. In a study of 245 patients undergoing methadone maintenance treatment, Crettol et al.[110] found that *CYP2B6*6/*6* carriers presented higher trough (S)-methadone plasma levels. Pilotto et al.,[111] in a study of 78 patients with nonsteroidal anti-inflammatory drug-related upper gastrointestinal bleeding, reported that the *CYP2C9*3* allele was associated with a significantly higher risk of bleeding, setting the *CYP2C9*1/*1* genotype as reference.

Uridine diphosphate glucuronosyltransferase

Uridine diphosphate glucuronosyltransferase (UGT), a phase II enzyme, catalyzes glucuronidation, which results in the addition of sugar to polar compounds and facilitates their metabolic elimination. Opioids, acetaminophen, and numerous NSAIDs are glucuronidated by UGTs.[112] The *UGT2B7* gene encodes UGT2B7, a primary hepatic enzyme responsible for the glucuronidation of morphine, and *G-840A*, the SNP of *UGT2B7*, is located in the gene's promoter region.[113] *G-840A* is tightly linked to five other promoter SNPs, *A-1248G, T-1241C, T-1054C, A-268G,* and *T-102C,* relative to the hepatic enzyme gene start site.[114] A recent study in patients with sickle cell disease reported that the presence of the *–840G* allele (*GG* and *GA* genotypes) was associated with significantly reduced morphine glucuronidation that caused variability in the hepatic clearance of morphine.[115]

Conclusions

Genetic approaches offer new opportunities to investigate the biological mechanisms underlying symptom development in patients with cancer. However, the nature and range of genetic modulation in cancer-related symptoms are not completely understood because of the limited number of genes and genetic variants that have been investigated to date. Studies of the genetics of symptoms, such as pain, are complicated by the fact that the genetic influences vary among modalities, such as the sexes, different SNPs/haplotapes, and different phenotypes.[116] In addition, findings from studies on genetic variation and treatment efficacy are limited because of small sample sizes, a limited number of gene candidates, and limitations in kinds of treatment. Consistent and clinically meaningful symptom phenotyping, which enables a more applicable interpretation of genetic profiles and more replicable associations between genetic factors and cancer-related symptoms, should be used in future studies. Finally, genome-wide association studies should be used to identify additional novel candidate genes, as such studies can scan the entire genome for millions of SNPs without hypothesizing specific biological pathways that might be associated with cancer-related symptoms.

References

1. Einfeld S, Hall W. Behavior phenotype of the fragile X syndrome. *Am J Med Genet* **43**(1–2):56–60, 1992.
2. Miller AH. Cytokines and sickness behavior: implications for cancer care and control. *Brain Behav Immun* **17**(Suppl 1):S132–S134, 2003.
3. Lee BN, Dantzer R, Langley KE, et al. A cytokine-based neuroimmunologic mechanism of cancer-related symptoms. *Neuroimmunomodulation* **11**(5):279–292, 2004.
4. Cleeland CS. Symptom burden: multiple symptoms and their impact as patient-reported outcomes. *J Natl Cancer Inst Monogr* **37**:16–21, 2007.
5. Clatworthy J, Buick D, Hankins M, Weinman J, Horne R. The use and reporting of cluster analysis in health psychology: a review. *Br J Health Psychol* **10**(Pt 3):329–358, 2005.
6. Nagin DS, Tremblay RE. Analyzing developmental trajectories of distinct but related behaviors: a group-based method. *Psychol Methods* **6**(1):18–34, 2001.
7. Zubieta JK, Heitzeg MM, Smith YR, et al. COMT val158met genotype affects mu-opioid neurotransmitter responses to a pain stressor. *Science* **299**(5610):1240–1243, 2003.
8. Diatchenko L, Slade GD, Nackley AG, et al. Genetic basis for individual variations in pain perception and the development of a chronic pain condition. *Hum Mol Genet* **14**(1):135–143, 2005.
9. Rakvåg TT, Ross JR, Sato H, Skorpen F, Kaasa S, Klepstad P. Genetic variation in the catechol-O-methyltransferase (COMT) gene and morphine requirements in cancer patients with pain. *Mol Pain* **4**:64, 2008.
10. Max MB, Wu T, Atlas SJ, et al. A clinical genetic method to identify mechanisms by which pain causes depression and anxiety. *Mol Pain* **2**:14, 2006.
11. Hunt R, Sauna ZE, Ambudkar SV, Gottesman MM, Kimchi-Sarfaty C. Silent (synonymous) SNPs: should we care about them? *Methods Mol Biol* **578**:23–39, 2009.
12. Nackley AG, Shabalina SA, Tchivileva IE, et al. Human catechol-O-methyltransferase haplotypes modulate protein expression by altering mRNA secondary structure. *Science* **314**(5807):1930–1933, 2006.
13. Kawaguchi Y, Tochimoto A, Hara M, et al. Contribution of single nucleotide polymorphisms of the IL1A gene to the cleavage of precursor IL-1alpha and its transcription activity. *Immunogenetics* **59**(6):441–448, 2007.
14. Gabriel SB, Schaffner SF, Nguyen H, et al. The structure of haplotype blocks in the human genome. *Science* **296**(5576):2225–2229, 2002.
15. National Institute of Environmental Health Sciences. Environmental Genome Project: NIEHS SNPs. Available from: URL: http://egp.gs.washington.edu/. Accessed Mar 21, 2010.
16. Johnson GC, Esposito L, Barratt BJ, et al. Haplotype tagging for the identification of common disease genes. *Nat Genet* **29**(2):233–237, 2001.
17. Stram DO, Haiman CA, Hirschhorn JN, et al. Choosing haplotype-tagging SNPS based on unphased genotype data using a preliminary sample of unrelated subjects with an example from the Multiethnic Cohort Study. *Hum Hered* **55**(1):27–36, 2003.
18. Wall JD, Pritchard JK. Haplotype blocks and linkage disequilibrium in the human genome. *Nat Rev Genet* **4**(8):587–597, 2003.
19. Chapman JM, Cooper JD, Todd JA, Clayton DG. Detecting disease associations due to linkage disequilibrium using haplotype tags: a class of tests and the determinants of statistical power. *Hum Hered* **56**(1–3):18–31, 2003.
20. Carlson CS, Eberle MA, Rieder MJ, Yi Q, Kruglyak L, Nickerson DA. Selecting a maximally informative set

of single-nucleotide polymorphisms for association analyses using linkage disequilibrium. *Am J Hum Genet* **74**(1):106–120, 2004.

21. Yang Y, Wang Y, Li S, et al. Mutations in SCN9A, encoding a sodium channel alpha subunit, in patients with primary erythermalgia. *J Med Genet* **41**(3):171–174, 2004.
22. Max MB. Assessing pain candidate gene studies. *Pain* **109**(1–2):1–3, 2004.
23. Armero P, Muriel C, Santos J, Sànchez-Montero FJ, Rodríguez RE, González-Sarmiento R. COMT (Val158Met) polymorphism is not associated to neuropathic pain in a Spanish population. *Eur J Pain* **9**(3):229–232, 2005.
24. Kim H, Lee H, Rowan J, Brahim J, Dionne RA. Genetic polymorphisms in monoamine neurotransmitter systems show only weak association with acute post-surgical pain in humans. *Mol Pain* **2**:24, 2006.
25. Hoggart CJ, Clark TG, De Iorio M, Whittaker JC, Balding DJ. Genome-wide significance for dense SNP and resequencing data. *Genet Epidemiol* **32**(2):179–185, 2008.
26. McCarthy MI, Abecasis GR, Cardon LR, et al. Genome-wide association studies for complex traits: consensus, uncertainty and challenges. *Nat Rev Genet* **9**(5):356–369, 2008.
27. Hindorff LA, Sethupathy P, Junkins HA, et al. Potential etiologic and functional implications of genome-wide association loci for human diseases and traits. *Proc Natl Acad Sci U S A* **106**(23):9362–9367, 2009.
28. Xu Z, Taylor JA. SNPinfo: integrating GWAS and candidate gene information into functional SNP selection for genetic association studies. *Nucleic Acids Res* **37**(Web Server issue):W600–W605, 2009.
29. Rakvåg TT, Klepstad P, Báár C, et al. The Val158Met polymorphism of the human catechol-O-methyltransferase (COMT) gene may influence morphine requirements in cancer pain patients. *Pain* **116**(1–2):73–78, 2005.
30. Ross JR, Riley J, Taegetmeyer AB, et al. Genetic variation and response to morphine in cancer patients: catechol-O-methyltransferase and multidrug resistance-1 gene polymorphisms are associated with central side effects. *Cancer* **112**(6):1390–1403, 2008.
31. Klepstad P, Rakvåg TT, Kaasa S, et al. The 118 A > G polymorphism in the human mu-opioid receptor gene may increase morphine requirements in patients with pain caused by malignant disease. *Acta Anaesthesiol Scand* **48**(10):1232–1239, 2004.
32. Reyes-Gibby CC, El Osta B, Spitz MR, et al. The influence of tumor necrosis factor-alpha -308 G/A and IL-6–174 G/C on pain and analgesia response in lung cancer patients receiving supportive care. *Cancer Epidemiol Biomarkers Prev* **17**(11):3262–3267, 2008.
33. Reyes-Gibby CC, Spitz M, Wu X, et al. Cytokine genes and pain severity in lung cancer: exploring the influence of TNF-alpha-308 G/A IL6–174G/C and IL8–251T/A. *Cancer Epidemiol Biomarkers Prev* **16**(12):2745–2751, 2007.
34. Campa D, Gioia A, Tomei A, Poli P, Barale R. Association of ABCB1/MDR1 and OPRM1 gene polymorphisms with morphine pain relief. *Clin Pharmacol Ther* **83**(4):559–566, 2008.
35. Klepstad P, Dale O, Skorpen F, Borchgrevink PC, Kaasa S. Genetic variability and clinical efficacy of morphine. *Acta Anaesthesiol Scand* **49**(7):902–908, 2005.
36. Dantzer R, Kelley KW. Twenty years of research on cytokine-induced sickness behavior. *Brain Behav Immun* **21**(2):153–160, 2007.
37. Bower JE, Ganz PA, Tao ML, et al. Inflammatory biomarkers and fatigue during radiation therapy for breast and prostate cancer. *Clin Cancer Res* **15**(17):5534–5540, 2009.
38. Wang XS, Shi Q, Williams LA, et al. Serum interleukin-6 predicts the development of multiple symptoms at nadir of allogeneic hematopoietic stem cell transplantation. *Cancer* **113**(8):2102–2109, 2008.
39. Reeve AJ, Patel S, Fox A, Walker K, Urban L. Intrathecally administered endotoxin or cytokines produce allodynia, hyperalgesia and changes in spinal cord neuronal responses to nociceptive stimuli in the rat. *Eur J Pain* **4**(3):247–257, 2000.
40. Song C, Horrobin DF, Leonard BE. The comparison of changes in behavior, neurochemistry, endocrine, and immune functions after different routes, doses and durations of administrations of IL-1beta in rats. *Pharmacopsychiatry* **39**(3):88–99, 2006.
41. Dominici R, Cattaneo M, Malferrari G, et al. Cloning and functional analysis of the allelic polymorphism in the transcription regulatory region of interleukin-1 alpha. *Immunogenetics* **54**(2):82–86, 2002.
42. Pociot F, Mølvig J, Wogensen L, Worsaae H, Nerup J. A TaqI polymorphism in the human interleukin-1 beta (IL-1 beta) gene correlates with IL-1 beta secretion in vitro. *Eur J Clin Invest* **22**(6):396–402, 1992.
43. di Giovine FS, Takhsh E, Blakemore AI, Duff GW. Single base polymorphism at -511 in the human interleukin-1 beta gene (IL1 beta). *Hum Mol Genet* **1**(6):450, 1992.
44. Tarlow JK, Blakemore AI, Lennard A, et al. Polymorphism in human IL-1 receptor antagonist gene

intron 2 is caused by variable numbers of an 86-bp tandem repeat. *Hum Genet* **91**(4):403–404, 1993.

45. Sakamoto K, Oka M, Yoshino S, et al. Relation between cytokine promoter gene polymorphism and toxicity of 5-fluorouracil plus cisplatin chemotherapy. *Oncol Rep* **16**(2):381–387, 2006.
46. Collado-Hidalgo A, Bower JE, Ganz PA, Irwin MR, Cole SW. Cytokine gene polymorphisms and fatigue in breast cancer survivors: early findings. *Brain Behav Immun* **22**(8):1197–1200, 2008.
47. Solovieva S, Leino-Arjas P, Saarela J, Luoma K, Raininko R, Riihimäki H. Possible association of interleukin 1 gene locus polymorphisms with low back pain. *Pain* **109**(1–2):8–19, 2004.
48. Bessler H, Shavit Y, Mayburd E, Smirnov G, Beilin B. Postoperative pain, morphine consumption, and genetic polymorphism of IL-1beta and IL-1 receptor antagonist. *Neurosci Lett* **404**(1–2):154–158, 2006.
49. Bianchi M, Maggi R, Pimpinelli F, et al. Presence of a reduced opioid response in interleukin-6 knock out mice. *Eur J Neurosci* **11**(5):1501–1507, 1999.
50. Boufidou F, Lambrinoudaki I, Argeitis J, et al. CSF and plasma cytokines at delivery and postpartum mood disturbances. *J Affect Disord* **115**(1–2):287–292, 2009.
51. Lutgendorf SK, Weinrib AZ, Penedo F, et al. Interleukin-6, cortisol, and depressive symptoms in ovarian cancer patients. *J Clin Oncol* **26**(29):4820–4827, 2008.
52. Jacobson CM, Rosenfeld B, Pessin H, Breitbart W. Depression and IL-6 blood plasma concentrations in advanced cancer patients. *Psychosomatics* **49**(1):64–66, 2008.
53. Bremmer MA, Beekman AT, Deeg DJ, et al. Inflammatory markers in late-life depression: results from a population-based study. *J Affect Disord* **106**(3):249–255, 2008.
54. Hogan D, Morrow JD, Smith EM, Opp MR. Interleukin-6 alters sleep of rats. *J Neuroimmunol* **137**(1–2):59–66, 2003.
55. Dugan LL, Ali SS, Shekhtman G, et al. IL-6 mediated degeneration of forebrain GABAergic interneurons and cognitive impairment in aged mice through activation of neuronal NADPH oxidase. *PLoS One 4(5):e5518*, 2009.
56. Fishman D, Faulds G, Jeffery R, et al. The effect of novel polymorphisms in the interleukin-6 (IL-6) gene on IL-6 transcription and plasma IL-6 levels, and an association with systemic-onset juvenile chronic arthritis. *J Clin Invest* **102**(7):1369–1376, 1998.
57. Bull SJ, Huezo-Diaz P, Binder EB, et al. Functional polymorphisms in the interleukin-6 and serotonin transporter genes, and depression and fatigue induced by interferon-alpha and ribavirin treatment. *Mol Psychiatry* **14**(12):1095–1104, 2009.
58. Oen K, Malleson PN, Cabral DA, et al. Cytokine genotypes correlate with pain and radiologically defined joint damage in patients with juvenile rheumatoid arthritis. *Rheumatology (Oxford)* **44**(9):1115–1121, 2005.
59. Karppinen J, Daavittila I, Noponen N, et al. Is the interleukin-6 haplotype a prognostic factor for sciatica? *Eur J Pain* **12**(8):1018–1025, 2008.
60. Sommer C, Petrausch S, Lindenlaub T, Toyka KV. Neutralizing antibodies to interleukin 1-receptor reduce pain associated behavior in mice with experimental neuropathy. *Neurosci Lett* **270**(1):25–28, 1999.
61. Utreras E, Futatsugi A, Rudrabhatla P, et al. Tumor necrosis factor-alpha regulates cyclin-dependent kinase 5 activity during pain signaling through transcriptional activation of p35. *J Biol Chem* **284**(4):2275–2284, 2009.
62. Wilson AG, Symons JA, McDowell TL, McDevitt HO, Duff GW. Effects of a polymorphism in the human tumor necrosis factor alpha promoter on transcriptional activation. *Proc Natl Acad Sci U S A* **94**(7):3195–3199, 1997.
63. Cerri AP, Arosio B, Viazzoli C, Confalonieri R, Vergani C, Annoni G. The -308 (G/A) single nucleotide polymorphism in the TNF-alpha gene and the risk of major depression in the elderly. *Int J Geriatr Psychiatry* **25**(3):219–223, 2010.
64. Jun TY, Pae CU, Chae JH, et al. Tumor necrosis factor-beta gene polymorphism may not be associated with major depressive disorder in the Korean population. *Psychiatry Clin Neurosci* **57**(1):31–35, 2003.
65. Matsushima K, Baldwin ET, Mukaida N. Interleukin-8 and MCAF: novel leukocyte recruitment and activating cytokines. *Chem Immunol* **51**:236–265, 1992.
66. Ahn SH, Cho YW, Ahn MW, Jang SH, Sohn YK, Kim HS. mRNA expression of cytokines and chemokines in herniated lumbar intervertebral discs. *Spine (Phila Pa* **1976**) 27(9):911–917, 2002.
67. Hull J, Thomson A, Kwiatkowski D. Association of respiratory syncytial virus bronchiolitis with the interleukin 8 gene region in UK families. *Thorax* **55**(12):1023–1027, 2000.
68. Babovic D, O'Tuathaigh CM, O'Connor AM, et al. Phenotypic characterization of cognition and social behavior in mice with heterozygous versus homozygous deletion of catechol-O-methyltransferase. *Neuroscience* **155**(4):1021–1029, 2008.
69. Sambataro F, Reed JD, Murty VP, et al. Catechol-O-methyltransferase valine(158)methionine

polymorphism modulates brain networks underlying working memory across adulthood. *Biol Psychiatry* **66**(6):540–548, 2009.

70. Mata I, Arranz MJ, Staddon S, Lopez-Ilundain JM, Tabares-Seisdedos R, Murray RM. The high-activity Val allele of the catechol-O-methyltransferase gene predicts greater cognitive deterioration in patients with psychosis. *Psychiatr Genet* **16**(5):213–216, 2006.
71. Han DH, Kee BS, Min KJ, et al. Effects of catechol-O-methyltransferase Val158Met polymorphism on the cognitive stability and aggression in the first-onset schizophrenic patients. *Neuroreport* **17**(1):95–99, 2006.
72. Weickert TW, Goldberg TE, Mishara A, et al. Catechol-O-methyltransferase val108/158met genotype predicts working memory response to antipsychotic medications. *Biol Psychiatry* **56**(9): 677–682, 2004.
73. Barnett JH, Scoriels L, Munafò MR. Meta-analysis of the cognitive effects of the catechol-O-methyltransferase gene Val158/108Met polymorphism. *Biol Psychiatry* **64**(2):137–144, 2008.
74. Benedetti F, Barbini B, Bernasconi A, et al. Acute antidepressant response to sleep deprivation combined with light therapy is influenced by the catechol-O-methyltransferase Val(108/158)Met polymorphism. *J Affect Disord* **121**(1–2):68–72, 2010.
75. Benedetti F, Colombo C, Pirovano A, Marino E, Smeraldi E. The catechol-O-methyltransferase Val(108/158)Met polymorphism affects antidepressant response to paroxetine in a naturalistic setting. *Psychopharmacology (Berl)* **203**(1):155–160, 2009.
76. Anttila S, Huuhka K, Huuhka M, et al. Catechol-O-methyltransferase (COMT) polymorphisms predict treatment response in electroconvulsive therapy. *Pharmacogenomics J* **8**(2):113–116, 2008.
77. Pert CB, Snyder SH. Opiate receptor: demonstration in nervous tissue. *Science* **179**(77):1011–1014, 1973.
78. Stein C. Peripheral mechanisms of opioid analgesia. *Anesth Analg* **76**(1):182–191, 1993.
79. Bidlack JM, Khimich M, Parkhill AL, Sumagin S, Sun B, Tipton CM. Opioid receptors and signaling on cells from the immune system. *J Neuroimmune Pharmacol* **1**(3):260–269, 2006.
80. McQuay H. Opioids in pain management. *Lancet* **353**(9171):2229–2232, 1999.
81. Bond C, LaForge KS, Tian M, et al. Single-nucleotide polymorphism in the human mu opioid receptor gene alters beta-endorphin binding and activity: possible implications for opiate addiction. *Proc Natl Acad Sci U S A* **95**(16):9608–9613, 1998.
82. Oertel BG, Kettner M, Scholich K, et al. A common human μ-opioid receptor genetic variant diminishes the receptor signaling efficacy in brain regions processing the sensory information of pain. *J Biol Chem* **284**(10):6530–6535, 2009.
83. Sia AT, Lim Y, Lim EC, et al. A118G single nucleotide polymorphism of human mu-opioid receptor gene influences pain perception and patient-controlled intravenous morphine consumption after intrathecal morphine for postcesarean analgesia. *Anesthesiology* **109**(3):520–526, 2008.
84. Chou WY, Wang CH, Liu PH, Liu CC, Tseng CC, Jawan B. Human opioid receptor A118G polymorphism affects intravenous patient-controlled analgesia morphine consumption after total abdominal hysterectomy. *Anesthesiology* **105**(2):334–337, 2006.
85. Landau R, Kern C, Columb MO, Smiley RM, Blouin JL. Genetic variability of the mu-opioid receptor influences intrathecal fentanyl analgesia requirements in laboring women. *Pain* **139**(1):5–14, 2008.
86. Zhang H, Shi YG, Woods JH, Watson SJ, Ko MC. Central kappa-opioid receptor-mediated antidepressant-like effects of nor-Binaltorphimine: behavioral and BDNF mRNA expression studies. *Eur J Pharmacol* **570**(1–3):89–96, 2007.
87. Blakely RD, De Felice LJ, Hartzell HC. Molecular physiology of norepinephrine and serotonin transporters. *J Exp Biol* **196**:263–281, 1994.
88. Lesch KP, Bengel D, Heils A, et al. Association of anxiety-related traits with a polymorphism in the serotonin transporter gene regulatory region. *Science* **274**(5292):1527–1531, 1996.
89. Heils A, Teufel A, Petri S, et al. Allelic variation of human serotonin transporter gene expression. *J Neurochem* **66**(6):2621–2624, 1996.
90. Caspi A, Sugden K, Moffitt TE, et al. Influence of life stress on depression: moderation by a polymorphism in the 5-HTT gene. *Science* **301**(5631):386–389, 2003.
91. Kosek E, Jensen KB, Lonsdorf TB, Schalling M, Ingvar M. Genetic variation in the serotonin transporter gene (5-HTTLPR, rs25531) influences the analgesic response to the short acting opioid Remifentanil in humans. *Mol Pain* **5**:37, 2009.
92. Schillani G, Capozzo MA, Aguglia E, et al. 5-HTTLPR polymorphism of serotonin transporter and effects of sertraline in terminally ill cancer patients: report of eleven cases. *Tumori* **94**(4):563–567, 2008.
93. Herken H, Erdal E, Mutlu N, et al. Possible association of temporomandibular joint pain and dysfunction with a polymorphism in the serotonin transporter gene. *Am J Orthod Dentofacial Orthop* **120**(3): 308–313, 2001.
94. King M, Su W, Chang A, Zuckerman A, Pasternak GW. Transport of opioids from the brain to the

periphery by P-glycoprotein: peripheral actions of central drugs. *Nat Neurosci* **4**(3):268–274, 2001.

95. Schinkel AH, Wagenaar E, van Deemter L, Mol CA, Borst P. Absence of the mdr1a P-Glycoprotein in mice affects tissue distribution and pharmacokinetics of dexamethasone, digoxin, and cyclosporin A. *J Clin Invest* **96**(4):1698–1705, 1995.
96. Thompson SJ, Koszdin K, Bernards CM. Opiate-induced analgesia is increased and prolonged in mice lacking P-glycoprotein. *Anesthesiology* **92**(5): 1392–1399, 2000.
97. Higgins CF. ABC transporters: physiology, structure and mechanism: an overview. *Res Microbiol* **152** (3–4):205–210, 2001.
98. Hoffmeyer S, Burk O, von Richter O, et al. Functional polymorphisms of the human multidrug-resistance gene: multiple sequence variations and correlation of one allele with P-glycoprotein expression and activity in vivo. *Proc Natl Acad Sci U S A* **97**(7):3473–3478, 2000.
99. Lötsch J, von Hentig N, Freynhagen R, et al. Cross-sectional analysis of the influence of currently known pharmacogenetic modulators on opioid therapy in outpatient pain centers. *Pharmacogenet Genomics* **19**(6):429–436, 2009.
100. Coller JK, Barratt DT, Dahlen K, Loennechen MH, Somogyi AA. ABCB1 genetic variability and methadone dosage requirements in opioid-dependent individuals. *Clin Pharmacol Ther* **80**(6):682–690, 2006.
101. Park HJ, Shinn HK, Ryu SH, Lee HS, Park CS, Kang JH. Genetic polymorphisms in the ABCB1 gene and the effects of fentanyl in Koreans. *Clin Pharmacol Ther* **81**(4):539–546, 2007.
102. Kim HS, Kim MK, Chung HH, et al. Genetic polymorphisms affecting clinical outcomes in epithelial ovarian cancer patients treated with taxanes and platinum compounds: a Korean population-based study. *Gynecol Oncol* **113**(2):264–269, 2009.
103. Qian W, Homma M, Itagaki F, et al. MDR1 gene polymorphism in Japanese patients with schizophrenia and mood disorders including depression. *Biol Pharm Bull* **29**(12):2446–2450, 2006.
104. Guengerich FP. Cytochrome p450 and chemical toxicology. *Chem Res Toxicol* **21**(1):70–83, 2008.
105. Stamer UM, Musshoff F, Kobilay M, Madea B, Hoeft A, Stuber F. Concentrations of tramadol and O-desmethyltramadol enantiomers in different CYP2D6 genotypes. *Clin Pharmacol Ther* **82**(1):41–47, 2007.
106. Zanger UM, Klein K, Saussele T, Blievernicht J, Hofmann MH, Schwab M. Polymorphic CYP2B6: molecular mechanisms and emerging clinical significance. *Pharmacogenomics* **8**(7):743–759, 2007.
107. de Leon J, Susce MT, Murray-Carmichael E. The AmpliChip CYP450 genotyping test: integrating a new clinical tool. *Mol Diagn Ther* **10**(3):135–151, 2006.
108. Desmeules J, Gascon MP, Dayer P, Magistris M. Impact of environmental and genetic factors on codeine analgesia. *Eur J Clin Pharmacol* **41**(1):23–26, 1991.
109. Wang G, Zhang H, He F, Fang X. Effect of the CYP2D6*10 C188T polymorphism on postoperative tramadol analgesia in a Chinese population. *Eur J Clin Pharmacol* **62**(11):927–931, 2006.
110. Crettol S, Déglon JJ, Besson J, et al. ABCB1 and cytochrome P450 genotypes and phenotypes: influence on methadone plasma levels and response to treatment. *Clin Pharmacol Ther* **80**(6):668–681, 2006.
111. Pilotto A, Seripa D, Franceschi M, et al. Genetic susceptibility to nonsteroidal anti-inflammatory drug-related gastroduodenal bleeding: role of cytochrome P450 2C9 polymorphisms. *Gastroenterology* **133**(2):465–471, 2007.
112. Armstrong SC, Cozza KL. Pharmacokinetic drug interactions of morphine, codeine, and their derivatives: theory and clinical reality, part I. *Psychosomatics* **44**(2):167–171, 2003.
113. Holthe M, Rakvåg TN, Klepstad P, et al. Sequence variations in the UDP-glucuronosyltransferase 2B7 (UGT2B7) gene: identification of 10 novel single nucleotide polymorphisms (SNPs) and analysis of their relevance to morphine glucuronidation in cancer patients. *Pharmacogenomics J* **3**(1):17–26, 2003.
114. Duguay Y, Báár C, Skorpen F, Guillemette C. A novel functional polymorphism in the uridine diphosphate-glucuronosyltransferase 2B7 promoter with significant impact on promoter activity. *Clin Pharmacol Ther* **75**(3):223–233, 2004.
115. Darbari DS, van Schaik RH, Capparelli EV, Rana S, McCarter R, van den Anker J. UGT2B7 promoter variant -840G>A contributes to the variability in hepatic clearance of morphine in patients with sickle cell disease. *Am J Hematol* **83**(3):200–202, 2008.
116. Mogil JS. Are we getting anywhere in human pain genetics? *Pain* **146**(3):231–232, 2009.

Section 2 Chapter 18

Cancer Symptom Mechanisms and Models: Clinical and Basic Science

Functional imaging of symptoms

T. Dorina Papageorgiou, Javier O. Valenzuela, and Edward F. Jackson

The brain is the stage upon which peripheral information is assembled and translated into perceptions, including consciousness of the symptoms produced by disease and treatment. The theme of this book is to bring together research findings from various scientific disciplines to help us understand why patients with cancer develop symptoms. Recent breakthroughs in functional imaging techniques – such as electroencephalography (EEG), positron emission tomography (PET), and functional magnetic resonance imaging (fMRI) – can help us investigate the localization of symptom expression in the brain. The abundance of literature on the functional imaging of pain, together with the growing number of studies of other cancer-related symptoms such as dyspnea (shortness of breath), nausea, loss of appetite, disturbed sleep, and fatigue, are beginning to help us understand how brain changes occur at the electrophysiological, hemodynamic, and metabolic levels. These functional imaging technologies have revolutionized basic and translational research and are directly applicable to clinical care.

What is unique about imaging cancer-related symptoms is that cancer is a dynamic process. First, tumor growth does not develop all at once but rather progresses over time, enabling us to examine symptoms as they develop. Second, the toxic nature of many cancer treatments results in the rapid development of symptoms in patients who are often symptom-free before the start of treatment. Finally, the dosage of symptom management drugs (such as analgesics, steroids, and antiemetics) used to control disease-related and treatment-related symptoms is continuously modified as the disease progresses. These features of cancer-related symptoms allow for longitudinal study of symptom development and management, which can be carried out by using noninvasive techniques currently available for brain mapping. Consequently, functional neuroimaging is helping us identify the brain networks involved in the development and expression of cancer symptoms.

Research findings are beginning to converge on how dissimilar symptoms, including pain, shortness of breath, and nausea, may display similar cortical and subcortical spatial patterns. Shared neuroanatomical substrates across symptoms may help explain why single symptoms, such as pain, rarely exist in isolation and why symptom clusters occur at the brain level. These potential functional similarities suggest avenues of exploration into existing or new interventions such as drug targeting, neurorehabilitation, and deep brain stimulation techniques, with the goals of modulating central nervous system and, in particular, cortical and subcortical pathways shared among certain symptoms and simultaneously attenuating the phenotypic expression of dissimilar symptoms.

The objectives of this chapter are to explore the spatial patterns of cortical and subcortical processing of symptoms and to investigate whether similar functional networks may underlie different symptoms. We will review our current knowledge of the anatomical regions and functional mechanisms of the physical symptoms that are highly prevalent in patients with cancer, investigate the similarities in spatial patterns that give rise to different symptoms, and suggest areas of future research in the functional imaging of cancer-related symptoms.

Functional imaging technologies

Brain mapping technologies can be largely divided into electrophysiological and metabolic/hemodynamic groups. The electrophysiological technologies include EEG, magnetoencephalography, and transcranial magnetic stimulation. The metabolic and hemodynamic technologies include PET, single-photon emission computed tomography, near-infrared spectroscopy, and fMRI. We focus primarily on studies using EEG, PET, or fMRI in this chapter.

EEG measures brain electrical signals of only a few microvolts from electrodes located on the scalp. The

Cancer Symptom Science: Measurement, Mechanisms, and Management, eds. Charles S. Cleeland, Michael J. Fisch, and Adrian J. Dunn.

various frequencies and distributions of specific EEG patterns change, providing us with two basic parameters: (1) amplitude, meaning how large the signal is; and (2) frequency, which describes the speed of the signal. There are three basic types of EEG patterns, which are defined solely in terms of frequency and are extremely reliable. (1) The α (alpha) pattern consists of large, rhythmic waves of about 8 to 12 Hz and can be observed when one is awake and relaxed (ie, not participating in a cognitive process). (2) The β (beta) pattern is described by lower-voltage variations ranging from about 18 to 30 Hz and occurs during an alert state; when beta activity reaches higher frequency variations of about 30–70 seconds it is referred to as γ (gamma) and is associated with the brain's ability to integrate the various stimuli into a coherent meaning. (3) The θ (theta) activity is in the 4 to 8 Hz range and has been observed during imagery, rapid-eye-movement (REM) sleep, problem solving, and attention. Although EEG recordings provide us with signals of excellent temporal resolution (milliseconds rather than seconds) from the cortical regions, selectivity for subcortical regions is difficult to identify and thus its usage has partially been integrated with imaging techniques, such as fMRI.

PET scanning uses a nuclear imaging technique that tracks biochemical and physiological processes. In PET, a short-lived radionuclide is injected into the patient's blood stream and decays by emitting positrons. The tracer compound becomes concentrated in metabolically active tissues (in the case of the radionuclide ^{18}F-fluorodeoxyglucose [FDG]) or tissues with elevated blood flow/volume (in the case of ^{15}O-H2). The positrons decay, yielding two gamma rays emitted 180 degrees apart; these are sensed by detectors and, in turn, a computer generates a three-dimensional functional image depicting areas of metabolic activity or blood flow/volume.

Functional MRI has been even more widely used than PET. The most common fMRI technique relies on the blood-oxygen-level-dependent (BOLD) signal intensity modulation to assess the hemodynamic response secondary to neuronal activation; ie, it reflects the downstream response to synaptic processing of a given area rather than its spiking output.[1] The BOLD signal is modulated by the oxyhemoglobin-to-deoxyhemoglobin ratio and is therefore dependent on cerebral blood flow and volume.[2,3] The advantages of fMRI over PET are that it does not require radioisotope injection, has better spatial resolution (millimeters) and temporal resolution (a few seconds compared with tens of seconds), and, more importantly, allows acquisition of multiple noninvasive scans within the same individual, even in a single imaging session.

Despite the difference in the ways that PET and fMRI acquire data, these two imaging tools produce similar results as to the brain-behavior relationships they generate.[4–6]

Lamina I spinothalamocortical pathway as a central afferent highway of symptoms

When represented in cortical and subcortical structures, symptoms can be thought of as interoceptive information, ie, cortical representations of a flow of bodily information coming from receptors from all organs and tissues. Exteroceptive information, in contrast, comes from outside the body via visual, auditory, and olfactory receptors.[7] Recent theories of interoception and emotion describe a central neural organization of bodily sensations.[7–9] In this model, small-diameter (Aδ- and C-type) primary afferent fibers innervating all tissues of the body convey peripheral information via the spinothalamocortical pathway to specific cortical structures, where they are processed and interpreted to reflect the physiological state and subjective feelings of disease that we call "symptoms" (Figure 18.1).

As discussed by Craig (on the basis of animal studies), when a homeostatic imbalance occurs, selective Aδ- and C-type primary afferent fibers expressing receptors specific for physiological parameters as diverse as body temperature, mechanical stress, local metabolism, cellular integrity, skin integrity from parasites and allergens, and mast cell and immune cell function become activated and relay this information monosynaptically to lamina I neurons of the spinal and trigeminal dorsal horns.[7,8] These modality-selective neurons project first to autonomic cell columns of the thoracolumbar spinal cord, forming a spinal "feedback loop" for sympathetic responses. They then reach the main homeostatic integration sites in the medulla and the midbrain, including the catecholaminergic cell columns and the parabrachial nucleus. The parabrachial nucleus is also a target of the nucleus tractus solitarius, which conveys parasympathetic vagal and glossopharyngeal afferent activity from gustatory and visceral stimuli. The parabrachial nucleus is the main brainstem homeostatic integration site and the core of a

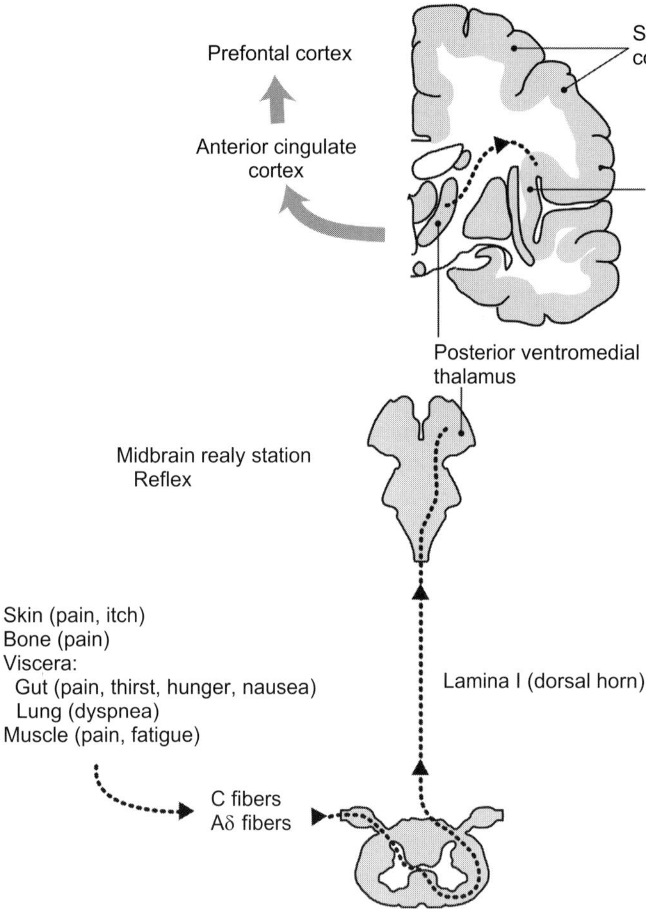

Figure 18.1. The spinothalamocortical pathway.

second loop of somatoautonomic reflexes aimed at regulating the balance of essential cardiovascular, respiratory, energetic, osmotic, and other basic homeostatic functions. From the parabrachial nucleus in the upper midbrain, lamina I and nucleus tractus solitarius neurons project to mesencephalic (periaqueductal gray [PAG]), diencephalic (hypothalamus), and telencephalic (amygdala) homeostatic control centers to drive the limbic system, primary (S1) and secondary (S2) somatosensory cortices, and motor cortex involved in goal-directed autonomic and behavioral responses.

In humans, lamina I neurons that reach the brainstem nuclei provide the first integrated anatomical substrate for the communication of homeostatic imbalances to the brain that give rise to symptoms. Integration at this level is exemplified by the observation that cordotomy of ascending lamina I neurons reduces not only pain, but also itching, thermal, and sensual sensations.[10] The next level of information relay is achieved through lamina I and nucleus tractus solitarius projections to the thalamus, which connects the spine and midbrain with the insula. PET and fMRI studies show activation of the insula in response to interoceptive stimuli as diverse as graded cooling, cold allodynia, itch, sensual touch, thermal pain, chronic pain, hunger, and dyspnea.[7] In addition, lesions of the anterior insula disrupt these sensations and other homeostatic functions.[11–15]

The insula and the anterior cingulate cortex (ACC) embody most of the limbic representations of the afferent information relayed by lamina I neurons regarding the physiological state of the body. PET studies have revealed a role for ACC activation in response to unpleasant heat pain during hypnosis[16] and to thermal grill illusions of pain that represent the urgency of thermal distress.[17] Therefore, the functions of the insula and ACC are related to decisions controlling internal homeostatic sensations with external motivational behaviors – ie, the two basic components of an emotional response.

The spinothalamocortical pathway described above provides a comprehensive anatomical substrate for the integration of sensations. Homeostatic imbalances that disrupt the body's condition are detected by specific receptors on small-diameter fibers and are quickly relayed through lamina I neurons to midbrain, and in turn, limbic, somatosensory, and somatomotor areas with the goal of restoring homeostatic functions that are essential for survival. The next section describes how symptoms common to patients with cancer, such as pain, shortness of breath (dyspnea), nausea, loss of appetite, fatigue, and disturbed sleep, may be associated with the spinothalamocortical pathway.

Brain spatial patterns of symptoms

Functional brain imaging studies have provided an important window into the cortical and subcortical spatial patterns observed across symptoms and after administration of agents to treat symptoms, such as analgesics. These studies suggest that during the expression of more than one symptom (ie, symptom clusters or constellations), dissimilar symptoms can activate similar brain regions and networks. To our knowledge, however, no functional brain studies of the symptoms of cancer have been carried out. We focus our review on imaging studies in healthy subjects and patient populations experiencing symptoms similar to those of cancer patients.

Studies of symptom expression

Pain

Most of what we know about the functional imaging of symptoms has developed only over the last two decades and is based on studies of pain in healthy subjects and in various patient populations with pain. Earlier studies by Melzack and Casey[18] offered a conceptual categorization of the pain experience as a function of potential behavioral needs: (1) sensory-discriminative (ie, "Where does it hurt?"); (2) affective-motivational (ie, "How bad is the threat?"); and (3) cognitive-evaluative (ie, "What needs to be done to escape the threat?"), suggesting that a cortical representation of pain might include separate areas for processing each of these needs. However, as discussed above, Craig[7] proposed a more integrative view of pain as a homeostatic emotion with sensory and motivational aspects. This conceptual model is particularly useful in clinical pain, which is dependent on the loss of homeostasis rather than on tissue damage, and suggests the possibility of overlap in the representation of the behavioral needs offered by Melzack and Casey.[18]

Experimentally induced acute pain. The experience of pain, including pain associated with cancer, can be temporally classified as acute, chronic, or breakthrough, a subclassification of chronic pain. Portenoy and Conn[19] give an exhaustive list of the temporal cortical correlates of pain syndromes in cancer. Although we are aware of no neuroimaging studies in acute pain syndromes in cancer, a plethora of functional imaging studies investigating the cortical and subcortical correlates of experimentally induced acute pain stimuli such as cutaneous insult, laser heat, cold thermode, capsaicin, electric shock, and thermal grill have been performed.[20–25] Studies of experimentally induced acute pain in healthy adults show that the most frequently activated regions are the brainstem nuclei, thalamus, ACC, insula, S1 and S2 cortices, and prefrontal cortex (PFC).

The brainstem nuclei activated in acute pain include the PAG, rostral ventromedial medulla, nucleus cuneiformis, ventral tegmental area, parabrachial nucleus, nucleus coeruleus, and the red nucleus. Bilateral activation of these nuclei can both facilitate and inhibit the nociceptive response.[26] The thalamus is also activated bilaterally in response to cognitive manipulations of pain, particularly the ventrolateral region associated with the sensory-discriminative aspect of nociception experienced after heat pain. Further, the reticular thalamus is involved in inhibitory pain pathways because of its downstream effect on the PAG and reticular formation. Therefore, thalamic responses to painful stimuli are part of both the discriminative and the attentional networks involved in pain processing.

The perigenual, middle, and posterior sections of the ACC are the pain regions most frequently associated with the affective-motivational dimension of pain. Apkarian et al.[25] showed that the ACC was activated in 81%, 94%, and 100% of fMRI, PET, and EEG pain studies, respectively. The insula and S2 cortex display concomitant increased activation during the application of acute pain, despite their functional differences: activation of the insula occurs as a consequence of negative affect, such as aversive conditioning,[27] whereas S2 activation, in particular Brodmann Area (BA) 3a, an overlapping region between the exteroceptive and interoceptive pain information systems, participates in the attentional processing of pain stimuli and has been observed with use of PET[28] and dipole modeling of brain electrical activity.[29] The S1 cortex is activated in response to moderately painful stimuli, but not by stimuli above a moderate pain threshold. This could be a consequence of increased attention to the stimulus and thus increased recruitment of cognitive regions as a compensatory mechanism. It follows, then, that S1 activation can be modulated via cognitive distraction methods that alter the perception of pain intensity rather than pain unpleasantness. Activation of higher-order cognitive regions, such as the PFC and posterior parietal lobe, predominantly of the right hemisphere, reflect the cognitive-evaluative component of pain in the context of pain stimulation or modulation.[30]

Somatic versus visceral pain. Nociceptive pain is further categorized into somatic and visceral pain. Although several functional imaging studies have investigated the cortical processing of somatic pain, these are laboratory-based rather than clinical pain studies. The functional imaging literature of visceral pain has not been so prolific as the literature of somatic pain.[20,21,23–25,27,31]

As discussed above, the anatomical processing of peripheral nociceptive information is via lamina I neurons of the dorsal horn of the spinal cord. Somatosensory inputs project via the lateral spinothalamic tract to two thalamic nuclei: (1) the posterior ventromedial nucleus, which in turn relays this information to the insular cortex; and (2) the ventrocaudal portion of the mediodorsal thalamic nucleus, which projects to the ACC. Visceral inputs, however, relay in the nucleus tractus solitarius and parabrachial nucleus and in turn project to the parvicellular ventromedial thalamic nuclei before reaching the agranular section of the insula (the anterior insula, or AI). Because of these anatomical processing differences between somatic and visceral pain, the former is localized precisely to the site of origin, whereas the latter often radiates and is perceived as originating from a larger area, and may even become more intense at one site. A common example of this "referred" sensation of visceral pain is the shoulder, abdominal, and back pain that occurs with pancreatic carcinoma. Referred pain is produced by the convergence of visceral afferents on spinal neurons that receive projections from somatic afferents, a phenomenon known as viscerosomatic spinal convergence.

Another difference between somatic and visceral pain is that somatic sensation activates cortical regions responsible for exteroception and spatial orientation, whereas visceral sensation primarily recruits cortical regions involved in interoception (Figure 18.2).[7] Thus, visceral sensation seems to activate primarily the limbic/paralimbic regions associated with unpleasantness, such as the ACC and AI. Increased rostral ACC activation is observed during esophageal distension (visceral pain), whereas activation of a more dorsal subregion is associated with somatic stimulation at the chest level (somatic stimulation).[32] Further, activation of the posterior ACC is decreased during rectal sensation (visceral pain), but is increased during stimulation of the foot or lower back (somatic sensation).[26] Recent studies suggest that negative emotional stimuli, or cognitive factors such as attention, can modulate visceral sensation at the cortical level, specifically in the insula and ACC. Although the insular cortex is a heterogeneous region, it is activated during both visceral and somatic pain. The AI, which has been associated with cognitive, affective, and autonomic responses, is most consistently activated during visceral sensation.

Neuropathic pain. Clinical neuropathy-induced cancer pain, discussed at length in Chapter 5, can result from neoplastic invasion, which can produce mass distortion or destruction of neural structures, or from therapy, such as radiotherapy or surgery. The pain sensation itself is a distortion of normal pain processing because usually innocuous stimuli, such as heat, cold, or touch, can become painful. The etiology of neuropathy-induced cancer pain encompasses a large variety of central or peripheral lesions or dysfunctions, such as chemotherapy-induced neurotoxicity. Of interest, although neuropathy-induced cancer pain can be mediated by a number of pathophysiological mechanisms, patients may present with similar symptoms, including spontaneous pain, which may be continuous or paroxysmal, and evoked pain, which may be allodynic (heat, cold, dynamic/static mechanical) or hyperalgesic (heat, cold, punctate mechanical).[33]

Most of the information about the cortical processing of neuropathic pain focuses on allodynia.[34–41] The term "allodynia" refers to pain evoked by a stimulus that does not normally induce pain, and the condition is characterized by dissociation between actual versus

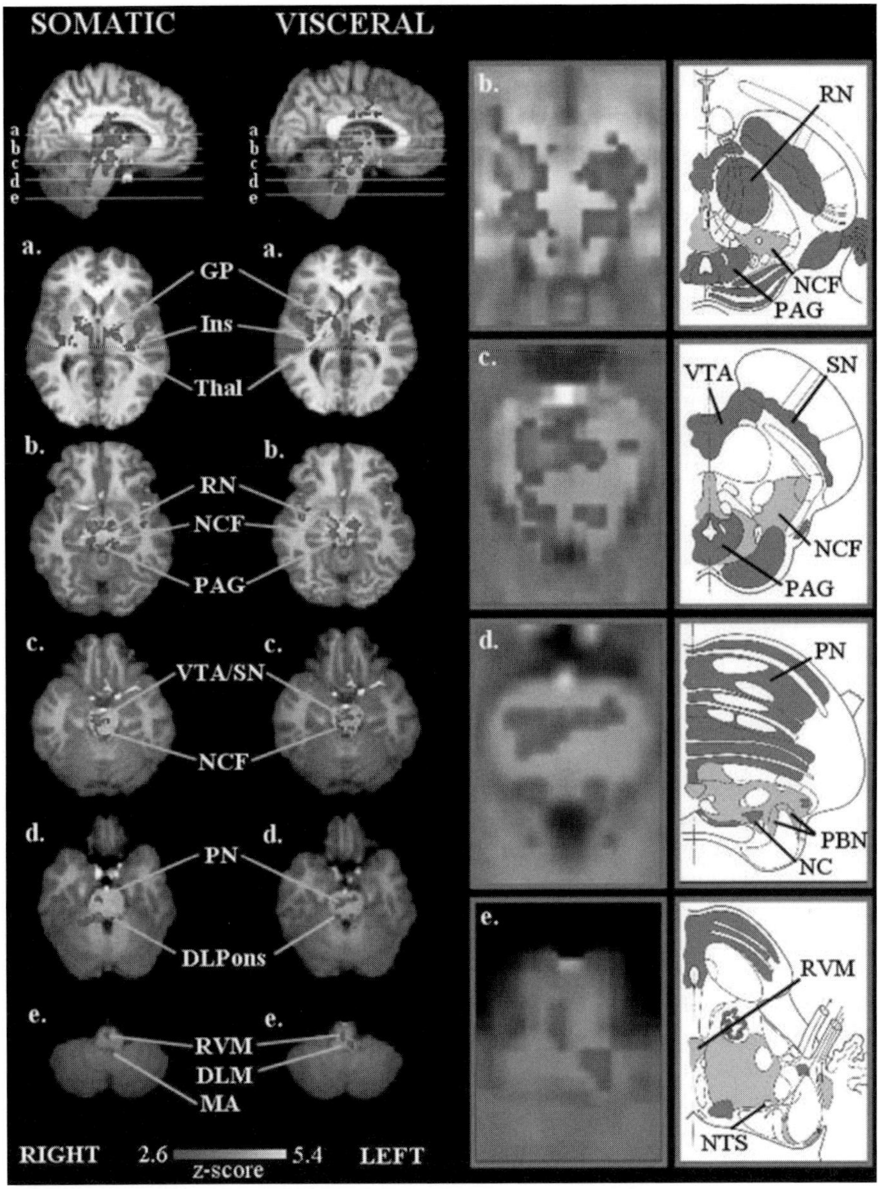

Figure 18.2. Differences and similarities in group activation maps for somatic and visceral pain. The sagittal slices show columns of activation within the brainstem in each group. Axial slices (a–e) correspond to the plane indicated in the sagittal slice. Regions commonly activated in whole-brain pain-imaging studies are significantly activated: thalamus (Thal) and posterior insula (Ins) bilaterally. Activation was also seen in the globus pallidus (GP) bilaterally in both groups. Significantly, activated brainstem nuclei included the red nucleus (RN), nucleus cuneiformis (NCF), periaqueductal gray (PAG), ventral tegmental area (VTA, which extended laterally into the substantia nigra [SN]), and the dorsolateral pons (DLPons) bilaterally. Bilateral activation of the pontine nuclei (PN) occurred in the visceral group but was limited to the right side in the somatic group. Activation in the region of the rostral ventromedial medulla (RVM) was also seen in both groups. In the visceral group alone, a region of activation occurred in the left dorsolateral medulla (DLM). The axial slices in the visceral group have been magnified and juxtaposed to drawings at the same anatomical location. See plate section for color version. Modified from Duvernoy (1995) with permission.
Source: Reprinted from the Journal of Neuroscience, vol. 25, Dunckley P, Wise RG, Fairhurst M, et al. A comparison of visceral and somatic pain processing in the human brainstem using functional magnetic resonance imaging, pp. 7333–7341, Copyright 2005, with permission from the Society for Neuroscience.

perceived stimulus intensity. Allodynia occurs as a consequence of impaired pain-transmitting pathways from the spinal cord to the brain, particularly the inputs to the medial thalamus and limbic regions, which primarily encode the affective-motivational component of pain.[42]

The regions most often activated across these studies are the ACC, AI, and S1 and S2 cortices. Two studies by Peyron et al.[35,36] showed increased posterior insula and S2 activation during stimulation of the allodynic side versus the control side of patients with neuropathic pain. Similarly, a study of clinical allodynia reported increased posterior insular activation, which may suggest the perceived intensity of the stimulus.[40] Witting et al.[41] reported activation of the AI in the hemisphere ipsilateral to brush-evoked stimulation in patients with allodynia, whereas Petrovic et al.[43] reported an absence of insular activation. These differences in AI activation among allodynia studies are most likely due to the patients' heterogeneity of neuropathic etiology, as a result of different relative contributions of deafferentation and reorganization along afferent pathways. ACC activation has also been reported during both capsaicin-induced and dynamic-mechanical allodynia. However, activation of the mid-ACC, which functions as an integrative site of pain perception and attentional processes, is quite variable across studies. Peyron et al.[36] reported enhanced ipsilateral mid-ACC activation during allodynic stimulation, whereas in a previous study,[35] no mid-ACC changes were reported but rather a decrease in the rostral and inferior ipsilateral (BA24/32) ACC. Likewise, in studies of patients with mononeuropathy in the lower extremities, correlations between mid-ACC activation and perceived pain intensity showed that the mid-ACC was not part of the "allodynic matrix" for those patients.[40,43]

The increased S1 activation observed in studies of neuropathy-induced cancer pain suggests that S1 extends its receptive fields outside the physiological somatotopic organization into the visual, auditory, language, and sensorimotor systems. Peyron et al.[35] reported increased bilateral S2 activation extending to the adjacent inferior parietal areas (BA39/40) in response to a non-noxious cold stimulus in allodynia patients with lateral-medullary infarct. However, when the same stimulus was applied to the unaffected side, the contralateral parietal region was activated. Similarly, extension of cortical activation from S2 to the adjacent parietal areas (BA39/40) has been previously reported in pain experiments in healthy subjects.[34] Petrovic et al.[43] suggested that S1 or S2 activation in pain studies could be the consequence of movement intention or preparation, which may in turn increase the activity in the motor cortex. However, it is not known how, or if, movement interacts with intense pain in S1 or S2 when attention is directed to the painful stimulus.

In conclusion, functional imaging studies suggest that the neural mechanisms of nociceptive versus neuropathic pain differ substantially between healthy subjects and patients with either central or peripheral neuropathy. This difference in mechanisms reflects the fact that the stimulus intensity and perceived intensity of nociceptive pain may be correlated, whereas in allodynic pain they are dissociated as a result of cortical and subcortical reorganization of afferent pathways, leading to aberrant activation of pain-related regions.

Dyspnea (shortness of breath)

Shortness of breath or air hunger is referred to clinically as dyspnea. Dyspnea is one of the cardinal symptoms of advanced cancer and can be caused by destruction of lung tissue due to disease or radiation, focal tumors in the cerebellum, or pulmonary toxicity associated with various chemotherapeutic agents (eg, busulfan, cyclophosphamide, or methotrexate). Dyspnea can also be caused by cancer-induced or treatment-related anemia, which reduces the amount of oxygen supplied to the lungs. Like pain, dyspnea is a subjective experience and adequate symptom control is therefore difficult to obtain.

We currently know of no studies that have used cortical imaging methods to examine cancer-related dyspnea. However, the cortical representation of air hunger induced in the laboratory has been studied in healthy persons[44–50] and in patients with congenital central hypoventilation syndrome (CCHS),[51–53] an autonomic nervous system-related disease characterized by alterations in blood pressure and reduced ventilatory responses to hypercapnia and hypoxia. Because dyspnea reflects motor deficits as a result of sensory losses, most imaging studies in dyspnea report activation of S1 and the supplemental motor area (SMA) and less activation of S2 and primary motor regions. Similarly, increased activation of frontal and PFC regions represents involvement of voluntary functions, such as vigilance/attention, which seems to provide a compensatory mechanism in an effort to sustain voluntary breathing. The cortical processing associated with the voluntary motor control of respiratory muscles seems to be achieved via activation of the association cortex, which, in turn, activates the motor cortex, thalamus, basal ganglia, and finally the cerebellum.

Despite these similarities in cortical motor function and compensation, studies of laboratory-induced and CCHS-induced dyspnea show some differences at the subcortical level. Decreased activation of thalamic and hypothalamic regions is noted in CCHS patients, whereas increased activation of these regions is observed in laboratory-induced dyspnea. Likewise, decreased activation of the ACC is observed in CCHS-induced dyspnea, resulting in aberrant afferent projections to the insula, whereas increased ACC and AI activation is observed in laboratory-induced dyspnea. Thus, laboratory-induced dyspnea, but not CCHS-induced dyspnea, seems to share common cortical and subcortical patterns with pain-induced brain substrates.

Nausea and vomiting

One of the physiological factors of nausea and vomiting (NV) is the vomiting reflex, which is not essential for survival but is advantageous for its anticipatory role in response to cognitive, visual, or olfactory stimulation in an effort to expel ingested toxins (such as chemotherapeutic agents) from the body. However, the difficulty in examining the cortical and subcortical imaging of NV is that vomiting inside a confined imaging system may result in aspiration, especially in a supine position, and thus medical ethics committees could oppose such a study. Additionally, examination of the cerebral representation of NV may be difficult, if not impossible, to examine in a single paradigm, since either nausea or vomiting should be imaged rather than the interplay of these two reflexes. Because of these difficulties in imaging NV, only one study by Miller et al[54] has investigated the cerebral representation of nausea via vestibular and drug induction using noninvasive magnetic source imaging. Activation of the inferior frontal gyrus was detected during the nausea state only, and not during various control sessions. This finding deserves further investigation because it may represent a new cortical target for antinausea drug delivery.

Another set of imaging studies focused on stimulating the vestibular system during circular vection, which also can help us understand the cortical and subcortical mechanisms of nausea. Vestibular activation can induce motion sickness, as a result of sensory conflict between vestibular and visual inputs.[55] A bilateral increase in medial parieto-occipital spatial pattern and simultaneous bilateral deactivation of the parieto-insular vestibular regions was reported in a PET circular vection study.[56] Another PET study suppressed visual motion with the subject's eyes closed and reported increased cerebral metabolism of the thalamus and vestibular regions, while the occipital lobe (BA17/18/19) was deactivated.[57] These studies suggest that a potential NV mechanism could be the generation of sensory conflict between visual, vestibular, and proprioceptive cortical systems.

A starting point in investigating the cerebral mechanisms of NV is to identify the lag in the temporal response between nausea and vomiting, and its supraspinal correlates of activation. The challenge in such a paradigm is that the stimulus has to be presented only once in an effort to identify the cortical response associated with the state of initiation of nausea rather than the state of vomiting. Nonetheless, these types of imaging studies are essential if we are to identify the cerebral representation of chemotherapy-induced NV with the long-term objective of targeting neuronal substrates for antinausea drug intervention.

Hunger, satiety, and appetite

The cortical regions most commonly activated across appetite and taste studies (presentation and ingestion of pleasant or unpleasant food stimuli) are the insula, particularly the AI, extending into the frontal operculum and part of the cortex (OFC).[58–63] The insular cortex is a multimodal integration center that is an important relay for the neuronal circuitry connecting the hypothalamus, other regions of the limbic system, and OFC and that responds to autonomic nervous system activation related to emotional states of feeding behavior. The OFC, in particular, besides becoming activated in response to visually rewarding stimuli, has been identified as the secondary gustatory cortex because of its role in assessing the reward value of food, which is reduced to zero when satiety is reached.[64] Various OFC regions are involved in eating and the olfaction of food (right caudal OFC) and in assessing pleasantness and unpleasantness of food taste (medial rostral and lateral OFC, respectively). Further, it has been shown that activation of the middle ACC occurs while perceiving both pleasant and unpleasant odors, whereas activation of the anterior part of the ACC is correlated with the subjective ratings of pleasant odors.[64,65]

Liu et al.[66] showed an enhanced response in the SMA after glucose ingestion, which suggests integration of sensory and visceral mechanisms, as well as affective responses associated with appetite, taste, and olfaction. However, this study also reported a decrease in the BOLD signal of the hypothalamus, which is a structure responsible for eating behavior and regulating plasma glucose concentration. These findings show that the cortical representation of eating and satiety in humans is quite complex and that currently, the link between these higher cognitive functions and the interoceptive signals that terminate a meal is unknown.

Fatigue

The cortical and subcortical processing of cancer-related fatigue, the most common symptom reported by cancer patients, has not yet been examined. However, some inferences can be made from studies done in healthy individuals and in patients with multiple sclerosis (MS) or chronic fatigue syndrome (CFS), as examples of peripheral or central nervous system-induced muscle weakness.

Functional MRI of healthy individuals exposed to fatiguing exercise showed a broad network of initial bilateral increased activation of S1, SMA, PFC, and cingulate cortex, which subsequently decreased to baseline levels.[67] The initial increase in the BOLD signal may suggest greater voluntary effort to maintain the required muscle output, and the subsequent decrease may indicate greater inhibition of spinal motor neurons that originate from the fatigued muscle. Another fMRI study in healthy subjects demonstrated a greater reduction in contralateral S1 activation during movement of the nonfatigued hand compared with the fatigued hand.[68] This group later showed that although reduction in activation was greater in S1, there was also reduced activation in the SMA, cerebellum, and primary visual (V1) cortex when a visually cued motor task was performed.[69] These studies demonstrate that fatiguing exercise involves not only motor substrates but also higher-order cognitive neuroanatomical substrates.

An ^{18}F-FDG PET study in patients with MS-associated fatigue showed decreased glucose metabolism in the lateral and medial PFC, the premotor cortex, SMA, and rostral putamen toward the lateral portion of the caudate nucleus, which suggests disruption of cortico-subcortical circuits.[70] This study also demonstrated a positive correlation between fatigue severity and increased activity in the cerebellar vermis and ACC in the MS-fatigued group compared with the MS nonfatigued group. Filippi et al.[71] examined the cortical processing of MS-fatigued patients on a simple motor task and reported an increase in the BOLD signal of the contralateral upper bank of the Sylvian fissure (a region in the S2 cortex), intraparietal sulcus, cingulate motor cortex, and SMA. A later fMRI study showed increased recruitment of S2, cerebellum, and parietal areas in MS patients without reversible fatigue after interferon β-1a treatment compared with those with reversible fatigue.[72] A more recent study[73] induced cognitive fatigue in MS patients by having them perform the Paced Auditory Serial Addition Task (PASAT), a task requiring attention; before and after the PASAT, a motor paradigm took place. The functional data obtained after the PASAT displayed increased selectivity for bilateral cingulate gyri, left S1 (BA3), and right superior and middle frontal gyri in comparison to healthy controls, where the spatial patterns and BOLD signal intensity were attenuated. Another study that examined cognitive fatigue over time using a modified version of the Symbol Digit Modalities Test, which was given four times to patients with MS, resulted in an increased spatial pattern in frontal, parietal, basal ganglia, and occipital regions.[74]

Motor-related fatigue studies suggest that recruitment of motor pathways as a consequence of SMA efferent projections to the brainstem and cervical cord may follow in response to the injured contralateral corticospinal tract present in MS-fatigued patients. Increased activation of the cerebellum, which is involved in motor imagery, learning, and planning, may also suggest that performance of a simple motor task by MS-fatigued individuals results in greater voluntary effort, which may serve as a compensatory mechanism for the reduced SMA activation. Cognitive-related fatigue results in increased spatial patterns and BOLD signal intensity in higher-order cognitive regions. This, however, may suggest increased hemodynamic or metabolic "effort" rather than a compensatory mechanism, since activation of higher-order cognitive regions continues to be robust.

CFS is characterized by persistent or relapsing physical and cognitive fatigue. Thus, investigating the brain mechanisms of CFS may help us form hypotheses relevant to the cortical processing of cancer-related fatigue. Structural imaging has demonstrated a significant correlation between frontal lobe white matter hyperintensities in CFS patients and decreased self-reported physical stamina. Functional imaging studies of CFS using visual motor tasks showed reduced cerebral blood flow of the superior temporal gyrus, visual cortices, inferior occipital cortex, and cerebellar declive, a region associated with the execution of saccades.[75,76] However, when CFS patients were tested on auditory tasks, findings showed increased spatial patterns in the ACC, dorsolateral PFC, middle and superior temporal lobes, as well as in the middle, superior, posterior, and inferior parietal lobe.[77–79]

When CFS patients did not undergo any fatiguing task and were imaged during rest, reduced cerebral blood flow was observed in the PFC, ACC, posterior cingulate cortex, and lateral and medial temporal and cuneus/precuneus regions.[80–82] A preliminary observation in reference to the cortical activation of CFS is a pattern of increased ACC and frontal/prefrontal activation during auditory tasks, which could imply a compensatory mechanism as a result of hypometabolism of these regions during rest. Further, a report by de Lange et al.[83] showed neuroplastic changes, specifically a moderate increase in the prefrontal (BA46/9) gray matter volume after cognitive behavioral therapy. This suggests the potential of reversing fatigue-related cerebral atrophy after effective behavioral rehabilitation.

Overall, the studies described above suggest that MS-related and CFS-related fatigue seem to be the consequence of abnormal cortical and subcortical processing in the frontal and somatomotor cortices, basal ganglia, and cerebellum. The cortical processing in patients with MS or CFS is characterized by recruitment of extensive cortical regions, as a result of greater effort exerted during the fatigued state.

Disturbed sleep

Sleep disturbance is a common symptom of cancer and cancer treatment (see Chapters 14 and 15). Before the advancement of functional neuroimaging, investigation of the normal and pathophysiological states of sleep was difficult because of EEG limitations in providing information about subcortical function. Nonetheless, EEG polysomnography led to the discovery of REM/stage-5 sleep, which has considerably advanced our understanding of the cortical mechanisms related to the regulation of sleep/wake cycles.

REM sleep in adults with sleep disturbances is characterized by increased cortical and subcortical activation similar to that observed during wakefulness, because beta waves are associated with day-to-day wakefulness. The main challenge in conducting an fMRI sleep study is that subjects must sleep in the fMRI scanning environment regardless of the considerable noise produced by the MR scanner while acquiring the image data. The first fMRI sleep study by Lovblad et al.,[84] which imaged five subjects during REM sleep using a silent MR sequence that recorded brain activation over many hours with simultaneous EEG acquisition, reported increased visual cortex activation and decreased lateral PFC activation compared with non-REM sleep. Functional imaging REM sleep studies showed increased limbic and occipital spatial patterns, which suggest the phenomenological properties of REM sleep related to the visual and emotional experience of dreaming. On the other hand, PET and EEG studies of non-REM sleep (also called slow-wave sleep stages 1–4) compared with wakefulness showed significant deactivation of the thalamus, frontal, OFC, and parietal cortices, brainstem, and basal ganglia – structures typically involved in motor, cognitive, and emotional processing.[85–91]

Primary insomnia, one of the most common sleep disturbance complaints not attributable to a medical or psychiatric condition, is defined as difficulty in initiating and/or maintaining sleep. The cortical and subcortical regions implicated in the neurocognitive model of primary insomnia include: (1) the ascending reticular activating system (ARAS, the center of arousal and motivation), the inputs of which project into cholinergic and aminergic brainstem regions related to the sleep and wake states, respectively; (2) the thalamus, which is deactivated not only during non-REM sleep but also in the transition from awake state to REM sleep in healthy subjects[92] (however, no differences in thalamic activation were observed in patients with primary insomnia while transitioning from the wake state to REM sleep, which may be suggestive of patients' difficulties falling and staying asleep and/or their perception of shallow sleep[93]); (3) the basal ganglia, deactivated during non-REM sleep, which suggests the inhibitory effect of nondisturbed sleep on voluntary movement, cognition, and emotion, due to their connections to limbic regions such as the thalamus, pons, and brainstem (however, increased caudate activation may lead to reciprocal thalamic excitation and in turn to hyperarousal, which may lead to insomnia); and (4) the frontal cortex, which has been observed as deactivated during

NREM sleep. The frontal metabolism of insomnia patients has been characterized by increased regional cerebral blood flow before onset of sleep; however, in these cases, worry and rumination may have been interfering with sleep initiation because increased dorsolateral PFC activation has been shown during anticipatory anxiety.

These findings suggest the involvement of two separate cortical and subcortical mechanisms in the neuropathology of primary insomnia: (1) the arousal network, which involves regions related to emotional and motor functions, such as the ARAS, thalamus-hypothalamus, and basal ganglia; and (2) a network of regions associated with higher-order cognitive structures, such as the frontal/OFC cortex. Future work is needed to determine the effect of interventions on altering activation in these networks to alleviate the sleep disturbances that patients with cancer experience.

Studies of analgesia

Functional imaging studies can enhance translational research by identifying new pharmacokinetic and pharmacodynamic parameters that could lead to drug development.[31,94–96] Our limited knowledge of the mechanism of action of analgesic drugs at the supraspinal level is primarily based on the cortical and subcortical processing data acquired from healthy adults. To our knowledge, there are no studies of the cortical effects of analgesics in cancer patients. In this section, we will review the central effects of analgesia on cerebral activation with and without the application of pain in healthy adults, as determined through functional neuroimaging.

The endogenous opioid system seems to affect not only the analgesic network but also several other cortical and subcortical circuits, such as those involved in mood, memory/attention, and learning, and thus can modulate chronic pain and other disorders such as depression, anxiety, and addictive behavior. Postmortem autoradiographic and PET studies have shown that the highest densities of μ-opioid receptors are found primarily in the medial thalamus, caudate nucleus, ACC, and PAG, the stimulation of which activates cholinergic, adrenergic, and dopaminergic systems.[97] To add to the complexity of the opioid system, its function is also affected by sex, genetic polymorphisms (eg, single nucleotide polymorphisms on the *COMT* gene), pain syndromes (eg, neuropathic pain), and long-term analgesic treatments that can modulate the opioid central sensitization system. Advances in this area should ultimately result in standardized functional imaging trials for early-phase evaluation of pharmacotherapies for pain.

Our review of functional imaging studies examining the effects of analgesia on brain activation and deactivation generated these observations: (1) decreased activation of the thalamus, insula, and posterior cingulate after administration of analgesia in the presence of pain stimulation,[98–103] which suggests that the effect of opioids administered during pain stimulation has a selective and specific effect on nociceptive processing and thus primarily involves brain regions associated with pain processing; (2) a decrease in the activation of temporal regions, which suggests that μ-opioids participate in the affective experience of auditory stimuli; and (3) increased OFC activation after administration of opioid analgesia in the absence of pain stimulation.[104–107] Middle and medial OFC regions have been implicated in the processes of positive reward, addiction, and attention, which suggests that the analgesic mechanisms of μ-opioid agonists can be associated with activation of regions other than those associated with the pain experience per se.

Discussion and future directions

Functional neuroimaging has in many respects revolutionized the study of cognitive neuroscience and is slowly becoming an important investigative tool in clinical research. Although we are aware of no functional imaging studies of symptoms in patients with cancer, current imaging findings in other patients and healthy subjects have provided important pieces of information on the brain regions activated across symptoms in a variety of diseases. Interestingly, these studies suggest that dissimilar symptoms seem to result from the activation of similar spatial patterns. For example, neuroimaging studies of pain and of dyspnea have shown that brain regions such as the ACC, OFC, insula, and somatosensory regions are involved in the processing of these symptoms (Figure 18.3). These findings suggest that selectivity for these brain spatial patterns may occur in the expression of different symptoms. However, our understanding of the functional connectivity across such symptoms has yet to be explored.

On the basis of brain spatial patterns generated by symptoms, we propose two categories of symptoms: (1) phasic symptoms that can be rapidly elicited, such

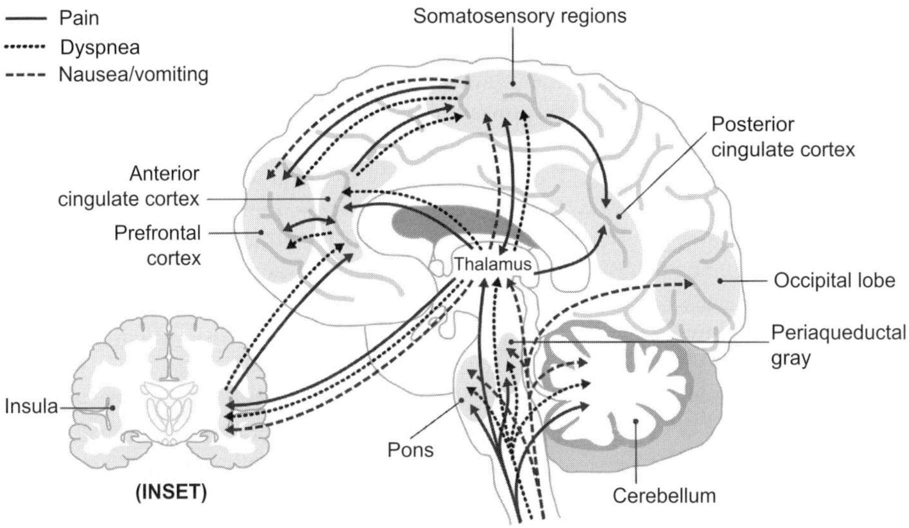

Figure 18.3. Common pathways in the processing of pain, dyspnea, and nausea/vomiting. Schematic of the mechanisms in the cortical and subcortical processing of phasic symptoms, such as pain, dyspnea, and nausea/vomiting, identified using functional imaging modalities. Because the insula cannot be localized midsagittally, it is depicted in a coronal section of the brain (inset). A preliminary review of the literature suggests that phasic symptoms seem to activate similar brain regions, such as the anterior cingulate cortex, orbitofrontal cortex (not shown), and insula.

as pain, dyspnea, nausea, and vomiting, and (2) state symptoms such as fatigue and sleep disturbance, the expression of which occurs over time. Because of the very limited amount of data available on the functional imaging of fatigue and sleep disturbances, proposing a conceptual model of state symptoms would be premature. However, on the basis of a plethora of functional imaging studies of pain and some on dyspnea, we propose a conceptual model of the cortical processing of phasic symptoms.

Phasic symptoms seem to be characterized by a hierarchy of control and interactive processes. Lower-order processing, which refers to the somatosensory and somatomotor functions, takes place when an incoming stimulus, such as a pain sensation, enters into conscious awareness. In turn, conscious awareness, reflected by higher-order control, modulates or overrides lower-order processing in an effort to control behavior. Mesulam[108] stated that conscious awareness seems to be associated with instinctive patterns of response, which are reflections of the evolving emergent patterns of learned behavior, thereby linking sensation to action. In the context of symptom interoception, when a pain stimulus is applied, the sensation of pain is relayed by local nociceptive afferents to lamina I neurons of the dorsal horn, which then decussate and, via long ascending fibers of the anterolateral portion of the spinal cord white matter, ascend to the brain. These fibers convey the nociceptive signal to the cerebral cortex, first to the thalamus, which in turn relays the information to the cingulate, insula, somatosensory cortices, and more posterior locations within the parietal lobe, and finally to the PFC. Subsequently, higher-order structures, such as the PFC, take over by inducing antinociceptive responses via long descending fibers that project down to various brainstem nuclei and, in turn, to the spinal gray matter. Thus, the sensation and perception of symptoms is a reflection of conscious awareness, mirrored by a set of cortical and subcortical neuronal substrates.

Therefore, we propose the following common elements among phasic symptoms at the brain level, as a function of higher-order and lower-order processing of conscious awareness (Figure 18.3): (1) the states of pain, dyspnea, and nausea/vomiting triggered by sensory, lower-level neuronal inputs seem to be modulated by higher-order representations, the goal of which is to inhibit the former responses; (2) the affective perception of pain and dyspnea is represented by higher-order cognitive and limbic spatial patterns of the ACC and insula, the latter also being a neurobiological substrate of motion sickness; (3) the ascending sensory pathways in the midbrain have been well identified to mediate the neural substrate of pain from the spinal cord to the brain, but these same pathways also seem to be related to the neural processing of dyspnea and motion sickness; and (4) inhibition of the ascending pathways is induced by the upregulation of descending pathways, which seem to be generated at the level of PFC regions and may reflect the voluntary act of "escaping" from pain, dyspnea, or nausea.

A major limitation in our ability to image cancer-related symptoms is our inadequate understanding of the complex pathology induced by the disease and/or its treatment, which together can generate highly variable brain spatial patterns. However, in spite of the heterogeneity of symptom pathophysiology, a unifying concept arises from the fact that most cancer-induced pathological conditions are inflammatory in nature, whether they result from the tumor, its treatment, or both. A goal for future studies is to examine the effects of inflammatory factors (eg, interleukin [IL]-6, IL-1β) in response to cancer and its treatment on brain spatial patterns. This will provide information on the cortical and subcortical processing of single or multiple symptoms experienced by patients with cancer. For example, Harrison et al.[109] investigated the effects of sickness behavior (behavioral and physiological changes such as decreased motivation, psychomotor retardation, fever, cognitive and affective changes) induced by peripheral inflammation on cognitive impairment and reported bilateral PFC and intraparietal sulci patterns, as well as increased BOLD signal at the level of the brainstem, thalamus, amygdala, cingulate, and AI in response to the inflammatory challenge administered.

Another crucial area for improvement is the methodology used for the study of neuronal response patterns induced by symptoms. The inconsistencies in the findings from studies examining symptoms may be partly explained by the use of various study paradigms, difficulties in accurately identifying subregions within the areas of interest, and the heterogeneous patient populations enrolled, such as in pain imaging studies. Ultimately, a powerful approach to address network identification is to increase the spatial and temporal resolution by integrating two or more neuroimaging techniques. One example of this approach is the fusion of fMRI or PET techniques with electrophysiological recordings, such as EEG or magnetoencephalography, which together allow the noninvasive localization of synaptic current flow changes in both space and time because of their complementary properties.[110–112] Thus, a multimodality imaging approach would help us obtain more precise, quantitative measurements of the coupling between a neuronal response and its associated hemodynamic or metabolic activity.

The motivation to integrate fMRI in clinical practice has been instrumental in the development of real-time fMRI (rt-fMRI), which has recently been evaluated for suitability as a neurofeedback tool with the goal of inducing plasticity and thus neurorehabilitation. Unlike conventional fMRI, which generates static activation maps in relation to time, rt-fMRI dynamically extracts the desired information, making it readily available during image acquisition. Most importantly, this technology allows customized treatment based on each patient's specific deficits and, in turn, the feedback signal can be modulated by optimization of strategy via learning. The focus of existing rt-fMRI implementations are based on either (1) localized approaches, meaning learning to regulate the level of activation in certain brain regions via their time-series fluctuations;[113–117] or (2) multivariate relationships in the data by using distributed brain state classification patterns.[118–121] This second supervised learning-based rt-fMRI approach has several advantages over localized strategies, in that no prior assumptions about functional localization and individual performance strategies are required; ie, the support vector machine algorithm learns these directly from the volunteer, and patients are therefore not required to be cognitively coached. Localized approaches, in contrast, rely heavily on coaching, which ultimately increases patient training time and level of effort. Nonetheless, recent studies by deCharms et al.,[114] which provide a compelling example of the utility of rt-fMRI neurofeedback for therapeutic applications, showed that when trained patients with chronic pain deliberately decreased activity in the rostral ACC, there was a corresponding decrease in pain perception, even after completion of the study.

Conclusion

As reviewed elsewhere in this book, animal and human studies strongly suggest that the etiological framework of various cancer symptoms, as a result of the tumor or its treatment, may be attributed to common biological mechanisms, such as inflammation. Identifying the pathways and mechanisms that form downstream of the brain is necessary, but this does not elucidate the networks occurring at the supraspinal level. Consequently, in an effort to eventually prevent, diagnose, and treat symptom burden in patients with cancer, it is essential that we identify the mechanisms of symptoms at the central nervous system level, in particular the cortical and subcortical pathways of aberrant activation or inhibition.

To further explore and better understand human brain function as it relates to cancer symptoms, it is important to make progress in the following areas: (1) integration of the spatial and temporal neural dynamics by further development of mapping techniques, which will help us investigate both local-scale (eg, synaptic transmission, axonal transport, neuronal) networks and larger-scale (eg, columns, sets of voxels) networks; (2) identification of brain networks for each symptom characterized by the anatomical substrates associated with a specific function in the expression of a symptom; and (3) refinement of the temporal properties (hemodynamic response as a consequence of the hemodynamic lag) of fMRI, as this modality is the most popular imaging technique because of its noninvasive nature, excellent spatial resolution, and ability to acquire multiple scans in a single imaging session.

References

1. Logothetis NK, Pauls J, Augath M, Trinath T, Oeltermann A. Neurophysiological investigation of the basis of the fMRI signal. *Nature* **412**(6843): 150–157, 2001.
2. Ogawa S, Menon RS, Tank DW, et al. Functional brain mapping by blood oxygenation level-dependent contrast magnetic resonance imaging: a comparison of signal characteristics with a biophysical model. *Biophys J* **64**(3):803–812, 1993.
3. Drake CT, Iadecola C. The role of neuronal signaling in controlling cerebral blood flow. *Brain Lang* **102**(2):141–152, 2007.
4. Ogawa S, Tank DW, Menon R, et al. Intrinsic signal changes accompanying sensory stimulation: functional brain mapping with magnetic resonance imaging. *Proc Natl Acad Sci U S A* **89**(13):5951–5955, 1992.
5. Bandettini PA, Jesmanowicz A, Wong EC, Hyde JS. Processing strategies for time-course data sets in functional MRI of the human brain. *Magn Reson Med* **30**(2):161–173, 1993.
6. DeYoe EA, Felleman DJ, Van Essen DC, McClendon E. Multiple processing streams in occipitotemporal visual cortex. *Nature* **371**(6493):151–154, 1994.
7. Craig AD. How do you feel? Interoception: the sense of the physiological condition of the body. *Nat Rev Neurosci* **3**(8):655–666, 2002.
8. Craig AD. Interoception: the sense of the physiological condition of the body. *Curr Opin Neurobiol* **13**(4): 500–505, 2003.
9. Damasio A. Feelings of emotion and the self. *Ann N Y Acad Sci* **1001**:253–261, 2003.
10. Craig AD. The functional anatomy of lamina I and its role in post-stroke central pain. In: Sandkühler J, Bromm B, Gebhart GF, eds. *Nervous System Plasticity and Chronic Pain*. Amsterdam: Elsevier, 2000:137–151. *Progress in Brain Research; vol. 129.*
11. Greenspan JD, Winfield JA. Reversible pain and tactile deficits associated with a cerebral tumor compressing the posterior insula and parietal operculum. *Pain* **50**(1):29–39, 1992.
12. Schmahmann JD, Leifer D. Parietal pseudothalamic pain syndrome: clinical features and anatomic correlates. *Arch Neurol* **49**(10):1032–1037, 1992.
13. Bassetti C, Bogousslavsky J, Regli F. Sensory syndromes in parietal stroke. *Neurology* **43**(10): 1942–1949, 1993.
14. Freund HJ. Somatosensory and motor disturbances in patients with parietal lobe lesions. *Adv Neurol* **93**:179–193, 2003.
15. Diserens K, Vuadens P, Michel P, et al. Acute autonomic dysfunction contralateral to acute strokes: a prospective study of 100 consecutive cases. *Eur J Neurol* **13**(11):1245–1250, 2006.
16. Rainville P, Duncan GH, Price DD, Carrier B, Bushnell MC. Pain affect encoded in human anterior cingulate but not somatosensory cortex. *Science* **277**(5328):968–971, 1997.
17. Craig AD, Reiman EM, Evans A, Bushnell MC. Functional imaging of an illusion of pain. *Nature* **384**(6606):258–260, 1996.
18. Melzack R, Casey KL. Sensory, motivational, and central control determinants of pain: a new conceptual model. In: Kenshalo DR, ed. *The Skin Senses: Proceedings of the First International Symposium on the Skin Senses*. Springfield IL: Thomas, 1968.
19. Portenoy RK, Conn M. Cancer pain syndromes. In: Bruera E, Portenoy RK, eds. *Cancer Pain: Assessment and Management*. Cambridge UK: Cambridge University Press, 2003:89–108.

20. Casey KL. Forebrain mechanisms of nociception and pain: analysis through imaging. *Proc Natl Acad Sci U S A* **96**(14):7668–7674, 1999.

21. Treede RD, Kenshalo DR, Gracely RH, Jones AK. The cortical representation of pain. *Pain* **79**(2–3):105–111, 1999.

22. Peyron R, Laurent B, García-Larrea L. Functional imaging of brain responses to pain: a review and meta-analysis (2000). *Neurophysiol Clin* **30**(5): 263–288, 2000.

23. Rainville P. Brain mechanisms of pain affect and pain modulation. *Curr Opin Neurobiol* **12**(2):195–204, 2002.

24. Porro CA. Functional imaging and pain: behavior, perception, and modulation. *Neuroscientist* **9**(5): 354–369, 2003.

25. Apkarian AV, Bushnell MC, Treede RD, Zubieta JK. Human brain mechanisms of pain perception and regulation in health and disease. *Eur J Pain* **9**(4): 463–484, 2005.

26. Dunckley P, Wise RG, Aziz Q, et al. Cortical processing of visceral and somatic stimulation: differentiating pain intensity from unpleasantness. *Neuroscience* **133**(2):533–542, 2005.

27. Peyron R, García-Larrea L, Grégoire MC, et al. Parietal and cingulate processes in central pain: a combined positron emission tomography (PET) and functional magnetic resonance imaging (fMRI) study of an unusual case. *Pain* **84**(1):77–87, 2000.

28. Casey KL, Minoshima S, Berger KL, Koeppe RA, Morrow TJ, Frey KA. Positron emission tomographic analysis of cerebral structures activated specifically by repetitive noxious heat stimuli. *J Neurophysiol* **71**(2):802–807, 1994.

29. Tarkka IM, Treede RD. Equivalent electrical source analysis of pain-related somatosensory evoked potentials elicited by a CO2 laser. *J Clin Neurophysiol* **10**(4):513–519, 1993.

30. Price DD. Psychological and neural mechanisms of the affective dimension of pain. *Science* **288**(5472):1769–1772, 2000.

31. Borsook D, Becerra LR. Breaking down the barriers: fMRI applications in pain, analgesia and analgesics. *Mol Pain* **2**:30, 2006.

32. Strigo IA, Duncan GH, Boivin M, Bushnell MC. Differentiation of visceral and cutaneous pain in the human brain. *J Neurophysiol* **89**(6):3294–3303, 2003.

33. Baron R. Mechanisms of disease: neuropathic pain: a clinical perspective. *Nat Clin Pract Neurol* **2**(2): 95–106, 2006.

34. Hsieh JC, Belfrage M, Stone-Elander S, Hansson P, Ingvar M. Central representation of chronic ongoing neuropathic pain studied by positron emission tomography. *Pain* **63**(2):225–236, 1995.

35. Peyron R, García-Larrea L, Grégoire MC, et al. Allodynia after lateral-medullary (Wallenberg) infarct: a PET study. *Brain* **121**(Pt 2):345–356, 1998.

36. Peyron R, Schneider F, Faillenot I, et al. An fMRI study of cortical representation of mechanical allodynia in patients with neuropathic pain. *Neurology* **63**(10):1838–1846, 2004.

37. Maihöfner C, Handwerker HO. Differential coding of hyperalgesia in the human brain: a functional MRI study. *Neuroimage* **28**(4):996–1006, 2005.

38. Maihöfner C, Handwerker HO, Birklein F. Functional imaging of allodynia in complex regional pain syndrome. *Neurology* **66**(5):711–717, 2006.

39. Ushida T, Ikemoto T, Taniguchi S, et al. Virtual pain stimulation of allodynia patients activates cortical representation of pain and emotions: a functional MRI study. *Brain Topogr* **18**(1):27–35, 2005.

40. Schweinhardt P, Glynn C, Brooks J, et al. An fMRI study of cerebral processing of brush-evoked allodynia in neuropathic pain patients. *Neuroimage* **32**(1): 256–265, 2006.

41. Witting N, Kupers RC, Svensson P, Jensen TS. A PET activation study of brush-evoked allodynia in patients with nerve injury pain. *Pain* **120**(1–2):145–154, 2006.

42. Hunt SP, Mantyh PW. The molecular dynamics of pain control. *Nat Rev Neurosci* **2**(2):83–91, 2001.

43. Petrovic P, Ingvar M, Stone-Elander S, Petersson KM, Hansson P. A PET activation study of dynamic mechanical allodynia in patients with mononeuropathy. *Pain* **83**(3):459–470, 1999.

44. Colebatch JG, Deiber MP, Passingham RE, Friston KJ, Frackowiak RS. Regional cerebral blood flow during voluntary arm and hand movements in human subjects. *J Neurophysiol* **65**(6):1392–1401, 1991.

45. Corfield DR, Fink GR, Ramsay SC, et al. Evidence for limbic system activation during CO2-stimulated breathing in man. *J Physiol* **488**(Pt 1):77–84, 1995.

46. Brannan S, Liotti M, Egan G, et al. Neuroimaging of cerebral activations and deactivations associated with hypercapnia and hunger for air. *Proc Natl Acad Sci U S A* **98**(4):2029–2034, 2001.

47. Liotti M, Brannan S, Egan G, et al. Brain responses associated with consciousness of breathlessness (air hunger). *Proc Natl Acad Sci U S A* **98**(4):2035–2040, 2001.

48. Parsons LM, Egan G, Liotti M, et al. Neuroimaging evidence implicating cerebellum in the experience of hypercapnia and hunger for air. *Proc Natl Acad Sci U S A* **98**(4):2041–2046, 2001.

49. Peiffer C, Poline JB, Thivard L, Aubier M, Samson Y. Neural substrates for the perception of acutely induced dyspnea. *Am J Respir Crit Care Med* **163**(4):951–957, 2001.

50. Evans KC, Banzett RB, Adams L, McKay L, Frackowiak RS, Corfield DR. BOLD fMRI identifies limbic, paralimbic, and cerebellar activation during air hunger. *J Neurophysiol* **88**(3):1500–1511, 2002.

51. Macey KE, Macey PM, Woo MA, et al. fMRI signal changes in response to forced expiratory loading in congenital central hypoventilation syndrome. *J Appl Physiol* **97**(5):1897–1907, 2004.

52. Macey PM, Woo MA, Macey KE, et al. Hypoxia reveals posterior thalamic, cerebellar, midbrain, and limbic deficits in congenital central hypoventilation syndrome. *J Appl Physiol* **98**(3):958–969, 2005.

53. Woo MA, Macey PM, Macey KE, et al. FMRI responses to hyperoxia in congenital central hypoventilation syndrome. *Pediatr Res* **57**(4):510–518, 2005.

54. Miller AD, Rowley HA, Roberts TP, Kucharczyk J. Human cortical activity during vestibular- and drug-induced nausea detected using MSI. *Ann N Y Acad Sci* **781**:670–672, 1996.

55. Bles W, Bos JE, Kruit H. Motion sickness. *Curr Opin Neurol* **13**(1):19–25, 2000.

56. Brandt T, Bartenstein P, Janek A, Dieterich M. Reciprocal inhibitory visual-vestibular interaction: visual motion stimulation deactivates the parieto-insular vestibular cortex. *Brain* **121**(Pt 9):1749–1758, 1998.

57. Wenzel R, Bartenstein P, Dieterich M, et al. Deactivation of human visual cortex during involuntary ocular oscillations: a PET activation study. *Brain* **119**(Pt 1):101–110, 1996.

58. Tataranni PA, Gautier JF, Chen K, et al. Neuroanatomical correlates of hunger and satiation in humans using positron emission tomography. *Proc Natl Acad Sci U S A* **96**(8):4569–4574, 1999.

59. O'Doherty J, Rolls ET, Francis S, et al. Sensory-specific satiety-related olfactory activation of the human orbitofrontal cortex. *Neuroreport* **11**(4):893–897, 2000.

60. Araújo IE. [Taste representation in the human cortex and the central control of appetite]. *Rev Bras Psiquiatr* **25**(Suppl 2):25–28, 2003.

61. Wang GJ, Volkow ND, Telang F, et al. Exposure to appetitive food stimuli markedly activates the human brain. *Neuroimage* **21**(4):1790–1797, 2004.

62. Simmons WK, Martin A, Barsalou LW. Pictures of appetizing foods activate gustatory cortices for taste and reward. *Cereb Cortex* **15**(10):1602–1608, 2005.

63. Porubská K, Veit R, Preissl H, Fritsche A, Birbaumer N. Subjective feeling of appetite modulates brain activity: an fMRI study. *Neuroimage* **32**(3):1273–1280, 2006.

64. Rolls ET. Smell, taste, texture, and temperature multimodal representations in the brain, and their relevance to the control of appetite. *Nutr Rev* **62** (11 Pt 2):S193–S204, 2004.

65. Rolls ET. Sensory processing in the brain related to the control of food intake. *Proc Nutr Soc* **66**(1):96–112, 2007.

66. Liu Y, Gao JH, Liu HL, Fox PT. The temporal response of the brain after eating revealed by functional MRI. *Nature* **405**(6790):1058–1062, 2000.

67. Liu JZ, Dai TH, Sahgal V, Brown RW, Yue GH. Nonlinear cortical modulation of muscle fatigue: a functional MRI study. *Brain Res* **957**(2):320–329, 2002.

68. Benwell NM, Byrnes ML, Mastaglia FL, Thickbroom GW. Primary sensorimotor cortex activation with task-performance after fatiguing hand exercise. *Exp Brain Res* **167**(2):160–164, 2005.

69. Benwell NM, Mastaglia FL, Thickbroom GW. Reduced functional activation after fatiguing exercise is not confined to primary motor areas. *Exp Brain Res* **175**(4):575–583, 2006.

70. Roelcke U, Kappos L, Lechner-Scott J, et al. Reduced glucose metabolism in the frontal cortex and basal ganglia of multiple sclerosis patients with fatigue: a 18F-fluorodeoxyglucose positron emission tomography study. *Neurology* **48**(6):1566–1571, 1997.

71. Filippi M, Rocca MA, Colombo B, et al. Functional magnetic resonance imaging correlates of fatigue in multiple sclerosis. *Neuroimage* **15**(3):559–567, 2002.

72. Rocca MA, Agosta F, Colombo B, et al. fMRI changes in relapsing-remitting multiple sclerosis patients complaining of fatigue after IFNbeta-1a injection. *Hum Brain Mapp* **28**(5):373–382, 2007.

73. Tartaglia MC, Narayanan S, Arnold DL. Mental fatigue alters the pattern and increases the volume of cerebral activation required for a motor task in multiple sclerosis patients with fatigue. *Eur J Neurol* **15**(4):413–419, 2008.

74. Deluca J, Genova HM, Hillary FG, Wylie G. Neural correlates of cognitive fatigue in multiple sclerosis using functional MRI. *J Neurol Sci* **270**(1–2):28–39, 2008.

75. de Lange FP, Kalkman JS, Bleijenberg G, et al. Neural correlates of the chronic fatigue syndrome: an fMRI study. *Brain* **127**(Pt 9):1948–1957, 2004.

76. Tanaka M, Sadato N, Okada T, et al. Reduced responsiveness is an essential feature of chronic fatigue syndrome: a fMRI study. *BMC Neurol* **6**:9, 2006.

77. Schmaling KB, Lewis DH, Fiedelak JI, Mahurin R, Buchwald DS. Single-photon emission computerized

tomography and neurocognitive function in patients with chronic fatigue syndrome. *Psychosom Med* **65**(1):129–136, 2003.

78. Lange G, Steffener J, Cook DB, et al. Objective evidence of cognitive complaints in Chronic Fatigue Syndrome: a BOLD fMRI study of verbal working memory. *Neuroimage* **26**(2):513–524, 2005.
79. Cook DB, O'Connor PJ, Lange G, Steffener J. Functional neuroimaging correlates of mental fatigue induced by cognition among chronic fatigue syndrome patients and controls. *Neuroimage* **36**(1):108–122, 2007.
80. Lewis DH, Mayberg HS, Fischer ME, et al. Monozygotic twins discordant for chronic fatigue syndrome: regional cerebral blood flow SPECT. *Radiology* **219**(3):766–773, 2001.
81. Yamamoto S, Ouchi Y, Onoe H, et al. Reduction of serotonin transporters of patients with chronic fatigue syndrome. *Neuroreport* **15**(17):2571–2574, 2004.
82. Siessmeier T, Nix WA, Hardt J, Schreckenberger M, Egle UT, Bartenstein P. Observer independent analysis of cerebral glucose metabolism in patients with chronic fatigue syndrome. *J Neurol Neurosurg Psychiatry* **74**(7):922–928, 2003.
83. de Lange FP, Koers A, Kalkman JS, et al. Increase in prefrontal cortical volume following cognitive behavioural therapy in patients with chronic fatigue syndrome. *Brain* **131**(Pt 8):2172–2180, 2008.
84. Lövblad KO, Thomas R, Jakob PM, et al. Silent functional magnetic resonance imaging demonstrates focal activation in rapid eye movement sleep. *Neurology* **53**(9):2193–2195, 1999.
85. Buchsbaum MS, Gillin JC, Wu J, et al. Regional cerebral glucose metabolic rate in human sleep assessed by positron emission tomography. *Life Sci* **45**(15):1349–1356, 1989.
86. Maquet P, Péters JM, Aerts J, et al. Functional neuroanatomy of human rapid-eye-movement sleep and dreaming. *Nature* **383**(6596):163–166, 1996.
87. Maquet P, Dive D, Salmon E, et al. Cerebral glucose-utilization during stage-2 sleep in man. *Brain Res* **571**(1):149–153, 1992.
88. Madsen PL, Schmidt JF, Holm S, Vorstrup S, Lassen NA, Wildschiødtz G. Cerebral oxygen metabolism and cerebral blood flow in man during light sleep (stage 2). *Brain Res* **557**(1–2):217–220, 1991.
89. Nofzinger EA, Mintun MA, Wiseman M, Kupfer DJ, Moore RY. Forebrain activation in REM sleep: an FDG PET study. *Brain Res* **770**(1–2):192–201, 1997.
90. Braun AR, Balkin TJ, Wesensten NJ, et al. Dissociated pattern of activity in visual cortices and their projections during human rapid eye movement sleep. *Science* **279**(5347):91–95, 1998.
91. Braun AR, Balkin TJ, Wesenten NJ, et al. Regional cerebral blood flow throughout the sleep-wake cycle: an H2(15)O PET study. *Brain* **120**(Pt 7):1173–1197, 1997.
92. Drummond SP, Brown GG, Salamat JS, Gillin JC. Increasing task difficulty facilitates the cerebral compensatory response to total sleep deprivation. *Sleep* **27**(3):445–451, 2004.
93. Nofzinger EA. What can neuroimaging findings tell us about sleep disorders? *Sleep Med***5**(Suppl 1):S16–S22, 2004.
94. Borsook D, Ploghaus A, Becerra L. Utilizing brain imaging for analgesic drug development. *Curr Opin Investig Drugs* **3**(9):1342–1347, 2002.
95. Schweinhardt P, Bountra C, Tracey I. Pharmacological FMRI in the development of new analgesic compounds. *NMR Biomed* **19**(6):702–711, 2006.
96. Lawrence J, Mackey SC. Role of neuroimaging in analgesic drug development. *Drugs R D* **9**(5):323–334, 2008.
97. Henriksen G, Willoch F. Imaging of opioid receptors in the central nervous system. *Brain* **131**(Pt 5): 1171–1196, 2008.
98. Adler LJ, Gyulai FE, Diehl DJ, Mintun MA, Winter PM, Firestone LL. Regional brain activity changes associated with fentanyl analgesia elucidated by positron emission tomography. *Anesth Analg* **84**(1):120–126, 1997.
99. Wise RG, Rogers R, Painter D, et al. Combining fMRI with a pharmacokinetic model to determine which brain areas activated by painful stimulation are specifically modulated by remifentanil. *Neuroimage* **16**(4):999–1014, 2002.
100. Becerra L, Harter K, Gonzalez RG, Borsook D. Functional magnetic resonance imaging measures of the effects of morphine on central nervous system circuitry in opioid-naive healthy volunteers. *Anesth Analg* **103**(1):208–216, table, 2006.
101. Papageorgiou TD. Blood-oxygen-level-dependent (BOLD) signal changes in total cortex and subcortex, pain, reward, and vigilance regions during mechanical pressure pain after morphine administration. *The University of Texas Health Science Center School of Public Health*, 2006.
102. Sprenger T, Valet M, Boecker H, et al. Opioidergic activation in the medial pain system after heat pain. *Pain* **122**(1–2):63–67, 2006.
103. Wagner KJ, Sprenger T, Kochs EF, Tölle TR, Valet M, Willoch F. Imaging human cerebral pain modulation by dose-dependent opioid analgesia: a positron emission tomography activation study using remifentanil. *Anesthesiology* **106**(3):548–556, 2007.

104. Firestone LL, Gyulai F, Mintun M, Adler LJ, Urso K, Winter PM. Human brain activity response to fentanyl imaged by positron emission tomography. *Anesth Analg* **82**(6):1247–1251, 1996.

105. Wagner KJ, Willoch F, Kochs EF, et al. Dose-dependent regional cerebral blood flow changes during remifentanil infusion in humans: a positron emission tomography study. *Anesthesiology* **94**(5): 732–739, 2001.

106. Iannetti GD, Zambreanu L, Wise RG, et al. Pharmacological modulation of pain-related brain activity during normal and central sensitization states in humans. *Proc Natl Acad Sci U S A* **102**(50): 18195–18200, 2005.

107. Leppä M, Korvenoja A, Carlson S, et al. Acute opioid effects on human brain as revealed by functional magnetic resonance imaging. *Neuroimage* **31**(2): 661–669, 2006.

108. Mesulam MM. From sensation to cognition. *Brain* **121**(Pt 6):1013–1052, 1998.

109. Harrison NA, Brydon L, Walker C, et al. Neural origins of human sickness in interoceptive responses to inflammation. *Biol Psychiatry* **66**(5):415–422, 2009.

110. Rosa MJ, Kilner J, Blankenburg F, Josephs O, Penny W. Estimating the transfer function from neuronal activity to BOLD using simultaneous EEG-fMRI. *Neuroimage* **49**(2):1496–1509, 2010.

111. Muzik O, Chugani DC, Zou G, et al. Multimodality data integration in epilepsy. *Int J Biomed Imaging* 2007:13963, 2007.

112. Iannetti GD, Niazy RK, Wise RG, et al. Simultaneous recording of laser-evoked brain potentials and continuous, high-field functional magnetic resonance imaging in humans. *Neuroimage* **28**(3):708–719, 2005.

113. deCharms RC, Christoff K, Glover GH, Pauly JM, Whitfield S, Gabrieli JD. Learned regulation of spatially localized brain activation using real-time fMRI. *Neuroimage* **21**(1):436–443, 2004.

114. deCharms RC, Maeda F, Glover GH, et al. Control over brain activation and pain learned by using real-time functional MRI. *Proc Natl Acad Sci U S A* **102**(51):18626–18631, 2005.

115. Posse S, Fitzgerald D, Gao K, et al. Real-time fMRI of temporolimbic regions detects amygdala activation during single-trial self-induced sadness. *Neuroimage* **18**(3):760–768, 2003.

116. Weiskopf N, Veit R, Erb M, et al. Physiological self-regulation of regional brain activity using real-time functional magnetic resonance imaging (fMRI): methodology and exemplary data. *Neuroimage* **19**(3):577–586, 2003.

117. Yoo SS, Jolesz FA. Functional MRI for neurofeedback: feasibility study on a hand motor task. *Neuroreport* **13**(11):1377–1381, 2002.

118. LaConte S, Strother S, Cherkassky V, Anderson J, Hu X. Support vector machines for temporal classification of block design fMRI data. *Neuroimage* **26**(2):317–329, 2005.

119. LaConte SM, Peltier SJ, Hu XP. Real-time fMRI using brain-state classification. *Hum Brain Mapp* **28**(10):1033–1044, 2007.

120. Papageorgiou T, Curtis WA, McHenry M, LaConte SM. Neurofeedback of two motor functions using supervised learning-based real-time functional magnetic resonance imaging. *Conf Proc IEEE Eng Med Biol Soc* **1**:5377–5380, 2009.

121. Papageorgiou TD, McHenry M, Lisinski JM, White JP, LaConte SM. Speech rate control using supervised learning-based real-time fMRI. *Neuroimage* **47**(1):S39–S41, 2009.

Section 2 Chapter 19

Cancer Symptom Mechanisms and Models: Clinical and Basic Science

High-dose therapy and posttransplantation symptom burden: striking a balance

Sergio A. Giralt and Loretta A. Williams

High-dose therapy (chemotherapy with or without radiotherapy) followed either by autologous or allogeneic hematopoietic stem cell transplantation (HSCT) has improved overall survival and disease-free survival for patients with various malignant and nonmalignant hematological disorders.[1] However, this therapeutic benefit has come at the expense of significant morbidity and occasional mortality.

Research focused on the first 3–4 weeks after the administration of high-dose therapy and HSCT (the acute phase) shows that most patients report multiple physical, affective, and cognitive symptoms.[2–7] Commonly reported physical symptoms during the acute phase include nausea, vomiting, diarrhea, decreased appetite, dry mouth, insomnia, weakness, and fatigue.[2,4,6,7] Cognitive symptoms, such as delirium, decreased concentration, and memory problems, also are common during the acute phase of transplantation.[5,8] Numerous studies have found that patients may continue to experience distressing symptoms, such as fatigue, pain, sleep disturbance, cognitive dysfunction, eye problems, dry mouth, taste changes, cough, shortness of breath, depression, anxiety, and sexual dysfunction, months or years after transplantation.[9–11]

In this chapter we examine the spectrum of symptoms produced by high-dose therapy combined with HSCT, the mechanisms underlying symptom development, and potential intervention strategies that can be used to ameliorate this symptom burden. Although HSCT can overcome the hematopoietic toxicities of cytoreductive therapies and allow patients to receive higher doses, other toxicities of high-dose therapy and HSCT may place a significant burden on patients. HSCT presents a challenge for health care providers and patients to find a balance between potentially curative therapy and the symptom burden caused by the therapy. Recognizing the symptom burden experienced by patients and identifying mechanisms responsible for these symptoms allows clinicians to more effectively decrease the burden of therapy and to offer this therapy in a safer manner to more patients.

Basic concepts of hematopoietic stem cell transplantation

Human HSCT was initially explored in the late 1950s and early 1960s in patients with terminal leukemia or severe bone marrow failure resulting from radiation exposure, disease, or both. Almost all of these patients died from complications related to their primary disease, graft failure, graft-versus-host disease (GVHD), or infections.[12,13] In 1968, the first successful allogeneic HSCT, in which a donor supplied the bone marrow stem cells, was performed in a patient with severe combined immunodeficiency.[14] In the 1970s Dr. E. Donnall Thomas and colleagues at the Fred Hutchinson Cancer Research Center in Seattle, Washington, reported the curative potential of this approach in patients with refractory leukemia. Since then, allogeneic HSCT has been used to treat thousands of patients with previously incurable diseases.[15]

In the early days of HSCT, it was thought that the curative effect of allogeneic transplantation was mediated primarily by the high doses of therapy administered to patients rather than by the transplanted cells. It was believed that the donor cells simply facilitated hematopoietic recovery within an acceptable period of time.[16] This concept of dose-intensity-as-cure led to the development of autologous HSCT, a treatment modality in which patients serve as their own stem cell donors after cytoreductive therapy. Autologous HSCT overcomes the hematopoietic toxicities of chemotherapy and radiation therapy, allowing patients to receive higher doses. It is now apparent, however, that the success of allogeneic HSCT relies on a powerful donor immune response against the host malignancy, a phenomenon known as graft-versus-tumor effect. This effect explains why the relapse rate is

Cancer Symptom Science: Measurement, Mechanisms, and Management, eds. Charles S. Cleeland, Michael J. Fisch, and Adrian J. Dunn.

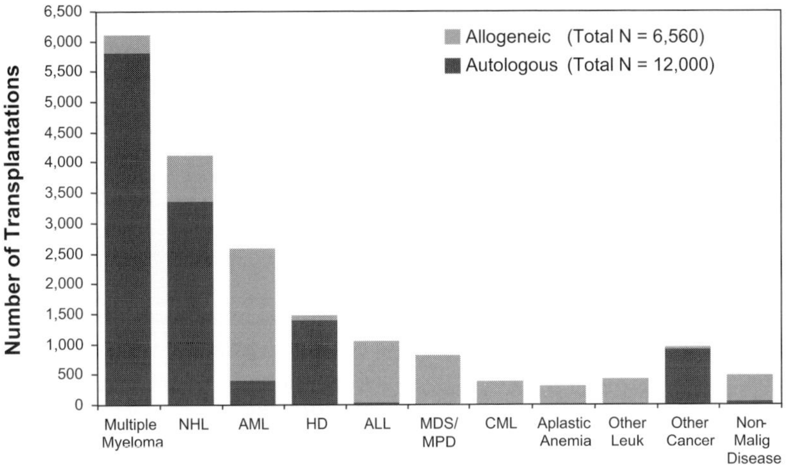

Figure 19.1. Indications for hematopoietic stem cell transplantation in North America, 2006 (HSCT). The most common indications for HSCT in North America in 2006 were multiple myeloma and lymphoma, accounting for 63% of all HSCTs. Multiple myeloma was the most common indication for autotransplantation and acute myeloid leukemia was the most common indication for allogeneic transplantation. Adapted from: Pasquini MC, Wang Z. Current uses and outcomes of hematopoietic stem cell transplantation: Part I – CIBMTR Summary Slides, 2009. *CIBMTR Newsletter [serial online]* 15(1):7–11, 2009.

usually significantly smaller after an allograft than after an autograft using the same conditioning regimen, because no graft-versus-tumor effect is operative in autologous HSCT.[15,17,18]

Notwithstanding, the effect of dose intensity on various hematopoietic and solid tumors has been demonstrated both *in vivo* and *in vitro*, and high-dose therapy supported by autologous HSCT has been shown to change the natural course of disease in diverse malignant and nonmalignant disorders. Autologous HSCT remains the most common form of transplantation performed in North America (Figure 19.1) and worldwide.[15]

The primary components of HSCT (Figure 19.2) include:

- Recipient
- Donor (in the autograft setting, the recipient and donor are the same)
- Preparative regimen
- Stem cell infusion
- GVHD prophylaxis in the allograft setting (including post-HSCT immunosuppression)
- Post-HSCT supportive care.

These components play a role not only in survival and disease outcomes, but also in the morbidity associated with HSCT, including post-HSCT symptom burden. Symptom burden during HSCT can be assessed using the M. D. Anderson Symptom Inventory (MDASI)[19] or other validated multisymptom measures.

Transplantation-related toxicities and symptoms

High-dose chemotherapy and radiotherapy are associated with extensive damage to normal tissues that undergo constant cell division and cell reproduction. Thus, the hematological and gastrointestinal (GI) systems are severely affected after high-dose therapy regimens. Pancytopenia and some degree of GI symptoms, which include sore mouth, sore throat, nausea, vomiting, and diarrhea, are seen in all recipients of high-dose therapy. However, despite the fact that all patients suffer similar degrees of pancytopenia, not all of them exhibit the same degree of GI symptom severity.

Severity and patterns of posttransplantation symptoms

Anderson et al.[2] conducted a prospective study of 90 patients with multiple myeloma or non-Hodgkin's lymphoma who were undergoing autologous HSCT. The most common symptoms reported at moderate to severe levels were lack of appetite, fatigue, and disturbed sleep (Figure 19.3). The intensity of symptoms was greatest at the time of white blood cell (WBC) nadir, and a significant proportion of patients continued to experience moderate to severe symptoms 30 days post-HSCT.[2,20] Campagnaro et al.[21] looked at only multiple myeloma patients undergoing autologous HSCT and found comparable results (Figure 19.4). For these patients, the most severe symptoms were fatigue, weakness, and lack of appetite.

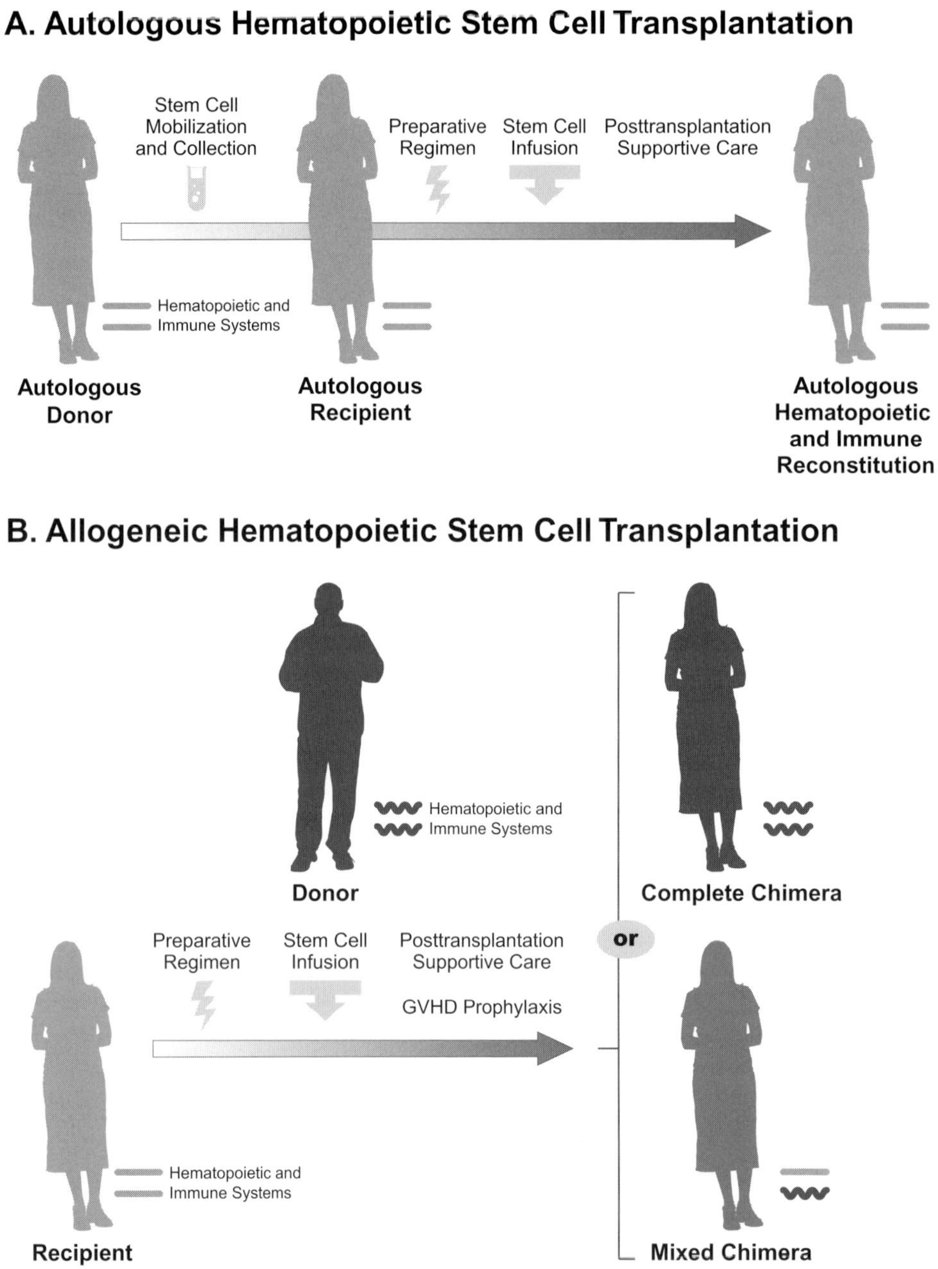

Figure 19.2. Components of hematopoietic stem cell transplantation GVHD indicates graft-versus-host disease.

Wang et al.[22] observed a similar constellation of symptoms in 30 patients undergoing allogeneic HSCT (Figure 19.5). The most severe symptoms experienced by these patients, including fatigue, drowsiness, and pain, occurred during WBC nadir. Twenty-six of the 30 patients developed GVHD post-HSCT. As shown in Figure 19.6, symptom severity dropped shortly after diagnosis of GVHD (Day 0), likely in response to treatment with corticosteriods, but some symptoms plateaued or even intensified thereafter.[23]

Several studies of patients undergoing autologous or allogeneic HSCT examined patients' neuropsycho-

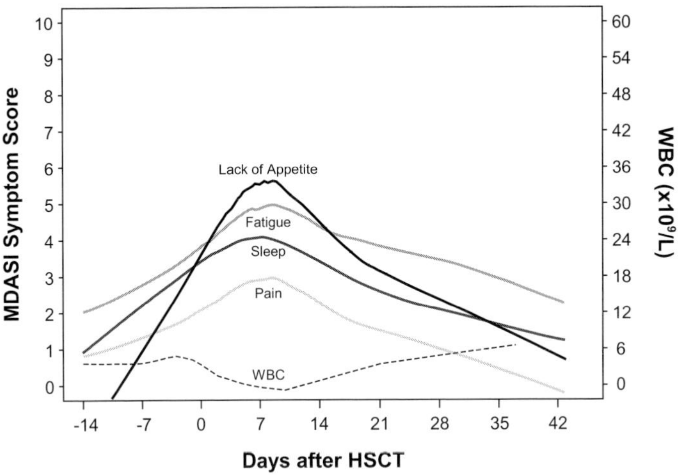

Figure 19.3. Symptom burden and white blood count of patients undergoing autologous transplantation for multiple myeloma or non-hodgkin's lymphoma. HSCT indicates hematopoietic stem cell transplantation; MDASI, M. D. Anderson Symptom Inventory; WBC, white blood cell count. *Source:* Adapted from: Anderson KO, Giralt SA, Neumann JL, et al. Symptom assessment following autologous transplantation: relation of symptom severity to laboratory measures [abstract]. American Society of Hematology 45th Annual Meeting and Exposition, San Diego CA, 12/2003. *Blood* 102(11):987A, 2003. Abstract 3672.

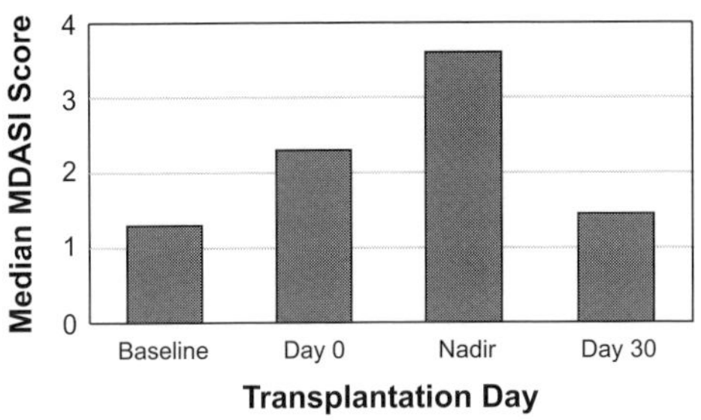

Figure 19.4. Symptom burden of patients undergoing autologous hematopoietic stem cell transplantation for multiple myeloma. MDASI indicates M. D. Anderson Symptom Inventory. Adapted from: Symptom burden after autologous stem cell transplantation for multiple myeloma.
Source: Campagnaro E, Saliba R, Giralt S, et al. *CANCER* 112(7). Copyright © 2008 American Cancer Society, Inc. Reprinted with permission of Wiley-Liss, Inc.

logical function before and during the acute phase of HSCT.[8,24,25] Results are contradictory as to whether a history of cranial radiation or central nervous system disease treated with intrathecal chemotherapy is associated with impaired neurocognitive functioning prior to HSCT.[8,24] Cognitive functioning, particularly memory, worsens over time after HSCT, but whether this deficit occurs within weeks or months is unclear.[8,25] Recently, the difference between objectively measured cognitive performance and patient-reported cognitive complaints has also been explored. Although cognitive complaints are correlated with other symptoms, such as fatigue, depression, anxiety, and poorer well-being, they are not significantly correlated with cognitive performance except for the patient's perception of other people noticing deficits.[26,27] Dyspnea and nausea have been correlated with impaired memory and attention both before and 3 months after allogeneic HSCT.[27]

Mechanisms of posttransplantation symptoms: the inflammatory cytokine theory

Recent research has focused on the biological mechanisms underlying the development of post-HSCT symptoms, in the belief that targeting the mechanisms that induce these symptoms could significantly improve HSCT-related morbidity and tolerance. Evidence from studies of both humans and animals suggests that inflammatory cytokines may significantly contribute to the development of symptoms.[28–33]

The role of inflammatory cytokines in the development of HSCT-related toxicities was initially explored within the context of allografting and the occurrence of acute GVHD.[34] Acute GVHD encompasses all of the reactions mediated by the donor immune system against host tissues. Acute GVHD may be initiated by tissue destruction in response to the preparative regimen or infection.[35] Tissue destruction results in the production of antigens, which are peptide macromolecules that elicit an immune response. Antigens are processed and presented by antigen-presenting cells, which display foreign antigens joined with the major histocompatibility complex (human lymphocyte antigen, or HLA) on their surfaces. T-cell activation occurs as long as the peptide–HLA complex is recognized by specific T cells with appropriate costimulatory molecules within a favorable cytokine environment. Activated T cells undergo clonal proliferation and mediate

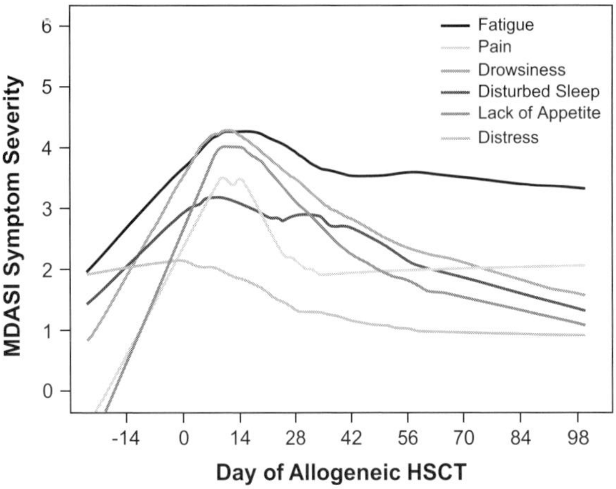

Figure 19.5. Symptom burden of patients undergoing allogeneic hematopoietic stem cell transplantation for acute myeloid leukemia or high-risk myelodysplasia. HSCT indicates hematopoietic stem cell transplantation; MDASI, M. D. Anderson Symptom Inventory.
Source: Adapted from: Wang XS, Cleeland CS, Williams LA, et al. Longitudinal assessment of inflammatory cytokines and symptom severity during 100 days of allogeneic BMT for AML/MDS patients [abstract]. American Society of Hematology 47th Annual Meeting, Atlanta GA. *Blood* 106(11):221B, 2005. Abstract 4569.

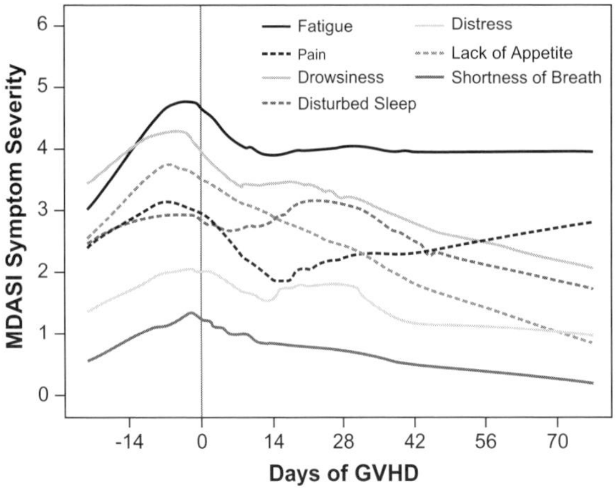

Figure 19.6. Symptom burden related to graft-versus-host disease in patients undergoing allogeneic hematopoietic stem cell transplantation for acute myeloid leukemia or high-risk myelodysplasia. GVHD indicates graft-versus-host disease; MDASI, M. D. Anderson Symptom Inventory.
Source: Adapted from: Giralt S, Cleeland CS, Reuben J, et al. Measuring multiple symptoms and inflammatory cytokines related to acute GVHD in AML/MDS patients under allogeneic BMT [abstract]. American Society of Hematology 47th Annual Meeting, Atlanta GA. *Blood* 106(11):412A, 2005.

further tissue destruction by inducing apoptosis or further inflammatory damage.

Although not fully understood, an important role for inflammatory cytokines in allogeneic transplantation outcomes is suggested by the results of clinical and laboratory research.[35] Evidence includes:

- Animal models showing that inhibition of tumor necrosis factor (TNF), a proinflammatory cytokine, abrogates GVHD[36];
- Correlation between TNF levels and transplant-related complications[37,37–39];
- Effects of the preparative regimen on TNF levels, and correlation between TNF levels and transplantation outcomes in animal models[37]; and
- Efficacy of anti-TNF agents and anti-interleukin (IL)-2 agents in treating and preventing GVHD.[40–44]

In the autograft setting, symptom burden has been correlated with laboratory values, specifically WBC count,[2] as well as cytokine measurements.[20] As demonstrated in Figure 19.3, the highest levels of symptom burden were associated with WBC nadir in autologous HSCT. In a later study, the same relationship between WBC count and symptom severity was found to occur in allogeneic HSCT (Figure 19.7).[7]

Studies attempting to correlate serum or tissue cytokine levels with GVHD or other autologous, or allogeneic HSCT-related outcomes have produced inconsistent results.[23,37,38,45–50] These inconsistencies may be due to the heterogeneity of the assays used, the short half-life of the cytokines studied, or the possibility that serum levels may be inappropriate measures of the cytokine milieu at the target tissue level.[23,37,38,45,46,49,50]

Nonetheless, in both the autologous and allogeneic HSCT settings strong correlations can be found between symptom burden and levels of various inflammatory cytokines, particularly IL-6 (Figures 19.7 and 19.8). These relationships provide a rationale for a link between laboratory abnormalities, inflammatory cytokines, and post-HSCT symptom burden, and have the potential to provide future targets for intervention. Accordingly, targeting inflammatory cytokines and their pathways may be a rational therapeutic approach for reducing post-HSCT symptom burden.

Risk factors for developing moderate to severe posttransplantation symptoms

Although the doses and types of agents administered to patients undergoing high-dose therapy are the most important contributors to the range and severity of post-HSCT toxicities and symptoms, the same

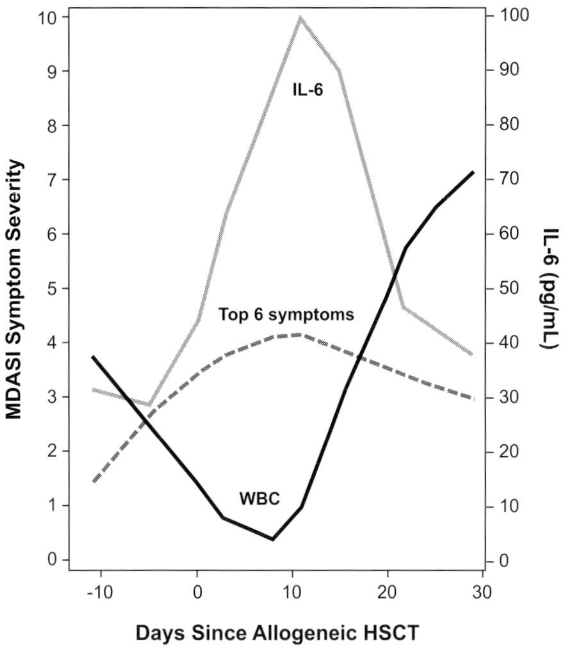

Figure 19.7. Relationship of symptom burden to white blood cell counts and interleukin-6 levels during allogeneic hematopoietic stem cell transplantation. Lowess curves depict the estimated severity levels of multiple symptoms and white blood cell count (WBC) during 30 days of allogeneic hematopoietic stem cell transplantation. The dotted line represents the mean of the six most severe symptoms reported by this patient group (pain, fatigue, disturbed sleep, dry mouth, lack of appetite, and drowsiness). HSCT indicates hematopoietic stem cell transplantation; MDASI, M. D. Anderson Symptom Inventory; IL-6, interleukin-6.
Source: Adapted from: Serum interleukin-6 predicts the development of multiple symptoms at nadir of allogeneic hematopoietic stem cell transplantation. Wang XS, Shi Q, Williams LA, et al. *CANCER* 113(8). Copyright © 2008 American Cancer Society, Inc. Reprinted with permission of Wiley-Liss, Inc.

conditioning regimen can elicit a remarkable degree of variation in symptom burden from one patient to the next. Defining the subset of patients who have the greatest risk for developing moderate to severe post-HSCT symptoms would allow targeted strategies to be developed to reduce the frequency and severity of symptoms for the most-severely affected patients.

Regimen-related factors

In recent years, reduced-intensity conditioning (RIC) regimens have been used with allogeneic HSCT to decrease toxicity and to allow more patients to take advantage of the treatment. It has been suggested that the best candidates for this approach are older patients and patients with several comorbid conditions and low disease burden.[51,52] RIC regimens have been shown to decrease clinician-assessed organ toxicity and regimen-related mortality.[53] It has been suggested that because RIC regimens cause less tissue damage, they may lead to lower levels of proinflammatory cytokines than conventional conditioning regimens during the first weeks or months after allogeneic HSCT.[54] This hypothesis is supported by the finding of lower C-reactive protein levels during the neutropenic phase in patients receiving RIC regimens compared with patients receiving conventional regimens.[48] Less organ toxicity and decreased proinflammatory cytokine levels suggest that RIC regimens may also produce less symptom burden.

Few studies have directly compared RIC regimens to conventional HSCT regimens or measured patient-reported symptom burden. One study compared health-related quality of life in patients receiving a RIC regimen and allogeneic HSCT with patients receiving high-dose chemotherapy and autologous HSCT.[55] At days 7 and 28 after HSCT, the patients receiving the RIC regimen had significantly lower physical symptom severity than the patients receiving the high-dose regimens with autologous HSCT. The RIC-regimen patients experienced milder symptoms overall during the first year than the autologous HSCT patients, but this difference was primarily due to lower symptom severity during the first six months post-HSCT. After six months, the overall symptom severity for the autologous HSCT patients declined, whereas the symptom severity for the RIC-regimen patients increased. In a study that compared the health-related quality of life of patients receiving RIC regimens and patients receiving conventional conditioning regimens for allogeneic HSCT, Bevans et al.[56] found no difference in physical functioning at several time points before and during the first year post-HSCT. However, this study did not assess patients during the first 30 days after HSCT, when symptom burden is highest.

Wang et al.,[7] in their study of multiple symptoms after allogeneic HSCT, did not find a difference in symptom burden between the 13 patients who received a RIC regimen versus the 17 patients who received a conventional regimen during the first 30 days post-HSCT. However, the patients who received the RIC regimen in this study were selected for this therapy because they were not good candidates for a conventional regimen. Bevans et al.[3] reported that patients scheduled to receive a conventional myeloablative conditioning regimen were more likely to report low symptom

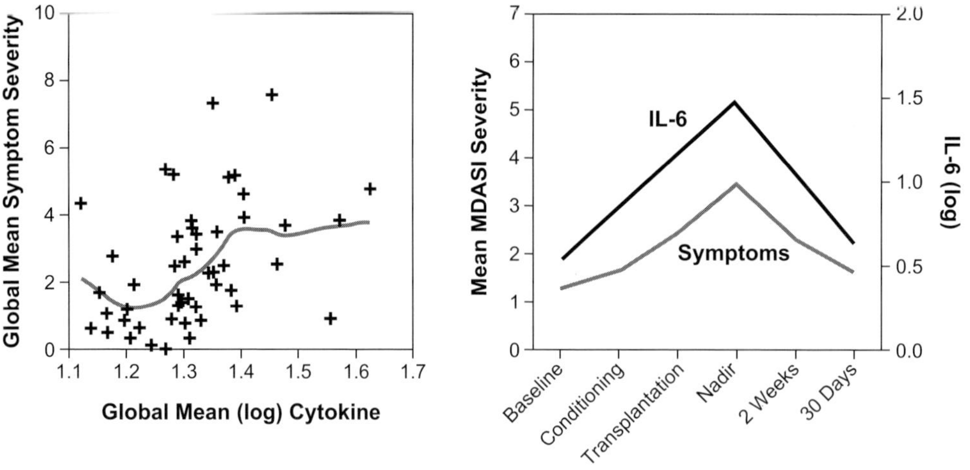

Figure 19.8. Relationship of interleukin-6 levels to symptom burden after autologous transplantation. Left panel: Lowess curve; right panel: linear curve. MDASI indicates M. D. Anderson Symptom Inventory; IL-6, interleukin-6.
Source: Adapted from: Wang XS, Giralt S, Mendoza TR, et al. Longitudinal assessment of inflammatory cytokines: symptom severity during autologous BMT [abstract]. American Society of Hematology 45th Annual Meeting and Exposition, San Diego CA. *Blood* 102(11):488B, 2003. Abstract 5681.

distress before the start of HSCT therapy; patients scheduled for a RIC regimen were more likely to report moderate or severe symptom distress at the same time. The symptom severity experienced during HSCT therapy by patients receiving a RIC regimen may be more disease-related, whereas the symptom severity reported by patients receiving a conventional regimen may be more regimen-related. Further research to define the effect of RIC regimens on symptom burden is needed.

Patient-related factors

Campagnaro et al.[21] reported on 64 patients with multiple myeloma who were undergoing autologous HSCT. Symptom burden at baseline was predictive of symptom burden at nadir ($P = 0.02$). Age, disease status, and comorbidities did not significantly influence post-HSCT symptom burden, and symptom burden during HSCT did not affect survival at up to 3 years post-HSCT. Individual symptoms clustered into four groups over the first 30 days after HSCT: symptoms that most patients reported as less severe 30 days post-HSCT than at baseline; symptoms that most patients reported as more severe 30 days post-HSCT than at baseline; symptoms that some patients reported as worsening while other patients reported as improving over the 30 days; and symptoms that were rarely reported during HSCT. Symptoms that were primarily effects of high-dose therapy, such as upper-GI toxicities, worsened over the 30 days post-HSCT, whereas affective symptoms, such as distress and sadness, decreased over the same time period.

Numerous non-HLA-encoded genetic single nucleotide polymorphisms (SNPs) that regulate myriad immune-mediated and nonimmune-mediated biological processes have been found to influence HSCT outcomes.[57] Among the most studied of these genetic polymorphisms are those associated with the inflammatory cytokines and their receptors.[57–65] Polymorphisms within the regulatory sequences of a cytokine gene may alter the amount of cytokine produced, the degree of receptor expression, the metabolism of drugs, or the response to infection.[65,65] The most important evidence for a role for cytokine gene polymorphisms in the setting of allogeneic HSCT is summarized in Table 19.1. How these polymorphisms affect symptom burden has not been well characterized, but they may explain some of the variability in post-HSCT symptom burden seen among patients who received the same conditioning regimen.

Reducing posttransplantation symptom burden

Current strategies

White blood cell recovery

A reduction in symptom burden is closely associated with hematological recovery and WBC count after

Table 19.1. Most common cytokine gene polymorphisms studied in the setting of allogeneic transplantation

Cytokine gene polymorphism	Proposed mechanism	Effect on transplantation outcomes
IL-6–174	Increased IL-6 production	Increase in acute and chronic GVHD
IFN-γ	Lower *in vitro* IFN-γ production	Increase in acute GVHD
IL-1α-889		Improved survival after unrelated donor transplant
IL-2-330 G/T	Upregulated TNF-α production	Increase in acute GVHD Severe toxic complications
IL-10–1064 (12–15)	Decreased IL-10 production	Increase in acute GVHD
IL-1RA VNTR	Downregulated IL-1	Increase in chronic GVHD

IL indicates interleukin; GVHD, graft-versus-host disease; IFN, interferon; TNF, tumor necrosis factor; IL-1RA VNTR, interleukin-1 receptor antagonist variable number of tandem repeats.

both autologous and allogeneic HSCT.[2,66] However, during allogeneic HSCT some individual symptoms, such as fatigue and weakness, persist after neutrophil recovery.[66] Strategies to enhance neutrophil recovery after autologous HSCT, such as hematopoietic growth factors and filgrastim-mobilized peripheral blood stem cells, have resulted in significant decreases in morbidity, cost, and health-resource utilization.[67,68] While it can be hypothesized that strategies to reduce the duration of neutropenia will significantly decrease symptom burden post-HSCT, this hypothesis has not been tested.

Antiemetics

Moderate to severe chemotherapy-induced nausea and vomiting can interfere significantly with patient functioning and can exacerbate other symptoms. Studies have shown that the introduction of 5-HT$_3$-receptor antagonists (ondansetron, granisetron, and tropisetron) combined with dexamethasone to control nausea improved complete response rates to some degree. In these studies, between 15% and 50% of patients had complete responses, which varied with the conditioning therapy administered, type of disease treated, and 5-HT$_3$-receptor antagonist used; however, the complete response rates for moderate to severe nausea consistently fell below the complete response rates for vomiting. Moderate to severe nausea continues to be problematic for patients and a major component of moderate to severe post-HSCT symptom burden.[69]

Treatments for oral mucositis

Mucosal damage causing mucositis, stomatitis, and diarrhea is an important source of post-HSCT symptom burden. Oral and esophageal mucositis during HSCT often becomes severe enough to require intravenous opioid analgesia. They can interfere with swallowing, which may lead to dehydration and weight loss, extend hospitalization, and require parenteral nutrition.[70]

Spielberger et al.[71] reported the results of a phase III randomized trial using recombinant keratinocyte growth factor (palifermin) before and after high-dose chemoradiotherapy as a method to reduce the incidence and severity of oral mucositis after autologous HSCT. The incidence and duration of grade 3 or 4 oral mucositis[72] was significantly less in the palifermin group than in the control group. Palifermin was associated with significant reductions in the incidence of grade 4 oral mucositis, patient-reported soreness of the mouth and throat, and the use of opioid analgesics. The palifermin recipients also reported better physical and functional well-being, as measured by the general Functional Assessment of Cancer Therapy, than did the control group patients.[71] An additional analysis showed that the cost of palifermin was balanced by a decrease in adverse outcomes and associated hospital expenses. Patients receiving palifermin had lower hospital costs (but not significantly so).[73] Additional small studies have confirmed the effectiveness of palifermin in decreasing oral mucositis in patients receiving melphalan prior to autologous HSCT.[74,75]

Several trials have reported a decrease in the incidence, severity, and duration of oral mucositis in patients undergoing allogeneic HSCT. [76–78] There has been some concern that palifermin might reduce graft-versus-tumor effects, but a small, double-blind, placebo-controlled trial showed no difference in engraftment, acute GVHD, or survival between palifermin recipients and patients receiving a placebo.[76] Further research is needed on the safety of palifermin in the allogeneic HSCT setting.

Oral cryotherapy (ice chips) has also been shown to significantly reduce the severity of oral mucositis, the need for opioid pain medication, and the use of intravenous nutrition after administration of high-dose melphalan.[79,80] None of these studies related the decrease in oral mucositis to overall symptom burden. In a multicenter study, cryotherapy was not found to be effective in decreasing the incidence, severity, or duration of mucositis caused by methotrexate for acute GVHD prophylaxis.[81]

Low-level laser therapy (LLLT) was shown in two small, randomized trials to decrease the severity of oral mucositis and mouth pain in patients undergoing either autologous or allogeneic HSCT.[82,83] The effect of reducing oral mucositis on total symptom burden was not measured in these trials. LLLT requires specialized equipment and personnel trained in administration. The optimum dose and schedule for the administration of LLLT in HSCT has not been determined.

Exercise

Several randomized, controlled trials have been conducted to look at the effect of exercise on physical functioning and symptoms post-HSCT. A program of exercise, relaxation, and psychoeducation improved physical performance after allogeneic HSCT[84] while decreasing the intensity of clusters of mucositis and gastrointestinal, cognitive, and functional symptoms.[85] Affective symptoms did not change with the intervention. Aerobic exercise, either biking or walking, during or after autologous HSCT has been found to increase physical performance and decrease the severity of diarrhea and pain.[86–88] During hospitalization for autologous HSCT, aerobic exercise stabilized patients' pretreatment levels of fatigue, whereas patients who did not exercise experienced an increase in fatigue.[87] After hospitalization for autologous HSCT, aerobic training decreased fatigue.[88]

Future directions

Notwithstanding these accomplishments in reducing post-HSCT symptom burden, moderate to severe symptoms that significantly interfere with patients' well-being remain extremely prevalent even after high-dose therapy regimens. Thus, more effective strategies aimed at targeting common pathways, or underlying mechanisms, of symptom development should be a foremost goal of future studies. As described in this chapter, one possible common pathway is proinflammatory cytokines.[29] Strong correlations between symptom burden and levels of proinflammatory cytokines observed in both autologous and allogeneic transplantation settings provide a rationale for a link between laboratory abnormalities, proinflammatory cytokines, and post-HSCT symptom burden. Targeting proinflammatory cytokines and their molecular pathways may be a rational therapeutic approach for reducing post-HSCT symptom burden. The effects of this approach on overall HSCT outcomes also requires exploration.

Conclusion

With the increasing use of high-dose therapy and HSCT as a curative strategy for various hematological malignancies, improving the tolerability of this therapy has become a critical area of research and investigation. Defining the biological underpinnings of why some patients have greater post-HSCT symptom burden than others will allow us to develop targeted interventions for all patients and risk-tailored therapies for at-risk patients. The ultimate goal is to provide the most effective therapy with minimum treatment burden.

References

1. Eapen M, Rocha V. Principles and analysis of hematopoietic stem cell transplantation outcomes: the physician's perspective. *Lifetime Data Anal* **14**(4):379–388, 2008.
2. Anderson KO, Giralt SA, Neumann JL, et al. Symptom assessment following autologous transplantation: relation of symptom severity to laboratory measures [abstract]. American Society of Hematology 45th Annual Meeting and Exposition, San Diego CA, 12/2003. *Blood* **102**(11):987A, 2003. Abstract 3672.
3. Bevans MF, Mitchell SA, Marden S. The symptom experience in the first 100 days following allogeneic hematopoietic stem cell transplantation (HSCT). *Support Care Cancer* **16**(11):1243–1254, 2008.
4. Danaher EH, Ferrans C, Verlen E, et al. Fatigue and physical activity in patients undergoing hematopoietic stem cell transplant. *Oncol Nurs Forum* **33**(3):614–624, 2006.
5. Fann JR, Alfano CM, Burington BE, Roth-Roemer S, Katon WJ, Syrjala KL. Clinical presentation of

delirium in patients undergoing hematopoietic stem cell transplantation. *Cancer* **103**(4):810–820, 2005.

6. Larsen J, Nordström G, Ljungman P, Gardulf A. Symptom occurrence, symptom intensity, and symptom distress in patients undergoing high-dose chemotherapy with stem-cell transplantation. *Cancer Nurs* **27**(1):55–64, 2004.
7. Wang XS, Shi Q, Williams LA, et al. Serum interleukin-6 predicts the development of multiple symptoms at nadir of allogeneic hematopoietic stem cell transplantation. *Cancer* **113**(8):2102–2109, 2008.
8. Ahles TA, Tope DM, Furstenberg C, Hann D, Mills L. Psychologic and neuropsychologic impact of autologous bone marrow transplantation. *J Clin Oncol* **14**(5):1457–1462, 1996.
9. Andrykowski MA, Bishop MM, Hahn EA, et al. Long-term health-related quality of life, growth, and spiritual well-being after hematopoietic stem-cell transplantation. *J Clin Oncol* **23**(3):599–608, 2005.
10. Edman L, Larsen J, Hägglund H, Gardulf A. Health-related quality of life, symptom distress and sense of coherence in adult survivors of allogeneic stem-cell transplantation. *Eur J Cancer Care (Engl)* **10**(2):124–130, 2001.
11. Kopp M, Holzner B, Meraner V, et al. Quality of life in adult hematopoietic cell transplant patients at least 5 yr after treatment: a comparison with healthy controls. *Eur J Haematol* **74**(4):304–308, 2005.
12. Thomas ED, Storb R, Clift RA, et al. Bone-marrow transplantation (second of two parts). *N Engl J Med* **292**(17):895–902, 1975.
13. Bortin MM. A compendium of reported human bone marrow transplants. *Transplantation* **9**(6):571–587, 1970.
14. Gatti RA, Meuwissen HJ, Allen HD, Hong R, Good RA. Immunological reconstitution of sex-linked lymphopenic immunological deficiency. *Lancet* **2**(7583):1366–1369, 1968.
15. Pasquini MC, Wang Z. Current uses and outcomes of hematopoietic stem cell transplantation: Part I – CIBMTR Summary Slides, 2009. *CIBMTR Newsletter* [serial online] **15**(1):7–11, 2009.
16. Fefer A, Buckner CD, Thomas ED, et al. Cure of hematologic neoplasia with transplantation of marrow from identical twins. *N Engl J Med* **297**(3):146–148, 1977.
17. Horowitz MM, Gale RP, Sondel PM, et al. Graft-versus-leukemia reactions after bone marrow transplantation. *Blood* **75**(3):555–562, 1990.
18. Weiden PL, Flournoy N, Thomas ED, et al. Antileukemic effect of graft-versus-host disease in human recipients of allogeneic-marrow grafts. *N Engl J Med* **300**(19):1068–1073, 1979.
19. Cleeland CS, Mendoza TR, Wang XS, et al. Assessing symptom distress in cancer patients: the M. D. Anderson Symptom Inventory. *Cancer* **89**(7):1634–1646, 2000.
20. Wang XS, Giralt S, Mendoza TR, et al. Longitudinal assessment of inflammatory cytokines: symptom severity during autologous BMT [abstract]. American Society of Hematology 45th Annual Meeting and Exposition, San Diego CA. *Blood* **102**(11):488B, 2003. Abstract 5681.
21. Campagnaro E, Saliba R, Giralt S, et al. Symptom burden after autologous stem cell transplantation for multiple myeloma. *Cancer* **112**(7):1617–1624, 2008.
22. Wang XS, Cleeland CS, Williams LA, et al. Longitudinal assessment of inflammatory cytokines and symptom severity during 100 days of allogeneic BMT for AML/MDS patients [abstract]. American Society of Hematology 47th Annual Meeting, Atlanta GA. *Blood* **106**(11):221B, 2005. Abstract 4569.
23. Giralt S, Cleeland CS, Reuben J, et al. Measuring multiple symptoms and inflammatory cytokines related to acute GVHD in AML/MDS patients under allogeneic BMT [abstract]. American Society of Hematology 47th Annual Meeting, Atlanta GA. *Blood* **106**(11):412A, 2005.
24. Andrykowski MA, Schmitt FA, Gregg ME, Brady MJ, Lamb DG, Henslee-Downey PJ. Neuropsychologic impairment in adult bone marrow transplant candidates. *Cancer* **70**(9):2288–2297, 1992.
25. Meyers CA, Weitzner M, Byrne K, Valentine A, Champlin RE, Przepiorka D. Evaluation of the neurobehavioral functioning of patients before, during, and after bone marrow transplantation. *J Clin Oncol* **12**(4):820–826, 1994.
26. Jacobs SR, Jacobsen PB, Booth-Jones M, Wagner LI, Anasetti C. Evaluation of the functional assessment of cancer therapy cognitive scale with hematopoietic stem cell transplant patients. *J Pain Symptom Manage* **33**(1):13–23, 2007.
27. Schulz-Kindermann F, Mehnert A, Scherwath A, et al. Cognitive function in the acute course of allogeneic hematopoietic stem cell transplantation for hematological malignancies. *Bone Marrow Transplant* **39**(12):789–799, 2007.
28. Cleeland CS, Bennett GJ, Dantzer R, et al. Are the symptoms of cancer and cancer treatment due to a shared biologic mechanism? *Cancer* **97**(11):2919–2925, 2003.
29. Dantzer R, Capuron L, Irwin MR, et al. Identification and treatment of symptoms associated with inflammation in medically ill patients. *Psychoneuroendocrinology* **33**(1):18–29, 2008.

30. Hart BL. Biological basis of the behavior of sick animals. *Neurosci Biobehav Rev* **12**(2):123–137, 1988.

31. Kelley KW, Bluthé RM, Dantzer R, et al. Cytokine-induced sickness behavior. *Brain Behav Immun* 17(Suppl 1):S112–S118, 2003.

32. Kent S, Bluthé RM, Kelley KW, Dantzer R. Sickness behavior as a new target for drug development. *Trends Pharmacol Sci* **13**(1):24–28, 1992.

33. Lee BN, Dantzer R, Langley KE, et al. A cytokine-based neuroimmunologic mechanism of cancer-related symptoms. *Neuroimmunomodulation* **11**(5):279–292, 2004.

34. Dickinson AM, Sviland L, Hamilton PJ, et al. Cytokine involvement in predicting clinical graft-versus-host disease in allogeneic bone marrow transplant recipients. *Bone Marrow Transplant* **13**(1):65–70, 1994.

35. Ferrara JL, Deeg HJ. Graft-versus-host disease. *N Engl J Med* **324**(10):667–674, 1991.

36. Piguet PF, Grau GE, Allet B, Vassalli P. Tumor necrosis factor/cachectin is an effector of skin and gut lesions of the acute phase of graft-vs.-host disease. *J Exp Med* **166**(5):1280–1289, 1987.

37. Holler E, Kolb HJ, Hintermeier-Knabe R, et al. Role of tumor necrosis factor alpha in acute graft-versus-host disease and complications following allogeneic bone marrow transplantation. *Transplant Proc* **25**(1 Pt 2): 1234–1236, 1993.

38. Holler E, Kolb HJ, Möller A, et al. Increased serum levels of tumor necrosis factor alpha precede major complications of bone marrow transplantation. *Blood* **75**(4):1011–1016, 1990.

39. Xun CQ, Thompson JS, Jennings CD, Brown SA, Widmer MB. Effect of total body irradiation, busulfan-cyclophosphamide, or cyclophosphamide conditioning on inflammatory cytokine release and development of acute and chronic graft-versus-host disease in H-2-incompatible transplanted SCID mice. *Blood* **83**(8):2360–2367, 1994.

40. Couriel DR, Hicks K, Giralt S, Champlin RE. Role of tumor necrosis factor-alpha inhibition with inflixiMAB in cancer therapy and hematopoietic stem cell transplantation. *Curr Opin Oncol* **12**(6):582–587, 2000.

41. Couriel D, Hicks K, Ippoliti C, et al. Infliximab for the treatment of graft-versus-host disease in allogeneic transplant recipients: an update [abstract]. American Society of Hematology 42nd Annual Meeting, San Francisco CA. *Blood* **96**(11):400A, 2000.

42. Holler E, Kolb HJ, Wilmanns W. Treatment of GVHD: TNF-antibodies and related antagonists. *Bone Marrow Transplant***12**(Suppl 3):S29–S31, 1993.

43. Holler E, Kolb HJ, Mittermüller J, et al. Modulation of acute graft-versus-host-disease after allogeneic bone marrow transplantation by tumor necrosis factor alpha (TNF alpha) release in the course of pretransplant conditioning: role of conditioning regimens and prophylactic application of a monoclonal antibody neutralizing human TNF alpha (MAK 195F). *Blood* **86**(3):890–899, 1995.

44. Przepiorka D, Kernan NA, Ippoliti C, et al. Daclizumab, a humanized anti-interleukin-2 receptor alpha chain antibody, for treatment of acute graft-versus-host disease. *Blood* **95**(1):83–89, 2000.

45. Engelberts I, Stephens S, Francot GJ, van der Linden CJ, Buurman WA. Evidence for different effects of soluble TNF-receptors on various TNF measurements in human biological fluids. *Lancet* **338**(8765):515–516, 1991.

46. Rowbottom AW, Norton J, Riches PG, Hobbs JR, Powles RL, Sloane JP. Cytokine gene expression in skin and lymphoid organs in graft versus host disease. *J Clin Pathol* **46**(4):341–345, 1993.

47. Artz AS, Wickrema A, Dinner S, et al. Pretreatment C-reactive protein is a predictor for outcomes after reduced-intensity allogeneic hematopoietic cell transplantation. *Biol Blood Marrow Transplant* **14**(11):1209–1216, 2008.

48. Fuji S, Kim SW, Fukuda T, et al. Preengraftment serum C-reactive protein (CRP) value may predict acute graft-versus-host disease and nonrelapse mortality after allogeneic hematopoietic stem cell transplantation. *Biol Blood Marrow Transplant* **14**(5):510–517, 2008.

49. Boosalis MG, Gray D, Walker S, Sutliff S, Talwalker R, Mazumder A. The acute phase response in autologous bone marrow transplantation. *J Med* **23**(3–4):175–193, 1992.

50. Ferrà C, de Sanjosé S, Gallardo D, et al. IL-6 and IL-8 levels in plasma during hematopoietic progenitor transplantation. *Haematologica* **83**(12):1082–1087, 1998.

51. Baron F, Storb R. Allogeneic hematopoietic cell transplantation following nonmyeloablative conditioning as treatment for hematologic malignancies and inherited blood disorders. *Mol Ther* **13**(1):26–41, 2006.

52. Harousseau JL. The allogeneic dilemma. *Bone Marrow Transplant* **40**(12):1123–1128, 2007.

53. Diaconescu R, Flowers CR, Storer B, et al. Morbidity and mortality with nonmyeloablative compared with myeloablative conditioning before hematopoietic cell transplantation from HLA-matched related donors. *Blood* **104**(5):1550–1558, 2004.

54. Alousi A, de Lima M. Reduced-intensity conditioning allogeneic hematopoietic stem cell transplantation. *Clin Adv Hematol Oncol* **5**(7):560–570, 2007.

55. Díez-Campelo M, Pérez-Simón JA, González-Porras JR, et al. Quality of life assessment in patients undergoing reduced intensity conditioning allogeneic as compared to autologous transplantation: results of a prospective study. *Bone Marrow Transplant* **34**(8):729–738, 2004.

56. Bevans MF, Marden S, Leidy NK, et al. Health-related quality of life in patients receiving reduced-intensity conditioning allogeneic hematopoietic stem cell transplantation. *Bone Marrow Transplant* **38**(2):101–109, 2006.

57. Dickinson AM, Middleton PG. Beyond the HLA typing age: genetic polymorphisms predicting transplant outcome. *Blood Rev* **19**(6):333–340, 2005.

58. Bogunia-Kubik K, Polak M, Lange A. TNF polymorphisms are associated with toxic but not with aGVHD complications in the recipients of allogeneic sibling haematopoietic stem cell transplantation. *Bone Marrow Transplant* **32**(6):617–622, 2003.

59. Cavet J, Middleton PG, Segall M, Noreen H, Davies SM, Dickinson AM. Recipient tumor necrosis factor-alpha and interleukin-10 gene polymorphisms associate with early mortality and acute graft-versus-host disease severity in HLA-matched sibling bone marrow transplants. *Blood* **94**(11):3941–3946, 1999.

60. Cavet J, Dickinson AM, Norden J, Taylor PR, Jackson GH, Middleton PG. Interferon-gamma and interleukin-6 gene polymorphisms associate with graft-versus-host disease in HLA-matched sibling bone marrow transplantation. *Blood* **98**(5):1594–1600, 2001.

61. Cullup H, Dickinson AM, Cavet J, Jackson GH, Middleton PG. Polymorphisms of interleukin-1alpha constitute independent risk factors for chronic graft-versus-host disease after allogeneic bone marrow transplantation. *Br J Haematol* **122**(5):778–787, 2003.

62. MacMillan ML, Radloff GA, DeFor TE, Weisdorf DJ, Davies SM. Interleukin-1 genotype and outcome of unrelated donor bone marrow transplantation. *Br J Haematol* **121**(4):597–604, 2003.

63. Middleton PG, Taylor PR, Jackson G, Proctor SJ, Dickinson AM. Cytokine gene polymorphisms associating with severe acute graft-versus-host disease in HLA-identical sibling transplants. *Blood* **92**(10):3943–3948, 1998.

64. Socié G, Loiseau P, Tamouza R, et al. Both genetic and clinical factors predict the development of graft-versus-host disease after allogeneic hematopoietic stem cell transplantation. *Transplantation* **72**(4):699–706, 2001.

65. Rocha V, Porcher R, Filion A, et al. Association of pharmacogenes polymorphisms with toxicities and GvHD after HLA-identical sibling bone marrow transplantation [abstract]. American Society for Hematology 45th Annual Meeting and Exposition, San Diego CA. *Blood* **102**(11):241A–242A, 2003. Abstract 848.

66. Williams LA, Wang XS, Cleeland CS, Mobley G, Giralt S. Assessment of symptoms and symptom burden before and after engraftment during allogeneic blood or marrow transplant (BMT) [abstract]. American Society for Blood and Marrow Transplantation 2006 BMT Tandem Meeting, Honolulu HI. *Biol Blood Marrow Transplant* **12**(2 Suppl 1):135, 2006. Abstract 389.

67. Smith TJ, Hillner BE, Schmitz N, et al. Economic analysis of a randomized clinical trial to compare filgrastim-mobilized peripheral-blood progenitor-cell transplantation and autologous bone marrow transplantation in patients with Hodgkin's and non-Hodgkin's lymphoma. *J Clin Oncol* **15**(1):5–10, 1997.

68. Duncan N, Hewetson M, Powles R, Raje N, Mehta J. An economic evaluation of peripheral blood stem cell transplantation as an alternative to autologous bone marrow transplantation in multiple myeloma. *Bone Marrow Transplant* **18**(6):1175–1178, 1996.

69. Anderson KO, Giralt SA, Mendoza TR, et al. Symptom burden in patients undergoing autologous stem-cell transplantation. *Bone Marrow Transplant* **39**(12):759–766, 2007.

70. Murphy BA. Clinical and economic consequences of mucositis induced by chemotherapy and/or radiation therapy. *J Support Oncol* **5**(9 Suppl 4):13–21, 2007.

71. Spielberger R, Stiff P, Bensinger W, et al. Palifermin for oral mucositis after intensive therapy for hematologic cancers. *N Engl J Med* **351**(25):2590–2598, 2004.

72. Miller AB, Hoogstraten B, Staquet M, Winkler A. Reporting results of cancer treatment. *Cancer* **47**(1):207–214, 1981.

73. Elting LS, Shih YC, Stiff PJ, et al. Economic impact of palifermin on the costs of hospitalization for autologous hematopoietic stem-cell transplant: analysis of phase 3 trial results. *Biol Blood Marrow Transplant* **13**(7):806–813, 2007.

74. Kobbe G, Hieronimus N, Graef T, et al. Combined use of palifermin and pegfilgrastim significantly reduces toxicity of high-dose therapy and autologous blood stem cell transplantation in patients with multiple myeloma [abstract]. American Society of Hematology 48th Annual Meeting and Exposition, Orlando FL, Dec 9–12, 2006. *Blood* **108**(11):406B–407B, 2006. Abstract 5260.

75. Luthi F, Berwert L, Frossard V, et al. Prevention of oral mucositis with palifermin in patients treated with high-dose chemotherapy and autologous stem cell transplantation. A single center experience [abstract]. American Society of Hematology 48th Annual Meeting and Exposition, Orlando FL, Dec 9–12, 2006. *Blood* **108**(11):843A, 2006. Abstract 2974.

76. Blazar BR, Weisdorf DJ, DeFor T, et al. Phase 1/2 randomized, placebo-control trial of palifermin to prevent graft-versus-host disease (GVHD) after allogeneic hematopoietic stem cell transplantation (HSCT). *Blood* **108**(9):3216–3222, 2006.

77. Langner S, Staber P, Schub N, et al. Palifermin reduces incidence and severity of oral mucositis in allogeneic stem-cell transplant recipients. *Bone Marrow Transplant* **42**(4):275–279, 2008.

78. Nasilowska-Adamska B, Rzepecki P, Manko J, et al. The influence of palifermin (Kepivance) on oral mucositis and acute graft versus host disease in patients with hematological diseases undergoing hematopoietic stem cell transplant. *Bone Marrow Transplant* **40**(10):983–988, 2007.

79. Lilleby K, Garcia P, Gooley T, et al. A prospective, randomized study of cryotherapy during administration of high-dose melphalan to decrease the severity and duration of oral mucositis in patients with multiple myeloma undergoing autologous peripheral blood stem cell transplantation. *Bone Marrow Transplant* **37**(11):1031–1035, 2006.

80. Tartarone A, Matera R, Romano G, Vigliotti ML, Di Renzo N. Prevention of high-dose melphalan-induced mucositis by cryotherapy. *Leuk Lymphoma* **46**(4):633–634, 2005.

81. Gori E, Arpinati M, Bonifazi F, et al. Cryotherapy in the prevention of oral mucositis in patients receiving low-dose methotrexate following myeloablative allogeneic stem cell transplantation: a prospective randomized study of the Gruppo Italiano Trapianto di Midollo Osseo nurses group. *Bone Marrow Transplant* **39**(6):347–352, 2007.

82. Antunes HS, de Azevedo AM, da Silva Bouzas LF, et al. Low-power laser in the prevention of induced oral mucositis in bone marrow transplantation patients: a randomized trial. *Blood* **109**(5):2250–2255, 2007.

83. Schubert MM, Eduardo FP, Guthrie KA, et al. A phase III randomized double-blind placebo-controlled clinical trial to determine the efficacy of low level laser therapy for the prevention of oral mucositis in patients undergoing hematopoietic cell transplantation. *Support Care Cancer* **15**(10):1145–1154, 2007.

84. Jarden M, Baadsgaard MT, Hovgaard DJ, Boesen E, Adamsen L. A randomized trial on the effect of a multimodal intervention on physical capacity, functional performance and quality of life in adult patients undergoing allogeneic SCT. *Bone Marrow Transplant* **43**(9):725–737, 2009.

85. Jarden M, Nelausen K, Hovgaard D, Boesen E, Adamsen L. The effect of a multimodal intervention on treatment-related symptoms in patients undergoing hematopoietic stem cell transplantation: a randomized controlled trial. *J Pain Symptom Manage* **38**(2):174–190, 2009.

86. Dimeo F, Fetscher S, Lange W, Mertelsmann R, Keul J. Effects of aerobic exercise on the physical performance and incidence of treatment-related complications after high-dose chemotherapy. *Blood* **90**(9):3390–3394, 1997.

87. Dimeo FC, Stieglitz RD, Novelli-Fischer U, Fetscher S, Keul J. Effects of physical activity on the fatigue and psychologic status of cancer patients during chemotherapy. *Cancer* **85**(10):2273–2277, 1999.

88. Dimeo FC, Tilmann MH, Bertz H, Kanz L, Mertelsmann R, Keul J. Aerobic exercise in the rehabilitation of cancer patients after high dose chemotherapy and autologous peripheral stem cell transplantation. *Cancer* **79**(9):1717–1722, 1997.

Section 3 Chapter 20

Clinical Perspectives In Symptom Management and Research

Promoting symptom research in cooperative groups

Lynne I. Wagner and David Cella

Established in the 1950s, the oncology cooperative group system is a national clinical trials network supported by the National Cancer Institute (NCI) as part of its National Cancer Program. Membership is composed of public and private institutions, and includes researchers, physicians, and health care professionals. This clinical-trials network is responsible for conducting hundreds of clinical trials each year for the treatment and prevention of all types of cancer, and in the area of cancer symptom management. Since its development in 1983, the NCI-funded Community Clinical Oncology Program links community cancer specialists, primary care physicians, and health care providers to oncology cooperative groups and academic cancer centers. The portfolio of research conducted in the Community Clinical Oncology Program has broadened to include symptom management and quality of life research. The relatively new discipline of symptom research is becoming an increasingly important research focus within the cooperative group system.

In this chapter we summarize key accomplishments of the cooperative groups that have cancer-control research-base funding. Factors that have facilitated the successful conduct of symptom research are described, including cooperative group organizational factors, member institution characteristics, and characteristics associated with research protocols.

Overview of the cooperative group system

The NCI-funded groups responsible for developing and implementing cancer prevention and control clinical trials are called Research Bases. The oncology cooperative group system includes eight Research Bases with NCI-funded cancer-control research (Table 20.1). Each of these cooperative groups leads a research program that includes cancer control and prevention research, and cancer symptom management trials. The organizational structure varies slightly by group. For some groups, one committee houses all symptom research; for other groups, symptom research is conducted through multiple committees (eg, in the Children's Oncology Group, the Nursing Research, Cancer Control, and Late-Effects Committees all contribute to its symptom research program). Table 20.1 lists the committee or committees that hold responsibility for symptom research in each cooperative group.

Benefits of conducting symptom research within oncology cooperative groups

Access to expertise and diverse patient populations

Cooperative group research enables access to a diverse, varied population of institutions, investigators, clinicians, and potential study participants. This access is particularly appealing for the conduct of trials examining cancer populations that are rare and that would, therefore, not be feasible within a single institution. Minority-based Community Clinical Oncology Programs provide access to cancer populations that are underserved and therefore typically difficult to reach for clinical investigation.

Cooperative group study concepts are investigator initiated and driven. Given the involvement of investigators from various disciplines who are often key leaders in their respective fields, cooperative group protocols are collaboratively developed by study teams with tremendous expertise and thus represent state-of-the-science research. Although support from industry is occasionally sought to support drug supply and distribution, representation from academic medical centers, community clinics and hospitals, statisticians, cooperative group staff, and the NCI provide a balanced, unbiased clinical trials mechanism. For this reason, cooperative group trials are often held in the highest esteem with regard to scientific integrity.

Cancer Symptom Science: Measurement, Mechanisms, and Management, eds. Charles S. Cleeland, Michael J. Fisch, and Adrian J. Dunn.
Published by Cambridge University Press.

Table 20.1. US Cancer cooperative groups with cancer control research base funding in 2009

Cooperative groups	Symptom research committees
Cancer and Leukemia Group B (CALGB)	Symptom Intervention Subcommittee
	Cancer Control and Health Outcomes Committee
Children's Oncology Group (COG)	Nursing Research Committee
	Cancer Control Committee
	Late Effects Committee
Eastern Cooperative Oncology Group (ECOG)	Symptom Management Committee
	Patient Outcomes and Survivorship Committee
Gynecologic Oncology Group (GOG)	Cancer Prevention and Control Committee
	Quality of Life Committee
National Surgical Adjuvant Breast and Bowel Project (NSABP)	Behavioral and Health Outcomes Committee
North Central Cancer Treatment Group (NCCTG)	Cancer Control Program
Radiation Therapy Oncology Group (RTOG)	Symptom Management Committee
Southwest Oncology Group (SWOG)	Symptom Control and Quality of Life Committee

Federal funding

The NCI sponsors cooperative group activities through funding of the groups' infrastructures. For some cooperative groups, such as the Eastern Cooperative Oncology Group, both symptom management and quality of life research is funded by the NCI's Division of Cancer Prevention. For other groups, such as the Radiation Therapy Oncology Group, funding for symptom management research is provided through the Division of Cancer Prevention, and funding for quality-of-life research is provided through the Cancer Therapy Evaluation Program.

Investigators are responsible for identifying a funding mechanism for study interventions; however, the costs of study coordination, accruing participants, and managing data are provided for through the cooperative group. In addition, the NCI offers additional symptom-research support to member institutions through awarding cancer control credits for activated protocols. This mechanism helps to defray costs of contributing to trial accrual. Investigators can leverage these resources to conduct research.

Intergroup cooperation

In 2007, at the direction of the Division of Cancer Prevention at NCI, a Symptom Management and Quality of Life (SxQOL) Intergroup committee was formed to promote intergroup collaboration and to minimize redundant clinical research protocols. The SxQOL Intergroup is chaired by interdisciplinary cancer specialists with demonstrated expertise in conducting symptom and quality-of-life research within the cooperative group system. Intergroup members include symptom management and quality-of-life committee chairs from each cooperative oncology group and from the six cancer centers that receive funding as a Community Clinical Oncology Program Research Base. The SxQOL Intergroup meets monthly via teleconference and annually for a face-to-face meeting to scientifically critique and prioritize proposed trial concepts and to discuss clinical research priorities in the area of symptom management and quality of life research. A report by Minasian et al.[1] provides a summary of NCI's scope of research in symptom management and health-related quality of life.

Major contributions to symptom research by oncology cooperative groups

Advances in therapy

The oncology cooperative group system has yielded significant contributions to the advancement of therapeutic approaches for most types of adult and pediatric cancers, and standard of care for the treatment of many cancers has been established on the basis of trial results.[2,3] As an illustration, the Eastern Cooperative Oncology Group protocol E3200 demonstrated significantly increased overall survival in previously treated patients with colorectal cancer who received bevacizumab and the chemotherapy regimen FOLFOX4 in comparison to FOLFOX4 alone or bevacizumab alone.[4] This practice-changing finding led to amendments to clinical trials for colorectal cancer to add bevacizumab as standard care and has led to the widespread use of bevacizumab in clinical settings, with corresponding improvements in disease outcomes.

Advances in symptom management

Significant contributions have occurred in the area of cancer symptom management research. Each of the eight oncology cooperative groups that has cancer-control research base funding is conducting symptom management research in some capacity. Key successes have been achieved by the cooperative groups in the last 10 years:

- ***The North Central Cancer Treatment Group (NCCTG)***, one of the most prolific groups with regard to symptom management clinical trials, has conducted more than 65 symptom-control trials targeting 13 symptoms associated with cancer and cancer treatment.[5] Von Gunten[6] recently acknowledged the NCCTG for "showing us the way" to the successful conduct of cooperative group symptom research. Key advances include: (1) finding effective nonhormonal approaches to manage hot flashes; (2) identifying megestrol acetate as helpful for anorexia cachexia and determining the most efficacious dose; (3) identifying oral cryotherapy as a preventive intervention for mucositis; and (4) finding that allopurinol mouthwash, which had become standard clinical practice without a solid evidence base, was in fact not effective in preventing 5-FU mucositis.
- ***Radiation Therapy Oncology Group (RTOG)*** trial 9714 demonstrated that a single 8-Gy treatment fraction was as effective as ten 30-Gy treatment fractions for palliating pain secondary to bone metastases, which helped to advance standard of care.[7]
- ***Southwest Oncology Group (SWOG)*** successes include: (1) a phase III trial evaluating two doses of megestrol acetate versus placebo for menopausal symptoms in women with breast cancer, which showed that 20 mg megestrol acetate was superior to 40 mg megestrol acetate plus placebo in reducing vasomotor symptoms;[8] and (2) a review of various contributions and experiences in conducting behavioral research in the SWOG, including symptom intervention trials.[9]
- The ***Children's Oncology Group (COG)*** activated the first behavioral intervention trial in the cooperative group system. Steady progress is being made toward the accrual goal for this trial (P Hinds, personal communication, 2009).
- The ***Clinical Community Oncology Program (CCOP)*** conducted 130 symptom management trials from 1987 to 2004. Symptom targets shifted over time, with pain, cachexia/anorexia, and stomatitis/mucositis being the most frequent targets from 1987 to 1994, stomatitis/mucositis, cachexia/anorexia, and nausea and vomiting being the most common targets from 1995 to 2000, and cachexia/anorexia, fatigue, hot flashes, and cognitive dysfunction being the most frequently targeted symptoms from 2001 to 2004.[10]

Advances in symptom measurement and patient self-report

Advancing measurement science is an equally important accomplishment in symptom research and complements symptom intervention research in that accurate assessment is a prerequisite for evaluating the efficacy of symptom treatment trials and quantifying the symptom burden associated with anticancer treatments. Key successes in this arena:

- ***The Gynecologic Oncology Group (GOG)*** moved measurement science forward in assessing abdominal discomfort and neurotoxicity. GOG trial 172 demonstrated significant superiority of intraperitoneal (IP) chemotherapy-versus-intravenous (IV) chemotherapy in median survival for advanced ovarian cancer; however, IP chemotherapy has not been fully embraced as standard of care due in part to toxicities.[11] At the time of GOG 172 protocol development, no instrument was available to assess abdominal discomfort from the patient's perspective, even though abdominal symptoms are commonly associated with ovarian cancer. The GOG Quality of Life committee utilized expert clinicians from the GOG to develop a 4-item abdominal discomfort subscale for the Functional Assessment of Cancer Therapy – Ovary (FACT-O), and this scale was validated among GOG 172 participants.[12] Administration of the

FACT/GOG-Abdominal Discomfort scale will provide valuable input from the patient's perspective on relief of disease-related symptoms, differences in response to treatment (eg, IV vs. IV/IP), and symptom burden associated with IP administration of chemotherapy.

- Further Gynecologic Oncology Group accomplishments include (1) advancing the patient-reported outcomes measurement of peripheral neuropathy through collaborating with GOG trial 177 investigators to validate a 4-item FACT/GOG-Neurotoxicity scale[13]; (2) using case examples of cooperative group treatment trials to demonstrate the importance of measuring symptom burden and quality of life from the patient's perspective in phase II treatment trials and phase III trials[14]; and (3) examining the role of assessing quality of life in symptom management trials and providing guidance on protocol design to best facilitate advancing the state of the science in symptom research.[10]
- The ***Eastern Cooperative Oncology Group (ECOG)*** completed a survey of 3016 adults with breast, lung, colorectal, or prostate cancer to identify the most common cancer-related and treatment-related symptoms (E2Z02). Providers were surveyed to establish practice patterns for the management of target symptoms. Initial results indicate that fatigue, sleep disturbance, and drowsiness are the most common moderate to severe symptoms and that lung cancer patients report the highest degree of symptom burden.[15] These results will be used to focus ECOG's symptom research program by guiding investigators to focus on the most important symptoms from the patients' perspective. Identifying priority symptoms from the patients' perspective will ensure a portfolio of protocols that have clinical relevance, thus facilitating successful accrual. The identification of efficacious interventions for these symptoms will significantly reduce the burden of cancer.

Factors contributing to successful symptom research within the cooperative groups

Symptom research committee leaders from US oncology cooperative groups were asked to identify the three to five most important factors contributing to a successful program of symptom management research within their group. Twelve factors reported by the committee leaders are summarized by cooperative group in Table 20.2 and fit three broad categories: factors related to the organizational structure of the cooperative group; factors related to group member institutions; and protocol-related factors.

Cooperative group organizational characteristics

Commitment from cooperative group leadership was commonly identified as critical to the successful conduct of a vibrant program of symptom research. Specifically, support from the group chair and executive leadership in terms of prioritizing the development of symptom management protocols, allocating funding, and providing the committee responsible for symptom research with the same level of resources as is provided to disease committees were described as factors that facilitate success. A symptom management expert should be included on the cooperative oncology group executive committee review of symptom concepts to ensure a fair review from an expert who understands priorities and science in the area, thus facilitating expeditious concept review and protocol development (W. McCaskill-Stevens, personal communication, 2009). Support from disease committee leaders is also helpful to the conduct of symptom research, not only through endorsing symptom trials, but also by inviting symptom researchers to have early input in disease committee protocol development to allow for the exploration of collaborative research opportunities. Additionally, support from biostatistics center staff is critical to the timely planning and development of symptom research protocols.

Two cooperative groups, NCCTG and the National Surgical Adjuvant Breast and Bowel Project (NSABP), provide support for dedicated staff at the home institution for the symptom committee chair, which has been cited as critical to the expeditious development of symptom protocols. Given the hundreds of steps involved in protocol development and the numerous individuals involved in the process from various organizations, having a specific, dedicated person to move protocol development forward and track progress through the system helps to avoid unnecessary delays and keeps progress on track (C. Loprinzi, personal communication, 2009). Von Gunten[6] concludes that leadership is perhaps the most likely characteristic that distinguishes the

Table 20.2. Factors contributing to the successful conduct of symptom management research[a]

	COG	ECOG	GOG	NCCTG	NSABP	RTOG	SWOG
Organizational factors							
Cooperative group leadership support	X	X			X		
Committee status		X					
Commitment from disease committees	X		X				X
Designated staff at academic institution base				X	X		
Support from all parties, including medical leadership, institutional staff, and biostatistics center staff			X		X		
Institutional factors							
Feedback from institutional members on symptom relevance				X			X
Feedback from institutional members on feasibility				X			X
Staff at institutions with designated responsibility to accrue to trials and monitor progress; financial support for staff		X	X				
Inspired data collectors who want to know the answer	X						
Protocol factors							
Financial support for intervention			X				X
Low complexity, low participation burden	X			X		X	
Addresses a symptom for which no treatment exists						X	

[a]Committee leaders asked to identify top 3–5 factors.
COG indicates Children's Oncology Group; ECOG, Eastern Cooperative Oncology Group; GOG, Gynecologic Oncology Group; NCCTG, North Central Cancer Treatment Group; NSABP, National Surgical Adjuvant Breast and Bowel Project; RTOG, Radiation Therapy Oncology Group; SWOG, Southwest Oncology Group.

NCCTG and its lead institution, the Mayo Clinic, from other cooperative groups in obtaining a track record of 20 successful years of symptom control research.

Member institution characteristics

According to the symptom research committee leaders, one of the most important factors contributing to the successful conduct of symptom research in the cooperative groups is the presence of staff at member institutions who have designated responsibility for activating symptom trials, identifying eligible patients for accrual, and monitoring trial progress and quality of data capture. This is particularly important for symptom trials that are not associated with a specific cancer type and that require surveillance for eligible patients based on symptom severity – for example, a trial for patients with any type of solid tumor who have moderate to severe fatigue. A system for routine screening of patients for level of symptom burden can also facilitate the identification of potentially eligible symptom trial participants. An additional factor that facilitates successful symptom research is a mechanism for institutional members to provide feedback on clinically relevant symptom targets and on the feasibility of symptom management concepts. At semi-annual ECOG and RTOG group meetings, the principal investigators from CCOP institutions meet with cancer control and symptom research leadership to discuss clinically relevant symptoms that might be targeted in upcoming trials and to review the portfolio of symptom trials in development and give input on feasibility of conducting such studies within the CCOP network.

Protocol characteristics

The symptom research committee leaders identified key protocol characteristics as critical to the successful conduct of symptom trials. Trials that address clinically relevant symptoms, such as common symptoms or symptoms that interfere with quality of life, are more likely to accrue patients quickly. Symptom management trials that evaluate a pharmacological or behavioral intervention require funding either for drug supply and distribution or to cover the costs of intervention delivery. Symptom trials that are most likely to be successful have low complexity with regard to intervention delivery and measurement of effect and have low burden for study participants. Successful protocols need to be "community friendly" (D. Bruner, personal communication, 2009) in that they cannot require access to technology that is not readily accessible to community hospitals. In addition, symptom trials should advance the science by evaluating an intervention for a symptom for which no standard treatment exists. The Southwest Oncology Group recently completed an online survey of Community Clinical Oncology Program members to identify important symptoms for future research to guide protocol development (C. Moinpour, personal communication, 2009).

Case example: developing a program of symptom research in ECOG

The development of a program of clinical research in symptom management within the Eastern Cooperative Oncology Group provides a case example to illustrate some of the factors described above. At an ECOG executive retreat in 1999, symptom management research was identified as a priority area for development. The ECOG Pain and Symptom Management Subcommittee was elevated to full committee status to reflect ECOG leadership's support and commitment to providing resources to cultivate a symptom research program. The committee name was changed to the Symptom Management Committee to reflect the leadership's broadened scope of areas for symptom research. Meetings with key ECOG opinion leaders, including Community Clinical Oncology Program principal investigators and chairs of ECOG disease committees, were held to solicit input on how to reinvigorate a symptom management research portfolio. The Symptom Management Committee was advised to identify institutions with a demonstrated track record of conducting symptom management research and to encourage their participation in ECOG. In addition, ECOG members noted that it is difficult to accrue to symptom management trials without dedicated staff to identify, recruit, and consent patients. As indicated in Table 20.2, one of the key factors to success in symptom management research is the availability of dedicated staff to accrue patients to open symptom trials.

In response to this feedback, the ECOG Symptom Management Consortium was formed as a formalized process to distribute funding to institutions that had demonstrated commitment to symptom management research. Institutional applications for membership in the Consortium were solicited and reviewed, while collaboration with a development professional garnered financial support for distribution among member institutions. Seven academic institutions and seven Community Clinical Oncology Programs were selected for Consortium membership, and each member institution was provided with funding to support approximately 50% of the 2-year salary for a clinical research nurse who would be dedicated to symptom management trial recruitment. The Symptom Management Consortium worked in parallel to the Symptom Management Committee to advance operational activities, while the Symptom Management Committee maintained a focus on scientific activities. Leadership from the Consortium and Committee collaborated closely, and decisions pertaining to operations and scientific priorities were made by consensus guided by members of the ECOG Executive Committee.

The Symptom Management Committee and Symptom Management Consortium recognized that success would also require a portfolio of clinically relevant symptom management trials. Simultaneous to the creation of the Consortium of dedicated investigators, the Committee solicited scientific concepts in the areas of depression, fatigue, and pain to form the basis for a portfolio of symptom management trials. The Eastern Cooperative Oncology Group trial E4Z02, "A phase III randomized placebo-controlled trial to determine efficacy of levocarnitine for fatigue in patients with cancer," was selected for focused development through ECOG and the NCI Division of Cancer Prevention. In addition, the NCI Office of Cancer Complementary and Alternative Medicine provided funding to support the supply and distribution of levocarnitine and placebo. This trial rapidly met its accrual goal due to multiple protocol-related factors. Because the symptom target, fatigue, is the most common cancer-related symptom, the trial had high clinical relevance for clinicians and patients. The intervention was easy to administer: levocarnitine or placebo were taken by patients at home in liquid form twice per day for 4 weeks. The low refusal rate indicated that levocarnitine and its mode of administration was acceptable to patients. The study assessments to measure primary and secondary endpoints consisted of patient-reported outcomes measures that were easy to administer to participants, did not require access to any novel technologies, and were not too time-consuming for patients to complete. A subgroup of study participants provided serum for the analysis of proinflammatory cytokines, which added complexity to the trial design; this correlative endpoint did not hinder accrual, however, and yielded interesting findings.[16]

Finally, Eastern Cooperative Oncology Group symptom management research activities have become self-sufficient through support from the NCI's Division of Cancer Prevention, which provides institutions with needed support to put patients on study by awarding cancer control credits for symptom trials.

Strategies for promoting symptom research within the oncology cooperative groups

The oncology cooperative groups employ a variety of strategies to promote symptom research within their respective groups. The lists presented below are comprehensive and all activities are not necessarily employed by every cooperative group.

Organizational strategies capitalize on some of the key factors contributing to successful symptom research, as mentioned above:

- Establish Symptom Management Committees to promote symptom research within the cooperative groups.
- Provide Symptom Management Committee liaisons to the disease committees to ensure key collaborations for symptom research; liaisons who become aware of disease protocols early in the process of protocol development can suggest correlative symptom research as an integral component of the trial design.
- Utilize between-meeting communication strategies, such as monthly conference calls and email distribution of conference call minutes to all Committee members, to maintain momentum toward research goals.

Other strategies focus on optimizing symptom clinical trials:

- Develop collaborations between symptom investigators and the disease committees early in concept development for treatment trials.
- Gain endorsement from the biostatistics and data centers and from members of the nursing committee early on in trial development, to facilitate training on data collection and monitoring of trial progress.
- Maintain regular communications with the disease committees, statistical center, and cooperative group leadership.

- When priority symptoms are identified, invite expert lecturers to present the latest research on the symptom of interest, including gaps in research and possible interventions.
- Recruit investigators from medical and radiation oncology and from the public health sciences to chair symptom studies.
- Strive to standardize instrumentation for assessing quality of life and symptom burden by promoting familiarity among clinical and research colleagues.
- Once symptom trials are complete, present findings in venues that typically value clinical treatment trial results to promote visibility and encourage ongoing enthusiasm for symptom research.

Challenges to the successful conduct of symptom research within the oncology cooperative groups

The successful completion of therapeutic and symptom management clinical trials and the cultivation of the science of patient-reported outcomes measurement in the cooperative group system is a complex and lengthy process. Comprehensive cancer centers and community oncology practices certainly face numerous barriers to the expeditious development and activation of clinical trials; however, oncology cooperative groups are confronted not only with those same barriers, but also with additional steps required to collaborate with multiple external agencies, which exacerbates the complexity of the process and lengthens the timeline for trial development.

Organizational and process challenges within the cooperative groups have been investigated in an effort to improve efficiency. Dilts et al.[17,18] examined the trial development and activation process in Cancer and Leukemia Group B (CALGB) and the Eastern Cooperative Oncology Group as an initial step toward developing a process improvement plan. The authors found that CALGB required 370 processes to go from an initial study idea to an open protocol, and ECOG required 481; these processes included work steps, decision points, and processing loops. The median number of calendar days from initial conception of the study to study activation was 784 for CALGB and 808 for ECOG. The National Cancer Policy Forum convened a workshop in July 2008 to outline the challenges of conducting cooperative group phase III cancer trials and to identify solutions.[19]

Organizational challenges

One of the key positive attributes of cooperative group research is the utilization of national experts from various disciplines and institutions to contribute to study design. However, this strength also presents a challenge in that consensus among coinvestigators, statisticians, and group administrators is required for trial development and conduct. The coordination of communication among all parties involved to achieve consensus can take weeks or months, depending on the complexity of trial design. The inclusion of various institutions, including academic medical centers and community practices, in the participation of research is a positive attribute in that it provides access to a heterogeneous cancer population typically not available to any single institution. This also creates a challenge in that institutions vary greatly with regard to their ability to access resources needed for study assessments and to deliver interventions, particularly those relying on sophisticated technology. For example, cognitive functioning has increasingly become a symptom of interest. To assess cognitive function using neuropsychological assessment as a study endpoint requires access to neuropsychological instruments, staff with specialized expertise in the administration and scoring of instruments, and availability of a distraction-free environment to administer study assessments, which may take several minutes to several hours to complete. This places extra demands on participating institutions that lack these needed resources to capture study endpoints. For pharmacological symptom interventions, obtaining funding for drug and drug distribution to potentially hundreds of participating institutions can pose a challenge (J. Walker, personal communication, 2009).

Institutions also vary in standard of care for common cancer symptoms, making it difficult to conduct research that does not accommodate these differing standards. For example, several randomized placebo-controlled trials were activated to establish the efficacy of methylphenidate for cancer-related fatigue. However, the trials could not meet accrual goals and were closed because many member institutions were already administering methylphenidate as standard care and would not put patients on trial because of the risk of randomizing fatigued patients to a placebo arm.

Process challenges

An additional challenge pertains to the length of time required for trial development and activation. Symptom research trials are often tied to a cooperative group treatment trial or to a particular group of patients with regard to disease and treatment characteristics. The ongoing and occasionally rapid evolution of cancer treatment can profoundly affect symptom research trials if target populations become unavailable. Due to the lengthy protocol development and activation process, the landscape of potentially eligible participants may significantly shift by the time a symptom trial is ready for accrual. For example, the Eastern Cooperative Oncology Group trial E1Z01 proposed to study an intervention for fatigue among men with hormone-refractory prostate cancer who were not receiving chemotherapy; however, the standard of care for men in this group changed during the time required to develop and activate this protocol, leaving a very small pool of potentially eligible participants.

Many symptoms, such as fatigue, pain, and distress, can only be described from the patient's perspective. Therefore, symptom research requires the collection of patient-reported outcomes data. Successful research is dependent upon the collection of quality data, with minimal missing data, to address study objectives and execute planned analyses. The North Central Cancer Treatment Group reports high compliance with collection of patient-reported outcomes data. According to Loprinzi (personal communication, 2009), the NCCTG obtains 80% to 90% compliance with data capture, which he attributes to ongoing monitoring of data submission compliance and the inclusion of patient-reported outcomes data compliance in member institutions' evaluations for ongoing group membership. Other groups, including the Eastern Cooperative Oncology Group and the Children's Oncology Group (P. Hinds, personal communication, 2009), have cited quality of patient-reported outcomes data as a challenge to conducting symptom research. ECOG has successfully improved patient-reported outcomes data capture by implementing a system to proactively notify institutions in advance of participant assessment due dates, monitoring data submission in "real time," and notifying institutions as soon as forms are late. In an ECOG quality-of-life correlative study of women with breast cancer (E1Z03), this approach has improved compliance to 98% at the primary assessment 3 months postrandomization, and to more than 90% 24 months postrandomization. The National Surgical Adjuvant Breast and Bowel Project tested a variety of methods to improve compliance with patient-reported outcomes data submission.[20]

Conclusions

Over the past 10 years, symptom research in the cooperative group system has become an increasingly important research focus. The eight cooperative groups with cancer control research base funding have yielded tremendous contributions in the area of symptom management, through building an evidence base for the management of cancer-related symptoms and improving symptom measurement. Although there are potential impediments to the conduct of symptom research in cooperative groups, the benefits of pursuing this line of work far outweigh the challenges. Continued accomplishments in symptom research through the oncology cooperative group mechanism hold promise for advancing the science of symptom care and, ultimately, for reducing the burden of cancer.

Acknowledgments

The authors express their appreciation to Drs. David Alberts, Deborah Bruner, Michael Fisch, Pamela Hinds, Stephanie Land, Charles Loprinzi, Worta McCaskill-Stevens, Carol Moinpour, Michele Naughton, Joan Walker, and Lari Wenzel for generously sharing their expertise, successes, and challenges in their respective oncology cooperative group committees.

References

1. Minasian LM, O'Mara AM, Reeve BB, et al. Health-related quality of life and symptom management research sponsored by the National Cancer Institute. *J Clin Oncol* **25**(32):5128–5132, 2007.
2. Herbst RS, Bajorin DF, Bleiberg H, et al. Clinical Cancer Advances 2005: major research advances in cancer treatment, prevention, and screening: a report from the American Society of Clinical Oncology. *J Clin Oncol* **24**(1):190–205, 2006.
3. Ozols RF, Herbst RS, Colson YL, et al. Clinical cancer advances 2006: major research advances in cancer treatment, prevention, and screening: a report from the American Society of Clinical Oncology. *J Clin Oncol* **25**(1):146–162, 2007.
4. Giantonio BJ, Catalano PJ, Meropol NJ, et al. Bevacizumab in combination with oxaliplatin, fluorouracil, and leucovorin (FOLFOX4) for previously treated metastatic colorectal cancer: results from the Eastern Cooperative Oncology Group Study E3200. *J Clin Oncol* **25**(12):1539–1544, 2007.

5. Loprinzi CL, Barton DL, Jatoi A, et al. Symptom control trials: a 20-year experience. *J Support Oncol* **5**(3):119–125, 128, 2007.
6. von Gunten CF. The right stuff to advance the science of comfort. *J Support Oncol* **5**(3):127–128, 2007.
7. Hartsell WF, Scott CB, Bruner DW, et al. Randomized trial of short- versus long-course radiotherapy for palliation of painful bone metastases. *J Natl Cancer Inst* **97**(11):798–804, 2005.
8. Goodwin JW, Green SJ, Moinpour CM, et al. Phase III randomized placebo-controlled trial of two doses of megestrol acetate as treatment for menopausal symptoms in women with breast cancer: Southwest Oncology Group Study 9626. *J Clin Oncol* **26**(10):1650–1656, 2008.
9. Gotay CC, Moinpour CM, Moody-Thomas S, et al. Behavioral science research in the cooperative group setting: the Southwest Oncology Group experience. *J Natl Cancer Inst* **92**(17):1381–1387, 2000.
10. Buchanan DR, O'Mara AM, Kelaghan JW, Minasian LM. Quality-of-life assessment in the symptom management trials of the National Cancer Institute-supported Community Clinical Oncology Program. *J Clin Oncol* **23**(3):591–598, 2005.
11. Walker JL, Armstrong DK, Huang HQ, et al. Intraperitoneal catheter outcomes in a phase III trial of intravenous versus intraperitoneal chemotherapy in optimal stage III ovarian and primary peritoneal cancer: a Gynecologic Oncology Group Study. *Gynecol Oncol* **100**(1):27–32, 2006.
12. Wenzel L, Huang HQ, Cella D, Walker JL, Armstrong DK. Validation of FACT/GOG-AD subscale for ovarian cancer-related abdominal discomfort: a Gynecologic Oncology Group study. *Gynecol Oncol* **110**(1):60–64, 2008.
13. Huang HQ, Brady MF, Cella D, Fleming G. Validation and reduction of FACT/GOG-Ntx subscale for platinum/paclitaxel-induced neurologic symptoms: a gynecologic oncology group study. *Int J Gynecol Cancer* **17**(2):387–393, 2007.
14. Wagner LI, Wenzel L, Shaw E, Cella D. Patient-reported outcomes in phase II cancer clinical trials: lessons learned and future directions. *J Clin Oncol* **25**(32):5058–5062, 2007.
15. Fisch M, Lee JW, Manola J, et al. Survey of disease and treatment-related symptoms in outpatients with invasive cancer of the breast, prostate, lung, or colon/rectum (E2Z02, the SOAPP study) [abstract]. American Society of Clinical Oncology 2009 Annual Meeting, Orlando FL, May 29–June 2, 2009. *J Clin Oncol* **27**(15 Suppl), 2009. Abstract 9619.
16. Rich TA, Fisch MJ, Manola J, et al. Analysis of cytokines in ECOG E4Z02: a phase III randomized study of l-carnitine supplementation for fatigue in patients with cancer [abstract]. American Society of Clinical Oncology 2009 Annual Meeting, Orlando FL, May 29–June 2, 2009. *J Clin Oncol* **27**(15 Suppl), 2009. Abstract 9635.
17. Dilts DM, Sandler AB, Baker M, et al. Processes to activate phase III clinical trials in a Cooperative Oncology Group: the Case of Cancer and Leukemia Group B. *J Clin Oncol* **24**(28):4553–4557, 2006.
18. Dilts DM, Sandler A, Cheng S, et al. Development of clinical trials in a cooperative group setting: the eastern cooperative oncology group. *Clin Cancer Res* **14**(11):3427–3433, 2008.
19. Patlak M, Nass SJ, Micheel C. *Multi-Center Phase III Clinical Trials and NCI Cooperative Groups: Workshop Summary*. Washington DC: National Academies Press, 2009.
20. Land SR, Ritter MW, Costantino JP, et al. Compliance with patient-reported outcomes in multicenter clinical trials: methodologic and practical approaches. *J Clin Oncol* **25**(32):5113–5120, 2007.

Section 3 Chapter 21

Clinical Perspectives In Symptom Management and Research

Practical aspects of symptom management in patients with cancer

Richard T. Lee and Michael J. Fisch

In addition to treating the patient's underlying malignancy, high-quality cancer care requires comprehensive symptom management. As stated by the Institute of Medicine,[1] one of the goals of symptom management for those at the end of life is to prevent or relieve all avoidable suffering. But what is suffering? According to Cassell, suffering occurs not merely in a body but in a person in whom intactness is threatened.[3] To reduce suffering, clinicians must come to understand their patients robustly. All patients have narratives of their illness that include their personal history, families, daily routines, and spirituality (Figure 21.1). In practical terms, thoroughly understanding patients' situations and helping them stay free of avoidable suffering is a lofty goal. To achieve that goal, clinicians must understand the definition of suffering (including what suffering might be considered unavoidable), know how to identify and monitor a patient's suffering over time, and be able to formulate a plan for preventing or eliminating that suffering.

In previous chapters, we outlined the current knowledge regarding many of the most common symptoms cancer patients experience. However, as is often the case in medicine, translating basic and clinical science into the daily practice of symptom management remains a challenge. The goal of relieving cancer patients of avoidable suffering is made more difficult because so few well-conducted, generalizable clinical trials investigating specific interventions for the management of symptoms and their functional disturbances have been performed. In this chapter, we highlight key aspects of practical symptom management in patients with cancer and provide examples from clinical cases to help clinicians achieve the best practice for symptom management. Although some of these topics may be well understood by seasoned clinicians, our hope is to discuss old and new ideas about symptom management to provide readers with an array of tools that can be used to manage cancer patients' symptoms.

The paucity of evidence in symptom management

Most symptom research lacks sufficient evidence-based information about the predisposing conditions, related pathophysiological insults, defining clinical features, and clinical consequences of symptom-specific diagnoses. Without this information, even expert clinicians cannot create succinct mental abstractions of their patients' symptoms or formulate "illness scripts" that facilitate the use of applicable clinical reasoning.[4] Unfortunately, clinical research is heavily weighted toward investigations directed at treating malignancies; conversely, the number of grants, investigators, and clinical trials directed at symptom management in cancer patients is strikingly low. Drug development for symptom management is still in its infancy, in part because the biological targets of symptoms are not well understood and the patient-reported outcome measures that might serve as appropriate primary endpoints for trials (and thus enable regulatory authorities to consider new drugs for specific symptom indications) remain controversial. Further, when clinical trials in symptom research are conducted, the interventions commonly involve either drugs that are actually approved for other indications, behavioral interventions that are difficult to reproduce and generalize, or dietary supplements and/or herbal remedies that are in the realm of integrative medicine.

A poor understanding of symptom biology, which contributes to the absence of preclinical models and a general lack of pilot research for symptom management, remains a key problem. A striking proportion of the randomized symptom trials, regardless of the intervention involved, have revealed treatment effects among participants to be small or nonexistent and rarely favor a particular intervention over other interventions and/or placebo. Without a firm understanding of symptom biology – the foundation of symptom

Cancer Symptom Science: Measurement, Mechanisms, and Management, eds. Charles S. Cleeland, Michael J. Fisch, and Adrian J. Dunn. Published by Cambridge University Press.

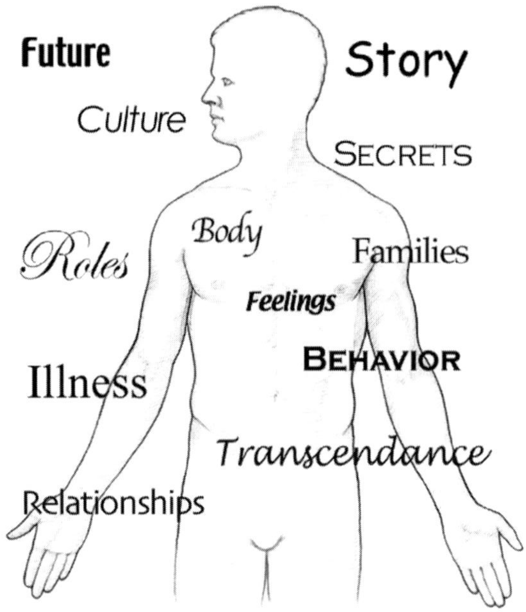

Figure 21.1. Components of a patient's narrative of illness.[2]
Source: Reprinted from Kantarjian H, Koller CA, Wolff RA. The M. D. Anderson Manual of Medical Oncology. New York: McGraw-Hill, Medical Publications Division, 2006. Reproduced with permission of the McGraw-Hill Companies, Inc.

management – the targeted selection of patients who are most likely to benefit from a given therapy is limited.

Methodological issues, including the heterogeneity of patient cohorts and the variation in the methods with which patients' symptoms are generally assessed and treated, provide an undertow for symptom-trials results to be negative. Trials that show positive results favoring certain interventions are often criticized for lacking an appropriate control group. Because the patient-reported outcome measures in interventional trials are subject to placebo effects and regression to the mean, a placebo control group is critical in symptom research studies, even when the intent is to explore the efficacy and feasibility of a new approach.

The overall result of these obstacles on the body of evidence in the area of symptom management is a poor foundation to guide practice. According to a National Institute of Health State-of-the-Science Panel, "Although research is producing increasingly hopeful insights into the causes and cures for cancer, efforts to manage the side effects of the disease and its treatments have not kept pace."[5]

Fortunately, advances in fields such as palliative medicine and integrative medicine have brought greater attention to symptom management in patients with cancer. This increased interest has been recognized by the National Cancer Institute, which now considers the elimination of suffering as part of its overall goal. The movement to eliminate suffering has been driven in part by the patients themselves, who have requested that improvements in health care be made to address quality-of-life issues and similar aspects of cancer care. This in turn has prompted quality-of-life and symptom management studies that may help provide new evidence for guiding symptom management in patients with cancer.

Establishing the doctor–patient relationship

From the Hippocratic Oath onward, the doctor–patient relationship has been considered key to any successful therapeutic relationship and transcends a mere textbook understanding of a patient's disease. Sir William Osler, the esteemed Canadian physician who established the medical residency and has been described as "The Father of Modern Medicine," remarked, "Care more for the individual patient than for the special features of the disease… Put yourself in his place… The kindly word, the cheerful greeting, the sympathetic look – these the patient understands."[6] As cancer treatment continues to evolve, with standards of care changing yearly, the doctor–patient relationship remains an

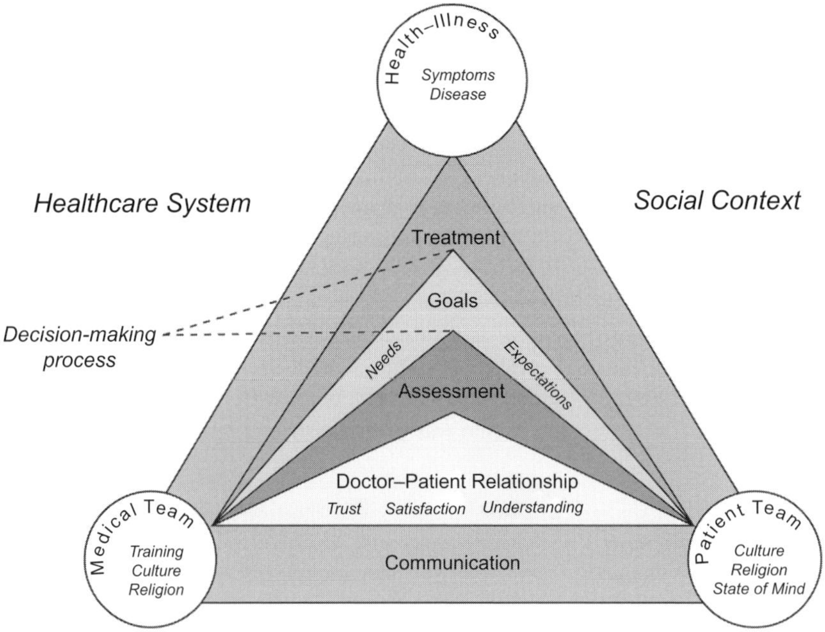

Figure 21.2. The Lee-Epner-Walsh Doctor–Patient-Health Model. See plate section for color version.

essential element of cancer care. Indeed, the doctor–patient relationship may even be considered critical in this instance because of the complex, interdisciplinary nature of cancer treatment.

As knowledge of the human body has grown, so too has the understanding of the doctor–patient relationship. A variety of key components, including communication, trust, decision making, and the establishment of care goals, contribute to a successful interaction. To provide clinicians with a framework in which to think about interacting with patients, we propose the doctor–patient-health model (Figure 21.2). Although this is not a complete or the only model, it creates a common point at which to think about the doctor–patient relationship and can be modified as each clinician considers appropriate.

The doctor–patient-health model begins when patients seek health advice from health care professionals. Clinicians must understand their patients' health concerns or their "state of illness," as described by Cassell.[7] To understand their patients' health concerns, clinicians must be able to communicate effectively, because communication is the mortar with which the doctor–patient relationship is built. The clinician, patient, and health–illness anchor the doctor–patient relationship, and through this relationship the healing process begins. Clinicians, through their words and nonverbal actions, can alleviate their patients' anxieties and fears and provide the hope of help. When clinicians communicate empathetically and effectively, their patients will often leave the office feeling better than they did at the start of their visit. Successful interactions will lead to important outcomes such as trust, understanding, and satisfaction for everyone involved.

Symptom assessment

Early in the doctor–patient relationship, some patients with cancer avoid discussing difficult subjects, including symptoms, for fear that they will be judged too weak or too damaged to undergo crucial therapy. Clinicians must reassure their patients that symptom management occurs alongside appropriate cancer therapy. Clinicians must also establish that, as health care providers, they are interested in responding to how the patient's symptoms really are – good or bad. Some patients try to avoid upsetting or disappointing their physicians, particularly if their physicians tend to show frustration when problems arise.

Given the current understanding of symptom biology and management, what does elegant symptom-directed care look like? In the context of multidisciplinary care, comprehensive assessments are collected and assimilated to provide a robust view of patients, their families, and their sources of suffering. In response to these assessments, the appropriate care plans are crafted, and most importantly, reassessed from time to time.

The multidisciplinary approach to cancer care enables multiple people to inform clinicians about a patient's spectrum of suffering. Patients often share different types of information with different members of the health care team; for example, a patient might discuss weight loss issues with a chaplain or reveal intimacy problems to a speech therapist. The information a patient chooses to disclose may be influenced as much by the clinician's personality or gender as it is by the specialty label on the clinician's white coat. No matter to whom the patient chooses to express certain information, this information provides valuable clues about the patient's suffering that can help guide treatment. To that end, communication among the health care team is key.

Reassessment

A cornerstone to successful, even elegant, symptom management in cancer patients is comprehensive assessment at multiple time points, which is, however, difficult to perform in a longitudinal fashion. The process of symptom reassessment is also a therapeutic tool in its own right, which occurs in part because patients perceive empathy, compassion, and a willingness to help them.

A validated symptom assessment tool can be used to assess patients' symptoms even before they visit the clinic. However, multi-item screening tools, symptom surveys, and quality-of-life-assessing instruments are rarely used in the routine care of cancer patients, although some research-oriented, symptom-directed clinics, such as pain or palliative care centers, are exceptions to this rule. In general, the most useful starting point in providing symptom management is pain assessment, in which the symptom's severity, location, timing, duration, and precipitating or relieving factors are ascertained. Assessing other symptoms generally follows a similar model.

Clinicians can use assessment instruments to "break the ice" with patients and establish a means for gathering patient information; however, these instruments are only one component of successful patient assessment. Skillful communication is another essential component that enables patients and clinicians to express their concerns to each other. One often-overlooked technique of effective communication is using silence to allow patients to find their own words to describe what they are experiencing as well as the impact and meaning of their experiences. For example, a patient may deny having pain, hurting, or aching in his back if the clinician asks about only pain, hurting, or aching, but the patient may admit to having a "tiredness" of the back if allowed to describe his symptoms himself. By not admitting to having pain, the patient may not be introduced to the appropriate pain management in the institution or may be considered ineligible for clinical trials of pain management interventions. However, by allowing the patient to describe what he is experiencing, the clinician may come to understand the patient's "tiredness" as an indication for opioid analgesia or imaging studies to evaluate for spinal cord compression.

Allowing patients to answer open-ended questions in writing or by email can also encourage patients to describe what they are experiencing in greater detail. Below is an example of a woman with an advanced pelvic malignancy whose email correspondence provided her treatment team with an augmented assessment that was useful in providing her care:

> Longevity. I really like to read about how Americans have longevity now. According to today's papers, everyone is living longer. Wow! It really makes me feel good to read about that. In fact, it makes me boil a little inside that I should be entitled to do that too, especially since longevity is one of the family inheritances I should have captured. My grandmother lived to be 101 years old, even with a cancer at age 80. Oh well, 51 is much too young to go away in this day and age, but what can I do about it. I guess confront God when I see him!!

In this example, the patient was experiencing spiritual pain associated with her mortality. Knowing this, her physician referred the patient to a spiritual counselor, which helped improve her overall condition.

Emotion is another key element of symptom management that is often overlooked and difficult to address. Fear, anxiety, acute grief, and other strong feelings can prevent patients from participating in meaningful interactions with their clinicians. For example:

> I accompanied my mother to a neurosurgery appointment in regards to her back pain. Not wanting to interfere with the visit, I minimized my involvement during the visit and allowed her to answer the questions from the physician. To my surprise, my mother answered multiple questions about her history and symptoms erroneously and needed to be corrected on several key questions. After the visit, I asked her about why she answered certain questions erroneously, and she admitted to being so anxious and nervous, that her responses became confused.

Strong emotions can alter perception and thinking. Patients with cancer often recount how, upon learning of their diagnosis, they became so overwhelmed with emotion that they could not remember the rest of their conversation with the clinician; they simply stopped remembering and processing information. To help put patients more at ease at the beginning of clinic visits, clinicians can initiate discussion by talking about nonmedical topics, such as the patients' families or hometowns. Any strong emotions patients experience during their visit should be acknowledged or named.[8] In doing so, the clinician begins the healing process by inferring that these emotions are important and part of the patient experience. In some cases, such emotions may take time to resolve, and follow-up visits will be required.

A rational, reproducible systematic approach to symptom assessment is impossible. Rather, clinicians must employ the "art of medicine" to undertake comprehensive, interdisciplinary care that focuses on managing their patients' underlying cancer and other medical conditions while preventing and relieving their suffering. In essence, this approach embraces the principles of palliative care rather than the principles of symptom management. Patients require unique, personalized approaches to finding a communication style and tools that optimize their relationship with their clinicians. For example, whereas the "power of silence" may be used effectively to garner information from some patients, it may incite an uncomfortable anxiety in others.

With each visit, clinicians need to not only assess their patients' symptoms but also determine whether the assessment itself can be improved upon. Indeed, no available assessment tools or techniques can capture the entirety of a person. For example, Balaban describes seeing an elderly woman at office visits who appeared to be younger than her stated age of 76 years; however, upon seeing the same patient at a local store, he found a much older-looking woman.[9] Clinicians must constantly remind themselves that they see patients for only an instant in which their patients have provided filtered versions of themselves. By obtaining information from their patients' families and friends about the patients' lives outside the hospital and clinic, clinicians are able to formulate more complete and natural assessments.

Masquerading symptoms

Although educational materials, treatment algorithms, and clinical trials use symptom labels (eg, "pain," "fatigue," "depression") to categorize specific patient complaints, patients often do not know exactly what is bothering them or why. Patients can only describe what they are experiencing, but clinicians may come to have a different understanding of the root cause of their patients' discomfort. Clinicians should be constantly aware of these symptom masquerades, which at first presentation appear to be a simple diagnosis, but instead are misleading symptoms of the actual etiology of the patients' pathological process. We offer two examples of the phenomenon of symptom masquerade.

Pain masquerading as fatigue

In the first example, a clinician reports on a visit with a man with hormone-refractory prostate cancer who was experiencing persistent severe fatigue:

> I had the opportunity to see Mr. X today. As you recall, he is the 77-year-old man with advanced prostate cancer, anemia, and profound and totally debilitating fatigue. He had bone metastases and bad fatigue at the time of diagnosis in 1998, and it has gotten very severe in recent months. He has been depressed but has not responded very much to sertraline and methylphenidate. In my opinion, he has severe chronic pain with overwhelming nociceptive input from osseous disease. He also has a personal history of fairly poor tolerance of pain. Unfortunately, he equates complaining about pain as "whining." For personal or cultural reasons, it is more acceptable to complain about fatigue than it is to use the language of pain. He has been on OxyContin for 8 weeks or so, but he hasn't been on a short-acting strong opioid and the dose escalation has been difficult because of his communication style. In essence, I think that his peculiar "fatigue factor" is chronic pain.

The patient's severe osseous pain was masquerading as fatigue. Mr. X was not being deceptive in saying that he was tired; he truly perceived the pain to be fatigue. Further, Mr. X's family also understood the pain to be fatigue. In Mr. X's case, the opioid was the pill used to treat the "fatigue," although it was explained to Mr. X that opioids are directed at the biology of pain and that they may help to resolve his terrible fatigue.

Identifying the correct etiology that is eliciting the patient's symptom is crucial to provide the best treatment options. Although Mr. X would have been eligible to participate in a trial of a psychostimulant for fatigue, the psychostimulant would not have been effective. Likewise, the patient would not have been eligible for any trials of pain management interventions in which pain expression was an entry criterion. In this case of Mr. X, from any angle, the clinical research treatment option is at a disadvantage because trials assume that masquerading symptoms are absent.

Anxiety masquerading as nausea

In the second example, a patient with thyroid cancer is unsuccessfully treated for nausea:

> A 71-year-old man with anaplastic thyroid cancer was hospitalized with pneumonia and severe nausea. His nausea did not resolve despite the intravenous use of corticosteroids, metoclopramide, ondansetron, and diphenhydramine. After comprehensive assessment, his nausea appears to have been driven by fear and dyspnea. The patient was given oxygen over his tracheostomy collar along with benzodiazepines and counseling. The patient's nausea resolved, allowing the discontinuation of all intravenous antiemetics.

Like fatigue, nausea is a poorly understood symptom with a complex biology involving multiple nervous system pathways and a variety of receptors. Like other symptoms, nausea is ultimately a functional disturbance that is manifested in the central nervous system. The medulla appears to be the clearing house for nausea-related stimuli, in the nucleus of the tractus solitarius and the reticular formation known as the "true vomiting center." The true vomiting center interacts with the cerebral cortex, vagal stimuli, the vestibular system, and the chemoreceptor trigger zone. These pathways involve an array of neurotransmitters, including histamine, acetylcholine, neurokinin-1, dopamine, serotonin, and cannabinoids.

Considering the above example, one can imagine how understanding the known anatomy and possible biology of nausea would not help resolve the nausea. Drugs, counseling, or other interventions could be used to mitigate many potential sources of input to the true vomiting center. The only way to mitigate chronic nausea is to comprehensively assess the patient, determine the cause of the nausea, and pursue time-limited therapeutic trials followed by further comprehensive, open-minded assessment. For very discrete causes of nausea, such as acute nausea due to noxious drugs, such as chemotherapy or anesthesia, focused clinical trials are possible and occasionally produce positive results. Yet chronic nausea remains difficult to treat and study, and the best clinical outcomes are driven more often by assessment than specific interventions.

Decision making and goals of care

Clinicians often initiate treatment planning before considering the goals of care for the patient. Prior to the 1960s, the doctor–patient relationship was primarily physician-focused and physician-driven. However, shared decision making and the patient-centered model of care have emerged over the past few decades. Today, most patients expect to be part of the decision making process. Consider the following:

> An 85-year-old Caucasian woman from a small farming town was diagnosed with breast cancer. After further work-up, it was determined to be an early stage cancer. After a lengthy discussion, the patient decided to forgo treatment, as she was concerned about her quality of life and self-image. Now 91 years old, the patient remains independent and actively maintains her garden.

In this example, to begin planning the patient's cancer treatment would have been premature. The patient was focused on managing her symptoms to achieve an acceptable quality of life, which included gardening – her favorite pastime. The patient's slow-growing cancer was unlikely to lead to her death, and an aggressive treatment plan may have negatively changed her self-esteem and quality of life. The decision-making process is a balance of preferences between the clinician and patient. Whereas some patients may demand to be the final decision maker in their care, other patients may prefer a more passive role, allowing the physician to direct therapy. In either case, the right personalized approach provides patients with a sense of ease about their goals of care and medical decisions.

Unmet needs

Many oncologists have increasingly demanding schedules in which clinical visits are often restricted to discussing treatment decisions with their patients. Although patients meet with their oncologists to discuss cancer treatment, it may be equally important for patients to discuss the treatment of symptoms that prevent them from working, such as pain. Unemployment may cause patients distress about supporting their family or paying health care bills. Engel's biopsychosocial model of health care, first published in Science more than 30 years ago, describes these domains of patient care and their importance in the treatment of all patients.[10] If clinicians do not address these needs, their patients may seek out other treatments for these symptoms, including complementary or alternative medicine. Although some of these therapies, such as massage, are considered harmless, others, such as the use of dietary supplements or herbal remedies, may have significant potential for harm. Without comprehensive assessment and appropriate attention given to all their needs – including the nonbiological ones – patients may perceive gaps in their care.

Goals of care

Although oncologists well realize the limitations of anticancer therapy and know that some tumors are particularly aggressive even in their earliest stages, it is still common for some oncologists to be overconfident in their ability to prevent and/or control suffering caused by severe symptoms. Indeed, some patients may accept the possibility of dying from their malignancy but ask their physicians to promise that their pain be controlled or their dignity preserved under all circumstances. While it is appropriate to commit to striving on the patient's behalf under all circumstances, clinicians must acknowledge that even these fundamental wishes cannot always be guaranteed. Clinicians should always beware of making promises, as symptom management can be humbling. For example:

> Mr. Y was a 68-year-old man with androgen-independent prostate cancer with extensive osseous disease. Despite prior radiation therapy for local control and systemic palliative therapy, the patient developed severe somatic and neuropathic pain due to sacral involvement. Medical pain management was unsatisfactory, despite several months of therapy and multiple attempts by pain management experts to treat the nociceptive pain and understand and treat the nonpain dimensions of his suffering. The patient ultimately underwent a midline dorsal myelotomy for neuroablative management of his pain. He experienced the expected postprocedure disabilities without meaningful improvement in his pain control. The patient died in an inpatient hospice 8 weeks later.

Promises of symptom control and dignity preservation are sometimes difficult to keep. Patents with chronic symptoms often become so fixated upon an unattainable result that they endure prolonged hospitalization or unnecessary procedures that prevent them from moving forward with their overall health care and life planning. Creating realistic goals provides patients with an opportunity to plan accordingly for the future. Indeed, symptoms that have persisted for years often involve physiological changes at the cellular level, and thus any "quick fix" for such symptoms is rare. Rather, a prolonged process of assessment and treatment followed by reassessment and treatment modification is likely the most effective process for addressing these symptoms.

Another approach is to encourage patients – especially patients with complex treatment profiles – to be active members of their health care team. Too often, patients and their families expect that the health care system will take care of everything, and their roles are diminished to those of passive spectators. When certain expectations are not met, neither the health care team nor the patient, but rather the disease process, is at fault. Having patients and family play an active role in decision making and treatment planning can provide patients with a sense of empowerment and responsibility, which often leads to a more powerful therapeutic relationship between patients and clinicians. Although the biological endpoint may remain the same, all parties experience an enhanced sense of success and satisfaction.

Treatment planning

Successful symptom management is a multistep process, and attributions of success are difficult. Commonly in medicine, when a discrete problem (eg, gout, cellulitis, or choledocholithiasis) is diagnosed, a specific intervention ameliorates the problem. However, managing symptoms usually involves some uncertainty as to the nature of the problem and the real cause of its improvement. This uncertainty is due in part to the natural progression of diseases. For example, migraine headaches, depression, radiation-related mucositis, and many other conditions have variable courses and often remit spontaneously. Although certain interventions can reduce the severity and duration of such conditions, it is difficult to know for sure just how effective a particular intervention is for an individual patient, especially when several interventions are involved simultaneously, as in the following case:

> Mr. W had progressive, refractory follicular thyroid carcinoma with pulmonary, osseous, ocular, and leptomeningeal involvement. He lived at home with his wife and three children. His medications included a short-acting opioid taken twice daily, an antidepressant, a serotonin-antagonist to control nausea, senna to reduce constipation, a long-acting benzodiazepine for anxiety, a proton-pump inhibitor to prevent gastritis, and thyroid and calcium supplementation. The patient presented to the clinic with progressive visual loss in his right eye with excessive tearing, moderate osseous pain in the left arm, left leg discomfort due to swelling, fatigue severity rated at level 7 on a 0–10 numerical rating scale, and nausea rated at level 8.

The patient was started on low-dose methadone to provide a long-acting oral opioid and given a time-limited therapeutic trial of dexamethasone to relieve pain and nausea. A patch was placed over his right eye. The clinician discussed the social and emotional aspects of the patient's situation with the patient and his wife and answered these patient questions[11]:

1. What is happening to me?
2. What is going to happen to me?
3. What can be done to help me?

Mr. W's care was enormously complex, and the reasons for his pain, fatigue, and nausea were not going to be easy to sort out. Mr. W would not have been eligible for most symptom-management trials on the basis of the complexity of his care and exposure to so many medications. If Mr. W had been eligible for a clinical trial related to symptom management, the staff probably would not have felt comfortable approaching him for consent during his first visit because of his distress level and the time needed to assess and treat him as an outpatient. Instead, simple interventions for Mr. W made a significant improvement in his symptoms. It remains unclear how the components of his care factored into the improvement of his symptoms, and some of the interventions may have been unnecessary or ineffective. Nonetheless, at follow-up 2 days later:

> Mr. W achieved good pain control and was less anxious, but he was dehydrated and constipated. Hypercalcemia was ruled out, and the patient was treated with intravenous fluids, metoclopramide, and an enema. His opioid dosing was adjusted slightly, and teaching about pain and symptom control was reinforced. The patient improved substantially within the following 3 days, and he was able to plan and enjoy a week-long family vacation before resuming aggressive palliative care. He died 3 months later.

Another limitation in applying existing knowledge about symptom management in the clinic is the overall heterogeneity of the patient populations studied. Fatigue research exemplifies this limitation. Any estimate of the prevalence of fatigue in mixed cohorts of patients varies depending on the nature of the patient population rather than reflecting the essence of cancer fatigue. Prue et al.[12] performed a literature review to identify interventional and noninterventional cohort studies in which adult cancer patients who experienced cancer-related fatigue while undergoing anticancer therapy were assessed with multidimensional cancer-related fatigue instruments. Forty such studies were identified. Only 32 of these studies were longitudinal; of the 29 longitudinal studies involving disease-specific cohorts, 24 included women only. The prevalence of fatigue in these studies was high – sometimes more than 90%. However, the type of cancer therapy (radiation, conventional-dose chemotherapy, high-dose chemotherapy) varied, some cohorts involved only men or only women, the timing of the fatigue assessments varied, and the rate of missing follow-up data was high. Moreover, these studies employed a dozen different multidimensional fatigue instruments. The variability in the instruments is particularly problematic because: (1) each instrument has a different cutoff point for clinically important fatigue and a different change score that might be considered clinically important; (2) the appropriate cutoff scores and clinically significant change scores are not well described for each instrument; and (3) none of the instruments is widely used in clinical practice, thus limiting the generalizability of their data. Lawrence et al.[13] completed a systematic review of cancer-related fatigue literature and reported that, depending on the population studied and the assessment methods used, the prevalence of cancer-related fatigue ranges from 4% to 91%. Thus, oncologists are profoundly limited in their attempts to describe cancer-related fatigue in their patients – not including the unknown proportion of patients who are improperly categorized as having or not having fatigue because of symptoms masquerading as fatigue.

Even when evidence supporting new clinical practice exists, the medical field is often slow to change. Many factors are involved in adopting new practice, including the level of medical urgency, complexity of the action, economic impact, previous experience and education, patient demands, attitudes toward the intervention, and external factors, such as laws.[14] Without an active desire to continually improve current practice patterns, health care practitioners are unlikely to integrate new therapies and techniques. Until sufficient information becomes available to guide symptom management, clinicians must extrapolate information from published clinical trials and balance how well the patient they are assessing may benefit from the available treatment options.

To treat or not to treat with anticancer therapies

High symptom burden in the presence of advanced cancer does not always preclude cancer treatment. A patient's performance status and level of symptom burden is an indicator of prognosis. In clinical trials of cytolytic chemotherapy for advanced solid tumors, most patients who benefit have excellent or good performance status, partly because performance status is often a predictive factor for treatment response and a reflection of the eligibility criteria. In practice, however, patients' treatment plans do not need to be based on a single visit or short span of assessment. Patients may undergo time-limited therapeutic trials to determine whether comprehensive assessment with appropriate symptom management interventions will yield improvements that allow for a more ambitious set of treatment choices or goals of care. The following case illustrates this point:

> Mr. K was a 74-year-old man with hepatitis C, cirrhosis, hypertension, and ischemic cardiomyopathy. He presented with back pain and was diagnosed with a 17-cm tumor in the left lobe of the liver and a thoracic vertebral metastasis due to hepatocellular carcinoma. His functional status was diminished, and he was bothered by severe pain, moderate dyspnea, moderate anxiety, and anorexia.
>
> With comprehensive, multidisciplinary assessment, his hypertension and cardiomyopathy were well managed. He started strong opioids for pain and dyspnea, a psychostimulant to control opioid-induced sedation, prokinetics and laxatives for bowel management, and an antidepressant along with supportive-expressive counseling. He improved and was able to undergo surgery to resect the liver tumor followed by palliative radiotherapy for local control of the painful vertebral metastases. By week 10, with excellent performance status and minimal symptom burden, outpatient chemotherapy was initiated.

While this example may seem extraordinary, the underlying point is worth emphasizing: it is not clear what is possible for any given patient until appropriate symptom control has been pursued over a series of visits. For some patients, comfort-oriented or hospice care is appropriate; however, more aggressive options may later become feasible. Generally, there is a lag between what is achievable in the context of expert multidisciplinary care under some circumstances and what is readily discernible in the medical literature on the basis of clinical trials.

Invasive pain-management procedures

A variety of experts are involved in symptom-directed care, particularly in the management of chronic cancer pain. Many anesthesiologists, orthopedic surgeons, neurosurgeons, and physical medicine and rehabilitation specialists have expertise in cancer pain-management procedures, including placing localized nerve blocks (such as celiac plexus blocks for visceral pain), injecting botulism toxin into muscles, implanting epidural or intrathecal pumps, performing vertebroplasties for compression fractures, and completing neuroablative procedures. At our institution, we are fortunate to have skillful and compassionate specialists who are able to apply these and similar procedures when appropriate; however, only small minorities of patients are viable candidates for these kinds of procedures, and the proportion of patients who obtain meaningful, durable, and complication-free responses is even smaller. Overall, less than 5% of the patients treated at our institution are considered appropriate candidates for such pain-management or palliative procedures, and less than half of those patients achieve a gratifying degree and duration of relief. Although physicians who commonly perform these procedures often report high success rates, a "perspective bias" must be considered, as the referring physicians will have already filtered the patients who undergo these procedures. In sum, although these procedures can benefit patients and play an important role in their symptom management, improvement tends to occur only in a minority of patients. Clinicians need to use these procedures judiciously and, as with any invasive therapy, carefully consider the risk–benefit ratio.

The barriers to the effective use of interventional procedures for the management of cancer pain are similar to those of medical pain management. Variations in patient assessment and the heterogeneity of patient cohorts make clinical trial data very difficult to obtain and interpret. Interventional care is generally expensive and not available in all settings because of personnel and resource limitations. Some interventions, such as the placement of implantable intrathecal opioid pumps, require ongoing monitoring and expertise that may restrict patients' choices of where to receive their care. For example, patients with implantable pumps may find that hospice enrollment is not an option in their region.

Polypharmacy and nonadherence

Mr. W's case illustrates a patient–care scenario in which a series of complex assessments and maneuvers were successful in managing a cancer patient's symptoms. Mr. W's case also underscores the hazards of polypharmacy. Mr. W was taking numerous medications, and there were clearly some overlapping toxicities and potential drug interactions. A patient taking a strong opioid such as methadone and a long-acting benzodiazepine may become excessively sedated. If the same patient were to develop oral candidiasis and begin taking fluconazole, the metabolism of methadone could be slowed because methadone and fluconazole share the same cytochrome 3A4 pathway of liver metabolism, with methadone as a substrate and fluconazole as an inhibitor. The net result could be an elevation of the methadone effect that requires assessment and possible dose reduction. Similarly, although many patients commonly use herbal remedies and dietary supplements, the belief that these natural products are always safe, while pervasive, is untrue. As studies continue to characterize these products, an increasing amount of information has surfaced regarding their side effects and potential medication interactions. Thus, patients' clinical histories must include all ingested products including prescription and over-the-counter drugs, herbal remedies, and dietary supplements.

Moreover, Mr. W could have struggled with persistent symptoms because of nonadherence. A patient prescribed methadone or any other strong, long-acting opioid for chronic pain may be reluctant to take the medication. This reluctance could be due to the patient's misunderstanding of the intent of the drug ("I thought that drug was used to treat heroin addicts"), fear of side effects ("I see that this drug causes constipation, and I'm already constipated"), fear of addiction ("My brother was addicted to cocaine, and I swore I'd never have that happen in my family"), or concerns about drug interactions ("My pharmacist warned me that this drug interacts with another medication I'm taking"). Reluctance to take the medication may also be due to the expense of the medication, the medication's lack of availability at local pharmacies, or diversion by family members. Patients may also be confused about how to take the medication because they are unable to read the pharmacy instructions because of visual barriers (as in the case of Mr. W and his progressive vision loss), language barriers, low literacy, or cognitive difficulties. The barriers to adherence take time to assess. To confront these issues openly without fear of being judged or abandoned, patients must trust their medical teams. The managing medical team must start a dialogue to understand reasons for poor adherence.

Generally, addressing polypharmacy and nonadherence requires more time than a busy outpatient oncologist can accommodate. As a result, patients' successful symptom management also often requires multidisciplinary input from nurses, pharmacists, and other midlevel providers.

Identifying guidelines and key resources in symptom management

The existing standards of care and guidelines for symptom management are overwhelmingly based on the consensus of panels of experts rather than empirical evidence. These expert panels have an eclectic makeup, with members from several disciplines whose expertise in symptom science ranges from basic science to measurement, biostatistics, epidemiology, primary care, and various subspecialties of internal medicine and other medical and nursing realms, such as surgery and radiation oncology. This multidisciplinary aspect of symptom science leads to significant variation in the language used to describe symptoms, heterogeneity in the design and conduct of clinical research, and a wide dissemination of findings in a variety of peer-reviewed journals and national meetings.

Not only does symptom management lack evidence-based guidelines, but a consensus among panels of experts is difficult to find and apply to the care of individual patients and their families. For example, the American Society of Clinical Oncology (ASCO) has developed high-quality educational materials for symptom management and palliative care.[15] Although ASCO has guidelines for some topics in supportive oncology, such as the use of antiemetics for chemotherapy-related nausea and the management of febrile neutropenia, no ASCO guidelines address pain management or other specific symptoms or topics in cancer communication. Similarly, the Multinational Association of Supportive Care in Cancer (MASCC), a professional organization more specifically focused on symptom management, has developed guidelines for using antiemetics to treat nausea and mucositis and has made significant contributions in febrile neutropenia-related research and education. However, additional MASCC guidelines for symptom management have not yet emerged. Consensus-based guidelines in the form of algorithms are available from the National Comprehensive Cancer Network (NCCN) for pain, fatigue, distress, and palliative care topics and specific symptoms, such as dyspnea, anorexia/cachexia, nausea/vomiting, constipation, and delirium.[16] A more widely accessible and education-oriented source of symptom management guidelines is available through the National Cancer Institute under the theme of "coping with cancer."[17] This information is developed and managed by a small panel of experts whose work is far less structured than that of the NCCN.

Overall, the paucity of effective guidelines and treatment algorithms for symptom management is not due to any lack of appreciation on the part of these professional organizations; rather, it reflects the lack of evidence in the field to serve as a foundation for evidence-based guidelines.

Summary

Attempts to reduce or eliminate suffering begin with the establishment of a doctor–patient relationship built upon good communication. From this foundation, clinicians should proceed with an open-minded, open-hearted, comprehensive assessment of the patient as a person. This assessment should be extended to patients' family members, as they also suffer, though in different ways than the patient. Symptoms require active, timely, and thoughtful management that is based on comprehensive assessment over time. Often, the treatment of patients who present with a multitude of symptoms is further complicated by symptom masquerades. Time-limited therapeutic trials are crucial to assessing the benefit of any treatment intervention and require early follow-up and continuity of care. Although multidisciplinary care creates additional work for clinicians, it also allows for multiple informants who help unveil the real and robust spectrum of patients' problems. In many patients whose care is especially challenging, the potential goals of care may not be clear at the onset of an episode of care in the face of symptom distress. Continued discussion and assessment helps clinicians communicate realistic goals to their patients without conveying undue expectations or fostering unmet needs.

The overwhelming majority of symptoms are managed with medical or behavioral interventions rather than interventional procedures. Whenever possible, the underlying causes of problems are treated on the basis of inferences or data regarding the pathophysiology of the disease. However, attribution of symptom problems as well as the real reasons for symptom improvement can be difficult to discern and is not of paramount importance. Patients should be screened for ubiquitous barriers to successful symptom control, such as polypharmacy and noncompliance.

Managing patients' suffering can be as humbling as a hurricane forecast, and the same can be said about symptom-related research. The most successful clinicians have an array of tools and adapt these to each individual patient. Health professionals and researchers should emphasize appropriate intentions of care and reflect compassion and skill in the context of safe and effective processes. As the understanding of cancer improves, treatment planning is becoming more complex and personalized. So too must be the approach to symptom management.

References

1. Field MJ, Cassel CK, Institute of Medicine, Committee on Care at the End of Life. *Approaching Death: Improving Care at the End of Life*. Washington DC: National Academy Press, 1997.
2. Kantarjian H, Koller CA, Wolff RA. *The M. D. Anderson Manual of Medical Oncology*. New York: McGraw-Hill, *Medical Publications Division*, 2006.

3. Cassell EJ. *The Nature of Suffering and the Goals of Medicine*, 2nd ed. New York: Oxford University Press, 2004.
4. Bowen JL. Educational strategies to promote clinical diagnostic reasoning. *N Engl J Med* **355**(21):2217–2225, 2006.
5. National Institutes of Health. Symptom management in cancer: pain, depression and fatigue: State-of-the-Science Conference Statement. *J Pain Palliat Care Pharmacother* **17**(1):77–97, 2003.
6. Cushing H. *The Life of Sir William Osler*. Oxford: The Clarendon Press, 1925.
7. Cassell EJ. Making the patient better–whatever the outcome. *J Support Oncol* **5**(2):58, 2007.
8. Back AL, Arnold RM, Baile WF, Tulsky JA, Fryer-Edwards K. Approaching difficult communication tasks in oncology. *CA Cancer J Clin* **55**(3):164–177, 2005.
9. Balaban DH. The show. *Ann Intern Med* **151**(2):139–140, 2009.
10. Engel GL. The need for a new medical model: a challenge for biomedicine. *Science* **196**(4286):129–136, 1977.
11. Cohen JJ. Remembering the real questions. *Ann Intern Med* **128**(7):563–566, 1998.
12. Prue G, Rankin J, Allen J, Gracey J, Cramp F. Cancer-related fatigue: a critical appraisal. *Eur J Cancer* **42**(7):846–863, 2006.
13. Lawrence DP, Kupelnick B, Miller K, Devine D, Lau J. Evidence report on the occurrence, assessment, and treatment of fatigue in cancer patients. *J Natl Cancer Inst Monogr* **32**:40–50, 2004.
14. Cleeland CS. Analgesic trials to clinical practice: when and how does it happen? In: Max MB, Portenoy RK, Laska E, eds. *The Design of Analgesic Clinical Trials*. New York: Raven Press, 1991:631–645. Advances in Pain Research and Therapy; vol. 18.
15. American Society of Clinical Oncology. Cancer.Net. Available from: URL: http://www.cancer.net. Accessed Feb 12, 2010.
16. National Comprehensive Cancer Network. Clinical recommendations: NCCN Clinical Practice Guidelines in Oncology™. Available from: URL: http://www.nccn.org/professionals/physician_gls/f_guidelines.asp. Accessed Feb 12, 2010.
17. National Cancer Institute. Coping with cancer: supportive and palliative care. Available from: URL: http://www.cancer.gov/cancertopics/coping. Accessed Feb 12, 2010.

Section 3 Chapter 22

Clinical Perspectives In Symptom Management and Research

The economics of cancer-related symptoms: valuing supportive-care interventions

Lesley-Ann Miller and Jane C. Weeks

Health care costs in the United States have been rising for years. Expenditures for health care in the United States grew 6.1% to $2.2 trillion in 2007, when US health care spending was about $7421 per person and accounted for 16.2% of gross domestic product.[1] These rising costs are due in part to the aging population, longer life spans, and greater prevalence of chronic illnesses.

Cancer is one of the most expensive health conditions. More than 1.4 million new cases of invasive cancer and another 1.0 million cases of basal cell and squamous cell skin cancer are projected to be diagnosed in 2008[2]; the overall cost of cancer in 2007, as estimated by the National Institutes of Health, was $219.2 billion, including $89.0 billion for direct medical costs (total of all health expenditures) and $18.2 billion for indirect morbidity costs (cost of lost productivity as a result of illness).[2]

The financial costs of cancer care are substantial, both from a societal perspective and from an individual perspective. Not only is cancer treatment expensive, but the economic burden of diagnosis and supportive care to meet patient needs throughout survival and at the end of life is also considerable. It is important to realize that over the years there has been an improvement in cancer survival, with 66% of patients with cancer surviving for at least five years.[2] The consideration that extended survival is only as good as the quality of the life it prolongs has engendered increased attention to economic factors related to the supportive care of patients with cancer.

Supportive care for patients with cancer encompasses a wide range of symptoms and conditions, ranging from less-severe issues such as nausea, vomiting, and anemia to more-severe and complex issues such as mucositis, febrile neutropenia, and pulmonary embolism. The treatments and costs for such supportive care are equally diverse. For example, the cost of treatment of febrile neutropenia in 2002 was estimated to be between $2200 and $12 100, depending on the site of care (inpatient or outpatient), and varying from one health care system to another.[3] Costs in 2002 dollars for treating mucositis were thought to exceed $47 000 for bone marrow transplant recipients[4] and $5000 per cycle for patients with solid tumors who developed postchemotherapy myelosuppression.[5] Further, new medical interventions – drugs, devices, and technology, for supportive care or otherwise – may substantially improve health outcomes, but often at considerable costs to the health care system and to patients individually.

The issue of cost related to health care is often a sensitive subject, as many clinicians believe that there is a conflict between consideration of health care costs and good clinical practice, or providing the best care for their patients. However, as supportive care therapies compete with cancer-preventive and cancer-treating interventions for the cancer-care dollar, consideration of costs is not necessarily unethical.[6] In fact, the clinical effectiveness of an intervention (or drug) is only part of the equation. Health systems operate in an environment of limited resources, which means that interventions should also be justified in economic terms. As the number of available therapeutic alternatives and the costs of such therapies continue to increase, economic analyses to inform decisions about resource allocation and cost-effectiveness of therapies for supportive care are crucial. Providing supportive care under limited health care budgets has become and will continue to be a major health care issue in the future.[7]

The rise of new interventions will require not only the standard evaluations of safety and efficacy, but also evaluations of the relative costs and benefits of the new interventions, if limited health care resources are to be used efficiently.[8,9] Economic evaluation may be performed using a variety of methods to assess the costs and consequences of comparative health care interventions. These types of evaluations may also have policy implications.

Cancer Symptom Science: Measurement, Mechanisms, and Management, eds. Charles S. Cleeland, Michael J. Fisch, and Adrian J. Dunn. Published by Cambridge University Press.

Types of economic evaluations

One of the major goals of economic research is to demonstrate the value and efficiency of various therapeutic products and services. There are many types of economic appraisals or evaluations to compare alternative therapeutic options in terms of both their costs and consequences. "Costs" refers to the economic resources consumed or expended, and "consequences" refers to the effects or outcomes.

Cost-minimization analysis

Cost-minimization analysis (CMA) is the evaluation of the costs of two or more alternative interventions that are demonstrated or assumed to be equivalent in terms of a given outcome or consequence. An example of CMA is the comparison of generic equivalents of the same drug. A generic medication must demonstrate that it is bioequivalent to the branded drug. Thus, only the cost of the medication itself needs to be compared since the outcomes should be the same.

Cost–benefit analysis

Cost–benefit analysis (CBA) is the comparison of the benefits that accrue from alternative interventions in dollars, with the costs to produce the benefits. The results from this type of analysis are in the form of the ratio of dollar costs to dollar benefits. CBA is usually used when comparing interventions where the outcomes are expressed in different units. Willingness-to-pay is a way to value health outcomes in monetary terms for cost–benefit analysis. This method quantifies or values individual (or societal) preferences for optimizing resources. It attempts to measure what people are willing to give up to get something needed, wanted, or desired.[10]

Cost-effectiveness analysis

Cost-effectiveness analysis (CEA) is the description and analysis of costs and of relevant outcomes that are expressed in natural units, for example, life-years gained. Competing interventions are compared on the basis of their relative cost-to-effectiveness ratios. CEA is used when differing therapies have a common outcome, but vary in terms of the difference in the magnitude of the effect. There are four different results that can be derived from a CEA:

(1) The new intervention is more costly and less effective than its comparator. For this result the intervention is said to be dominated by its comparator. That is, it produces worse outcomes at a higher cost.
(2) The new intervention is less costly and more effective than its comparator. For this result the intervention is said to dominate its comparator. It produces better outcomes for less money.
(3) The new intervention is less costly and less effective than its comparator. It produces fewer health benefits than the standard of care, but at a lower cost.
(4) The new intervention is more costly and more effective than its comparator. It produces more health benefits than the standard of care, but at a higher cost.

For CEA, the difference in mean cost between the two interventions (new intervention cost minus comparator cost) is divided by the difference in mean effectiveness (new intervention effectiveness minus comparator effectiveness) to get an incremental cost-effectiveness ratio (ICER).

$$\text{CER} = \frac{\Delta\text{Cost}}{\Delta\text{Effects}} = \frac{\text{Cost of New Intervention} - \text{Cost of Comparator}}{\text{Effects of New Intervention} - \text{Effects of Comparator}}$$

This ratio indicates the additional cost for obtaining one additional unit of the outcome of interest for the new intervention, compared with the comparator. The ICER is often compared with some preselected threshold value to determine whether the new intervention is lower than that threshold and thus considered to be cost effective.[11]

Cost-utility analysis

Cost-utility analysis (CUA) is the description and analysis of costs and of relevant outcomes that are measured in terms of quantity and quality of life, that is, quality-adjusted survival, in quality-adjusted life years (QALYs). The QALY concept is discussed in detail below. CUA can be used to evaluate various disease states and interventions, because the endpoint is not dependent on the condition and transcends disease states. For example, one could compare the cost per QALY for coronary artery bypass surgery versus the cost per QALY for using erythropoietin-stimulating agents in the treatment of anemia. Table 22.1 lists examples of how these evaluations are calculated. Table 22.2 shows results of a hypothetical intervention.

Table 22.1. Summary of types of economic evaluations

Study type	Cost measure	Benefit measure	Unit of analysis
Cost-minimization	Dollars	Assumed identical	Dollars
Cost–benefit	Dollars	Dollars	No units
Cost–effectiveness	Dollars	Life year (LY) or other unit of effectiveness	Cost/LY or other unit of effectiveness
Cost-utility	Dollars	QALY	Cost/QALY

QALY indicates quality-adjusted life years.

Table 22.2. Example of hypothetical intervention

Strategy	Cost	LYs gained	Utilities	QALYs gained	Benefit
New intervention	$100000	2.0	0.8	1.6	$70000
Comparator	$60000	1.0	0.7	0.7	$25000

LY indicates life years; QALY, quality-adjusted life years.

For this hypothetical scenario,

$$\text{Cost–benefit} = \frac{\$100000 - \$60000}{\$70000 - \$25000} = 0.89$$

$$\text{Cost-effectiveness ratio} = \frac{\$100\,000 - \$60\,000}{2.0 - 1.0}$$
$$= \$40\,000 \,/\, \text{life year(LY)}$$

$$\text{Cost-utility ratio} = \frac{\$100\,000 - \$60\,000}{1.6 - 0.7}$$
$$= \$44\,444 \,/\, \text{QALY}$$

Cost considerations

Perspective of the evaluation

Economic evaluations must clearly state the study perspective to be explored. The study perspective indicates the viewpoint from which the study is conducted, usually that of the key decision makers, and may include: society; third-party payers; patients; or employers, among others. According to the US Panel on Cost-Effectiveness in Health and Medicine, economic evaluations taking the societal perspective should include all the costs and consequences of health care interventions no matter who accrues them.[12] Although the societal perspective is usually recommended in most textbooks of economic evaluation, it is generally agreed that the choice of perspective depends on the purpose of the evaluation.[13] For the purposes of resource allocation, government officials may be interested in costs and benefits of a new intervention to the society at large, whereas decision makers in a managed-care organization are more likely to be interested in only the costs and benefits that would be associated with patients enrolled in their organization.

Types of costs

Costs to be included in economic evaluations can be categorized into direct and indirect costs. Direct costs include medical and nonmedical costs that are directly related to the health care intervention. Examples of direct medical costs are: drug costs or treatment costs; the cost of emergency room visits; physician visits; hospitalizations; and the cost of diagnostic testing. Examples of direct nonmedical costs are: cost for travel to hospital or clinic; and childcare or babysitting costs while the patient gets the intervention.

Indirect costs refer to time consumed by patients and their caregivers as a result of the intervention. Indirect costs may also refer to the labor-market consequences of illnesses or interventions. Examples of indirect costs are: time off from work; lost productivity due to illness or death (whether for the patient or the patient's caregiver); and cost to employers due to employee replacement or turnover.

As mentioned previously, the type of costs to be included in the economic evaluation depends on the study perspective and purpose. For example, studies using a societal perspective should include both direct and indirect costs to capture the full economic impact of the new intervention. On the other hand, studies using the managed-care or payer perspective often exclude indirect costs, as the payer's primary concern is usually the financial consequence to their particular health plan.

Time horizon

The time horizon is the duration of time being considered when evaluating clinical strategies. The time horizon should encompass the entire decision process being modeled. All events and resulting effects, both clinical and economic, should be considered within the time horizon when a clinical problem or situation is being modeled. When comparing more than one intervention, the time horizon over which the outcomes are evaluated must be the same across all potential intervention strategies in order to make a fair and appropriate comparison.

The time horizon should be explicitly stated at the outset of an economic evaluation. However, no particular time horizon can be generally recommended since the time horizon for each study should be matched to the intervention and outcomes being studied.

There are situations in which a very narrow time horizon should be used: when making decisions about acute or short-term events, it may be appropriate to use a time horizon of a few hours or days. For chronic or long-term events, a longer time horizon would be appropriate.

Discounting

The effects of time should be included in any economic evaluation with a time horizon longer than a year. Future costs and outcomes should be discounted, which would adjust for differences in preferences for money and health outcomes over time. For example, most people prefer to have money now than 5 years from now; the money they have now could be spent today, or it could be put in a bank to earn interest and be worth more in 5 years. In economic evaluations that measure costs and outcomes in different units, such as cost-effectiveness and cost-utility analyses, the general recommendation is to discount costs as well as outcomes.[11]

Inflation adjustment also needs to be considered in economic evaluations. This entails making sure that all costs included in the evaluation represent values from the same year. If an evaluation uses cost data from different years – for example, drug costs from one year and emergency room visit costs from another year – an appropriate price index (such as the Bureau of Labor Statistics Consumer Price Index for Medical Care) needs to be applied to standardize these cost values to the same year.

Sensitivity analysis

Often, cost-effectiveness and cost-utility economics evaluations will be conducted with the aid of decision analytical models. Decision analytical models are valuable in situations in which the estimate of the input parameter(s) (costs and/or outcomes) is imprecise. The key to the power of decision analysis is sensitivity analysis, a technique by which one can discover whether a particular input parameter is important in determining the preferred strategy. This tool helps to identify the sources of uncertainty that can affect the study's conclusions.

Sensitivity analysis is used to test the robustness of the conclusions of an evaluation. Given an imprecise estimate and a reasonable guess about the lowest and highest possible values of that input parameter, a one-way sensitivity analysis is performed by first inserting the lowest value of the range and conducting the evaluation then repeating that process substituting the highest value of the range. If the optimal strategy or intervention is the same in both calculations, the decision is not sensitive to the value of this particular input parameter. N-way sensitivity analyses can also be undertaken, as can probabilistic sensitivity analysis, whereby the parameter estimate is described by a distribution and a value for that parameter is randomly selected for repeated evaluations.

The quality-adjusted, life-year concept

Because health care interventions may affect both quantity and quality of life, having a measure that captures both dimensions is essential. The QALY, which weights each interval of survival time by a utility value reflecting quality of life during that interval, is such a measure.

Utilities and quality-adjusted life years

Utilities are numerical weights assigned to each health state. They are a quantitative measure of the strength of an individual's preference for a particular health state or outcome. By convention, utilities are rated on a scale of 0–1, where 0 represents death and 1 represents a state of full or perfect health (Figure 22.1).

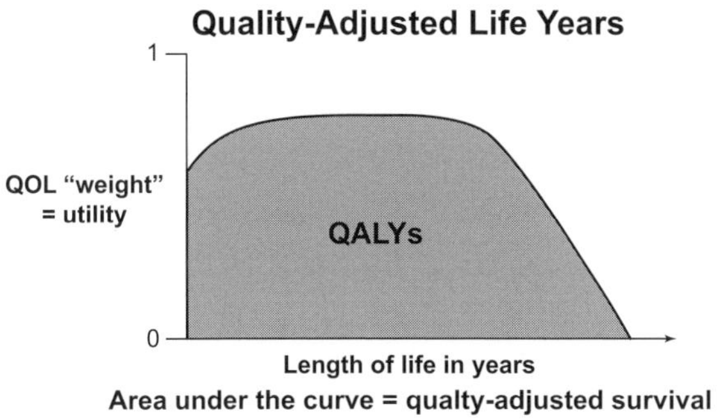

Figure 22.1. QALY equals the area under the curve of utility over time

Utilities can be estimated for disease health states and for health states brought on by the effects of an intervention or by side effects or adverse events resulting from the intervention. They can be generated by assessing a hypothetical health condition or a person's own health condition.

Three methods are commonly used to directly measure utility weights[14]: visual analogue scale (VAS), time trade-off (TTO), and standard gamble (SG):

(1) The VAS asks respondents to rate a hypothetical health state or their current health state on a "feeling thermometer," with 0 corresponding to death, and 1 corresponding to perfect health. This measurement technique does not require the individual to trade-off quality and/or quantity of life.

(2) The TTO method asks the respondent the number of years in perfect health that would be equivalent to the given number of years in the specified health state being valued. For example, the respondent is asked the years of life (y) in perfect health that would be equivalent to living for 20 years with severe pain. The QALY-weight for severe pain is then equal to y/20, meaning that the respondent is willing to give up a (20 – y)/20 proportion of their remaining life span to improve their quality of life.

(3) The SG method asks the respondent to indicate the risk of death they are willing to accept to move from the specified health state being valued to perfect health. For example, the respondent is given two options: a current condition of severe pain for 20 years with certainty; or a surgery (the gamble) that gives the respondent a probability (p) of living in normal health for 20 years, and a probability (1 – p) of immediate death. The probability (p) at which the respondent is indifferent between the two options is the utility for the severe pain. Of the three methods, the SG is preferred by economists because it is based on the von Neumann–Morgenstern utility theory.[15]

There are also indirect utility measures such as the EQ-5D and the SF-6D, which are simple, self-administered questionnaires that contain a descriptive multiattribute health-state classification system capable of generating a composite score or index reflecting the preference value associated with a given health state.

Utilities are integral to cost–utility analyses, as they provide weights for calculating QALYs and a means of quantifying relative value of one state of health compared with another in the context of decision making. A QALY is calculated by assigning the utility or quality weight to each heath state, assessing the duration of time in each health state, and then multiplying and summing. For example, if a person lives for 7 years, with 3 years in a compromised health state valued at 0.7 and 4 years in full health valued at 1.0, their total QALYs $(3 \times 0.7) + (4 \times 1.0) =$ 6.1 QALYs.

Curative vs. life-extending vs. supportive-care interventions

In exploring gains in QALYs for various types of interventions, with curative interventions, there are significant gains in QALYs by way of increase in both length and quality of life (Figure 22.2). With life-extending interventions, QALY gains are predominately due to extensions in length of life (Figure 22.3). In contrast, with supportive care or palliative interventions that have little effect on length of life, QALY gains are mostly due to improvements in quality of life (Figure 22.4).

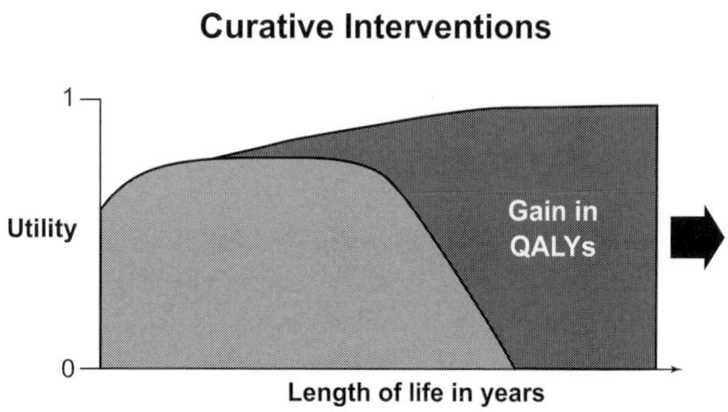

Figure 22.2. QALY gains with curative interventions

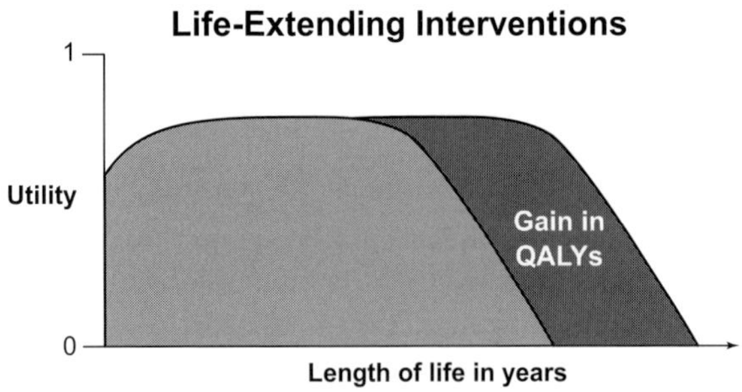

Figure 22.3. QALY gains with life-extending interventions

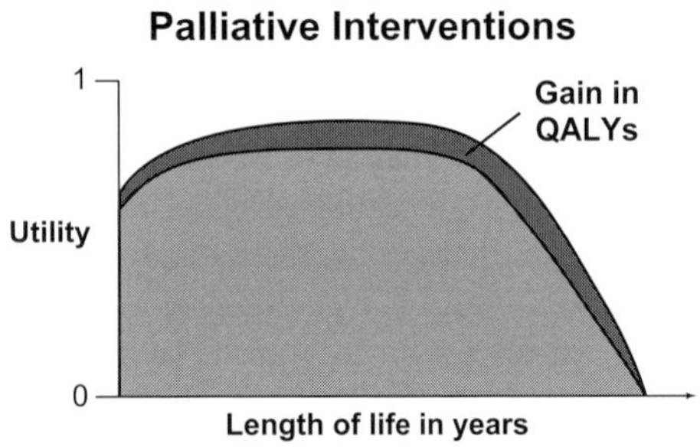

Figure 22.4. QALY gains with supportive care or palliative interventions

Cost per quality-adjusted life year and league tables

QALYs provide a common currency to assess the extent of the benefits gained from a variety of interventions in terms of quality of life and survival for patients. QALYs are used to assess the effectiveness of interventions and are combined with the costs incurred to provide the interventions to generate cost-utility ratios. Similar to the aforementioned ICER, a cost-utility ratio is the difference between the costs of two interventions divided by the difference in the QALYs they produce.

$$\text{Cost–utility ratio} = \frac{\text{Cost of Intervention A} - \text{Cost of Intervention B}}{\text{No. of QALYs produced by intervention A} - \text{No. of QALYs produced by intervention}}$$

The cost per QALY ratio can be compared with ratios from other interventions, as shown in Table 22.3. The construction and use of such QALY league tables showing the relative value of a variety of interventions has generated considerable discussion and debate, and they should be used with caution. The fact that the various studies included in such tables have been carried out at different times and in various locations and settings, and have used different methods of utility elicitation, must be considered.

Cost per QALY is currently our best measure of value per health care dollar, but it has limitations. The philosophical roots of cost-effectiveness analysis lie in utilitarianism. The focus is on the "greatest good for the greatest number" rather than how fairly those goods are distributed across individuals. An intervention that yields 0.5 QALYs for each of 20 individuals is valued exactly the same as one that yields 10 QALYs for a single individual. Cost-utility analyses consider only the absolute and not the proportional increases in length or quality of life provided by an intervention. In other words, an intervention that slightly prolongs the life of patients with a rapidly terminal illness will be valued the same as one that adds the same number of QALYs (after appropriate discounting) among healthier patients even if the proportional increase in life expectancy is substantial in the first case and only modest in the second. For these reasons, few people advocate using cost-effectiveness analysis results as the sole basis for making decisions about how best to allocate health care resources. Data on the costs and benefits of competing uses for health care resources measured in standard units across conditions can certainly inform the decision-making process, but the final decisions must also reflect societal judgments about distributional considerations.

Applications to symptom management and supportive-care treatments in cancer

There is considerable uneasiness in the supportive-care community about the prospect of using the cost-per-QALY metric to evaluate short-term treatment or interventions (such as supportive or palliative care) that enhance the quality but not the length of life. The concern is that even a highly effective new agent for preventing nausea and vomiting, for example, will not yield substantial incremental QALYs simply because the symptoms it alleviates occur only for the relatively short period during which active therapy is ongoing.

That in turn will lead to the undervaluing of those interventions compared with therapies having long-term impacts (ie, treatments that increase life expectancy by years).[22]

But is this really a limitation of the method? It can be argued that interventions that save lives should be valued more highly by society than those that relieve transient symptoms. However, it is important to recognize that cost-effectiveness analysis involves a consideration of both the incremental benefit and the incremental cost, and an intervention that relieves symptoms may be just as cost-effective as a life-prolonging one so long as the cost is proportional to the benefit. A new antiemetic drug produces only short-term quality-of-life improvements, but it is also given only a limited number of times. The cost-effectiveness ratio for this agent could easily fall within the "reasonable" range so long as the price is not extremely high. Greater attention to this ratio could lead to lower prices for these very useful agents, to the great benefit of both patients and taxpayers.

There is a real challenge in applying the cost-effectiveness framework to supportive care interventions, but it is practical rather than theoretical. The QALY benefits from symptom relief come primarily from improvements in quality rather than length of life. Preferences for a given health state vary substantially across individuals, making it challenging to measure changes in utilities induced by health care interventions, especially when those changes are rather modest. Currently available measurement strategies are theoretically robust and valid, but they may not be especially responsive to small differences or changes. Thus, further research examining the value of changes in quality of life in the context of supportive care is needed.

Strategies to improve the value for money in supportive care interventions

In oncology, new therapeutic regimens are usually associated with substantial costs. Given that drugs continue to be more and more expensive, it will be important to justify the costs of these new therapies relative to their benefits. Since we do not live in a society of unlimited resources, it is important to assess the value of new therapeutic interventions in order to prioritize various health care expenditures.

If efforts to contain costs are to succeed, health care providers must be active participants in these efforts. One way that providers can contribute is to ensure that costly supportive-care therapies are limited to those who are most likely to benefit. Risk-based prescribing of antiemetics and choice of setting of care in febrile neutropenia are excellent examples of reducing excess care and reserving high-cost, complex care for those most likely to benefit.[77] Guidelines have been successful in implementing such strategies.[23] Evidence-based guidelines should incorporate economic as well as clinical outcomes, particularly when multiple, therapeutically similar strategies are available. Cost-effectiveness analyses can inform decision makers of the trade-off between costs and outcomes (clinical as well as humanistic) of alternative therapies. Results from these analyses can be used to determine whether a higher acquisition cost of a newer agent is justifiable

Table 22.3. Example of QALY league table

Intervention	Cost/QALY
Adjuvant chemotherapy with cyclophosphamide-methotrexate-fluorouracil vs. no treatment in 50-year-old women with lymph-node positive breast cancer	\$13 000[16]
Anthracycline-based adjuvant trastuzumab regimen vs. conventional chemotherapy (without trastuzumab) alone for node-positive, HER2-positive breast cancer	\$39 000[17]
Annual vaccination vs. antiviral therapy for influenza in working adults	\$41 000[18]
Pamidronate vs. no pamidronate for breast cancer metastasis to bone	\$108 000[19]
HercepTest immunohistochemical assay, confirmed with fluorescence *in situ* hybridization followed by trastuzumab and chemotherapy for patients with positive test results and chemotherapy alone for patients with negative test results vs. no test, chemotherapy alone for metastatic HER2-positive breast cancer	\$125 000[20]
Gemcitabine plus erlotinib vs. gemcitabine alone for advanced pancreatic cancer	>\$430 000[21]

QALY indicates quality-adjusted life years; HER2, human epidermal growth factor receptor 2.

when considering its clinical superiority and the resulting resource consumption or costs avoided.

It is important for health care providers to consider the economic impact on patients when making treatment decisions. Providers should select the most cost-effective treatment, keeping in mind that what is important is the incremental cost difference for any additional benefit – which means most cost-effective may not be least expensive.

Conclusions

In summary, economic analysis involves comparing the costs and benefits of a medical care intervention with one or more other interventions. The difference between the four types of analyses described in this chapter lies in how costs are defined and outcomes are measured, as summarized in Table 22.1.

Clinicians are in a unique position to understand the health benefits of therapies and to observe the costs of these therapies. It is not in the patient's best interest to have oncologists excluded from the process of determining the cost-effectiveness of new cancer therapies. If clinicians, other cancer health care providers, and cancer researchers do not actively participate in assessing the relative costs and benefits of new oncology interventions, others – such as policy makers and politicians – will make these cost-effectiveness conclusions. Finally, vigilant cost-effectiveness and cost-utility studies are needed for many supportive-care conditions and treatments to inform clinical decision making.

References

1. Department of Health & Human Services, Centers for Medicare & Medicaid Services. National health expenditure data: Historical. Available from: URL: http://www.cms.hhs.gov/NationalHealthExpendData/02_NationalHealthAccountsHistorical.asp. Accessed Aug 11, 2009.
2. American Cancer Society. Cancer facts and figures 2008. Available from: URL: http://www.cancer.org/downloads/STT/2008CAFFfinalsecured.pdf. Accessed Aug 11, 2009.
3. Elting LS, Cantor SB. Outcomes and costs of febrile neutropenia: adventures in the science and art of treatment choices. *Support Care Cancer* **10**(3):189–196, 2002.
4. Sonis ST, Oster G, Fuchs H, et al. Oral mucositis and the clinical and economic outcomes of hematopoietic stem-cell transplantation. *J Clin Oncol* **19**(8):2201–2205, 2001.
5. Elting LS, Cooksley C, Chambers M, Martin C, Manzullo E, Rubenstein E. Outcomes of oral mucositis among cancer patients [abstract]. Multinational Association of Supportive Care in Cancer (MASCC) 14th International Symposium, Boston MA, June 23–26, 2002. *Support Care Cancer* **10**(4):363, 2002. Abstract 34.
6. Drummond M, Stoddart G, Labelle R, Cushman R. Health economics: an introduction for clinicians. *Ann Intern Med* **107**(1):88–92, 1987.
7. Elting LS, Shih YC. The economic burden of supportive care of cancer patients. *Support Care Cancer* **12**(4):219–226, 2004.
8. Trueman P, Drummond M, Hutton J. Developing guidance for budget impact analysis. *Pharmacoeconomics* **19**(6):609–621, 2001.
9. Taylor RS, Drummond MF, Salkeld G, Sullivan SD. Inclusion of cost effectiveness in licensing requirements of new drugs: the fourth hurdle. *BMJ* **329**(7472):972–975, 2004.
10. Arbuckle RB, Adamus AT, King KM. Pharmacoeconomics in oncology. *Expert Review of Pharmacoeconomics & Outcomes Research* **2**(3):251–260, 2002.
11. Drummond MF, Sculpher MJ, Torrance GW, O'Brien BJ, Stoddart GL. *Methods for the Economic Evaluation of Health Care Programmes*, 3rd ed. New York: Oxford University Press, 2005.
12. Russell LB, Gold MR, Siegel JE, Daniels N, Weinstein MC. The role of cost-effectiveness analysis in health and medicine. Panel on Cost-Effectiveness in Health and Medicine. *JAMA* **276**(14):1172–1177, 1996.
13. Gold MR. *Cost-Effectiveness in Health and Medicine.* New York: Oxford University Press, 1996.
14. Froberg DG, Kane RL. Methodology for measuring health-state preferences – II: Scaling methods. *J Clin Epidemiol* **42**(5):459–471, 1989.
15. Gafni A. The standard gamble method: what is being measured and how it is interpreted. *Health Serv Res* **29**(2):207–224, 1994.
16. Norum J. Adjuvant cyclophosphamide, methotrexate, fluorouracil (CMF) in breast cancer – is it cost-effective? *Acta Oncol* **39**(1):33–39, 2000.
17. Kurian AW, Thompson RN, Gaw AF, Arai S, Ortiz R, Garber AM. A cost-effectiveness analysis of adjuvant trastuzumab regimens in early HER2/neu-positive breast cancer. *J Clin Oncol* **25**(6):634–641, 2007.
18. Rothberg MB, Rose DN. Vaccination versus treatment of influenza in working adults: a cost-effectiveness analysis. *Am J Med* **118**(1):68–77, 2005.

19. Hillner BE, Weeks JC, Desch CE, Smith TJ. Pamidronate in prevention of bone complications in metastatic breast cancer: a cost-effectiveness analysis. *J Clin Oncol* **18**(1):72–79, 2000.

20. Elkin EB, Weinstein MC, Winer EP, Kuntz KM, Schnitt SJ, Weeks JC. HER-2 testing and trastuzumab therapy for metastatic breast cancer: a cost-effectiveness analysis. *J Clin Oncol* **22**(5):854–863, 2004.

21. Miksad RA, Schnipper L, Goldstein M. Does a statistically significant survival benefit of erlotinib plus gemcitabine for advanced pancreatic cancer translate into clinical significance and value? *J Clin Oncol* **25**(28):4506–4507, 2007.

22. Shih YC, Halpern MT. Economic evaluations of medical care interventions for cancer patients: how, why, and what does it mean? *CA Cancer J Clin* **58**(4):231–244, 2008.

23. Bennett CL, Weeks JA, Somerfield MR, Feinglass J, Smith TJ. Use of hematopoietic colony-stimulating factors: comparison of the 1994 and 1997 American Society of Clinical Oncology surveys regarding ASCO clinical practice guidelines. Health Services Research Committee of the American Society of Clinical Oncology. *J Clin Oncol* **17**(11):3676–3681, 1999.

Section 4 Chapter 23

Symptom Measurement

Symptom measurement by patient report

Charles S. Cleeland and Tito R. Mendoza

The symptoms of both cancer and cancer treatment (eg, pain, fatigue, poor appetite, sleep disturbance, and cognitive impairment), like the symptoms of other chronic diseases, can significantly impair a patient's quality of life, comfort, and ability to function. The inability to tolerate treatment-related symptoms often preempts full and effective treatment, and residual symptoms of treatment may limit the functioning of those who are otherwise cured of the disease.

Reducing the severity and impact of symptoms is naturally an endpoint for clinical trials that include symptom-focused interventions. In contrast, symptom management during clinic visits requires planning that is based on the clinician's having the best possible information about the patient's symptom status. Because clinicians and patients commonly face choices among treatments that are similarly effective for tumor control and prolonging survival, differences in the patient's symptoms during the survival period have become critical variables in making individualized treatment choices and in developing new therapies. Thus, having the ability to compare treatment-related symptoms provides an additional benchmark for appraising various cancer treatments. Policy planning and quality assurance also depend on information about the extent and severity of symptoms. All of these objectives require symptom measurement, the focus of this chapter.

Although symptoms are based on complex biological and behavioral phenomena, as subjective experiences their measurement is typically restricted to self-report. This chapter presents a status report on characterizing and measuring cancer-related symptoms by asking the patient about them using single items, single-symptom multi-item measures, and multisymptom questionnaires.

Symptoms and patient-reported outcomes

Symptom assessment by patient report

A symptom report is the patient's statement of their sensation or perception of disturbance in normal function that is caused by disease or treatment of disease. Because a symptom can only be known through the patient's *subjective* report, it is by definition a patient-reported outcome (PRO) and can be classified on the basis of its severity and its perceived impact on function. The term "PRO" encompasses all clinical and clinical-research information obtained from patients responding to questions. In contrast, a sign or laboratory value, such as elevated white blood cell count or reduced hemoglobin, is *objective* evidence of the presence of a disease or toxicity of therapy.

Measuring PROs is today a highly dynamic area of both discussion and investigation. Several factors have contributed to this dynamism. First, realizing the importance of accurately representing the patient's response to both disease and treatment, the National Institutes of Health (NIH), as part of its Roadmap Program, has made a significant investment in attempting to increase the measurement precision of patient self-report questionnaires.[1] Second, the US Food and Drug Administration (FDA) has issued guidance for the pharmaceutical industry entitled *Patient-reported outcome measures: use in medical product development to support labeling claims*, which describes how self-report measures are to be used for making claims about the effectiveness of agents for which approval is being sought.[2] Third, there is increasing recognition in the general public, along with policy debate, that the relative impact of therapy on symptoms and functional status may influence the selection of one treatment over another. In 2002, the NIH convened a State-of-the-Science Conference on Symptom Management (http://consensus.nih.gov) to review the current state of knowledge, provide recommendations, and identify potential future projects to help patients with cancer by treating their pain, depression, and fatigue.[3] A key issue was the need for refinement and utilization of symptom-report measures.

Cancer Symptom Science: Measurement, Mechanisms, and Management, eds. Charles S. Cleeland, Michael J. Fisch, and Adrian J. Dunn.

Desirable properties of a symptom measure

The ideal symptom assessment measure should be brief and easy to complete, so as to place minimal burden on ill respondents. Brevity is particularly important if the symptom measure is used repeatedly to monitor changes in symptoms over time. A symptom measure must also be easy to understand, so that a patient with limited educational background can complete it with minimal assistance. Availability in multiple languages is important, especially in settings where patients come from diverse linguistic and ethnic groups. In addition, a good symptom assessment measure should be applicable in both clinical and research settings. Finally, the scores derived from the measure need to intuitively "mean something" for both the patients reporting symptoms and the clinicians and researchers making decisions about them.

Relationship of symptom reports to other patient-reported outcomes

Patient-reported outcomes can take a variety of forms, including measures of symptom severity and functional impact. Symptom reports are a subset of a larger domain of patient perceptions about health status referred to as health-related quality of life (HRQOL). A consensus among health researchers is that HRQOL is a multidimensional construct comprising at least four dimensions: physical function (eg, daily activities, self care); psychological function (eg, emotional or mental state, mood); social role function (eg, social interactions, family dynamics); and disease-related or treatment-related symptoms (eg, pain, nausea).[4] Most HRQOL measures therefore include questions that evaluate the severity of at least some symptoms. Commonly used HRQOL measures, including the Medical Outcomes Study Short Form-36 (SF-36),[5] the Functional Assessment of Cancer Therapy (FACT),[6] and the European Organisation for Research and Treatment of Cancer Quality of Life Questionnaire (EORTC QLQ-C30),[7] address major symptoms such as pain, depression, fatigue, and nausea. In the EORTC QLQ-C30, 18 of 30 items are self-reported symptoms. HRQOL measures also ask questions about various dimensions of patient perception, such as societal role function and concerns about social support. In most conceptualizations of HRQOL, symptoms can be viewed as the patient report closest to the physical and psychological perceptions of the disease process and the immediate effects of treatment on these perceptions.[8]

An approach to measuring symptoms

We cannot put pain, fatigue, or nausea in a petri dish or weigh them on a scale, even though we "know" that these symptoms are real and that some people seem to experience them more frequently and severely than do others. Symptoms are only known by what people tell us. Statements about symptoms (such as, "I am in terrible pain") are reports of experiences that have common meaning, as each receiver of the report will have generally shared an experience somewhat like the reporter (ie, the patient) is describing. Without that background, the receiver of the report would not be able to attach much meaning to it. In other words, a person who has never experienced pain might find a pain report hard to comprehend.

We can share information about our symptoms because others have experienced them as well and have used similar language to describe the experience. Most of this language is very general, however, and does not help us quantify how much or how little of the symptom is being experienced. Symptom measurement depends on shaping our understanding of this common language to maximize the precision of the communication between the person experiencing the symptom and the people who need to know about it. In the true sense, self-reported symptoms are "constructs," internal bodily and mental states that we cannot know in an objective manner, as we can height or weight. For an in-depth review of psychological constructs see the classic paper by Cronbach and Meehl.[9] The measurement of such constructs as symptoms depends on the science of psychometrics, a specialized tradition that has its roots in the measurement of educational achievement, public opinion, and psychological states. The primary domain of psychometrics is measuring the precision of self-report.

Many investigators are suspicious of subjective reports as real scientific data, and this had led to persistent efforts to find objective symptom measures. In fact, there are multiple biological correlates of symptom report, including changes in autonomic function and various laboratory-determined values and changes reflected in brain imaging methods. To some, these physiological measures are a more satisfying portrayal of the "real" nature of symptoms than are subjective reports, and they supposedly minimize known sources of measurement variability in symptom reporting, such as social or environmental expectations, mood state, or personality characteristics. Nonetheless, the veracity and relevance of physiological measures are dependent on symptom self-report. As illustrated in other chapters in this book, understanding the associations between physical events and self-report is critical if we are to make any headway in understanding the mechanistic basis of symptoms. There is currently no substitute for self-report in understanding symptoms.

Symptom burden: the impact of cancer-related symptoms

Considerable progress has been made in some aspects of symptom measurement. We have found that the task of measuring multiple symptoms is helped conceptually by introducing the concept of symptom burden, which, in cancer, is the subjective counterpart of tumor burden and has parallels with the concept of disease burden. Symptom burden encompasses not only the severity of each of the patient's symptoms, but also the overall effect of the symptoms on the patient's daily functioning. Thus, we define symptom burden as the combined impact of all symptoms (related to disease, therapy, or both) on the ability of people to function as they did before the onset of the disease or therapy.[8] Although the term "symptom burden" has most often been used for cancer, it has also been applied to the study of other chronic illnesses, such as diabetes, asthma, and HIV infection.[10–12]

Symptom interference with functioning

As symptoms become more severe, they exert increasing impact on how patients feel and function, such that rating only the severity of a symptom may miss crucial information that should be included even in the most abbreviated symptom assessment. Like the symptoms themselves, the dimensions of function affected by symptoms are also constructs. Pain, for example, is liable to influence a variety of social, emotional, functional, and even spiritual domains; the degree of influence will depend on the individual. If one were to carry this to the extreme, one could attempt to find all the feelings and functions that were diminished for a patient as pain increased and to try to capture a representation of all of these dimensions when measuring pain – an impractical measurement goal.

A good clinician will attempt to get as broad a perspective on what impact a symptom will have on various aspects of the person's life, but it is impossible to capture these multiple dimensions in a symptom assessment tool. The evolving compromise is to get an estimate of a more global dimension – usually, how much the symptoms interfere with or distress the patient. In our own approach, we have asked the patient to estimate how much symptoms interfere with common feelings and functions.[13] Others have asked patients how much distress is caused by a symptom that is also being rated for its severity. For example, patients are asked to rate its severity, frequency, and distress for each symptom item in the Memorial Symptom Assessment Scale (MSAS).[14] For pain, an emerging consensus suggests that the measurement of symptom interference is important,[15] and this probably applies to other symptoms as well.

Finally, patients may be asked to estimate the frequency or duration of a symptom during a period of time, on the basis of the assumption that a symptom that is present for a few hours (or minutes) during a day (or week) will likely have less impact on the patient than a symptom that is present chronically. Although this assumption makes sense intuitively, it needs to be examined in clinical studies.

This relationship between symptom severity and impact is not necessarily a linear function, and the correlations of the dimensions of symptom impact with severity are not perfect. For example, an increase of one point at the lower end of a severity scale has only a modest impact on a patient's functional status. Similarly, once the symptom becomes severe, additional one-point increases in severity have relatively little impact on changes in function, as the impact is already high.[16,17]

Symptom clusters

By its very nature, symptom burden results from a composite of multiple symptoms experienced simultaneously. Studies documenting the multiplicity of symptoms experienced by cancer patients[13,18–20] have shown that pain, fatigue, sleep disturbance, emotional distress, and poor appetite co-occur almost universally. The term "symptom cluster" refers to two or more symptoms following the same time course in response to disease or treatment.[21,22] Certain severe symptoms, such as pain, fatigue, difficulties with concentration, and disturbed sleep, appear together in sick patients across various diseases and treatments. Possible biological mechanisms that may cause symptoms to occur together are the subject of many chapters in this book.

Considerations in measuring symptoms

Types of instruments

Single-item measures

The simplest assessment of a symptom is to have the patient rate its severity using a single item. For example, a patient may be asked to rate their pain on a 0–10 scale with 0 defined as "no pain" and 10 defined as "pain as bad as you can imagine" or "the most severe pain." Single-symptom items have at times been combined to create multisymptom measures (described below) of common symptoms experienced by patients with cancer, such as nausea, distress, fatigue/tiredness, and appetite loss – eg, the M. D. Anderson Symptom Inventory (MDASI)[13] or the Edmonton Symptom Assessment Scale (ESAS).[23,24] Several of the more-complex HRQOL measures represent some symptoms as single items. Single-item measures have been shown to be sensitive to clinically relevant parameters and to treatment effects and are often reported in the clinical trials literature; some have been recommended as outcome measures for use in clinical trials for some symptoms, such as pain severity.[25]

Single-symptom questionnaires have their detractors. Certain standard psychometric assays used with PROs – for example, estimations of internal consistency – are not available for single-item measures. Some would contend that more than one item is required to represent any symptom because symptoms are constructs, which, by definition, require more than one item for full representation. Nevertheless, single items tend to correlate highly with single-symptom, multi-item measures.[26]

The relative trust in single items depends on the conceptual complexity of the symptoms they address. Most would have little trouble accepting single items to represent such symptoms as nausea, vomiting, and shortness of breath. In contrast, the use of single items for other symptom constructs, such as fatigue (where the single item might be "rate the severity of your tiredness/fatigue") are hotly debated. Some contend that such a single item cannot capture the multidimensionality of fatigue, with its physical, mental, and affective components. A practical reality is that, in clinical assessment, the probability that patients will be asked more than one question about each symptom is slim, especially when these questions need to be asked repeatedly to monitor clinical status over time.

Single-symptom, multi-item measures

Numerous multiple-item assessment tools have been developed to measure a single symptom, such as pain, fatigue, or sleep disturbance. Only a subset of these measures have been specifically developed for and validated in patients with cancer. Multi-item measures directed at single symptoms illustrate the idea that a symptom, such as pain, really is a construct, and that the adequate representation of this construct needs to sample two or more dimensions of the construct (eg, both symptom severity and symptom interference, as discussed above). These dimensions need to be mapped to subsets of items that will represent those dimensions. Factor analysis is typically used to determine which items map to the corresponding underlying constructs by examining factor loadings, guided by the principle of simple structure. In the next sections, we discuss several examples of single-symptom, multi-item measures (see also Table 23.1).

Pain assessment instruments. A measure of pain should reflect (1) important aspects of what a person with pain experiences; and (2) how pain is expected to change as a result of the study to be conducted or the treatment to be administered. These issues have been the focus of a long-standing working group called the Initiative on Methods, Measurement, and Pain Assessment in Clinical Trials (IMMPACT, see http://www.immpact.org). The collective publications of this working group, available on its website, are an important resource for persons planning symptom trials. IMMPACT has specified domains of measurement that should be considered in a clinical pain study, such as pain severity, pain interference, and effects of the treatment on other symptoms, including mood. One single-symptom, multi-item measure that assesses these recommended dimensions is the Brief Pain Inventory (BPI).[27,28]

The BPI has become one of the more widely used measurement tools for assessing clinical pain. Initially developed for use with cancer patients, the BPI allows patients to rate (1) the severity of their pain; and (2) the degree to which their pain interferes with common dimensions of feeling and function. The BPI has been shown to be an appropriate measure for pain caused by a wide range of clinical conditions.

Although the BPI is a single-symptom measure, it was designed to measure two dimensions of pain: pain severity and pain's interference with function. Many investigators have found that two dimensions of pain

Table 23.1. Commonly used single-symptom and multiple-symptom scales and instruments

Pain	Fatigue	Multiple symptoms
Single-item NRS	Single-item NRS	Single-item NRS
Single-item VAS	Brief Fatigue Inventory[32]	European Organisation for Research and Treatment of Cancer QLQ C30[7]
Single-item VRS	Cancer Fatigue Scale[34]	Rotterdam Symptom Checklist[43]
Brief Pain Inventory[17]	Fatigue Symptom Inventory[35]	M. D. Anderson Symptom Inventory[13]
McGill Pain Questionnaire[92] Short-form McGill Pain Questionnaire[31]	Functional Assessment of Cancer Therapy – Anemia Subscale[36,93]	Symptom Distress Scale[44]
Medical Outcomes Study SF-36 bodily pain scale[5]	Lee Fatigue Scale[37]	The Memorial Symptom Assessment Scale[14]
European Organisation for Research and Treatment of Cancer QLQ-C30 bodily pain scale[7]	Multidimensional Fatigue Inventory[38]	Symptom Monitor[45]
	The Piper Fatigue Scale[39]	Edmonton Symptom Assessment System[23]
	Schwartz Cancer Fatigue Scale[40]	

NRS indicates numerical rating scale; VAS, visual analog scale; VRS, verbal rating scale.

self-report account for most of the variability in the way patients describe pain. Beecher[29] called these dimensions "pain" and "reaction to pain"; Clark and Yang[30] called them "sensory-discriminative" and "attitudinal." Following Beecher, we called these dimensions "sensory" and "reactive."[28] To capture the sensory construct, the BPI asks patients to rate the severity of their pain now, at its worst, at its least, and on average using 0–10 scales. To capture the reactive construct, patients are asked to rate how much pain interferes with such everyday functions as general activity, mood, walking ability, normal work activities, relations with other people, sleep, and enjoyment of life.

Other tools that are commonly used for pain assessment in cancer are the Short-Form McGill Pain Questionnaire (recently revised),[31] the bodily pain subscale of the SF-36,[5] and the EORTC QLQ-C30 pain scale.[7]

Fatigue assessment instruments. Fatigue, the most common symptom described by patients with cancer, is endemic during cancer treatment and in advanced disease. Substantial debate is being waged over how best to measure fatigue, which many agree is multidimensional, having physical, mental, and, perhaps, emotional components. It has been argued that single-item fatigue measures and short single-symptom, multi-item measures are too simplistic to represent the complex construct of fatigue; conversely, measures that attempt to capture the complexity of fatigue have many more items and take longer to complete, making them more burdensome for longitudinal administration than the shorter measures.

The Brief Fatigue Inventory (BFI)[32] is a single-symptom, multi-item measure that evolved from the Brief Pain Inventory. The BFI is useful for rapid assessment of fatigue severity in clinical screening and clinical trials. We developed the BFI along the lines of the BPI and examined its psychometric properties in inpatients and outpatients with cancer and in a comparison sample of community-dwelling adults. As with the BPI, the BFI asks patients to rate their fatigue or tiredness on three items assessing fatigue severity and six items assessing how much fatigue interferes with daily functioning. Although our aim in constructing the BFI was to capture both fatigue severity and interference, several studies have demonstrated that the underlying structure of the BFI items suggests a single dimension underlying all items. This single-factor result for the BFI is consistent with the report of Lai et al.[33] that, on the basis of results from 555 patients with cancer who responded to 72 fatigue items, cancer-related fatigue can be considered unidimensional.

Other single-symptom, multi-item measures for fatigue include the Cancer Fatigue Scale,[34] Fatigue Symptom Inventory,[35] the FACT Fatigue Scale,[36] Lee Fatigue Scale,[37] Multidimensional Fatigue Inventory,[38] the revised Piper Fatigue Scale,[39] and the Schwartz Cancer Fatigue Scale.[40]

Item banks for individual symptoms. The Patient-Reported Outcomes Measurement Information System (PROMIS) is an NIH-funded initiative tasked with developing a more fluid, yet consistent, measurement system for PROs. PROMSIS is developing and testing a large bank of items that measure PROs and is creating a computerized adaptive testing system that allows for efficient, psychometrically robust assessment of PROs in clinical research.[41] PROMIS is using item response theory (IRT) to generate a list of patient self-report questions based on initial cues.

Although the PROMIS measures represent a major advance in the development of PROs because of item banking and its methodical IRT approach, much work remains to be done to provide evidence for the utility of the PRO measures that would lead to clinicians' acceptance of their use.

Multisymptom measures

A theme of this book is that many symptoms commonly occur together and that they may very well share biological mechanisms. As mentioned above, these co-occurring symptoms have been labeled "symptom clusters." The definition of a true symptom cluster is evolving with the development of multiple-symptom measures, several of which have been designed for use with cancer patients. An ideal multisymptom assessment tool should include the symptoms that occur most frequently and are most distressing to patients. At the same time, the assessment should be short, easy to understand, and applicable in both clinical and research settings. Given that symptoms have an adverse impact on function and activity, symptom measures should also assess the interference with different activities caused by these symptoms, as viewed from the patients' perspective.

Multisymptom inventories can be used to identify symptoms that are prevalent and distressing across various cancers and treatments. For example, the M. D. Anderson Symptom Inventory (MDASI) is a brief measure of the severity and impact of cancer-related symptoms regardless of cancer or treatment type.[13,42] The MDASI was developed on the basis of our previous efforts to assess the severity and interference of single symptoms, including the development of the Brief Pain Inventory and the Brief Fatigue Inventory.[28,32] The MDASI asks patients to rate the severity of 13 symptoms that are common in patients with cancer once treatment begins: fatigue; disturbed sleep; pain; drowsiness; poor appetite; nausea; vomiting; shortness of breath; numbness; difficulty remembering; dry mouth; distress; and sadness. Patients rate each symptom's presence and greatest severity in the previous 24 hours on an 11-point (0–10) scale, with 0 representing "not present" and 10 representing "as bad as you can imagine." The MDASI also contains six items that assess the degree to which symptoms have interfered with aspects of the patient's life in the previous 24 hours: general activity; mood; walking ability; normal work (including work outside the home and housework); relations with other people; and enjoyment of life. Each interference item is also rated on an 11-point scale, with 0 signifying "did not interfere" and 10 signifying "interfered completely."

Other most commonly used multisymptom assessment tools include the EORTC QLQ-C30,[7] the Rotterdam Symptom Checklist,[43] the Symptom Distress Scale,[44] the MSAS,[14] the ESAS,[23] and the symptom monitor.[45]

Length of the instrument: thoroughness versus assessment burden

The dynamic tension inherent in symptom assessment is to deploy instruments that gather enough information to adequately represent the symptom without overwhelming the patient with too many questions. As noted above, there is ongoing debate over whether single-item symptom measures and single-symptom, multi-item measures are robust enough to represent the complex constructs of certain symptoms (such as pain and fatigue), or whether longer, multiple-symptom measures with several items per symptom would more thoroughly describe the symptoms. Multiple items are somewhat more stable over time and may better represent the extremes of the symptom's severity at its lowest and highest levels. At issue is the degree of assessment burden – the cost in time and complexity of asking multiple as opposed to single items, especially in longitudinal studies.

It may be that precision at the extremes of symptom severity do not contribute much to clinical decision making or trial evaluation, as change within units of these extremes may not be very clinically meaningful. For example, reduction of fatigue from "extremely severe" to "very severe" may not be of much interest to patients or contribute to the evaluation of treatment effectiveness. However, if asked, patients might well say that a significant reduction in their single-item rating of fatigue or tiredness would be meaningful indeed. Although symptom measurement research is finally beginning to incorporate patient views of outcomes (sometimes called qualitative research), substantially more such research is needed.

The debate as to whether a single symptom severity rating item is "good enough" will go on for some time. The adequacy of single items for symptoms such as fatigue, distress, and sadness certainly needs more study. Clinicians are not yet convinced that patient-reported outcomes – even simple single-symptom items – contribute to patient care, and this attitude does not seem to be changing.[46] Perhaps the computer-administered item bank being developed by the PROMIS is one answer to the dilemma: a limited number of items for each symptom might be more satisfying psychometrically than single items. In any event, the debate will continually be driven by the practicality of the use of symptom PROs in the clinical situation.

Response options

Types of response scales

Symptom assessment involves asking the patient to rate the intensity of a given symptom, or the degree to which that symptom interferes with function, using some type of response scale that frames the patient's answer. The simplest type of scale is a dichotomous one that asks the patient to indicate the presence or absence of a particular symptom. Yes/no responses, however, provide little information about the characteristics of a symptom. Most response scales included in symptom measures ask patients to rate a symptom on a graded scale that provides information about intensity, frequency, or distress. The intensity (severity) and other characteristics of a symptom (eg, frequency or level of distress or interference caused by the symptom) can be rated using various response options, the most common of which are visual analogue scales (VAS), verbal rating scales (VRS), and numerical rating scales (NRS).

Visual Analogue Scale. The VAS usually consists of a horizontal or vertical straight line, often about 10 cm in length or height. One end of the line represents the absence of the symptom and the other end represents an extreme of severity, such as "as bad as you can imagine" or "as severe as can be." The patient is asked to place a mark across the line indicating how much of the scale is equivalent to the severity (or frequency, unpleasantness, etc.) of the symptom.

Verbal rating scales. Verbal rating scales, sometimes called verbal descriptor scales, are categorical scales that ask patients to choose a verbal descriptor that best describes a symptom. A simple VRS might include "none," "mild," "moderate," and "severe."

Numerical rating scales. Many symptom measures use NRS that ask patients to rate their symptoms by assigning a number to the severity of the symptom. The scales typically range from 0–5, 0–10, or 0–100. Numerical scales usually are presented horizontally, with a verbal anchor given for each end of the scale, but with the intervening numbers not described. For example, the "0" end of a symptom scale assessing pain may be defined as "no pain," and the other end may be defined as "pain as bad as you can imagine" or "very severe pain."

Choice of response scale

The NRS, VAS, and VRS have been employed extensively in symptom research. Each response scale has its own advantages and shortcomings. For example, the VAS requires that patients understand the analogue concept, often necessitates considerable instruction and supervision from clinical or research staff, and requires additional time for scoring of the patients' responses by measuring the line. Gagliese et al.[47] reported that VAS has a high rate of unscorable data and tends to be less accurate. However, Breivik et al.[48] found that both VAS and NRS are equally sensitive to changes in pain intensity.

The VRS assume that patients have approximately the same meaning in mind when choosing the descriptor that best describes their symptom. This assumption is questionable given that patients come from diverse educational, cultural, and linguistic backgrounds.[17,49] Nonetheless, Lund et al.[50] favored using the VRS in pain intensity assessments because of its high test–retest reliability, and Li et al.[51] found that the VRS had low error rates compared with either the NRS or VAS.

The NRS is generally considered easier than the VAS for patients to understand. The use of numbers instead of words may remove some sources of cultural and linguistic variation that might occur with verbal descriptor scales.[49,52] Hollen et al.[53] reported that NRS scores adequately reproduced VAS scores and went further by adopting the NRS in the Lung Cancer Symptom Scale to replace the original VAS. In fatigue assessment, when the 42-item Piper Fatigue Scale was first developed, it was available in both 0–100 VAS and 0–10 NRS versions.[54] The much shorter revised Piper Fatigue Scale uses the NRS version because the NRS resulted in fewer missing data, whereas the increased measurement sensitivity supposedly provided by the VAS was not clinically significant.[39] The Lee Fatigue

Scale,[37] which originally used a VAS, was rescaled to a 0–10 NRS in its subsequent version.[55]

Number of response options

The number of response options (eg, a 5-point scale vs. an 11-point scale) and the degree to which scale descriptors (eg, mild vs. moderate) affect patient responses has been examined.[56–58] The literature is conflicting on whether variations in response-option format produce measurement error or bias; some studies[59–62] have reported that response format has a consequential effect, whereas others[63,64] suggest that it has a marginal effect. Preston and Colman[65] conducted a study to compare the reliability, validity, discriminating power, and respondent preferences of a 5-item questionnaire assessing quality of service using 11 different response categories (2, 3, 4, 5, 6, 7, 8, 9, 10, 11, and 101 response options), with the order randomly presented. They found that on several indices of reliability, validity, and discriminating power, the 2-point, 3-point, and 4-point scales performed poorly. The most reliable were scales with 7–10 response categories. The most discriminating scales had 6 or more response categories. Respondent preferences were highest for the 10-point scale, closely followed by the 7-point and 9-point scales. Aside from this study, there has been very little qualitative testing of response options, a neglected component of symptom measurement research.

In the end, a good test of the best response option is to pilot test the ease of use and meaningfulness of the option in the population targeted for study. It would also be helpful to examine the distributions of responses using the response format selected to ensure that the potential spectrum of responses are adequately represented.

Psychometric validity

Any measure, whether of weight, blood pressure, or hematocrit, must demonstrate stability, or reproducibility, across various time points (reliability), present an accurate representation of something important for us to know about (validity), and be able to reflect changes in that something that are meaningful (sensitivity). Patient reported outcomes, including symptom reports, also must meet similar standards of measurement. The science of psychometrics provides methods for making judgments about these attributes as they pertain to self-report measures. Much of psychometric methodology comes from educational and psychological testing and is summarized in the periodically updated Standards for Educational and Psychological Testing of the American Psychological Association.[66] The Standards, which outline the principles that are the core of any validation process, are required reading for those wishing to understand how self-report measures function or how to develop new self-report measures. Much of what is incorporated in the FDA guidance for patient-reported outcomes[2] is based on these standards.

Because symptom reports are constructs – Paul Meehl somewhat facetiously called such constructs "useful fictions"[9] – the validation of an instrument is never complete. There will never be a perfectly validated symptom self-report measure. Validation is an incremental process in which we learn more about an instrument's characteristics each time it is used. Over time, each measurement tool develops a "dossier" of information that allows a potential user to make judgments about whether or not its measurement characteristics suit the intent of her or his study.

Reliability

Test–retest reliability. If patients are asked to rate their symptoms more than once within a short time frame and there is no reason that symptoms should be expected to change, symptom-rating values should be very similar each time. As a frame of reference, the correlations between the ratings of the same item at these various times are considered adequate if they equal or exceed 0.70.[67] This type of consistency in measurement is known as "test–retest reliability." Because the symptoms of patients with cancer can change fairly rapidly, test–retest reliability is best assessed in patients whose symptoms and disease status are relatively stable during the time of measurement.

Internal consistency reliability. Another measure of reliability is internal consistency, or the degree to which individual items in a measure correlate with the total score to which the item contributes. One of the most widely used measures of internal consistency reliability is the Cronbach alpha.[68] The Cronbach alpha can be thought of as the average correlation calculated from all possible combinations of items when split into two half-tests; its value generally increases if items correlate highly among themselves.

Ideally, a symptom measure will be only as lengthy as necessary to characterize the symptoms of interest. Item redundancy can increase the length of a measure and the effort required to complete it, and should thus be avoided.

Because highly intercorrelated items are likely to be redundant and may not provide additional information about the construct being measured, only moderate inter-item correlations are desirable when selecting the final set of items for a measure.[69] Performing cluster analysis and dropping items that respondents perceive to be highly similar is another way of addressing this issue.[13]

Validity

Content validity. Self-report measures need to be more than just stable or consistent. The term "validation" is sometimes used broadly to include all the steps used to evaluate a self-report instrument. However, in a more technical psychometric sense, "validity" refers to evidence that the assessment instrument is actually capturing the concept or concepts it is designed to measure. An assessment instrument has content validity if it appears to measure the construct of interest. Cronbach and Meehl[9] suggested that if an instrument measures what it is intended to measure, it has logical relationships with other constructs. For example, a measure of pain should reflect salient aspects of what a person with pain experiences.

Content validity is related to face validity, which reflects the judgment of stakeholders who will use the measurement tool (health care professionals and patients) that the instrument appropriately represents what it is intended to measure. Clinicians have long been consulted on item selection, but the incorporation of patient input into the measurement process is becoming a new standard of validation not stressed in the APA standards.[66] The FDA's guidance imposes the common-sense criteria that a PRO measurement needs to "make sense" to the patients who will be asked to complete the measure, and should incorporate symptoms relevant to the disease/treatment to be evaluated.[2,70] This typically involves patient interviewing and commenting at several steps in the item-development process, a method known as "qualitative research" or "cognitive debriefing." If a new measurement tool is being created, this partially ensures that the items and scales are meaningful and understood by patients.[71] If an existing assessment tool is to be used in a study, cognitive debriefing supports the appropriateness of using the tool in that particular study or trial. For an illustration of how qualitative methods are used to develop a symptom measure, see Wang et al.[72] The FDA guidance recommends that cognitive debriefing studies be included in the medical product's dossier to support labeling claims.[2]

Convergent validity. Convergent validity indicates whether scores agree with results from a similar-but-independent measure. Convergent-related validity is determined by correlating the new assessment measure with a known "gold standard" for assessing the variable of interest (the symptom). Unfortunately, few gold standards are available for measuring symptoms. Some studies of convergent validity have used previously validated measures of the symptom or symptom-specific subscales from validated HRQOL measures, such as the pain items from the SF-36 or the fatigue subscale of the Profile of Mood States, to estimate measurement convergence.

Known-group validity. Known-group validity refers to the ability of the instrument to differentiate between groups in a predictable way. For example, cancer patients with poor performance status or late-stage disease should demonstrate higher symptom burden on the measurement instrument compared with patients who have good performance status or early-stage disease, respectively. Similarly, patients undergoing aggressive therapy should have higher severity levels of treatment-related symptoms (such as fatigue) later on in their treatment, compared with pretreatment symptom severity.

Sensitivity to change

Whereas known-group validity is cross-sectional in nature, a measure's sensitivity is assessed repeatedly over the time that symptoms are expected to change. A symptom measure should be able to demonstrate change in the expected direction with treatments known to be effective for the symptom; for example, pain severity ratings should improve when the patient receives appropriate analgesics for pain. Similarly, patients undergoing aggressive cancer therapy are expected to experience worsening symptoms as they progress through their treatment regimen, and a symptom assessment tool should be able to detect those expected changes.

Interpreting patient-reported symptom data

The minimum clinically important difference

Widespread use of an instrument depends on how well clinicians and researchers can use and interpret scores derived from the tool. Once a tool's validity has been established, the next step is to determine the instrument's minimal clinically important difference (MCID; or minimally important difference, MID) in symptom scores. With large enough sample sizes, very small differences in symptom ratings can be statistically significant, yet offer little value to patients and health care providers making treatment decisions. Determining the MCID in the field of health-related quality-of-life can facilitate the interpretability of symptom scores. Two approaches are used to determine the MCID: distribution-based methods and the anchor-based methods.[73] One approach is not preferred over the other, and one clinical significance consensus panel[74] suggested that the procedures within each method are not sufficient by themselves but are complementary, especially when their respective results are consistent.

Using distribution-based methods

Distribution-based methods compare the change in symptom scores seen in a clinical trial to measures of variability in score distributions, such as the standard deviation, the effect size, or the standard error of measurement (SEM). For effect sizes, variability of symptom reports at baseline for all trial patients is typically used. However, estimates of variability can potentially vary from one study to another depending on the heterogeneity of the patient sample.

One approach for the distribution-based method is to set the MCID as one-half standard deviation of the symptom scores at baseline.[75,76] Cohen's effect-size guidelines, which attach values to the magnitude of an effect, can also be used to aid interpretation of symptom scores.[77] The SEM can be calculated to further minimize the impact of population heterogeneity. This is computed as the baseline standard deviation multiplied by the square root of (1 minus the reliability of the symptom scores); for any longitudinal study, either of two estimates of reliabilities, internal consistency and test–retest reliability, can be used. Wyrwich et al.[78] demonstrated that a criterion of 1 SEM was closely related to the anchor-based approach when determining the MCID for the Chronic Respiratory Questionnaire and the Chronic Heart Failure Questionnaire.

Using anchor-based methods

As the name implies, this method requires the use of an "anchor," which typically is a question or set of questions designed to compare the patient's judgment of degree of change in a variable (eg, a rating of health status) that is logically associated with the change. The anchor can either be individual-focused (single anchor) or population-focused (multiple anchors). Both approaches require that the anchor by itself is interpretable and that the anchor is related to symptoms. An example of the single-anchor method might be an item stating, "Compared with your last treatment, how do you rate your symptom now?" with possible response options of "better," "no change," or "worse." The average symptom score that falls into each value of this item constitutes an MCID. This strategy is consistent with approaches used in developing MCIDs for the Chronic Heart Failure Questionnaire.[79] For the multiple-anchor method, this procedure can be extended by using candidate variables such as disease severity, disease progression, response to treatment, or treatment discontinuation.

Using cut points to determine treatment responders

Categorizing symptoms as mild, moderate, or severe may be useful for interpreting clinically significant changes in symptom levels in the clinic and in determining the amount of change that constitutes a response to treatment in a clinical trial. Serlin et al.[80] showed how cancer "pain at its worst" measured on a 0–10 NRS can be categorized into mild (1–4), moderate (5–6), or severe (7–10) levels using cut points determined by multivariate analysis of variance. Previous studies have shown that patients whose pain is moderate to severe (ie, 5 or greater on the 0–10 NRS) report significantly greater pain-related interference with function than do patients with mild or no pain. The derivation of cut points has also been applied to fatigue using the 0–10 NRS scale of the Brief Fatigue Inventory. Several researchers have employed this methodology using "average pain" rather than "pain at its worst" and with noncancer disease conditions (eg, diabetic neuropathy,[81] low back pain[82]). Cut-point-defined categories such as mild, moderate, and severe are a simple way for clinicians to assess patient symptoms within the practice setting.

This cut-point method can also be used to compare treatment groups in clinical trials.[83,84] For example, a responder can be defined as a patient whose "pain at its worst" changed from moderate or severe at intake to none or mild at follow-up after an intervention.

Longitudinal analysis and the area under the curve

Assessing change over time is a complex problem in symptom measurement.[85,86] The natural history of symptoms can be assessed using both summative and individual symptom measures (prevalence, severity,

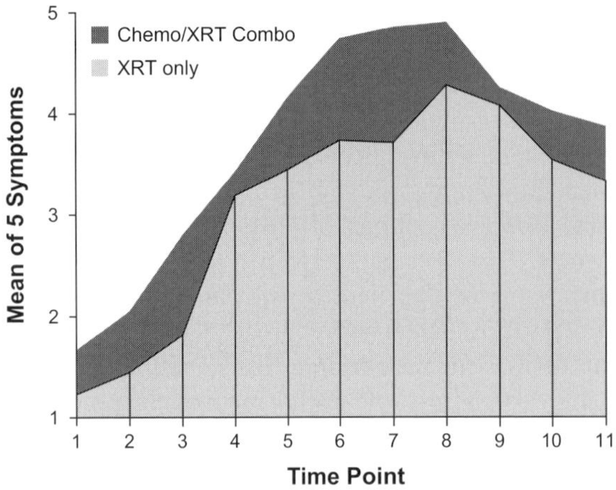

Figure 23.1. Example of area under the curve by treatment type. The area under the curve (AUC) is calculated using trapezoidal approximation. In the figure, vertical lines are drawn across the AUC for radiation treatment (XRT) only to illustrate the trapezoidal configuration; normally, they are not shown. The area of each trapezoid is derived by multiplying half of the base with the sum of the two heights, where the base is the number of days between two symptom assessments and the two heights correspond to the two mean symptom scores computed at each of those assessment time points. The AUC is the sum of the area of these trapezoids.

and patterns of symptoms). A more detailed discussion of fitting longitudinal models is given in Chapter 24.

An alternative to longitudinal modeling is to summarize the extent of symptom burden over the course of a study using area under the curve (AUC). The AUC is a single number summarizing the severity of symptoms over a period of time. For example, the AUC values for each patient cohort can be the mean value of symptoms over the observation period. A more detailed discussion of how to calculate the AUC is given in Chapter 25.

An application of AUC as a summary measure of symptom burden is to demonstrate how the AUC varies depending on treatment type. Figure 23.1 presents the AUC comparisons for five symptoms (pain, fatigue, disturbed sleep, lack of appetite, and difficulty swallowing) in cancer patients being treated with chemotherapy and radiation (CXRT; n = 83) and radiotherapy alone (XRT; n = 69). Across 10 weeks, patients undergoing CXRT, the more toxic option, demonstrated significantly larger AUC than patients receiving XRT (CXRT = 198.9 vs. XRT = 156.1, $P < 0.021$).

Technological solutions for gathering symptom data

Historically, the principal mode of gathering symptom ratings from patients has been for them to fill in their ratings on paper forms, or for staff to read the questions aloud and record the patient's responses on paper forms (so-called "paper-and-pencil" administration). This can be cumbersome in the clinic because of the lack of private space in which patients can respond and the need to score the measures and transform the scores to a clinically useful format. At home, patients are often asked to fill out patient symptom diaries, but may forget to do these at appropriate times and may "guesstimate" the severity of their ratings over several days – sometimes called the "waiting room" or "parking lot" effect.

Many of the issues inherent in paper-and-pencil administration can be addressed through computer technology. A variety of innovative data-collection methods are now available. Developments in computer and communications technology offer new opportunities for the assessment of patient symptoms, allowing great flexibility in the collection of data regardless of time or venue.

Presenting symptom questionnaires on tablet PCs connected to the Internet is one solution for clinic or hospital administration. The tablets can be programmed to present questions in an easily readable format that can be responded to using a touch-sensitive screen. Questions can also be presented in an audio-recorded format to patients with reading problems. The tablets (or server) can be programmed to detect inconsistent responses and to coach the patient in completing the questionnaire. At any time, scores can be sent to the server to be scored, summarized, and formatted in a useful display for clinic use, and can then become part of the electronic medical record. As with any symptom assessment, caution must be taken to ensure that the symptom-rating process is relatively private and that family members do not intervene in or take over the task of making the ratings on the patient's behalf.

Away from the clinic, patients can rate their symptoms using a computer and the Internet. Personal digital assistants (PDAs) can be synchronized with the Internet or telephone to download data for specific time points. Many patients with cancer, however, are not computer literate or may not have ready access to a computer; PDAs can be misplaced or be difficult to use, and patients may forget to transmit data.

Telephone-based interactive voice response (IVR) technology provides an exciting option for two-way communication between patient and health care provider that is acceptable to most patients. Telephone systems have been widely used in outpatient health care settings for communicating with patients, identifying symptoms that need medical attention, and following patients after treatment.[87] However, traditional telephone communication requires considerable staff time and is not feasible for assessing symptoms on a regular basis. In contrast, IVR systems provide an effective way to gather reliable, valid data from patients whose symptoms need to be monitored closely while the patient is away from the clinic or hospital. IVR technology combines touch-tone telephones, computers, and the Internet with NRS questionnaires, so that a patient can respond to spoken instructions using the telephone's keypad – for example, a patient might be asked to rate his or her pain at its worst in the last day from 0 (no pain) to 10 (pain as bad as you can imagine). An IVR system designed to assess the special needs of cancer patients receiving chemotherapy was reported to be acceptable to patients, who were able to use it accurately and reliably.[88]

Information obtained via an electronic data-capture system can be deployed in a number of ways. As protected patient information, it is sent directly to a secure server for processing to the patient's medical file and to study investigators for analysis. The electronic data-capture system can be configured to compare the data against preset symptom severity levels, and to trigger an alert to health care providers for any symptom that exceeds its severity threshold. Such alerts can be sent in a variety of formats, including to a pager or fax, or via email. Further, electronic systems can be programmed to present additional questions via branching routines when a symptom rating exceeds the preset threshold. For example, a pain rating of 4 or greater may trigger additional questions about the characteristics of the pain, such as its temporal pattern, location, and quality. This feature, sometimes referred to as computer adaptive testing, allows gathering of additional data that may be useful for either clinical or research purposes and reduces patient response time when the symptom is not present or present at very low levels.

Although we still are learning about potential method differences in item presentation, most studies have shown relative equivalency between computer or IVR acquisition and acquisition by traditional paper-and-pencil methods.[89] Some studies have shown, however, that there may be systematic differences between questions asked in electronic format and questions presented in person by clinic staff, with a bias for patients reporting less severe symptoms when asked about them by a person.[90]

Symptom measurement in context

The choice of a symptom measurement tool, or the decision to develop a new one, will be framed by its intended use – in the clinic, or in a clinical trial – and by consideration of what knowledge is needed about the status of individual or multiple symptoms over time. Many symptom measures are available to suit a variety of needs but require critical thinking about how they will be used and possible effects of their use.

Symptom measurement in the clinic

In the clinic, issues of practicability, ease of administration, level of patient (assessment) burden, scoring, and interpretability are paramount. Since 2001, the Joint Commission on Accreditation of Health Care Organizations has required the assessment of pain (usually a single 0–10 rating of pain severity), but not of other prominent cancer-related symptoms, such as fatigue. Additionally, evidence obtained over time from multiclinic surveys indicates that use of patient-reported outcomes measures, including symptom lists, have not increased in the last few years.[91]

Initial assessments are typically conducted using a multisymptom measure like the MDASI or the ESAS. If patients are very symptomatic, additional measures that address specific symptoms in more detail may be added as part of the patient evaluation. Some specialty clinics use this sequential administration of symptom measures using paper-and-pencil measures, but computer adaptive testing with branching routines that gather more information about specific identified symptoms may greatly improve clinical symptom assessment in support of symptom-treatment decisions.

Symptom measurement in clinical trials

Selection of symptom assessment methods for clinical research and clinical trials that are designed to evaluate symptoms as outcomes has a much different set of requirements than does selection of symptom measures for the management of individual patients. The designer of a clinical trial with symptom outcomes must select, before the trial starts, instruments that will be used consistently for all patients who participate in the trial. Ultimately, the questions asked by the trial will dictate the selection of the symptom measures, and responses to the instruments selected must be summarized to communicate clearly what happened during the trial. This will require the development of a measurement plan.

Labeling claims, as described in the FDA guidance on patient-reported outcomes,[2] provide an excellent framework for thinking about assessment design (see Chapter 28). What are we able to say about the treatment once the trial is completed? Does the treatment reduce symptoms that are present (eg, shortness of breath in lung cancer) or prevent symptoms normally expected to occur (eg, neuropathy from certain cancer treatments)? Will the treatment have rapid effects on symptoms, requiring repeated assessments over a short time period, perhaps even every hour? Or will the treatment have more gradual effects on the symptom, such as the pain reduction associated with palliative radiotherapy? In the first example, repeated use of a single-item symptom is probably the only choice, whereas in the second example, assessment will be less frequent and more items can be administered.

Conclusions

Many issues involved in symptom assessment for clinical practice and for clinical trials have yet to be resolved, thus forming a rich agenda for future research. Nonetheless, it can no longer be argued that we cannot use patient report to represent patients' symptoms with a relatively high degree of precision or to meet the standards of "assay sensitivity" that are expected of standard clinical assessments and laboratory tests.

Changes in symptom status as measured by patient report are critical for clinical care and for implementation of clinical guidelines for symptom control. Quality assurance and clinical effectiveness research increasingly demand assessment of symptom status as a representation of what the patient experiences in a clinical trial or clinical encounter. Finally, progress in understanding the underlying biobehavioral mechanisms underlying symptom expression, a major theme of this book, is dependent on our ability to capture variations in symptom severity and impact on the basis of what patients can report to us.

References

1. Patient-Reported Outcomes Measurement Information System. Welcome to PROMIS. Available from: URL: http://www.nihpromis.org. Accessed Oct 30, 2009.
2. US Food and Drug Administration, Center for Drug Evaluation and Research, Center for Biologics Evaluation and Research, Center for Devices and Radiological Health. Guidance for industry. Patient-reported outcome measures: use in medical product development to support labeling claims. Available from: URL: http://www.fda.gov/downloads/Drugs/GuidanceComplianceRegulatoryInformation/Guidances/UCM071975.pdf. Accessed Dec 18, 2009.
3. Patrick DL, Ferketich SL, Frame PS, et al. National Institutes of Health State-of-the-Science Conference statement: symptom management in cancer: pain, depression, and fatigue, July 15–17, 2002. *J Natl Cancer Inst* **95**(15):1110–1117, 2003.
4. de Haes JC. Quality of life: conceptual and theoretical considerations. In: Watson M, Greer S, Thomas C, eds. *Psychosocial Oncology*. Oxford: Pergamon Press, 1988:61–70.
5. Ware JE, Jr., Sherbourne CD. The MOS 36-item short-form health survey (SF-36). I. Conceptual framework and item selection. *Med Care* **30**(6): 473–483, 1992.
6. Cella DF, Tulsky DS, Gray G, et al. The Functional Assessment of Cancer Therapy scale: development and validation of the general measure. *J Clin Oncol* **11**(3):570–579, 1993.
7. Aaronson NK, Ahmedzai S, Bergman B, et al. The European Organization for Research and Treatment of Cancer QLQ-C30: a quality-of-life instrument for use in international clinical trials in oncology. *J Natl Cancer Inst* **85**(5):365–376, 1993.
8. Cleeland CS. Symptom burden: multiple symptoms and their impact as patient-reported outcomes. *J Natl Cancer Inst Monogr* **37**:16–21, 2007.
9. Cronbach LJ, Meehl PE. Construct validity in psychological tests. *Psychol Bull* **52**(4):281–302, 1955.
10. Ciechanowski PS, Katon WJ, Russo JE, Hirsch IB. The relationship of depressive symptoms to symptom reporting, self-care and glucose control in diabetes. *Gen Hosp Psychiatry* **25**(4):246–252, 2003.
11. Paton NI, Chapman CA, Chan SP, et al. Validation of the Medical Outcomes Study HIV Health Survey as a measure of quality of life in HIV-infected patients in Singapore. *Int J STD AIDS* **13**(7):456–461, 2002.
12. Adams BK, Cydulka RK. Asthma evaluation and management. *Emerg Med Clin North Am* **21**(2):315–330, 2003.

13. Cleeland CS, Mendoza TR, Wang XS, et al. Assessing symptom distress in cancer patients: the M. D. Anderson Symptom Inventory. *Cancer* **89**(7):1634–1646, 2000.
14. Portenoy RK, Thaler HT, Kornblith AB, et al. The Memorial Symptom Assessment Scale: an instrument for the evaluation of symptom prevalence, characteristics and distress. *Eur J Cancer* **30A**(9):1326–1336, 1994.
15. Turk DC, Dworkin RH, Allen RR, et al. Core outcome domains for chronic pain clinical trials: IMMPACT recommendations. *Pain* **106**(3):337–345, 2003.
16. Wang XS, Mendoza TR, Gao SZ, Cleeland CS. The Chinese version of the Brief Pain Inventory (BPI-C): its development and use in a study of cancer pain. *Pain* **67**(2–3):407–416, 1996.
17. Cleeland CS. Pain assessment in cancer. In: Osoba D, ed. *Effect of Cancer on Quality of Life*. Boca Raton: CRC Press, Inc., 1991:293–305.
18. Portenoy RK, Thaler HT, Kornblith AB, et al. Symptom prevalence, characteristics and distress in a cancer population. *Qual Life Res* **3**(3):183–189, 1994.
19. Grond S, Zech D, Diefenbach C, Bischoff A. Prevalence and pattern of symptoms in patients with cancer pain: a prospective evaluation of 1635 cancer patients referred to a pain clinic. *J Pain Symptom Manage* **9**(6):372–382, 1994.
20. Donnelly S, Walsh D, Rybicki L. The symptoms of advanced cancer: identification of clinical and research priorities by assessment of prevalence and severity. *J Palliat Care* **11**(1):27–32, 1995.
21. Dodd MJ, Miaskowski C, Paul SM. Symptom clusters and their effect on the functional status of patients with cancer. *Oncol Nurs Forum* **28**(3):465–470, 2001.
22. Barsevick AM, Whitmer K, Nail LM, Beck SL, Dudley WN. Symptom cluster research: conceptual, design, measurement, and analysis issues. *J Pain Symptom Manage* **31**(1):85–95, 2006.
23. Bruera E, Kuehn N, Miller MJ, Selmser P, Macmillan K. The Edmonton Symptom Assessment System (ESAS): a simple method for the assessment of palliative care patients. *J Palliat Care* **7**(2):6–9, 1991.
24. Philip J, Smith WB, Craft P, Lickiss N. Concurrent validity of the modified Edmonton Symptom Assessment System with the Rotterdam Symptom Checklist and the Brief Pain Inventory. *Support Care Cancer* **6**(6):539–541, 1998.
25. Dworkin RH, Turk DC, Farrar JT, et al. Core outcome measures for chronic pain clinical trials: IMMPACT recommendations. *Pain* **113**(1–2):9–19, 2005.
26. Wolfe F. Fatigue assessments in rheumatoid arthritis: comparative performance of visual analog scales and longer fatigue questionnaires in 7760 patients. *J Rheumatol* **31**(10):1896–1902, 2004.
27. Cleeland CS, Ryan KM. Pain assessment: global use of the Brief Pain Inventory. *Ann Acad Med Singapore* **23**(2):129–138, 1994.
28. Cleeland CS. Measurement of pain by subjective report. In: Chapman CR, Loeser JD, eds. *Issues in Pain Measurement*. New York: Raven Press, 1989:391–403. Advances in Pain Research and Therapy; vol. 12.
29. Beecher HK. *Measurement of Subjective Responses: Quantitative Effects of Drugs*. New York: Oxford University Press, 1959.
30. Clark WC, Yang JC. Applications of sensory decision theory to problems in laboratory and clinical pain. In: Melzack R, ed. *Pain Measurement and Assessment*. New York: Raven Press, 1983:15–25.
31. Dworkin RH, Turk DC, Revicki DA, et al. Development and initial validation of an expanded and revised version of the Short-form McGill Pain Questionnaire (SF-MPQ-2). *Pain* **144**(1–2):35–42, 2009.
32. Mendoza TR, Wang XS, Cleeland CS, et al. The rapid assessment of fatigue severity in cancer patients: use of the Brief Fatigue Inventory. *Cancer* **85**(5):1186–1196, 1999.
33. Lai JS, Crane PK, Cella D. Factor analysis techniques for assessing sufficient unidimensionality of cancer related fatigue. *Qual Life Res* **15**(7):1179–1190, 2006.
34. Okuyama T, Akechi T, Kugaya A, et al. Development and validation of the cancer fatigue scale: a brief, three-dimensional, self-rating scale for assessment of fatigue in cancer patients. *J Pain Symptom Manage* **19**(1):5–14, 2000.
35. Hann DM, Jacobsen PB, Azzarello LM, et al. Measurement of fatigue in cancer patients: development and validation of the Fatigue Symptom Inventory. *Qual Life Res* **7**(4):301–310, 1998.
36. Cella D. The Functional Assessment of Cancer Therapy-Anemia (FACT-An) Scale: a new tool for the assessment of outcomes in cancer anemia and fatigue. *Semin Hematol* **34**(3 Suppl 2):13–19, 1997.
37. Lee KA, Hicks G, Nino-Murcia G. Validity and reliability of a scale to assess fatigue. *Psychiatry Res* **36**(3):291–298, 1991.
38. Smets EM, Garssen B, Bonke B, de Haes JC. The Multidimensional Fatigue Inventory (MFI) psychometric qualities of an instrument to assess fatigue. *J Psychosom Res* **39**(3):315–325, 1995.
39. Piper BF, Dibble SL, Dodd MJ, Weiss MC, Slaughter RE, Paul SM. The revised Piper Fatigue Scale: psychometric evaluation in women with breast cancer. *Oncol Nurs Forum* **25**(4):677–684, 1998.

40. Schwartz AL. The Schwartz Cancer Fatigue Scale: testing reliability and validity. *Oncol Nurs Forum* **25**(4):711–717, 1998.

41. Garcia SF, Cella D, Clauser SB, et al. Standardizing patient-reported outcomes assessment in cancer clinical trials: a patient-reported outcomes measurement information system initiative. *J Clin Oncol* **25**(32):5106–5112, 2007.

42. Kirkova J, Davis MP, Walsh D, et al. Cancer symptom assessment instruments: a systematic review. *J Clin Oncol* **24**(9):1459–1473, 2006.

43. de Haes JC, van Knippenberg FC, Neijt JP. Measuring psychological and physical distress in cancer patients: structure and application of the Rotterdam Symptom Checklist. *Br J Cancer* **62**(6):1034–1038, 1990.

44. McCorkle R, Young K. Development of a symptom distress scale. *Cancer Nurs* **1**(5):373–378, 1978.

45. Hoekstra J, Bindels PJ, van Duijn NP, Schadé E. The symptom monitor. A diary for monitoring physical symptoms for cancer patients in palliative care: feasibility, reliability and compliance. *J Pain Symptom Manage* **27**(1):24–35, 2004.

46. Donaldson MS. Taking stock of health-related quality-of-life measurement in oncology practice in the United States. *J Natl Cancer Inst Monogr* **33**:155–167, 2004.

47. Gagliese L, Weizblit N, Ellis W, Chan VW. The measurement of postoperative pain: a comparison of intensity scales in younger and older surgical patients. *Pain* **117**(3):412–420, 2005.

48. Breivik EK, Björnsson GA, Skovlund E. A comparison of pain rating scales by sampling from clinical trial data. *Clin J Pain* **16**(1):22–28, 2000.

49. Cleeland CS, Serlin RC, Nakamura Y, Mendoza TR. Effects of culture and language on ratings of cancer pain and patterns of functional interference. In: Jensen TS, Turner JA, Wiesenfeld-Hallin Z, eds. *Progress in Pain Research and Management*. Seattle: IASP Press, 1997:35–51. Proceedings of the 8th World Congress on Pain; vol. 8.

50. Lund I, Lundeberg T, Sandberg L, Budh CN, Kowalski J, Svensson E. Lack of interchangeability between visual analogue and verbal rating pain scales: a cross sectional description of pain etiology groups. *BMC Med Res Methodol* **5**:31, 2005.

51. Li L, Liu X, Herr K. Postoperative pain intensity assessment: a comparison of four scales in Chinese adults. *Pain Med* **8**(3):223–234, 2007.

52. Cleeland CS. Assessment of pain in cancer: measurement issues. In: Foley KM, Bonica JJ, Ventafridda V, eds. *Proceedings of the Second International Congress on Cancer Pain*. New York: Raven Press, 1990:47–55. Advances in Pain Research and Therapy; vol. 16.

53. Hollen PJ, Gralla RJ, Kris MG, McCoy S, Donaldson GW, Moinpour CM. A comparison of visual analogue and numerical rating scale formats for the Lung Cancer Symptom Scale (LCSS): does format affect patient ratings of symptoms and quality of life? *Qual Life Res* **14**(3):837–847, 2005.

54. Piper BF. Piper fatigue scale available for clinical testing. *Oncol Nurs Forum* **17**(5):661–662, 1990.

55. Miaskowski C, Lee KA. Pain, fatigue and sleep disturbances in oncology outpatients receiving radiation therapy for bone metastasis: a pilot study. *J Pain Symptom Manage* **17**(5):320–332, 1999.

56. Bogen K. *The effect of questionnaire length on response rates – a review of the literature. Proceedings of the Survey Research Methods Section*. Alexandria VA: American Statistical Association, 1996:1020–1025.

57. Sloan JA, Berk L, Roscoe J, et al. Integrating patient-reported outcomes into cancer symptom management clinical trials supported by the National Cancer Institute-sponsored clinical trials networks. *J Clin Oncol* **25**(32):5070–5077, 2007.

58. Sloan JA, Aaronson N, Cappelleri JC, Fairclough DL, Varricchio C. Assessing the clinical significance of single items relative to summated scores. *Mayo Clin Proc* **77**(5):479–487, 2002.

59. Cleopas A, Kolly V, Perneger TV. Longer response scales improved the acceptability and performance of the Nottingham Health Profile. *J Clin Epidemiol* **59**(11):1183–1190, 2006.

60. Arnould B. Patient-reported outcomes and clinical practice. From measurement instruments to decision tools: much more than a simple change in format. *Patient-Reported Outcomes Newsletter* **36**:21–24, 2006.

61. Cheung YB, Goh C, Thumboo J, Khoo KS, Wee J. Quality of life scores differed according to mode of administration in a review of three major oncology questionnaires. *J Clin Epidemiol* **59**(2):185–191, 2006.

62. Cheung YB, Wong LC, Tay MH, et al. Order effects in the assessment of quality of life in cancer patients. *Qual Life Res* **13**(7):1217–1223, 2004.

63. Brundage M, Feldman-Stewart D, Leis A, et al. Communicating quality of life information to cancer patients: a study of six presentation formats. *J Clin Oncol* **23**(28):6949–6956, 2005.

64. Grassi M, Nucera A, Zanolin E, Omenaas E, Anto JM, Leynaert B. Performance comparison of Likert and binary formats of SF-36 version 1.6 across ECRHS II adults populations. *Value Health* **10**(6):478–488, 2007.

65. Preston CC, Colman AM. Optimal number of response categories in rating scales: reliability, validity, discriminating power, and respondent preferences. *Acta Psychol (Amst)* **104**(1):1–15, 2000.

66. American Educational Research Association, American Psychological Association, National Council on Measurement in Education, Joint Committee on Standards for Educational and Psychological Testing. *Standards for Educational and Psychological Testing*, 2nd ed. Washington, DC: American Educational Research Association, 1999.

67. Litwin MS. *How to Measure Survey Reliability and Validity: 7 (Survey Kit)*. Thousand Oaks CA: Sage Publications, 1995.

68. Nunnally JC, Bernstein IH. *Psychometric Theory, 3rd ed.: McGraw-Hill Series in Psychology*. New York: McGraw-Hill, 1994.

69. Crocker LM, Algina J. *Introduction to Classical and Modern Test Theory*. Pacific Grove CA: Wadsworth Publishing Co., 2006.

70. Turner RR, Quittner AL, Parasuraman BM, Kallich JD, Cleeland CS. Patient-reported outcomes: instrument development and selection issues. *Value Health* **10**(s2):S86–S93, 2007.

71. Willis GB, Reeve BB, Barofsky I. Invited Paper C: The use of cognitive interviewing techniques in quality of life and patient-reported outcomes assessment. In: Lipscomb J, Gotay CC, Snyder C, eds. *Outcomes Assessment in Cancer: Measures, Methods and Applications*. Cambridge UK: Cambridge University Press, 2004:610–622.

72. Wang XS, Williams LA, Eng C, et al. Validation and application of a module of the M. D. Anderson Symptom Inventory for measuring multiple symptoms in patients with gastrointestinal cancer (the MDASI-GI). *Cancer*. In press.

73. Revicki D, Hays RD, Cella D, Sloan J. Recommended methods for determining responsiveness and minimally important differences for patient-reported outcomes. *J Clin Epidemiol* **61**(2):102–109, 2008.

74. Guyatt GH, Osoba D, Wu AW, Wyrwich KW, Norman GR. Methods to explain the clinical significance of health status measures. *Mayo Clin Proc* **77**(4):371–383, 2002.

75. Norman GR, Sloan JA, Wyrwich KW. Interpretation of changes in health-related quality of life: the remarkable universality of half a standard deviation. *Med Care* **41**(5):582–592, 2003.

76. Sloan JA, Dueck A. Issues for statisticians in conducting analyses and translating results for quality of life end points in clinical trials. *J Biopharm Stat* **14**(1):73–96, 2004.

77. Cohen J. *Statistical Power Analysis for the Behavioral Sciences*, 2nd ed. Hillsdale, NJ: Lawrence Earlbaum Associates, 1988.

78. Wyrwich KW, Tierney WM, Wolinsky FD. Further evidence supporting an SEM-based criterion for identifying meaningful intra-individual changes in health-related quality of life. *J Clin Epidemiol* **52**(9):861–873, 1999.

79. Guyatt G, Walter S, Norman G. Measuring change over time: assessing the usefulness of evaluative instruments. *J Chronic Dis* **40**(2):171–178, 1987.

80. Serlin RC, Mendoza TR, Nakamura Y, Edwards KR, Cleeland CS. When is cancer pain mild, moderate or severe? Grading pain severity by its interference with function. *Pain* **61**(2):277–284, 1995.

81. Zelman DC, Gore M, Dukes E, Tai KS, Brandenburg N. Validation of a modified version of the brief pain inventory for painful diabetic peripheral neuropathy. *J Pain Symptom Manage* **29**(4):401–410, 2005.

82. Keller S, Bann CM, Dodd SL, Schein J, Mendoza TR, Cleeland CS. Validity of the brief pain inventory for use in documenting the outcomes of patients with noncancer pain. *Clin J Pain* **20**(5):309–318, 2004.

83. Cleeland CS, Portenoy RK, Rue M, et al. Does an oral analgesic protocol improve pain control for patients with cancer? An intergroup study coordinated by the Eastern Cooperative Oncology Group. *Ann Oncol* **16**(6):972–980, 2005.

84. Wong GY, Schroeder DR, Carns PE, et al. Effect of neurolytic celiac plexus block on pain relief, quality of life, and survival in patients with unresectable pancreatic cancer: a randomized controlled trial. *JAMA* **291**(9):1092–1099, 2004.

85. Cleeland CS, Wang XS. Measuring and understanding fatigue. *Oncology* **13**(11A):91–97, 1999.

86. Sprangers MA, Moinpour CM, Moynihan TJ, Patrick DL, Revicki DA. Assessing meaningful change in quality of life over time: a users' guide for clinicians. *Mayo Clin Proc* **77**(6):561–571, 2002.

87. Korcz IR, Moreland S. Telephone prescreening enhancing a model for proactive healthcare practice. *Cancer Pract* **6**(5):270–275, 1998.

88. Given CW, Sikorskii A, Tamkus D, et al. Managing symptoms among patients with breast cancer during chemotherapy: results of a two-arm behavioral trial. *J Clin Oncol* **26**(36):5855–5862, 2008.

89. Abernethy AP, Herndon JE, Wheeler JL, et al. Improving health care efficiency and quality using tablet personal computers to collect research-quality, patient-reported data. *Health Serv Res* **43**(6):1975–1991, 2008.

90. Sikorskii A, Given CW, Given B, Jeon S, You M. Differential symptom reporting by mode of

administration of the assessment: automated voice response system versus a live telephone interview. *Med Care* **47**(8):866–874, 2009.

91. Velikova G, Booth L, Smith AB, et al. Measuring quality of life in routine oncology practice improves communication and patient well-being: a randomized controlled trial. *J Clin Oncol* **22**(4):714–724, 2004.

92. Melzack R. The McGill Pain Questionnaire: major properties and scoring methods. *Pain* **1**(3):277–299, 1975.

93. Yellen SB, Cella DF, Webster K, Blendowski C, Kaplan E. Measuring fatigue and other anemia-related symptoms with the Functional Assessment of Cancer Therapy (FACT) measurement system. *J Pain Symptom Manage* **13**(2):63–74, 1997.

Section 4
Chapter
24

Symptom Measurement

Longitudinal models for symptoms

Diane L. Fairclough

When we study symptoms over time, we have a number of goals. One goal may be to characterize the average trajectory of symptom severity over time. Often we are asking questions such as: Do symptoms change over time? If so, what factors (eg, treatment) modify that trajectory? We also may be interested in characterizing the impact of symptoms and answering questions such as: Which symptoms have the greatest impact on subjects? How do changes in symptoms affect patient reports of health status and quality of life? How does the level of severity influence that impact? Finally, the goals of the investigation may be to characterize between-subject and within-subject variation, to answer questions such as: Are there groups of symptoms that change within individuals in a similar manner? Are there biological factors (eg, cytokines) that change in conjunction with the development of symptoms? For example, we might be interested in the relationship of inflammatory cytokines to fatigue, pain, and other symptoms of cancer and cancer treatment.

These questions differ from traditional analysis, in which we would typically test whether the average change in symptoms is a function of biological factors by examining the mean scores for groups of subjects with high versus low values of the biological factors. When our interest becomes focused on change and variation at the level of the individual rather than the group, we might be interested in questions such as: Do individuals with generally higher levels of interleukin (IL)-6, an inflammatory cytokine strongly associated with lung cancer, report more pain? After adjusting for initial levels of the biological factors and symptoms, do individuals whose levels of IL-6 increase report increasing levels of pain? Do variations in IL-6 over time predict similar variations in the levels of reported pain?

Data from two studies will be used to illustrate how longitudinal models can be used to answer these questions. Study 1 was a prospective longitudinal study of 64 patients with locally advanced (stage II–IIIB) non-small cell lung cancer (NSCLC).[1] Symptoms were measured using the lung cancer module of the M. D. Anderson Symptom Inventory (MDASI) administered before, weekly for 12 weeks during, and after concurrent chemoradiation therapy (CXRT). The core MDASI includes 13 symptom items: fatigue; sleep disturbance; pain; drowsiness; poor appetite; nausea; vomiting; shortness of breath; numbness; difficulty remembering; dry mouth; distress; and sadness. Two additional symptoms (cough and sore throat) are included in the MDASI-lung module used in this study. The severity of these symptoms during the previous 24 hours is assessed on a 0–10 scale, with 0 being "not present" and 10 being "as bad as you can imagine." The MDASI also contains six symptom interference items that describe how much symptoms have interfered with different aspects of the patient's life during the past 24 hours: general activity; mood; walking ability; normal work (including both work outside the home and housework); relations with other people; and enjoyment of life. The interference items are rated on a 0–10 scale, with 0 being "did not interfere" and 10 being "interfered completely." A component (mean) score of all six symptom interference items was used for presenting the burden of cancer-related symptoms.

Study 2 was a pilot study of 18 adult patients with stage III NSCLC undergoing concurrent CXRT.[2] The study included weekly assessments of serum levels of cytokines and self-reported symptoms using the MDASI. The questions of interest were whether levels of inflammatory cytokines (focusing on IL-6) and symptoms (focusing on pain) (1) covaried over time in these patients stimulated by CXRT; and (2) increased over time during therapy.

Modeling the average trajectory

The most traditional approach for modeling the average trajectory of symptoms over time utilizes polynomial models. This is illustrated by the fourth-degree polynomial used to model the changes in fatigue over time in Study 1 during therapy (Figure 24.1). This model is:

$$Y_{ij} = \beta_0 + \beta_1 t_{ij} + \beta_2 t_{ij}^2 + \beta_3 t_{ij}^3 + \beta_4 t_{ij}^4 + e_{ij} \quad \text{(Model 1)}$$

where Y_{ij} is the j-th measure of the outcome for the i-th subject and t_{ij} is the time of that measurement. The residual errors, e_{ij}, are assumed to be correlated within subjects but uncorrelated among subjects.

Although polynomial models can be useful in graphical presentations of change, it is very difficult to interpret the estimated parameters (βs) except for the simplest models that include only intercept and slope terms. A practical alternative is a piecewise linear model that approximates a linear rate of change over intervals of time. In Figure 24.1, the rate of change (or slope) is allowed to change at weeks 1, 2, and 4. The model is:

$$Y_{ij} = \beta_0 + \beta_1 t_{ij} + \beta_2 t_{ij}^{[1]} + \beta_3 t_{ij}^{[2]} + \beta_4 t_{ij}^{[4]} + e_{ij} \quad \text{(Model 2)}$$

where $t_{ij}^{[k]}=\max(0,\ t - k)$ allows the slope to change when $t_{ij} = k$. The parameters of this model are interpreted as the change in the slope after $t_{ij} = k$. For example, β_2 is the change in the slope after one week of therapy. If $\beta_2 = 0$, then the inference is that the rate of change between weeks 0 and 1 is equal to the change between weeks 1 and 2. If $\beta_2 \neq 0$, then the rate of change between weeks 1 and 2 is estimated as the sum of the initial slope (β_1) plus the change in the slope after one week (β_2).

This strategy was applied to all of the symptom measures in Study 1, where the change was assumed to be linear over four periods: the first two weeks on therapy, the second three weeks on therapy, the last three weeks on therapy, and the first four weeks off therapy.[1] Based on the MDASI's 0–10 rating scale, the mean rates of change in fatigue over the four periods were 0.45 (SE, 0.16), 0.01 (SE, 0.13), 0.73 (SE, 0.16) and −0.22 (SE, 0.08), respectively. This suggests that the most rapid increases in fatigue occurred during the early and late phases of therapy, and that fatigue decreased after therapy was discontinued. This model was extended to all the symptom measures to identify four qualitatively different trajectories, as illustrated in Figure 24.2.

Often we are interested in how various factors, such as therapy and patient characteristics, modify these trajectories. In a randomized trial with a treatment group and a control group, the question of primary interest would be how therapy (Tx) modifies these average symptom trajectories. The model would then be expanded by adding interactions of indicators of treatment arm with time. If we assume that the rates are linear over the first 4 weeks and

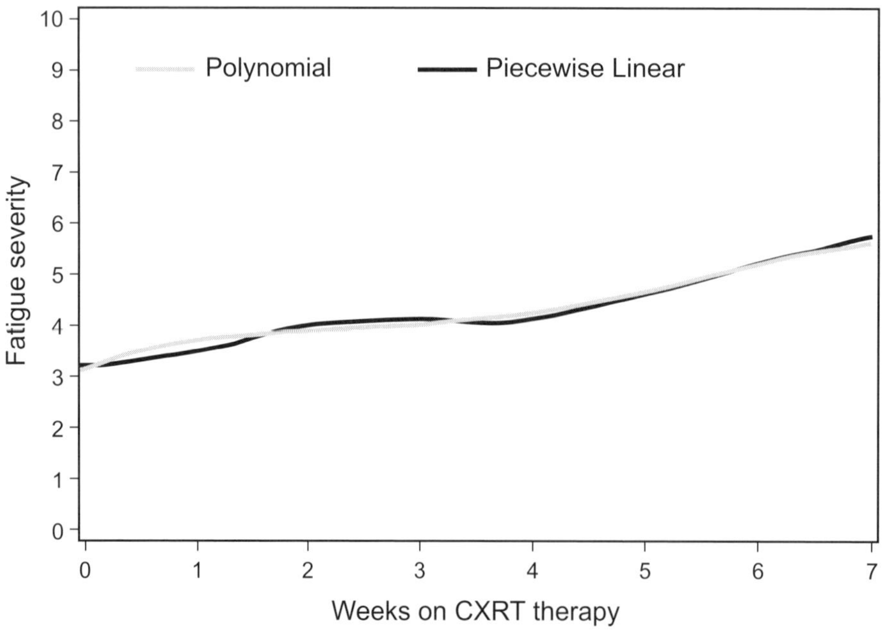

Figure 24.1. Predicted trajectories in fatigue for patients with NSCLC over a 7-week course of CXRT using a fourth-degree polynomial and piecewise linear regression.

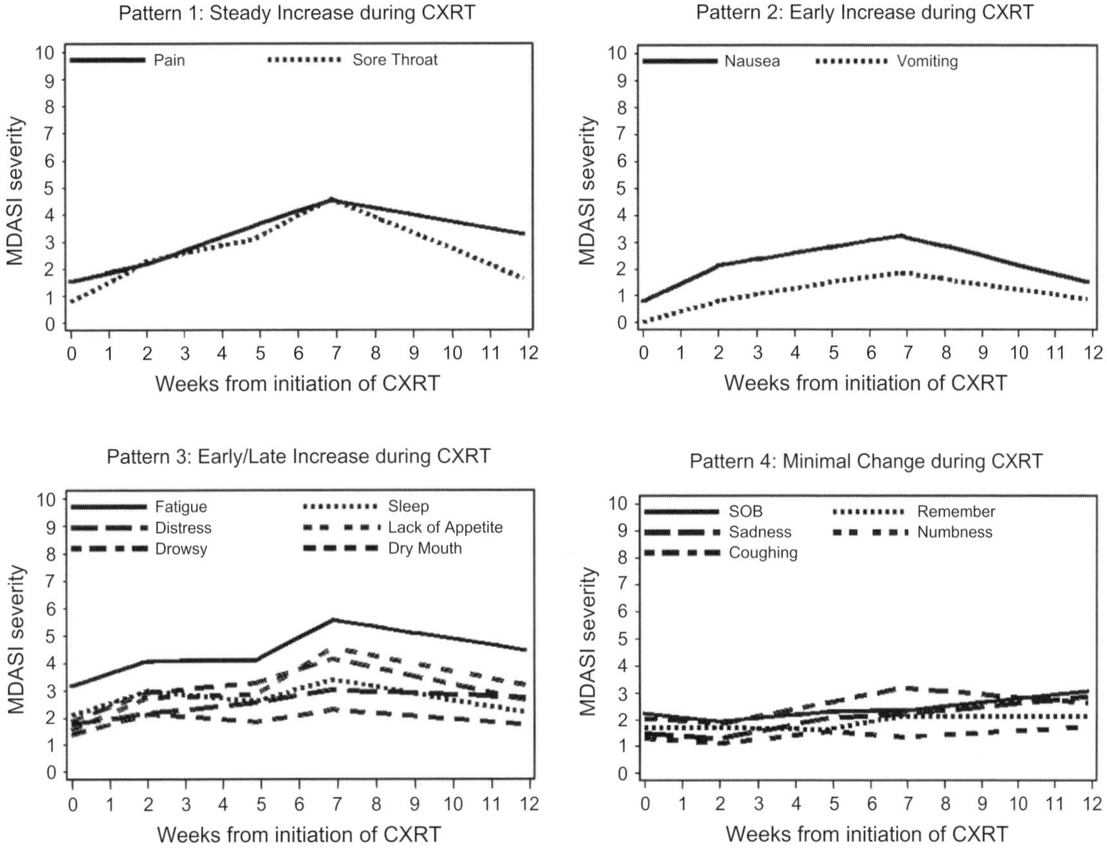

Figure 24.2. Patterns of change in symptoms in patients with NSCLC over a 7-week course of CXRT. MDASI indicates M. D. Anderson Symptom Inventory; SOB, shortness of breath.
Source: Wang XS et al: *J Clin Oncol* 24(27), 2006: 4485–4491. Reprinted with permission.

after 4 weeks, we would propose the following model:

$$Y_{ij} = \beta_0 + \beta_1 t_{ij} + \beta_2 t_{ij}^{[4]} + \beta_3 Txt_{ij} + \beta_4 Txt_{ij}^{[4]} + e_{ij}$$

(Model 3)

where $Tx = 0$ for the reference group and $Tx = 1$ for the experimental group. If a test of the null hypothesis $\beta_3 = 0$ was rejected then we would infer that the experimental treatment modified the symptom trajectory during the first 4 weeks relative to the reference group. Similarly, if a test of the null hypothesis $\beta_3 + \beta_4 = 0$ was rejected, we would infer that the experimental treatment modified the change in the outcome after the first 4 weeks.

In observational studies such as Study 1, we are often interested in whether various patient characteristics (X_i), such as age and previous therapy, modify the trajectory of symptoms after adjusting for the overall impact of that characteristic. Making similar assumptions about changes over time, we would propose the following model:

$$Y_{ij} = \beta_0 + \beta_1 t_{ij} + \beta_2 t_{ij}^{[4]} + \beta_3 X_i + \beta_4 X_i t_{ij} + \beta_5 X_i t_{ij}^{4} + e_{ij}$$

(Model 4)

In this model, β_3 estimates the effect of the patient characteristic on the outcome before treatment. Tests of $\beta_4 = 0$ and $\beta_4 + \beta_5 = 0$ assess the impact of the patient characteristic on symptom severity during and after the first 4 weeks of treatment, respectively.

Impact of symptoms on quality-of-life measures

Similar models can be extended to answer questions about how specific symptoms interfere with other outcomes, such as the patient's assessment of quality of life or ability to perform usual activities. The questions of clinical interest are, Which symptoms have the greatest contribution to the patient's rating of interference? Does that impact vary over the severity of the symptom? In Study 1, patients used the MDASI to rate how severely their symptoms interfered with several components of daily living. The measure of interference increased over the course of treatment without any evidence of differences over the course of therapy; thus, the reference model includes two parameters for the average trajectory:

$$Y_{ij} = \beta_0 + \beta_1 t_{ij} + e_{ij} \qquad \text{(Model 5)}$$

To assess the impact of specific symptoms, one could assume that the impact of severity of a selected symptom was linear over the entire range of the patient's assessment of severity:

$$Y_{ij} = \beta_0 + \beta_1 t_{ij} + \beta_2 X_{ij} + e_{ij} \qquad \text{(Model 6)}$$

where X_{ij} is the measure of the symptom severity at the j-th assessment. β_2 is the estimated change in the outcome for a unit change in the symptom and β_1 is the estimated change over time, assuming that the severity of the symptom is constant. If the value of β_1 in Model 6 is closer to 0 than in Model 5, the data suggests that the symptom explains the increase in the outcome over time. This is illustrated in Study 1, where in the absence of any symptoms as explanatory variables the measure of interference increased at a mean rate of 0.27 units per week (SE, 0.04). When the patient's assessment of fatigue is included in the model, the estimate change in interference over time is reduced roughly by half, to 0.12 units per week. The estimated mean change in the measure of interference for every unit change in fatigue was 0.47 points (SE, 0.03). While strong causal inferences are not possible in observational studies, these results suggest that fatigue is strongly associated with the impact of therapy over the course of treatment and that interventions to ameliorate fatigue may be of potential clinical benefit.

It is recognized that scales assessing the severity of symptoms may not have a linear relationship to their impact on the patient's well-being. To illustrate this, the impact of the severity of specific symptoms can be assessed over specific intervals of the rating scale. To facilitate interpretation, one can use the strategy of a piecewise linear regression, as described previously for time. For example, we can estimate the change in the outcome over prespecified ranges of the severity of the symptom. Symptom severity scores measured by the MDASI have a potential range of 0–10. In the following example, that range has been divided into four intervals: 0–3, 3–5, 5–7, and 7–10.

$$Y_{ij} = \beta_0 + \beta_1 t_{ij} + \beta_2 t_{ij}^{[1]} + \beta_3 t_{ij}^{[2]} + \beta_4 t_{ij}^{[4]} + e_{ij} \qquad \text{(Model 7)}$$

where $X_{ij}^{[k]} = \max(0, X_{ij} - k)$. $\hat{\beta}_2$ is the estimate of the change in the interference score for every unit change in the symptom score over the range of 0–3. $\hat{\beta}_2$ is the estimate of the change in the symptom interference relationship over the range of 3–5 relative to $\hat{\beta}_2$. If $\hat{\beta}_3 = 0$, then we infer that the symptom interference relationship is the same over the entire range from 0 to 5. Otherwise, the change in the interference score for every unit change in the symptom score over the range of 3–5 is estimated by $\hat{\beta}_2 + \hat{\beta}_3$. The same logic is extended to the ranges of 5–7 and 7–10 in the symptom severity score.

The results of this analysis are summarized in Table 24.1 and provide some interesting suggestions for clinical practice. One observation is that some symptoms, such as fatigue, have a greater impact on the patient's function and that the impact varies across the range of the severity. Another observation is that, for most of the symptoms, scores in the lower range have less impact on function than scores in the higher range; however, symptoms such as sadness and distress have a significant impact even in the lower range of scores.

Between-subject and within-subject variation

What possible strategies could be considered to answer questions about the associations between symptoms or between symptoms and biological factors, as in Study 2? The simplest is examination of cross-sectional correlations of the two measures, Y and X, in N subjects, $r = \Sigma z_{Xi} z_{Yi}/(N - 1)$, where i indicates the i-th individual, $\bar{X}$ and S_x are the mean and standard deviation of the measure X, $z_{Xi} = (X_i - \bar{X})/s_x$ and $z_{Yi} = (Y_i - \bar{Y})/s_y$. This approach is simple to implement and interpret, but it does not assess how changes in one measure are associated with the changes in another measure. An alternative approach is to examine the correlation of changes in the two measures over a fixed period of time, but the results would be limited to

Table 24.1. Predicted change in interference scores per unit change in symptom severity[a]

Symptom	Range of symptom score on 0–10 scale			
	0–3	3–5	5–7	7–10
Increasing impact on interference with increasing symptom severity				
Fatigue	0.12	0.50[b]	0.50[b]	0.91[b]
Sleep	0.18[b]	0.18[b]	0.18[b]	0.70[b]
Nausea	0.26[b]	0.26[b]	0.26[b]	0.66[b]
Sore throat	0.12[c]	0.12[c]	0.38[b]	0.38[b]
Constant impact on interference over symptom severity of 3–10				
Shortness of breath	0.20[d]	0.49[b]	0.49[b]	0.49[b]
Drowsiness	0.15[c]	0.49[b]	0.49[b]	0.49[b]
Lack of appetite	0.14[c]	0.39[b]	0.39[b]	0.39[b]
Pain	0.05	0.35[b]	0.35[b]	0.35[b]
Coughing	0.08	0.22[b]	0.22[b]	0.22[b]
Decreasing impact on interference with increasing symptom severity				
Sadness	0.61[b]	0.61[b]	0.15	0.15
Distress	0.49[b]	0.49[b]	0.49[b]	−0.03
Constant impact on interference over 0–10				
Difficulty remembering	0.48[b]	0.14	0.53[b]	0.53[b]
Dry mouth	0.31[b]	0.31[b]	0.31[b]	0.31[b]
Vomiting	0.32[b]	0.32[b]	0.32[b]	0.32[b]
Numbness	0.25[b]	0.25[b]	0.25[b]	0.25[b]

[a]Wang XS et al. *J Clin Oncol* 24(27), 2006: 4485–4491. Reprinted with permission.
[b]$P < 0.001$
[c]$P < 0.05$
[d]$P < 0.01$

rates of change. One might also consider examining the correlation of estimates of intercept and slope obtained from separate simple linear regressions of longitudinal assessments. However, a number of methodological questions arise, such as, Do you weight all subjects equally when there is variation in the number of observations per subject or the length of follow-up? One might also consider using the approach described in the preceding section (Models 6 and 7) with one measure as the dependent variable, Y_{ij}, and the other as a time-varying covariate, X_{ij}. The interpretation focuses on the average change in the outcome.

To answer some of the questions posed in the introduction, we might consider a model with two levels of variation. The first component would be the average levels of the two scores, X and Y, for the i-th subject, which vary among individuals around the mean for the entire sample. In Study 2, for example, if the deviations of X and Y are positively correlated, then the patients with higher levels of IL-6 are more likely to report higher levels of pain. The corresponding models might appear as: $X_{ij}=\mu_X+d_{Xi}+e_{Xit}$ and $Y_{ij}=\mu_Y+d_{Yi}+e_{Yit}$ where d_{Xi} and d_{Yi} indicate the difference between the mean scores (μ_X and μ_Y) and the average score for the i-th individual. In this model, d_{Xi} and d_{Yi} are allowed to be correlated. We are also interested in general trends over time in levels of cytokines and symptoms. Thus, we might expect that increasing (or decreasing) levels of specific cytokines would be correlated with increasing levels of symptoms. To model this, we would add another component corresponding to between-subject variation in the rates of change of slopes. This is illustrated in Figure 24.3,

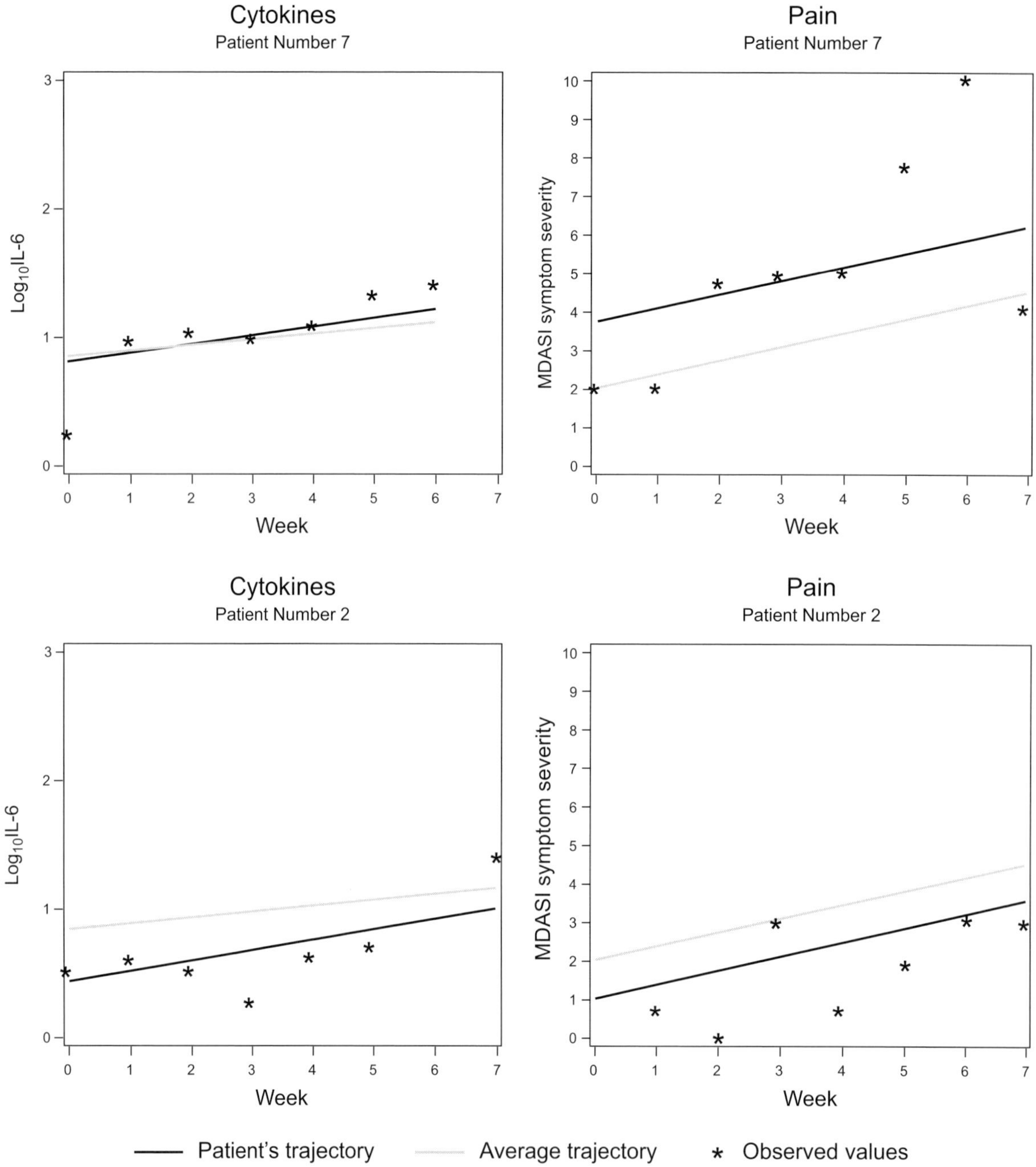

Figure 24.3. Between-subject and within-subject variations in pain and $\log_{10}$ IL-6 levels for two patients. MDASI indicates M. D. Anderson Symptom Inventory. In each panel, the difference between the light and dark lines represents the between-subject variation and the difference between the stars and the dark line represents the within-subject variation.
Source: Adapted from Fairclough DL, Wang XS. Understanding the correlations between biologic and symptom measures over time. In: Lenderking WR, Revicki DA, editors. *Advancing Health Outcomes Research Methods and Clinical Applications.* McLean, VA: Degnon Associates; pp. 177–190, 2005. Used with permission of the International Society for Quality of Life Research.

where the solid line indicates the mean scores across all patients and the dashed line indicates the average scores for an individual patient. The corresponding models would appear as:

$$X_{ij} = \beta_{0X} + \beta_{1X}t_{ij} + d_{0Xi} + d_{1Xi}t_{ij} + e_{Xij} \qquad \text{(Model 8a)}$$

and

$$Y_{ij} = \beta_{0Y} + \beta_{1Y}t_{ij} + d_{0Yi} + d_{1Yi}t_{ij} + e_{Yij} \qquad \text{(Model 8b)}$$

where d_{0Xi} and d_{0Yi} indicate the deviation of the intercepts for each subject from the overall intercept and d_{1Xi} and d_{1Yi} indicate the deviations of the rates of change for each subject from the overall slope. The relationship between the two measures, X and Y, is modeled by the correlation of d_{0Xi} with d_{0Yi}, and d_{1Xi} with d_{1Yi}.

After we have accounted for the variation in the average levels of the two measures between subjects, it is possible that the weekly within-subject variation in the cytokines may be associated with concurrent changes in symptoms. Specifically, we may see correlations between the residual variation of the cytokines, e_{Xij}, and the residual variation in the reported symptoms, e_{Yij}. In Figure 24.2, this would correspond to the actual values, represented by the stars, being higher than the dashed lines at approximately the same time. Visual inspection of these plots also suggests that measures that are closer together will be more strongly correlated with each other than those that are further apart. One possibility is an autoregressive error structure (AR(1)) where the correlation between measures, $\xi^{|t-t'|}$, decreases as the absolute value of the time between measures, $|t-t'|$, increases.

In Study 2, the variation among subjects in the initial baseline levels of IL-6 and pain severity (measured before the therapy) are weak ($\hat{\rho}_1 = 0.077$). However, there is a strong between-subjects correlation of the rate of change in log IL-6 levels and pain severity ($\hat{\rho}_S = 0.85$), and a moderate correlation of the within-subject variation between the two measures over time ($\hat{\rho}_w = 0.30$).

Missing data

The methods that have been previously presented[3,4] all rely on the assumption that data are missing at random (MAR) given the observed data and covariates.[5] When patients experiencing mobility or mortality drop out of studies or miss assessments, estimates of change over time may be biased if subjects who experience the most severe symptoms are those with missing data. Estimates of change within groups are mostly likely to be affected, such that the estimated trajectories are overly positive and best characterize the changes in the subgroup of patients who remain on study. There has been extensive research over the last 15 years in statistical methods to minimize these biases. The major barrier is that we are missing the information (the missing values) that would allow use to determine which model is correct or most closely approximates the true scores. As a result, we have to rely on assumptions. The best strategy is prevention; designing trials in a manner so as to minimize missing data. If that is not possible, the next best strategy is to collect auxiliary or surrogate data that are strongly correlated with the outcome of interest. Jointly modeling the outcomes of interest with the auxiliary data[6–9] may satisfy the assumption of MAR given the observed outcome, the auxiliary data, and covariates.

Summary

In longitudinal studies that incorporate assessments of symptoms and other patient-reported outcomes, there may be a wealth of untapped information that might shed light on the relationships that occur among symptoms and between symptoms and other biological factors such as cytokines. The illustrations in this chapter highlight only a few of the various procedures that are widely available.

References

1. Wang XS, Fairclough DL, Liao Z, et al. Longitudinal study of the relationship between chemoradiation therapy for non-small-cell lung cancer and patient symptoms. *J Clin Oncol* **24**(27):4485–4491, 2006.

2. Wang XS, Shi Q, Mao L, Cleeland CS, Liao Z. Association between inflammatory cytokines and the development of multiple symptoms in patients with non-small cell lung cancer undergoing chemoradiation therapy [abstract]. American Society of Clinical Oncology 44th Annual Meeting, Chicago IL, May 30–June 3, 2008. *J Clin Oncol* **26**(15 Suppl), 2008.

3. Jennrich RI, Schluchter MD. Unbalanced repeated-measures models with structured covariance matrices. *Biometrics* **42**(4):805–820, 1986.

4. Laird NM, Ware JH. Random-effects models for longitudinal data. *Biometrics* **38**(4):963–974, 1982.
5. Little RJA. Modeling the drop-out mechanism in repeated-measures studies. *Journal of the American Statistical Association* **90**(431):1112–1121, 1995.
6. Fairclough DL, Gagnon D, Papadopoulos G. Planning analyses of quality-of-life studies: a case example with migraine prophylaxis. *J Biopharm Stat* **14**(1):31–51, 2004.
7. Schluchter MD. Methods for the analysis of informatively censored longitudinal data. *Stat Med* **11**(14–15):1861–1870, 1992.
8. Vonesh EF, Greene T, Schluchter MD. Shared parameter models for the joint analysis of longitudinal data and event times. *Stat Med* **25**(1):143–163, 2006.
9. deGruttola V, Tu XM. Modeling progression of CD4-lymphocyte count and its relationship to survival-time. *Biometrics* **50**(4):1003–1014, 1994.

Section 4 Chapter 25

Symptom Measurement

Bayesian adaptive design: a novel approach to test the effectiveness of symptom-reducing agents using patient-reported outcomes

Valen E. Johnson and Tito R. Mendoza

Better symptom management, in cancer as well as in other diseases, has been hampered by the lack of a strong clinical-trial evidence base for guiding symptom management practice. The 2001 Institute of Medicine report *Improving Palliative Care for Cancer*[1] reviewed the paucity of clinical research that might present a basis for evidence-based symptom management. A 2003 NIH State of the Science review[2] concluded that symptoms, especially pain, fatigue, and depression, were undermanaged in cancer care and recommended an increased effort to develop evidence that would support the rational use of both biological and behavioral interventions for symptom management.

Various barriers have hindered the development of evidence-based methods for controlling treatment-related symptom burden, despite the availability of adequate symptom measurement methods. For example, the control of treatment-related symptoms almost always involves the use of combined treatment modalities, which are difficult to evaluate using traditional randomized clinical trial methods, where single symptoms are typically managed with single agents (eg, pain controlled with a single analgesic). When clinicians do treat multiple symptoms, they are likely to prescribe multiple agents based on anecdotal experience or the patient's perceived needs, rather than on evidence-based research.[1] Further, many of the agents that might be effective in the control of treatment-related symptom burden are generic or off-patent drugs that will never receive clinical research support from the pharmaceutical industry because there is no financial incentive to support clinical trials testing their effectiveness for symptom control.

Typical approaches for evaluating combined symptom therapies, such as factorial designs, require large sample sizes, especially when there are many competing agents to account for main effects and all possible combinations of these agents. An alternative to the classic randomized clinical trial approach for developing clinical evidence in support of effective symptom management is a Bayesian adaptive randomization design. An adaptive Bayesian design offers the potential for rapid assessment of the efficacy of several potential treatments. Patient outcomes can be assessed as the trial progresses, with the possibility of incorporating historical information and synthesizing results of new information to eliminate interventions or combinations of interventions that do not show promise. Adaptive designs can also exploit the fact that most treatments expected to benefit symptoms are known *a priori* to have minimal toxicities, a feature that is rarely the case in the development of combined curative therapies for cancer.

A major hurdle for the development of adaptive designs – the lack of computational power and algorithms necessary for performing this type of trial – has been overcome.[3,4] The maturity of the adaptive testing approach has been acknowledged by the US Food and Drug Administration, which recently published a guidance supporting the efficiency of the adaptive approach in the testing and labeling of medical devices.[5] A major tertiary cancer center has used the Bayesian approach as a standard in designing clinical trials.[6] Developments in web-based software for data collection and implementation of relational databases have facilitated quick and relatively easy access to information needed to continuously update interim data.

Although there is an increased recognition of the potential utility of Bayesian methodology for testing of medical devices (as evidenced by the FDA guidance[5]), the application of such methodology is lacking in the design and analysis of symptom outcomes. Exceptions to this include an adaptive randomization study using joint efficacy/toxicity outcomes[7] and a study of acute ischemic stroke measured using the Scandinavian Stroke Scale.[8] However the outcomes in these trials were physician or clinician-rated rather than patient-reported. To

Cancer Symptom Science: Measurement, Mechanisms, and Management, eds. Charles S. Cleeland, Michael J. Fisch, and Adrian J. Dunn.

our knowledge, no adaptive designs have been used when patients' ratings of their symptoms are the outcome of interest.

In this chapter, we describe the basic principles that underlie Bayesian adaptive randomization and discuss general issues that arise when incorporating this technique into the design of clinical trials. We then describe a clinical trial that uses Bayesian adaptive randomization to test the effectiveness of combinations of four symptom interventions for patients with head and neck cancer.

Symptom intervention versus cancer treatment

Randomized clinical trials of symptom interventions differ from clinical trials of cancer treatment therapies in a number of ways, each of which has important implications for the design of their trials. In contrast to cancer therapies:

- Symptom interventions tend to be nontoxic, and are often not associated with severe adverse events. This remains the case even when they are administered in combination with other treatments.
- Because symptom burden is often multifaceted, multiple symptom interventions may be required to alleviate distinct aspects of patient distress.
- Efficacy of randomized clinical trials of symptom interventions must be gauged according to patient-reported outcome (PRO) instruments, rather than more traditional, physician-reported clinical outcome measures.
- PRO measures are usually recorded on essentially continuous (and often even multidimensional) scales. Such measures naturally support more sophisticated statistical analyses.

These features of symptom interventions can be exploited to design clinical trials that quickly identify efficacious treatments and combinations of treatments. Further, the mechanism that facilitates such designs – Bayesian adaptive randomization – increases the probability that effective treatments are administered to patients who participate in the resulting clinical trials. Adopting a Bayesian adaptive randomization is particularly important in trials that enroll a significant proportion of the at-risk patient population.

Bayesian adaptive randomization

Classic phase II and III randomized clinical trials are designed so that a predetermined number of patients receive either a standard treatment (control group) or one or more trial agents (treatment groups). The number of patients assigned to treatment and control groups is determined before the start of the trial to guarantee that the trial has a specified level of statistical significance and power. Significance levels are generally based on a test of a null hypothesis that there is no difference between standard and trial treatments, while statistical power calculations are premised on prior assumptions regarding the magnitude of the desired treatment effect(s).

Staged designs incorporate interim analyses of patient outcomes before the mandated termination of the trial. Most staged designs involve one interim examination of data and are therefore called two-stage designs. Staged trials may be terminated during an interim analysis for at least two reasons. When evidence collected early in the trial convincingly demonstrates a beneficial treatment effect, the trial can be declared a success and is terminated early. Alternatively, if data available at the time of an interim analysis suggests that there is only a small probability that the trial will be successful after all patients have been accrued, then the trial may be stopped early for futility and deemed a failure. To control Type 1 error (the probability that an ineffective trial agent is declared superior to the standard treatment) in staged trials, more stringent end-of-trial success criteria are required for classic multistage designs than for single-stage designs. In both standard single-stage and multi-stage designs, the number of patients assigned to each treatment group during each stage of the trial does not deviate from the original trial design as patient outcome data is accrued.

In contrast to classical designs, Bayesian adaptive designs change the probabilities that patients are assigned to treatments according to the outcomes of patients who have previously entered the trial.

An illustration of a Bayesian adaptive design

To illustrate the operation of a simple adaptive design, consider an example in which the probability that a patient is "cured" after receiving the standard treatment is denoted by p and the probability that a patient is cured after receiving a trial agent is denoted by q. In general, neither the value of p or q is known. Within the Bayesian paradigm, uncertainty about the unknown values of p and q is represented by a probability distribution. Before observing any trial data, these probability distributions are called "prior distributions." For example, one might assume that the prior distributions assigned to p and q are uniform on the interval (0, 1); that is, all values of p and q are assumed to be equally likely. After observing trial data, the updated probability distributions that represent uncertainty regarding the values of p and q are called "posterior distributions."

Suppose now that an adaptive trial is underway, and that x of m patients treated with the standard treatment were cured, and that y of n patients treated with the trial agent are cured. A new patient has just entered the trial, and we wish to assign this patient to either the standard or trial therapy.

As an example, suppose that $x = 3$ and $m = 6$, or in other words that 50% of the first six patients assigned to the standard treatment were cured. Also, suppose that $y = 5$ and $n = 6$, or that 83% of the first six patients assigned to the trial agent were cured. From these data and the assumption of uniform prior distributions for p and q, the posterior distributions for p and q can be calculated from Bayes' theorem. The density functions describing these distributions are pictured in Figure 25.1.

Adaptive randomized assignment of the next (13th) patient entering the trial to a treatment is based on the (current) posterior probability that $q > p$. This probability is equal to the probability that

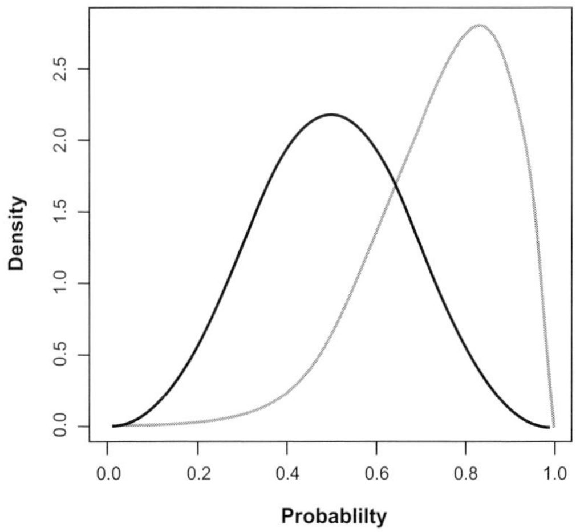

Figure 25.1. Depiction of posterior probability densities that result from a uniform prior and three out of six successes (left) and five out of six successes (right).

a value drawn at random from the posterior density of q is greater than a value drawn at random from the posterior density of p. Let r denote the value of that probability, which in this particular case is calculated to be 0.87.

A number of rules have been proposed for using the value of r to assign a treatment to the newly enrolled patient. The rule used here simply assigns the new patient to the experimental treatment group with probability identically equal to r. Other rules might be based on assigning the next patient to the experimental treatment group according to some function of r, for example with probability proportional to $\sqrt{r}$.

The advantage of adaptive randomized assignment of patients to treatments is based on the fact that patients have a higher probability of being assigned to the treatment currently judged to be most successful. In this example, if the 13th patient is assigned to the experimental treatment and is cured, the probability that the 14th patient is also assigned to the experimental treatment would increase to 0.90.

Stopping rules, operating characteristics, and sample-size calculations

The previous section describes the principle that underlies randomization procedures used in Bayesian adaptive designs. Other important aspects of these designs concern the rules that specify termination of the trial. Typically, these rules require that the posterior probability that one treatment is better than all others exceeds a certain threshold, or that enrollment of patients has reached a specified maximum. For example, a Bayesian adaptive randomization trial might be stopped when any one of the following conditions occurs:

- The posterior probability that one trial agent is more effective than all others exceeds a specified threshold. In the example above, such a stopping rule might require that $\Pr(q > p|data) > 0.95$, or, in other words, that there be a 95% chance the experimental treatment is better than the standard treatment, given all available patient outcomes.
- The probability that no trial agent is more effective than the standard therapy exceeds a specified threshold. That is, in the example above one might stop and declare the trial a failure if $\Pr(q < p|data) > 0.8$.

- Patient enrollment reaches the maximum trial limit.
- The trial period expires.

A criterion must also be specified for declaring a treatment or treatments to be a success if the trial is stopped for either of the last two reasons.

A trial's operating characteristics describe the frequentist properties of a trial under a variety of assumptions regarding the true state of nature (eg, the true, but unknown, values of p and q). These properties include the Type 1 error rate and the power of the trial in hypothetical replications of the trial. In the example described above, the operating characteristics of the trial might be summarized in a table that provided, for a variety of assumed values of p and q, (1) the probability that the trial agent was declared superior to the standard treatment; (2) the probability that the standard treatment was declared superior to the trial agent; and (3) the average number of patients enrolled before trial termination. In general, operating characteristics of adaptively randomized clinical trials must be determined through numerical simulation.

The numerical computations required to determine a trial's operating characteristics can also be used to calculate the (frequentist) power of a trial as a function of sample size and specified treatment effects. In this regard, sample-size calculations performed for Bayesian adaptive randomized designs are conceptually similar to the calculations used to determine sample sizes required for classic designs. The trial designer specifies the desired power for the trial (often 80%) and the values of treatment efficacy for both standard and experimental agents, and then repeatedly simulates outcomes of the trial until he finds a sample size that provides the desired power. Bayesian adaptive trials provide additional flexibility in determining sample sizes because their stopping rules can also be modified as part of this optimization process.

A Bayesian adaptive randomized clinical trial for symptom intervention in patients with head and neck cancer

To illustrate the basic concepts described in the previous sections, we describe how we plan to apply them in the conduct of an actual Bayesian adaptive trial designed to test the utility of single and combination treatments for symptoms encountered in response to radiation therapy for head and neck cancer. Patients undergoing treatment for head and neck cancer typically report symptoms of fatigue, pain, sleep disturbance, difficulty swallowing, and lack of appetite; many of these symptoms are associated with mucositis.

The goal of this trial is to test the premise that a single trial agent or combination of trial agents is successful in reducing treatment-related symptom burden. Four trial agents will be evaluated in 200 patients with head and neck cancer during this study:

- Minocycline, an agent that exhibits strong suppression of proinflammatory cytokines. Preclinical data suggests that minocycline protects against the development of neuropathy due to chemotherapy and other neural insults and has demonstrated a high degree of safety when administered to patients suffering from other types of cancer.
- Curcumin (diferuloylmethane) is a polyphenol derived from the rhizomes of *Curcuma longa* and is the main constituent of the yellow spice turmeric. It has been shown to be safe and has demonstrated anti-inflammatory properties.
- Modafinil, originally developed for the treatment of narcolepsy, is a wakefulness-promoting agent that acts as a psychostimulant. It has also been shown to potentially improve wakefulness in cancer patients and patients suffering from other medical conditions.
- Bupropion, an antidepressant of the aminoketone class, is a nonselective inhibitor of the dopamine and norepinephrine transporters that is unrelated to tricyclic, tetracyclic, or selective serotonin reuptake inhibitors or other known antidepressant agents. Bupropion is also an antagonist at neuronal nicotinic acetylcholine receptors, and as such it is widely used to support smoking cessation. In addition to its antidepressant effects, bupropion is known to have anti-inflammatory effects, specifically the suppression of tumor necrosis factor-α.

Outcome variable: area under the curve

The primary outcome variable in this study will be the combined area under the curve (AUC). The AUC is a single number expressing the approximate combined area of two or more trapezoids calculated over a period of time; the area of a trapezoid is derived by multiplying half of the base (the distance between two assessment time points) by the sum of the two heights (the scores at each of the two time points). In this study, the AUC will summarize the severity of fatigue, difficulty swallowing, lack of appetite, pain, and disturbed sleep during the first 10 weeks after the initiation of radiation therapy. The base of each trapezoid will be the number of days between two symptom-assessment time points, and the two heights will correspond to the two mean symptom scores (mean of the five symptoms) computed at each of those assessment time points. Given a weekly assessment schedule over a 10-week period, the AUC for this study will be the sum of the area of 10 trapezoids. Missing data between administrations will be interpolated by fitting fewer trapezoids and will be extrapolated with regression models.

The five symptoms – fatigue, difficulty swallowing, lack of appetite, pain, and disturbed sleep – were chosen because they were the most prevalent and most severe symptoms in this particular group of patients; they will be measured using the head and neck cancer module of the M. D. Anderson Symptom Inventory (MDASI)[9–11] MDASI scores will be collected using an interactive voice response (IVR) system, which solicits patient responses using the MDASI's 11-point rating scale collected using touch-tone telephone keys. A response of 0 indicates the absence of the queried symptom, and a response of 10 signifies the highest level of the given symptom.

We denote the AUC value collected for the *i*-th patient by *auc(i)*. Because *auc(i)* represents the average of a large number of ordinal variables, by the central-limit theorem we assume that its value can be considered to be approximately normally distributed. Based on preliminary data, a conservative estimate of the standard deviations of the AUC values for this variable is 130.

The Bayesian adaptive randomized clinical trial design for this study will entail two phases, a factorial lead-in component and an adaptive component (Figure 25.2). During the first phase, we will assign patients to treatments according to a factorial design. The purpose of the factorial component is to obtain initial estimates of the efficacy of all combinations of treatments. Note that with four trial agents, there are $2^4 = 16$ possible treatment combinations. With two patients per treatment combination, we will be able to obtain treatment effects and the associated variance estimates for each of the 16 possible treatments. Hence, the factorial component requires 32 patients. On the basis of data collected during the factorial component of the design, we will implement adaptive randomization treatment allocation for the next 168 patients.

The primary advantage of this factorial component is the efficiency with which main treatment effects and second-order interactions between treatments can be evaluated. Ignoring higher-order interactions between treatments, this means we can estimate the main effects of each treatment with the same precision as we would in a two-arm trial involving only that treatment.

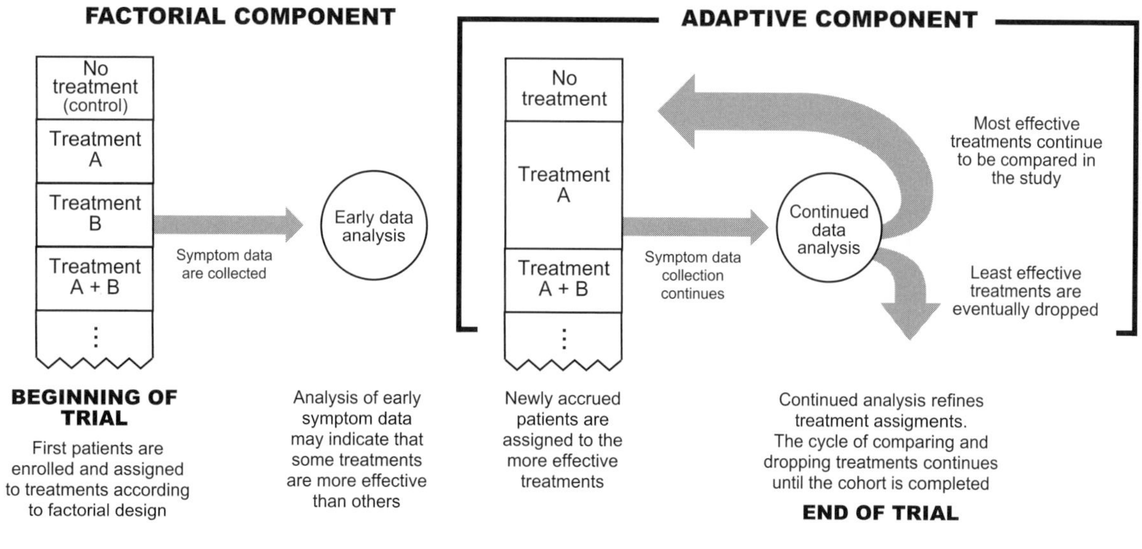

Figure 25.2. Study schema for an adaptive clinical trial

Similar gains in efficiency will also be accrued in evaluating second-order synergies among treatments. As a consequence, we anticipate substantially reducing the number of patients who are assigned to ineffective treatments.

Success of treatments will be judged according to the average predicted AUC, penalized for the number of treatments administered. A penalty is imposed on treatment administration to account for the inconvenience and cost of providing treatment, as well as to avoid treatments that are estimated to provide only marginal patient benefit. The trade-off between the cost of treatment administration and treatment benefit was assessed using the following reasoning. On the basis of our previous experience with these patient groups, we defined an effective treatment to be a treatment that results in a 0.35 average reduction in each of the five MDASI symptom variables collected for the patient cohort. The AUC values for the cohort are approximately equal to the sum of the five symptom scores observed over the 10-week observation period. Thus, we expect effective treatments to decrease the average AUC score for a patient by 0.35×10 weeks $\times 7$ days $= 25$. In contrast, we define treatments that do not achieve even 40% of this effect to be ineffective and not worth the cost and inconvenience associated with their administration. Thus, a cost of 10 AUC units is imposed on the administration of each intervention. This penalty term represents approximately 7% of the estimated standard deviation of the combined AUC measurement for a single patient.

We will stop the trial for futility if the posterior probability that no treatment is effective exceeds 0.99. Alternatively, if the posterior probability that one treatment is better than all others exceeds 0.99, then we will also stop the trial early and declare that treatment to be superior. If the trial enrolls all 200 patients, we will report the treatment that has the lowest posterior mean AUC to be superior.

Factorial component

Four treatments – minocycline, curcumin, modafinil, and bupropion – will be tested alone and in combination for their ability to reduce the value of patient AUC. An initial factorial design will be used to estimate treatment effects for all 16 combinations of treatments and will be replicated twice to obtain both estimates of treatment effects and the variability of these estimates. Because 16 patients are required for a single replication of the factorial design for four treatments, 32 patients will be used during the factorial component of the study.

According to a complete factorial design, the first 16 patients to enter the trial are randomly assigned to one of the 16 treatment regimens. As shown in Table 25.1, each treatment agent will be administered either alone or in some combination to 8 of the 16 patients, and will not be administered to the remaining eight patients. Evaluation of the main effects of each treatment can thus be estimated as the difference in the means between the two groups. That is, each of the four main treatment effects is based on the difference in the means of two groups of eight patients.

Issues with symptom intervention-related toxicity

The efficiency of such factorial designs extends also to trials that contain more than four trial agents. It is important to note, however, that factorial designs like the one described in Table 25.1 cannot typically be employed in curative cancer trials where each trial agent is associated with significant toxicity. Factorial designs are only appropriate when there is medical evidence that demonstrates the safety of each trial agent in combination with other trial agents.

This design is particularly useful when there is also an interest in estimating the synergies between treatments. When subsets of treatments are thought to interact to cause adverse reactions, the use of fractional factorial designs can be contemplated. Fractional factorial designs involved a selected subset, or fraction, of treatments or treatment combinations of a full factorial design. Using the sparsity-of-effects principle, a reasonable approach is to select main effects and the first-order interactions. An alternative and perhaps more practical approach is to include Phase I toxicity design in the conduct of the study.

To address the issue of whether combinations of the proposed symptom agents might potentially harm patients, we will incorporate a Phase I toxicity design. Phase I trials typically include successive cohorts with 3–6 patients per cohort to find the maximum tolerated dose (MTD). A cohort is a small group of patients. Instead of finding the MTD, we will use standard 3 + 3 criteria (three or six patients per dose paradigm) for determining whether any treatment or treatment combination produces either grade 3 or 4 toxicities in the first six patients assigned to each treatment combination. That

Table 25.1. Patient assignment to treatments for factorial component with four trial agents

Intervention	**Patient**															
	1	2	3	4	5	6	7	8	9	10	11	12	13	14	15	16
Curcumin	0	x	0	0	0	x	x	x	0	0	0	x	x	x	0	x
Modafinil	0	0	x	0	0	x	0	0	x	x	0	x	x	0	x	x
Minocycline	0	0	0	x	0	0	x	0	x	0	x	x	0	x	x	x
Bupropion	0	0	0	0	x	0	0	x	0	x	x	0	x	x	x	x
Intervention	**Patient**															
	17	18	19	20	21	22	23	24	25	26	27	28	29	30	31	32
Curcumin	0	x	0	0	0	x	x	x	0	0	0	x	x	x	0	x
Modafinil	0	0	x	0	0	x	0	0	x	x	0	x	x	0	x	x
Minocycline	0	0	0	x	0	0	x	0	x	0	x	x	0	x	x	x
Bupropion	0	0	0	0	x	0	0	x	0	x	x	0	x	x	x	x

In this design, patients are assigned in random order to 1 of the 16 treatments indicated by columns in the table. For example, a patient assigned to the 7th or 23rd treatment column would be assigned to both curcumin and minocycline, but would not receive modafinil or bupropion.

is, if more than one symptom intervention-related toxicity (grade 3 or 4) is observed in the first six patients assigned to any treatment combination, that treatment combination will be deleted from the study. The presence of grade 3 or 4 toxicities will be counted against all higher-order treatment combinations whenever at least one toxicity is observed for a specified treatment. For example, if at least one grade 3 or 4 treatment toxicity is attributed to a patient who receives curcumin and modafinil, then toxicities observed in patients who received (curcumin, modafinil, minocycline), (curcumin, modafinil, bupropion), or (curcumin, modafinil, minocyline, bupropion) will also be counted toward the number of patients experiencing toxicities with the combination of only curcumin and modafinil. Similarly, the presence of grade 3 or 4 toxicities will also be counted against lower-order treatment combinations when the treating physician determines that the toxicity could have been the result of one of the component treatments alone. For example, the observation of grade 3 diarrhea in a patient assigned to curcumin and modafinil might also be counted against the single-agent treatment of curcumin, since curcumin is known to be associated with the occurrence of diarrhea.

The determination of whether a patient's grade 3 or 4 toxicity was caused by the symptom-treatment combination (rather than by the primary chemotherapy agent) will be performed by the principal investigator in consultation with the treating physician. A list of adverse events known to be associated with primary treatments has been compiled.

After six patients have been assigned to a treatment, that treatment will be dropped from further study if the posterior probability that the toxicity is greater than 0.33 exceeds 0.5. A beta (0.5, 0.5) density will be used as the prior density in this calculation. The resulting toxicity exclusion boundaries are 2/6, 3/9, 4/12, 5/15, or 6/16.

Although each specific combination of treatments will be assigned to only two patients, each of the four primary treatments will be received by 16 patients. For example, 16 patients will receive curcumin alone or in combination with other treatments. Thus, if curcumin causes toxicity in any of these 16 patients, that toxicity will be counted against curcumin in all patients who experienced toxicity because of it, whether or not the patient experiencing toxicity was assigned other treatments. Sixteen patients are therefore available to assess the safety of curcumin. Similarly, eight patients will be available to assess the safety of each two-way combination of treatments, four patients will be available to assess the safety of each three-way combination of treatments, and two patients will be available to assess the safety of the four-treatment combination. Toxicity reports collected during the factorial component will be retained for use in the follow-on adaptive trial where, in combination with the stopping boundaries described above, the safety assessment of treatments assigned during the adaptive trial can be completed.

With regard to safety assessment, an advantage of this factorial lead-in study and follow-on adaptive trial is that we may avoid assessments of treatments combinations that are not deemed to be efficacious. For example, if one of the study drugs does not demonstrate efficacy, the number of patients assigned to treatment combinations including that drug is likely to be limited. As a consequence, it may become unnecessary to evaluate the safety profiles of combinations of treatments involving that drug. For example, the lack of efficacy of one or more treatments or treatment combinations may obviate the requirement to evaluate the safety of assigning all four treatments to a single patient, since this treatment will not be considered for assignment to any more than the two patients assigned to it during the factorial component.

Bayesian adaptive component

After the factorial component is completed, we will enter the Bayesian adaptive randomization component of the trial, in which we will randomly assign patients to treatments according to current estimates of each treatment's efficacy. In this phase of the study, subjects will be assigned to treatments according to the probability that each treatment results in the lowest predicted combined symptom AUC measurement. This adaptive assignment scheme represents a randomized version of "pick the winner"[12] and provides assurance that effective treatments are not completely disallowed because of early trial failures.

To obtain predictive probabilities for values of patient's AUC for each treatment combination, we assume that the statistical properties of the response variable *auc(i)* can be described by a linear model expressible as:

$$auc_i = \beta_0 + \beta_1 Ind(T_1) + \beta_2 Ind(T_2) + \beta_{1,2} Ind(T_1 T_2) + \ldots + \beta_{1,2,3,4} Ind(T_1 T_2 T_3 T_4) + \varepsilon_i \qquad \text{(Equation 25.1)}$$

In this equation, $Ind(T_1, T_2)$ denotes the assignment of treatments/interventions 1 and 2 to patient i, and $\beta_{1,2}$ represents the average effect of this treatment on the symptom AUC score. Similar notation applies to other treatment combinations. Note that the parameter $\beta_{1,2}$ represents the additional or synergistic treatment effect of treatments 1 and 2 when these treatments are assigned together, over and above the effects that these treatments have alone (ie, $\beta_1 + \beta_2$). The term ε denotes interpatient variability in reported AUC values and is assumed to be approximately normally distributed, with mean 0 and variance σ^2. *A priori*, we assume noninformative priors for the values of the regression coefficients β and σ^2.

The factorial component of the trial's adaptive design will provide a joint posterior distribution on the values of the regression coefficients β and patient variance parameter σ^2. After completion of the factorial lead-in, each new patient will be assigned to a treatment according to the probability that the given treatment, plus the penalty associated with the administration of the treatment, results in a lower predicted mean symptom AUC for that patient. In other words, we will sample a value of the vector β from its current posterior distribution, and we will assign the new patient to the treatment for which sum of the linear predictor and the penalty term is a minimum. By sampling β from its (current) posterior, we implicitly account for the uncertainty associated with its value based on data collected up to that point in the trial. If uncertainty about the efficacy of treatments and combinations of treatments is still high after the initial 32 patients have been treated and assessed, then each combination of treatments will receive approximately the same probability of assignment to the next patient. As the trial progresses, the uncertainty associated with the value of each treatment will be reduced, and effective treatments will be allocated a higher probability of being assigned to each new patient.

Simulating the operating characteristic of the trial

An important validation step in the design phase of a Bayesian adaptive trial involves assessment of the performance of the trial when it is repeatedly simulated while holding the values of model parameters fixed. To perform such simulations, parameters are arbitrarily assigned values that represent hypothesized treatment benefits. Based on these assigned values, the outcomes for patients can be simulated from the statistical model assumed for the outcome variable. In this hypothetical trial, a linear model is assumed for patient outcomes, so the mean response predicted for a patient is easily calculated based on given values of the regression coefficients β from

Equation 25.1 above. To account for interpatient variability, a random error with variance σ^2 is added to the predicted mean value to obtain a simulated value for a patient's AUC value.

Using such a procedure, statistical experiments can be performed by simulating patient responses for arbitrary treatment combinations. For this design, that means that the first 32 patients are assigned to treatments according to two replications of the factorial design provided in Table 25.1. After simulating an *auc(i)* value for each of these patients, the joint posterior distribution for β and σ^2 can be estimated using responses from the factorial component (pretending that the actual values of β and σ^2 are not known). Next, an additional 168 patients are sequentially assigned to treatments according to the adaptive randomization scheme described above, and AUC values are simulated for these patients as well. The posterior distribution is re-estimated after each AUC value is simulated, and randomization probabilities for patients are based on all data available at the time of their entry into the trial. After 200 patient AUC values and treatment assignments have been simulated in this way, conclusions from the trial will be recorded and the next trial replicate performed.

Table 25.2 illustrates the results from four experiments in which 1000 trials were simulated in this way. All values of the regression parameter β not listed in the first column of the table were assumed to be equal to zero. For example, in the second row of the table (β_1=-25), only the first treatment was assumed to have an effect on symptom burden, and the effect of this treatment on symptom burden was to reduce the AUC of the 10-week MDASI scores by 25 units. For 1000 replications of a trial in which the first treatment had this effect, the probability that treatment 1 was judged to be the only effective treatment was 0.98. The third column of the table lists the proportion of patients, on average, who received the most effective treatment(s) during the trial. For the second row of the table, on average 175/200 patients received only treatment 1 – the optimal treatment. Note that of the 25 patients who did not receive treatment 1, 16 would have enrolled in the trial during the lead-in factorial component, before adaptive randomization began. Similarly, the third row of the table reports results when the only effective treatment occurred when both treatments 1 and 2 were assigned to a patient (neither being effective alone), and the fourth row of the table provides results when both treatment 1 and the combination of treatments 1 and 2 had the beneficial effect of a 25-point average reduction in AUC.

Sample size calculations and statistical size of the trial

Tables of operating characteristics also can be used to summarize both the power of a design and the level of significance associated with the null hypothesis of no treatment effect. Referencing again row two of Table 25.2, if the only effective treatment is the first treatment and the effect of the first treatment is to reduce the 10-week AUC measurement by 25 units on average, then entries in this row imply that the frequentist power of this trial for detecting the optimal treatment is 0.98.

The statistical significance of this trial design can be inferred from the first row of Table 25.2. In the simulated trials represented in this row, no treatments were effective. At the end of these trials, the treatment that predicted the lowest mean patient AUC was "no treatment" in 96% of the simulated trials; that is, the probability that "no treatment" was declared the best treatment at the end of the trial was 0.96. The size of the test associated with the null hypothesis is $\alpha = 1 - 0.96 = 0.04$. Thus, the significance level of the proposed adaptive trial is 4%.

The power of the trial in detecting several treatment effects is listed in the remaining rows of column 2. For example, if a single treatment reduces patients' AUC value by 25 units on average, there is a 98% chance that this treatment will be declared effective at the end of the trial. The power for detecting this treatment effect is

Table 25.2. Operating characteristics of the trial

Treatment	Probability that correct therapy is chosen	Average number of patients who receive optimal therapy
No effective treatment	0.96	123/200
$\beta_1 = -25$	0.98	175/200
$\beta_{1,2} = -25$	0.97	150/200
$\beta_1 = \beta_{1,2} = -25$	0.98	159/200

thus 0.98. The other entries in this column have a similar interpretation. The third-row entry shows that the trial has 97% power in detecting an efficacious interaction effect of 25 units even when the associated individual treatments are ineffective; the fourth row demonstrates that the trial has 98% power in detecting a single treatment effect and a synergistic effect with this treatment when both effects are 25 units in magnitude.

Reporting study results

According to our trial design, randomization will continue until 200 patients are accrued (32 during the factorial component and 168 during the adaptive component). The results of Bayesian analyses will be summarized using posterior credible intervals. Because we have assumed noninformative priors for the regression coefficients in our model, these credible intervals will exactly match the corresponding non-Bayesian confidence intervals. That is, the 95% credible intervals we estimate at the end of the trial for treatment effects will exactly match the 95% confidence intervals using the same trial data.

Our final report of the best treatment or treatment combination will be determined according to the posterior mean estimate of the treatment/treatment combination effects on symptom reduction at the conclusion of the trial. This will also correspond to the usual, non-Bayesian least-squares estimates. Rather than using traditional *P* values for comparing treatment arms, Bayesian methods use posterior probabilities and credible intervals to quantify the magnitude of treatment effects, providing an intuitive way to think about outcomes of clinical studies. The interpretation of posterior credible intervals from within the Bayesian paradigm is slightly different from the more traditional frequentist (non-Bayesian) interpretation. For example, the Bayesian 95% credible interval is interpreted as an interval that contains the true effect size with probability 0.95. As an illustration, in a recent Bayesian adaptive trial examining single-agent versus combined cancer treatment as its primary focus, the authors reported that "given the data, the posterior probabilities that gemcitabine-docetaxel was superior for progression-free and overall survival were 0.98 and 0.97, respectively."[13]

Conclusion

Bayesian statistical methods are increasingly being used in clinical research because the Bayesian approach is ideally suited to adapting study treatment to information that accrues during a trial, potentially allowing for smaller, more informative trials and for patients to receive better treatment during the course of study.[4,5] Bayesian methodology provides a mechanism for updating what is known as results accumulate during a trial. Such updating can be incorporated completely, explicitly, and prospectively. Accumulating results can be assessed periodically, with the possibility of adapting randomization probabilities to favor better-performing therapies and changing the trial population to focus on patient subsets that are responding better to the experimental therapies. An important use for the Bayesian approach is to calculate the predictive probability distribution of future results on the basis of current results. Such analyses also allow for the use of historical information and for synthesizing results of relevant trials.

Several successful adaptive oncology trials have demonstrated the effectiveness of this approach for reducing the number of patients receiving inferior therapy during the course of curative trials.[13–15] Recent innovative applications of Bayesian adaptive designs include the development of targeted therapies in lung cancer,[16] joint modeling of efficacy and toxicity of monoclonal antibody regimens,[7] and the use of short-term response for survival clinical trials.[17]

The benefits of taking a Bayesian approach to clinical trial design include efficiency, better treatment of patients in the trial, and greater precision regarding primary endpoints, all positive attributes when relieving symptom distress is the study focus.

References

1. Foley KM, Gelband H. *Improving Palliative Care for Cancer*. Washington DC: National Academy Press, 2001.
2. National Institutes of Health. Symptom management in cancer: pain, depression and fatigue: State-of-the-Science Conference Statement. *J Pain Palliat Care Pharmacother* **17**(1):77–97, 2003.
3. Thall PF, Wathen JK. Practical Bayesian adaptive randomisation in clinical trials. *Eur J Cancer* **43**(5):859–866, 2007.
4. Spiegelhalter DJ, Abrams KR, Myles JP. *Bayesian Approaches to Clinical Trials and Health Care Evaluation*. Chichester: Wiley, 2004.
5. US Food and Drug Administration, Center for Devices and Radiological Health. Draft guidance for

industry and FDA staff. Guidance for the use of Bayesian statistics in medical device clinical trials. Available from: URL: http://www.fda.gov/downloads/MedicalDevices/DeviceRegulationandGuidance/GuidanceDocuments/ucm071121.pdf. Accessed Jun 9, 2009.

6. Biswas S, Liu DD, Lee JJ, Berry DA. Bayesian clinical trials at the University of Texas M. D. Anderson Cancer Center. *Clin Trials* **6**(3):205–216, 2009.

7. Ji Y, Bekele BN. Adaptive randomization for multiarm comparative clinical trials based on joint efficacy/toxicity outcomes. *Biometrics:e*-pub ahead of print, 2009.

8. Krams M, Lees KR, Hacke W, Grieve AP, Orgogozo JM, Ford GA. Acute Stroke Therapy by Inhibition of Neutrophils (ASTIN): an adaptive dose-response study of UK-279,276 in acute ischemic stroke. *Stroke* **34**(11):2543–2548, 2003.

9. Cleeland CS, Mendoza TR, Wang XS, et al. Assessing symptom distress in cancer patients: the M. D. Anderson Symptom Inventory. *Cancer* **89**(7):1634–1646, 2000.

10. Rosenthal DI, Mendoza TR, Chambers MS, et al. Measuring head and neck cancer symptom burden: the development and validation of the M. D. Anderson Symptom Inventory, head and neck module. *Head Neck* **29**(10): 923–931, 2007.

11. Rosenthal DI, Mendoza TR, Chambers MS, et al. The M. D. Anderson symptom inventory-head and neck module, a patient-reported outcome instrument, accurately predicts the severity of radiation-induced mucositis. *Int J Radiat Oncol Biol Phys* **72**(5): 1355–1361, 2008.

12. Berry DA, Fristedt B. *Bandit Problems: Sequential Allocation of Experiments (Monographs on Statistics and Applied Probability)*. London: Chapman and Hall, 1985.

13. Maki RG, Wathen JK, Patel SR, et al. Randomized phase II study of gemcitabine and docetaxel compared with gemcitabine alone in patients with metastatic soft tissue sarcomas: results of sarcoma alliance for research through collaboration study 002 [corrected]. *J Clin Oncol* **25**(19):2755–2763, 2007.

14. Giles FJ, Kantarjian HM, Cortes JE, et al. Adaptive randomized study of idarubicin and cytarabine versus troxacitabine and cytarabine versus troxacitabine and idarubicin in untreated patients 50 years or older with adverse karyotype acute myeloid leukemia. *J Clin Oncol* **21**(9):1722–1727, 2003.

15. Kantarjian H, Oki Y, Garcia-Manero G, et al. Results of a randomized study of 3 schedules of low-dose decitabine in higher-risk myelodysplastic syndrome and chronic myelomonocytic leukemia. *Blood* **109**(1):52–57, 2007.

16. Zhou X, Liu S, Kim ES, Herbst RS, Lee JJ. Bayesian adaptive design for targeted therapy development in lung cancer – a step toward personalized medicine. *Clin Trials* **5**(3):181–193, 2008.

17. Huang X, Ning J, Li Y, Estey E, Issa JP, Berry DA. Using short-term response information to facilitate adaptive randomization for survival clinical trials. *Stat Med* **28**(12):1680–1689, 2009.

Section 5 Chapter 26

Government and Industry Perspectives

Promoting cancer symptom science research

Ann O'Mara and Maria Sgambati

Federal support for research on cancer symptoms has steadily increased since 1975, partly in response to national policy statements that have made effective symptom control a priority across the course of the disease, not just at the end of life. The Institute of Medicine (IOM) of the National Academy of Sciences lists the control of cancer pain as one of its top 20 priorities for improving health care.[1] The 2001 IOM report *Improving Palliative Care for Cancer*[2] and the 2002 National Institutes of Health (NIH) State-of-the-Science Conference report *Symptom Management in Cancer Pain, Depression, and Fatigue*[3] both highlighted the paucity of data on the epidemiology, underlying mechanisms, and effective treatments for the most prevalent disease-related and treatment-related symptoms of cancer. The 2001 IOM report called for a significant increase in symptom-directed research, noting that symptom control and palliative care are critical components in comprehensive cancer management. Severe symptoms can result in the postponement or cessation of potentially curative therapies, and poorly managed symptoms are a major source of distress and impaired physical and social functioning for patients and families. For many patients and survivors, effective symptom management is almost as important as tumor control.

Symptoms such as pain, cognitive impairment, depression, fatigue, appetite loss/cachexia, and sleep disorders are not unique to cancer, nor are the studies of their etiologies and treatments unique to one scientific or professional discipline. Investigators seeking NIH support for cancer symptom research must keep these principles in mind, because more than one of the Institutes and Centers (ICs) within the NIH are engaged in the scientific review and financial support of cancer-related symptom research. Further, the NIH is but one of many federal and nonfederal sources that provide support for cancer research.

In this chapter we will (1) identify the primary NIH ICs currently supporting cancer symptom research; (2) briefly describe the NIH review process for applicants seeking funding; (3) summarize the various NIH funding mechanisms that support this area of research; (4) review trends in NIH support since 1980 for cancer symptom research in the areas of pain, cognitive impairment, depression, fatigue, appetite loss/cachexia, and sleep disorders; (5) highlight symptom management clinical trials that have been implemented through the National Cancer Institute's clinical trials network, specifically the Community Clinical Oncology Program (CCOP); and (6) identify other federal and nonfederal sources of support for cancer research.

Primary NIH institutes and centers supporting cancer symptom research

A common misperception among seasoned and junior investigators seeking NIH support for cancer symptom research is that both scientific review and funding decisions occur within the same Institute or Center. In reality, most scientific reviews are conducted by one of the Integrated Review Groups (IRGs) located within the NIH Center for Scientific Review, which is a separate entity from the ICs that make funding decisions.

Every IRG is composed of a number of study sections, each with its specific areas of science. Similarly, each IC has its own unique mission and specific area of science, usually disease-specific, such as the National Cancer Institute (NCI) or the Institute for Allergies and Infectious Diseases (NIAID). However, it is not uncommon for one or more IRGs and ICs to encompass overlapping areas of science. For example, beyond the customary NCI support, cancer pain could also potentially be reviewed in one of four study sections and receive support from several of the 15 ICs. Because so many ICs support pain and sleep research, the NIH established the Trans-NIH Pain Consortium and the Trans-NIH Sleep Research

Cancer Symptom Science: Measurement, Mechanisms, and Management, eds. Charles S. Cleeland, Michael J. Fisch, and Adrian J. Dunn.

Coordinating Center to enhance these areas of research and to promote collaboration among researchers across the ICs with programs and activities addressing pain and sleep.[4,5]

The overlap between the IRGs and the ICs is shown in Table 26.1, which outlines the IRG study sections that currently review and the ICs that currently support research in pain, fatigue, cognitive impairment, depression, anorexia, and sleep disorders. The authors recognize that this is far from being a comprehensive list of cancer symptoms and the choice of these six symptoms, which are meant to be representative rather than exhaustive, was guided by several factors. These factors include: (1) data presented on the symptoms referenced in the IOM report,[1] the State-of-the Science report,[3] and the report by Cleeland et al[6]; (2) the prevalence of research studies in these symptom areas in the various NCI portfolios; and (3) the recognition that these symptoms can cross disease entities and therefore might be of interest to multiple ICs.

The NIH grant review process

Grant review at the NIH is a two-step process designed to provide a fair review of every application and to prevent a conflict of interest by separating an application's scientific merit (the IRG review) from its implications for the policy of a particular IC (the IC Advisory Council review).[7] Receipt of the grant application at the NIH Center for Scientific Review initiates a general sequence of events:

- The application is assigned to a study section in the most appropriate IRG to assess its scientific and technical merit. The application also will be assigned to the IC best suited to fund the application (more than one IC may be assigned, as appropriate). Given the array of IRGs and ICs with an interest in cancer symptom research and the expertise to review a given application, investigators seeking NIH funding are encouraged to consider (1) which study group might best review the project; and (2) how the project dovetails with one or more ICs' missions and goals. The investigator may request assignment to a specific study section or IC in a cover letter attached to the grant application, unless the application is being made in response to a specific Request for Applications (RFA) or Funding Opportunity Announcement (FOA). Applicants should be aware that ICs vary in their requirements for submission and review and should contact the particular IC before submitting their projects.
- Information about the application becomes available online at the NIH Commons, including the NIH institute(s) to which the application has been assigned for possible funding, the 12–14-character assignment number indicating the funding mechanism being applied for, the IRG or study section that will review the application, and the name and contact information of the Scientific Review Officer who will manage the study section. To learn more about the NIH Commons and to apply for an account, visit http://commons.era.nih.gov/commons.
- The Scientific Review Officer will assess appropriateness of assignment, completeness of application, adherence of application to guidelines, and scientific and technical expertise needed to fairly and appropriately review the application. Each application is assigned to three reviewers approximately 6 weeks before the study section meeting, and at least two of them provide confidential, preliminary written critiques and scores to the Center for Scientific Review. These assigned reviewers will lead the discussions at the meeting.
- Before the study section meets, the Center for Scientific Review gives the reviewers a list of applications that were initially scored in the lower half. If all reviewers agree, these applications are "streamlined," which means they will not be discussed at the meeting. Applicants whose applications are streamlined may resubmit an improved application that addresses the reviewers' critiques.
- At the study section meeting, assigned reviewers and discussants present their evaluations, and outside opinions are read. After a general discussion, reviewers mark their priority scores privately on scoring sheets, which are later tabulated by the Center for Scientific Review.
- Priority scores and percentile rankings become available via the NIH Commons within a few days of the meeting. A summary statement will be posted to the Commons approximately 1 month later and will include (1) the written

Table 26.1. NIH Scientific Review and Institute and Center support of cancer-related symptoms

Symptom	Scientific Review (IRGs)[a]	Funding (ICs)[b,c]
Pain	1. Integrative, Functional, Cognitive Neuroscience	Trans-NIH Pain Consortium created to coordinate activities of 15 ICs supporting research (http://painconsortium.nih.gov/members.html)
	2. Risk, Prevention, and Health Behavior	
	3. Surgical Sciences, Biomedical Imaging, and Bioengineering	
	4. Health of the Population	
Fatigue	1. Musculoskeletal, Oral, and Skin Sciences	1. National Institute of Nursing Research
	2. Oncological Sciences	2. National Institute of Mental Health
	3. Health of the Population	3. National Institute of Allergies and Infectious Diseases
	4. Risk, Prevention, and Health Behavior	4. National Center for Complementary and Alternative Medicine
Cognitive impairment	1. Health of the Population	1. National Institute of Aging
	2. Risk, Prevention, and Health Behavior	2. National Institute of Nursing Research
		3. National Institute of Mental Health
		4. National Institute of Neurological Disorders and Stroke
Depression/affective impairment	1. Biobehavioral and Biobehavioral Processes	1. National Institute of Aging
	2. Risk, Prevention, and Health Behavior	2. National Institute of Nursing Research
	3. Molecular, Cellular, and Developmental Neuroscience	3. National Institute of Mental Health
Anorexia/ cachexia	1. Endocrinology, Metabolism, Nutrition, and Reproductive Sciences	1. National Institute of Nursing Research
	2. Oncological Sciences	2. National Institute of Arthritis and Musculoskeletal and Skin Diseases
	3. Integrative, Functional, and Cognitive Neuroscience	
Sleep disorders	1. Brain Disorders and Clinical Neuroscience	Trans-NIH Sleep Research Coordinating Center created to coordinate activities of 12 ICs supporting research
	2. Health of the Population	(http://www.nhlbi.nih.gov/health/prof/sleep/sleep-05.htm)
	3. Integrative, Functional, and Cognitive Neuroscience	

IRG indicates Integrated Review Group; IC, Institutes and Centers.
[a]For more information on each of the review groups: http://cms.csr.nih.gov/PeerReviewMeetings/CSRIRGDescription.
[b]Institutes and Centers are in addition to NCI support.
[c] For more information on each of the ICs: http://www.nih.gov.

critiques produced by the assigned reviewers; (2) the Scientific Review Officer's summary of the study section's discussion; (3) study section recommendations; and (4) administrative notes of special consideration.

- After the review, the assigned IC takes charge and the IC program officer becomes the primary point of contact.
- In a second level of peer review, IC Advisory Councils may consider the study section's

recommendations and determine the relevance of the proposed research to IC priorities and public health needs – ie, whether to fund the application. Principal investigators are notified of funding status within 6–10 months.

NIH funding mechanisms for biomedical research

Over the years, the NIH has developed several mechanisms to fund specific types of research projects. These funding mechanisms are assigned an alphanumeric identification code (eg, K23, R01) and can take the form of a grant, a cooperative agreement, or a contract. Each has specified rules and policies governing the roles of the grantee and the funding source (NIH). The remainder of this section will focus on the grants and cooperative agreements that are most likely to support cancer symptom research; information about other funding mechanisms can be found at various NIH websites.[8]

Grants

A grant is broadly defined as an award for an approved activity for which the IC anticipates no substantial programmatic involvement with the recipient during performance of the financially assisted activities.[9] Most investigators are familiar with the R01,[10] the oldest grant mechanism used by the NIH. The R01 supports a discrete, specified project to be performed by the investigator and can be funded up to $500 000 annually in direct costs. Funding can cover one to five budget periods. R01 grants can be investigator initiated or can be submitted in response to an FOA. A number of R01 FOAs that are specifically focused on symptoms are available.[11] R mechanisms with lesser amounts of support and shorter budget periods include the R03 (smaller research project)[12] and the R21 (exploratory/developmental project)[13] grants.

Closely related to the R mechanisms are the P mechanisms.[8] In general, these mechanisms support multidisciplinary teams or several aspects of one discipline conducting multiple interdependent research projects directed toward a well-defined research program goal. P mechanisms do not have a dollar limit unless specified in an FOA. The P01 (research program project) grant supports integrated, multiproject research efforts involving multiple independent investigators who share knowledge and common resources. Each project must contribute to or be directly related to the common theme of the entire research effort, thus forming a synergistic system of research activities and projects. The P50 (specialized center) grant supports a broad spectrum of multidisciplinary activities addressing a specific disease or biomedical problem area, including both basic and clinical research and development efforts and related ancillary support activities, such as protracted patient care. P50-supported centers may serve as regional or national resources for special research purposes. Other P mechanisms (eg, P20, P30) support the activities of large program projects and centers by funding administrative support, planning, shared resources, and facilities. These grants are integrated with the center's component projects or program projects but are funded independently.

Career development awards (F, K, and T mechanisms) support the training of individuals at the predoctoral level and beyond. F mechanisms[14] are fellowship programs, K mechanisms[15] are research career programs, and T mechanisms[16] are training programs. Many of these (eg, F32, K07, K08, K12, K23, K25, and T32) are particularly helpful to new or junior investigators who have recently completed their doctorates, as they provide protected time for the grantee to gain additional knowledge and skills and to pursue their program of research. The K07 (academic career) award, for example, supports development activities for junior candidates who are interested in developing academic and research expertise, and leadership activities for more-senior individuals who are interested in improving the curricula and research capacity within an academic institution. A subset of the K07, the NCI-funded Cancer Prevention, Control, Behavioral, and Population Sciences Career Development Award, supports individuals with health professional or science doctoral degrees who are not fully established investigators and who want to pursue research careers in the cancer prevention, control, population, or behavioral sciences. Other career development awards (eg, F33, K05, and K24) are targeted to established investigators who need protected time to broaden their scientific background or to act as mentors for new investigators.

The omnibus NIH Pathway to Independence (PI) Award (K99/R00) provides an opportunity for promising postdoctoral scientists to receive both mentored and independent research support from the same award. The initial phase provides 1 or 2 years of mentored support for highly promising, postdoctoral research scientists, followed by up to 3 years of support contingent on securing an independent research position. Award recipients will be expected to compete successfully for independent R01 support from the NIH during the career transition award period.

Cooperative agreements

Cooperative agreements, designated by the letter U (U01, U10), are used when the IC anticipates substantial federal programmatic involvement with the recipient during performance of the award.[17] The most widely known example is the U10 grant, which is awarded to cancer cooperative groups, such as the Cancer and Leukemia Group B (CALGB) and the Children's Oncology Group (COG). Each of the funded groups works with NCI staff to identify important questions in cancer research and to design clinical trials to answer these questions.

Further discussion of these and other granting mechanisms are beyond the scope of this chapter. Visit http://www3.cancer.gov/admin/gab/2005GPB/GPB05-HighRes.pdf for more information about the NCI grants process.

Federally supported projects in cancer symptom science

The NIH RePORTER (Research Portfolio Online Reporting Tools Expenditures & Results; *http://www.projectreporter.nih.gov/reporter.cfm*) is a publicly accessible and searchable database of federally funded biomedical research projects conducted at universities, hospitals, and other research institutions. The database, which dates back to 1972, includes projects funded by the NIH, the Substance Abuse and Mental Health Services Administration (SAMHSA), the Health Resources and Services Administration (HRSA), the Food and Drug Administration (FDA), the Centers for Disease Control and Prevention (CDCP), the Agency for Health Care Research and Quality (AHRQ), and the Office of the Assistant Secretary of Health (OASH). The RePORTER interface allows users to search for scientific concepts and emerging trends and techniques and to identify specific projects and investigators.

To examine the overall federal cancer symptom research portfolio, the authors performed searches of the RePORTER's predecessor database, CRISP (Computer Retrieval of Information on Scientific Projects). Searches were kept as broad as possible to fully capture the funding patterns over the past three decades.

Search parameters and inclusion criteria

For the data presented here, CRISP database searches were conducted by three time periods (by decade: 1980–1989; 1990–1999; and 2000–2007). Although CRISP contains information dating back to 1972, the number of grants in the cancer symptoms of interest from the years 1972–1979 was small, so these years were not included.

Several factors can be modified using search fields in the CRISP database. Search terms were selected for "cancer AND [specific symptom]." The six symptoms searched for were (1) pain; (2) depression/affective impairment; (3) appetite loss/cachexia; (4) fatigue; (5) cognitive impairment; and (6) sleep disorder/insomnia. For the symptoms with two sets of terminology (eg, "appetite loss" or "cachexia"), separate searches were conducted, duplicates removed, and the results combined. For type of award, only new grants were selected, so that an investigator's project was counted only once during its funding period. If an investigator was awarded a competitive renewal, it was counted as a new grant. The search was not limited by type of grant mechanism or institute.

The initial items from these searches, listed in Table 26.2, were then reviewed to determine if they accurately represented research on cancer symptoms. Grants were excluded if they were conference-related grants (U13 or R13) or if they were NIH intramural grants (Z01). Grants were also excluded if they were part of the currently funded CCOP cooperative agreements or the predecessor project, the Community Hospital Oncology Program, which was funded in the 1980s. Projects from these funding mechanisms are discussed later in this chapter. If the same grant appeared under more than one symptom (for example, the grant "Fatigue, Pain and Sleep Problems during Radiation" appeared under all three symptom searches), that grant was counted under each symptom.

For clinical studies, grants were excluded if they appeared to focus on the study of a designated symptom in a population other than the cancer population. For instance, if a study on diabetic neuropathy came up in the search only because cancer-related neuropathy might have been mentioned in the abstract or thesaurus terms in CRISP, the grant was not counted. Grants were excluded if the symptom term was used only to reference an anticipated side

Table 26.2. Initial and final numbers[a] of NIH grants found in CRISP for selected cancer symptoms, by decade

	1980–1989		1990–1999		2000–2006	
	Initial	Final	Initial	Final	Initial	Final
Pain	105	48	175	107	312	145
Depression/affective impairment	85	38	99	33	230	104
Appetite loss/cachexia	45	17	33	18	45	19
Fatigue	12	4	51	19	137	93
Cognitive impairment	2	2	11	1	32	21
Sleep disorder/insomnia	4	2	3	6	49	22

CRISP indicates Computer Retrieval of Information on Scientific Projects database.
[a]See text for explanation of how initial and final numbers were determined.

effect from a chemotherapy protocol (eg, a study of a new biological agent where fatigue might be an anticipated side effect). Grants for studies of depression or affective disorders where caregivers were the primary focus were not included in the final numbers. Basic science projects that appeared to be correlated with or that could eventually contribute to clinical studies in the symptom of interest (eg, studies of methadone receptor expression in animal models) were retained.

In cases where it was not clear if a grant should be counted or not, we adjudicated these items. When possible, individual abstracts for each study were reviewed to determine inclusion. However, in a number of cases, no abstract was available in CRISP and we adjudicated the inclusion or exclusion of a grant on the bases of whether the grant was funded solely by NCI (versus other NIH institutes) and our knowledge of the symptom research field and the researchers. If we were still uncertain, we used internal NIH grants databases to locate further information.

Results of the CRISP search

The data are presented in Figure 26.1 and Table 26.2. Both basic science and clinical research grants are listed in CRISP, but because the database does not have a way to sort for these, the grants are presented as a total number. Further discussion will relate only to the final grant numbers.

The increase in number of grants funded for pain, depression/affective impairment, appetite loss/cachexia, fatigue, cognitive impairment, and sleep disorder/insomnia from the first decade to the last decade (for which there are only data to 2006) ranged from 12% to 2225%. The least change was seen in the category of appetite loss/cachexia, which essentially did not change over the past three decades in terms of absolute number of grants. The largest increase in terms of absolute number of grants was seen in the category of pain: whereas only 48 new grants closely related to cancer pain were funded from 1980 to 1989, 145 new grants were funded in the years 2000–2006, representing a 200% increase between the two time periods. The largest relative increase has been in the category of fatigue. The number of new grants funded in cancer fatigue grew from four in 1980–1989 to 93 in 2000–2006, a 2225% increase.

Several factors have contributed to these increases. Between 1999 and 2003, the NIH experienced a doubling of its budget, which had a significant impact on the number of submitted and awarded grants. For example, in 1995 the NIH awarded nearly $4.7 billion for R01 grants; by 2005 that amount had more than doubled to nearly $10.7 billion.[18] During the same time period, increasing attention to cancer-related symptoms brought them to the forefront. Publication of the 2001 IOM report *Improving Palliative Care for Cancer*[2] and the 2002 NIH State-of-the-Science Conference report *Symptom Management in Cancer Pain, Depression, and Fatigue*[3] emphasized the lack of available data on the epidemiology and underlying mechanisms of, and effective treatments for, the most prevalent disease-related and treatment-related symptoms of cancer.

There are at least a couple of limitations to the data presented here. First, the authors acknowledge that

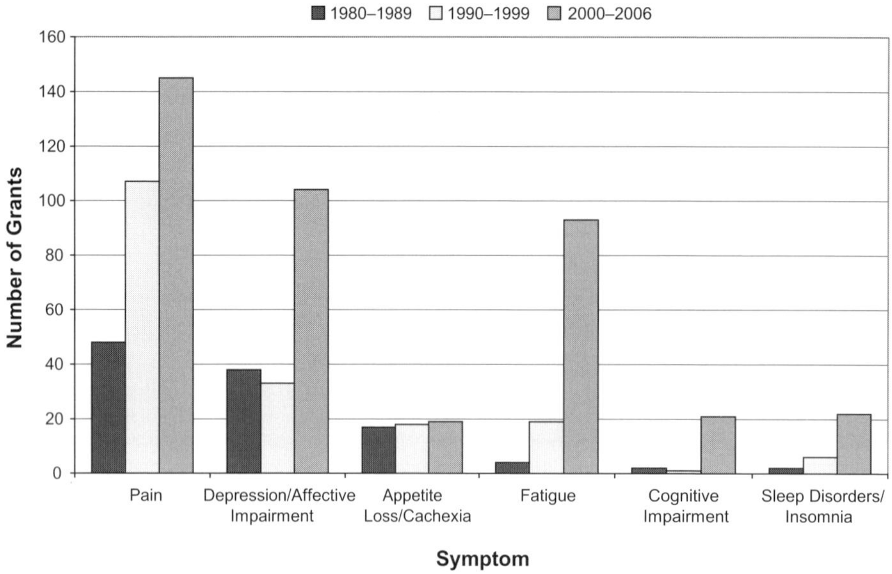

Figure 26.1. Number of NIH grants, by symptom and decade

Table 26.3. Current NCI-funded research bases (as of mid-2008)

Cancer cooperative groups	Cancer centers
1. Children's Oncology Group	1. H. Lee Moffitt Cancer Center
2. Cancer and Leukemia Group B	2. The University of Texas M. D. Anderson Cancer Center
3. Eastern Cooperative Oncology Group	3. University of Rochester Cancer Center
4. North Central Cancer Treatment Group	4. Wake Forest University Cancer Center
5. Radiation Therapy Oncology Group	
6. Southwest Oncology Group	
7. National Surgical Adjuvant Breast & Bowel Project	
8. Gynecologic Oncology Group	

the adjudication process had a degree of subjectivity to it. For this reason, both the initial and final search numbers are included in this report and the process for excluding grants has been described. Second, CRISP does not sort basic science projects from clinical science projects, so this presentation of the data necessarily groups these together, making it difficult to discuss how many clinical projects have actually resulted.

The Community Clinical Oncology Program as a venue for symptom trials

In 1983, recognizing the need to increase accrual for cancer clinical trials beyond the academic centers, the NCI established the Community Clinical Oncology Program,[19] which is funded through the U10 mechanism. In addition to expanding access to cancer treatment trials, the CCOP created a network for designing and conducting clinical trials for cancer prevention, symptom management, and palliative care. As of mid-2008, 12 research bases comprising eight cancer cooperative groups and four NCI Designated Cancer Centers (Table 26.3) are funded for this purpose. Sixty-one physician practices across the country are funded to accrue patients to these trials and to NCI-approved disease treatment trials. NCI provides support for (1) full-time and part-time administrative personnel, clinical research associates, data managers, and study assistants; (2) salary support for the principal investigator;

(3) supplies and services directly related to study activities (eg, processing and sending material for pathology review, processing and sending port films for radiation therapy quality control); and (4) appropriate travel to meetings directly related to study activities.[20]

Many of the symptom management protocols conducted in the early years of the CCOP were observational or descriptive, as little was known about the incidence, prevalence, or severity of cancer-related symptoms and virtually nothing was known about how to prevent or ameliorate these symptoms. One of the most important findings from one of the protocols supported by the CCOP in those early years was the 1994 Cleeland et al study of pain in 1308 outpatients with metastatic cancer who were being treated in 54 locations affiliated with the Eastern Cooperative Oncology Group.[6] More than a decade later, data from this study continue to be cited as a demonstration of the continuing problems in cancer pain management.

Historical and current CCOP symptom management trials

Using internal NCI databases, we investigated the history and current status of symptom management trials conducted through the CCOP. Since 1988, 72 studies have been conducted in the specific areas of pain, cognitive impairment, depression, fatigue, appetite loss/cachexia, and sleep disorders; however, no studies on sleep disorders, cognitive impairment, and depression/affective disorders were conducted in the 1980s and 1990s (Table 26.4). In marked contrast, between 2000 and mid-2008 a total of 45 studies in these scientific areas were opened. Of note is the significant percentage (75%) of pain studies focusing on neuropathic pain opened between 2000 and 2006. This strong interest can be attributed to the widespread use of agents, such as the taxanes, that have neurotoxicity as a side effect. Table 26.5 depicts the array of interventions that were or are being tested from 2000 to 2007.

Because behavioral interventions tend to be labor intensive and the CCOP RFA does not allow for reimbursement of patient care expenses,[20] most CCOP-sponsored protocols are testing pharmacological interventions.

Other federal and nonfederal sources of support

Locating sources of support to conduct cancer symptom research outside of the NIH can be a daunting experience. To find additional federal sources, the best place to start is http://www.grants.gov. A recent search of the site using the search term "cancer symptom" identified the US Department of the Army as a potential source for conducting cancer symptom management research. The agency listed programs in breast, ovarian, and prostate cancer, each describing research issues in symptom management and quality of life.

A Google search of the terms "funding cancer research" and "funding cancer symptom research" yielded six well-recognized foundations and societies that support cancer research. Among these, the American Cancer Society, the Oncology Nursing Society, and the Susan B. Komen Foundation listed specific research interests (symptoms, cancer control, psychosocial support, and survivorship) that could fit within the spectrum of cancer symptom management. Non-NIH and nonfederal sources are listed with their 2008 URLs in Table 26.6. Another resource for identifying potential

Table 26.4. Growth in CCOP protocols, by decade[a]

Symptom protocol	1983–1989	1990–1999	2000–2006	Grand total
Pain/neuropathy	8	9	12	29
Sleep disorders	0	0	2	2
Appetite loss/cachexia	1	6	9	16
Fatigue	0	3	13	16
Cognitive impairment	0	0	8	8
Depression/affective impairment	0	0	1	1
Total	9	18	45	72

CCOP indicates Community Clinical Oncology Program.
[a]*Source:* CCOP database of approved and open protocols.

Table 26.5. Types of interventions tested in CCOP clinical trials, 2000–2006[a]

Symptom (n)	Type of Intervention[b]
Pain (12)	Amifostine; glutamic acid; alpha-lipoic acid; spinal drug delivery system; gabapentin; lamotrigine; lidocaine patch; intravenous calcium & magnesium; vitamin E; cryoblation; cognitive-behavioral
Insomnia (2)	Valeriana officinalis; yoga
Anorexia/cachexia (9)	Megace; thalidomide; creatine; cyproheptadine hydrochloride; etanercept; docetaxel/infliximab; Juven®; oxandrolone
Fatigue (13)	Extended-release methylphenidate; valeriana; erythropoietin; levocarnitine; cognitive-behavioral; panax quinquefolius; modafinil; coenzyme Q10
Cognitive impairment[c] (8)	*Gingko biloba*; methylphenidate; donepizil; vitamin E; amphetamine/dextroamphetamine XR
Depression (1)	St. John's Wort; sertraline

CCOP indicates Community Clinical Oncology Program.
[a]*Source:* CCOP database of studies.
[b]Same agent may be used in several studies.
[c]Two studies are observational.

Table 26.6. Additional federal and nonfederal sources of support

Federal agency	Web Address
Department of the Army (USAMRAA)	http://www.grants.gov/search/basic.do, keyword=USAMRAA
Nonfederal organizations	
American Cancer Society	http://www.cancer.org/Research/ResearchProgramsFunding
American Association for Cancer Research	http://www.aacr.org/home/scientists/research-funding-fellowships.aspx
Cancer Research Institute	http://www.cancerresearch.org/criprogs.html
Lance Armstrong Foundation	http://www.livestrong.org/What-We-Do/Our-Actions/Professional-Tools-Training/For-Communities/Community-Awards
Oncology Nursing Society	http://www.ons.org/Awards/FoundationAwards
Susan G. Komen Cancer Foundation	http://cms.komen.org/komen/GrantsProgram/index.htm

nonfederal funding opportunities is the Foundation Center, which was established in 1956 and maintains a database on US grant makers and their grants.[21]

Summary

The study of cancer-related symptoms is a multidisciplinary endeavor and NIH support for this area of research can be found among many Institutes and Centers. Various funding mechanisms can be used to support this area of research, most notably the R mechanisms and the career development awards. Since the 1980s, significant growth in NIH support for the study of cancer-related pain, fatigue, sleep disorders, anorexia/cachexia, cognitive impairment, and depression/affective impairment has occurred. Outside the federal arena, the most often cited source of support is the American Cancer Society, which has a number of funding mechanisms to support both research and career development.

References

1. Institute of Medicine. *Priority Areas for National Action: Transforming Health Care Policy*. Washington DC: The National Academies Press, 2003.
2. Foley KM, Gelband H. *Improving Palliative Care for Cancer*. Washington DC: National Academy Press, 2001.

3. Patrick DL, Ferketich SL, Frame PS, et al. National Institutes of Health State-of-the-Science Conference Statement: Symptom Management in Cancer: Pain, Depression, and Fatigue, July 15–17, 2002. *J Natl Cancer Inst* **95**(15):1110–1117, 2003.
4. National Institutes of Health, NIH Pain Consortium. Purpose. Available from: URL: http://painconsortium.nih.gov/purpose.html. Accessed Oct 1, 2008.
5. National Institutes of Health, National Heart Lung and Blood Institute. Annual Report of the Trans-NIH Sleep Research Coordinating Committee, Fiscal Year 2005. Available from: URL: http://www.nhlbi.nih.gov/health/prof/sleep/sleep-05.htm. Accessed Oct 2, 2008.
6. Cleeland CS, Gonin R, Hatfield AK, et al. Pain and its treatment in outpatients with metastatic cancer. *N Engl J Med* **330**(9):592–596, 1994.
7. National Institutes of Health, Center for Scientific Review. The peer review process. Available from: URL: http://cms.csr.nih.gov/AboutCSR/OverviewofPeerReviewProcess.htm. Accessed Oct 8, 2008.
8. National Institutes of Health, Office of Extramural Research. Types of extramural programs. Available from: URL: http://grants.nih.gov/grants/funding/funding_program.htm. Accessed Oct 2, 2008.
9. National Institutes of Health, Office of Extramural Research. Glossary and acronyms: G. Available from: URL: http://grants1.nih.gov/grants/glossary.htm#G. Accessed Oct 2, 2008.
10. National Institutes of Health, Office of Extramural Research. NIH research project grant program (R01). Available from: URL: http://grants1.nih.gov/grants/funding/r01.htm. Accessed Oct 2, 2008.
11. National Institutes of Health, National Cancer Institute. Funding opportunities in symptom management and palliative care research. Available from: URL: http://www.cancer.gov/researchandfunding/announcements/symptommanagement. Accessed Oct 2, 2008.
12. National Institutes of Health, Office of Extramural Research. NIH small grant program (R03). Available from: URL: http://grants1.nih.gov/grants/funding/r03.htm. Accessed Oct 2, 2008.
13. National Institutes of Health, Office of Extramural Research. NIH exploratory/developmental research grant award (R21). Available from: URL: http://grants1.nih.gov/grants/funding/r21.htm. Accessed Oct 2, 2008.
14. National Institutes of Health, Office of Extramural Research. F kiosk: information about Ruth L. Kirschstein NRSA individual fellowship funding opportunities. Available from: URL: http://grants1.nih.gov/training/F_files_nrsa.htm. Accessed Oct 8, 2008.
15. National Institutes of Health, Office of Extramural Research. K kiosk: information about NIH career development awards. Available from: URL: http://grants1.nih.gov/training/careerdevelopmentawards.htm. Accessed Oct 2, 2008.
16. National Institutes of Health, Office of Extramural Research. About grants: activity codes search results: T. Available from: URL: http://grants1.nih.gov/grants/funding/ac_search_results.htm?text_curr=T&Search_Type=Activity. Accessed Oct 8, 2008.
17. National Institutes of Health, Office of Extramural Research. Glossary and acronyms: C. Available from: URL: http://grants1.nih.gov/grants/glossary.htm#C. Accessed Oct 2, 2008.
18. National Institutes of Health. Frequently asked questions about the NIH extramural budget. Available from: URL: http://grants.nih.gov/grants/financial/QA_Doubling_Period.doc. Accessed Oct 2, 2008.
19. National Cancer Institute, Division of Cancer Prevention. Community Clinical Oncology Program (CCOP): history and accomplishments. Available from: URL: http://dcp.cancer.gov/programs-resources/programs/ccop/about/history. Accessed Oct 8, 2008.
20. National Institutes of Health, Office of Extramural Research. Funding opportunities and notices: RFA-CA-07–025: Section II – award information. Available from: URL: http://grants.nih.gov/grants/guide/rfa-files/RFA-CA-07–025.html#SectionII. Accessed Oct 8, 2008.
21. Foundation Center. Welcome grantmakers. Available from: URL: http://foundationcenter.org/grantmakers. Accessed Oct 8, 2008.

Section 5 Chapter 27

Government and Industry Perspectives

Developing symptom management drugs

Joanna M. Brell and Lori M. Minasian

The experience of cancer might be described as a symptom continuum that begins at diagnosis, when cancer-related symptoms provide the first indication of disease, and continues throughout treatment to either death or survivorship. Morbidity from cancer-related symptoms is highly prevalent and has generally been managed by tumor eradication. Treatment of the malignancy, however, is associated with significant treatment-related symptoms and toxicities that can, in themselves, be disabling or life threatening. Typically, treatment toxicities have been managed by decreasing anticancer therapy doses or discontinuing the therapy altogether, but this approach is potentially detrimental to the patient's longevity. Now, decades after the first chemotherapies were administered, there is recognition of the need for balance between surviving the cancer and surviving the treatment.

Perhaps understandably, the primary focus in oncology drug development has been therapeutic drugs, with relatively less effort spent on supportive-care drugs. As a result, the number of approved high-impact agents for managing symptoms has not paralleled recent advances in cancer therapeutics, even though the evolution in anticancer treatments has engendered a spectrum of treatment-related toxicities. This chapter focuses on the development of specific drugs to reduce the toxicities and symptoms produced by cancer therapies. Issues in the assessment of symptoms and the measurement of response to treatment, as well as the design of symptom management trials, will be discussed.

Defining the problem

The rate of cancer survivorship in the United States is trending upward. In response to screening, early detection, and therapeutic advances, US cancer survivors numbered approximately 11 million in 2009. Some malignancies are highly curable or have an excellent long-term prognosis. For example, female breast cancer survivors comprise 23% of all cancer survivors.[1] In pediatric acute lymphocytic leukemia, the 5-year overall survival rate is greater than 80%, with approximately 50 000 survivors in 2009. Approximately 90% of patients with Hodgkin's lymphoma survive for at least 5 years.

These advances come with a price, however. The treatment plans for these diseases are extensive and often involve a multimodal approach. Patients and survivors must contend not only with acute toxicities during therapy, but also with possible long-term problems posttreatment (Table 27.1). For example, approximately two-thirds of deaths 10 years after a Hodgkin's diagnosis are related to therapy-induced morbidities, including cardiovascular disease and second primary cancers, and not to cancer recurrence.[2] Some of the issues faced by cancer survivors pertain to altered health-related quality of life (HRQOL), a concept that captures the patients' experiences in all aspects of their health. Among broader ramifications are (1) for patients, the inability to participate in the workforce, denial of health insurance coverage, and learning/cognitive impairments, especially in children; and (2) for the medical system, the burdens associated with long-term disability.

The magnitude of this situation warrants discovery of approaches to ameliorate acute and chronic treatment-related toxicity and to maximize aspects of HRQOL without compromising the effectiveness of treatment. These approaches will depend on the development and testing of novel agents for symptom control and supportive care. New paradigms for clinical trial design in symptom drug development may emerge by paralleling the principles used in therapeutic-agent development.

The science of cancer symptom control faces daunting, but attainable, tasks:

- Unwind complex symptoms into discrete, biological entities.

Cancer Symptom Science: Measurement, Mechanisms, and Management, eds. Charles S. Cleeland, Michael J. Fisch, and Adrian J. Dunn.
Published by Cambridge University Press.

Table 27.1. Examples of possible chronic toxicities from example anticancer treatments[40,41]

Possible toxicity	Treatment
Cardiomyopathy	Doxorubicin
Left ventricular dysfunction	Trastuzumab
Congestive heart failure	Mitoxantrone
Coronary artery vasospasm	5-fluorouracil
	Capecitabine
Coronary artery disease	Radiation therapy
Infertility	Alkylating agents
	Surgery
	Radiation therapy
Sexual dysfunction	Most hormones
Teratogenicity	Most anticancer therapies given in the first trimester of pregnancy
Pulmonary fibrosis	Bleomycin
Interstitial lung disease	Erlotinib
Cataracts	Tamoxifen
Bone demineralization	Aromatase inhibitors
Prolonged myelosuppression	Alkylating agents
	Temozolomide
Peripheral neuropathy	Platinums
	Taxanes
	Vinca alkaloids
	Proteasome inhibitors
Cerebellar toxicity	Cytosine arabinoside
Leukoencephalopathy	Methotrexate
Organic brain syndrome	Radiation therapy
Cerebrovascular accidents	Bevacizumab
Polyradiculopathy	Intrathecal methotrexate
	Cytosine arabinoside
Diabetes/pancreatic insufficiency	Pancreatic resection
Renal dysfunction	Cisplatin
Hepatic dysfunction	Imatinib
	Vinorelbine
	Methotrexate
Lumenal strictures	Radiation therapy
Secondary malignancies	Topoisomerase inhibitors
	Alkylating agents

- Explore the biological processes for key pathways leading to symptoms and treatment toxicities.
- Consider novel therapies to interfere with these pathophysiological targets.
- Discern the most advantageous methods for translating subjective, experienced sensations into reproducible and measurable data.
- Design trials with hypothesis-driven assessment of therapies and meaningful endpoints.

Exploring the biology of symptoms

The pathophysiology of symptoms is as complex as tumor biology and requires the same discipline, attention to detail, and funding support. Understanding the pathophysiology of the observable components of symptoms should facilitate the discovery of symptom management drugs, the initial development of which is a physiology-driven process to discern mechanisms of action. The biological sciences have produced volumes on the pathophysiology of some symptoms; however, as with early therapeutic developments in oncology, the focus on translational research is a relatively recent development and as such has delayed arrival of these discoveries to clinical practice.

Barriers to biological symptom research

The seemingly slow progress in symptom management research for drug development appears to be related to several barriers, as shown in Table 27.2. First, in contrast to the number of animal models available for cancer therapeutic drug discovery, there is a dearth of preclinical models for cancer symptoms. Small animal models (mainly murine) can somewhat recapitulate human symptoms like pain from neuropathy and cachexia with muscle wasting. Other types of models commonly utilized in therapeutic trials, such as tissue cultures, gene and protein microarrays (for instance, using skeletal muscle), and mathematical or computer-generated models, have not yet been widely considered in symptom management. Methods for correlating physical signs with the patient's perception of suffering are lacking.

A second barrier lies in the evaluation of agents without a known mechanism of action. In many clinical settings, physicians have taken an empirical approach and tried a variety of readily available agents, driven by the immediacy of reducing patient suffering. Working from "bedside to bench," researchers have studied interventions based upon patient reports of

Table 27.2. Barriers to research in symptom-management drug development

Lack of physiological data for symptoms with observable components
Few agents developed specifically for symptom control
Use of the empirical/experience-based approach to identifying potential agents
Presence of multiple, multifactorial symptoms, which complicate development of a single agent
Patients with high symptom burden, who may be unable to take part in clinical trials

agents that were effective for them or that showed efficacy in noncancer situations. Some patients, in an attempt to find agents with a presumed lack of additional toxicity, have used herbs and alternative medications for symptom palliation[3]; subsequent evaluations of these agents indicated no noteworthy success. Following the empirical pathway approach to research has been a barrier to the "bench to bedside" method of drug development.

Additionally, given the primary goal of tumor eradication, symptom management science was not originally on the research forefront. Because symptoms are subjective, rapidly changing, and fluid in intensity, finding a particular drug for a precise problem has been a considerable challenge in symptom drug development. Care must be taken to separate symptoms related to disease burden from other symptom-causing factors, such as treatment toxicity, physical function, financial concerns, and other issues.[4]

Further complicating assessment is the typical cancer patient who does not experience just one symptom. Often, symptoms occur together in a cluster, suggesting a mutual pathophysiology.[5,6] Symptom clusters have diverse manifestations that are interrelated with a host of environmental and psychosocial factors, resulting in varying degrees of functional impairment for patients. A key step in symptom-cluster research is the dissection of cancer-specific symptoms from therapy-induced side effects, each of which may involve entirely different management approaches.

For example, cancer-related fatigue is multifactorial and often associated with sleep disorders, depression, and treatment-related toxicities such as anemia. The difficulties inherent in attempting to tease apart the complex interplay of symptoms in a cluster is illustrated by a randomized controlled clinical trial that tested paroxetine in patients with fatigue during chemotherapy, hypothesizing that this 5-hydroxytryptamine (5-HT, or serotonin) reuptake inhibitor would attenuate the symptoms of both fatigue and depression.[7] Regardless of the presence of depression at baseline, no improvement in fatigue levels was found in the paroxetine group compared with the placebo group; however, the placebo group experienced more depression. Thus, a shared mechanism of action for fatigue and depression was not confirmed for central nervous system serotonin.[7] Either the similarities of these clustered symptoms come through other pathways, or else they are two distinct entities that must be approached separately.

Another inadvertent barrier is related to the patients themselves. Patients with advanced cancer, who can be quite ill with uncontrolled symptoms, can be one of the most challenging patient populations to study. Patients with less-advanced symptoms are able to participate in descriptions of their symptoms and in clinical trials, whereas information from those with a high symptom burden cannot always be obtained. In drug or other intervention trials, the differences between patient groups with more-subtle symptoms may be difficult to measure; if this is the case, small-to-moderate-sized trials may give negative results.

Biological pathways to cancer-related symptoms

Preclinical models may be of benefit in discerning the mechanisms underlying cancer-related symptoms. There is an animal model that displays certain behaviors after inflammatory cytokine administration that is very similar to human malignancy and other illnesses such as systemic infection. These animals are less active and exhibit diminished food intake and reduced social behaviors,[8] a phenomenon known as "sickness behavior."[9] Sickness behavior is the focus of much active research.

The interrelationships between serum inflammatory cytokines, neuroendocrine cortisol response, hypothalamic-pituitary-adrenal axis function, CNS catecholamine/neurotransmitter production, and signaling pathways secondary to malignancy and its therapy have been proposed as the complex mechanism causing sickness behavior.[10] Cytokine production is a known phenomenon of many diseases, including cancer, and there is evidence of cytokine elevations in animal models and patients with conditions such as depression and fatigue (see Chapters 8–11). A systematic approach to dealing with the intricacies of this model would allow researchers to assess neuro-immune function in malignancy, monitor appropriate biological targets, and then correlate the targets with clinical symptoms.[10]

Mechanistic understanding of symptom production will lead to discovery of targets that are "druggable." In other words, if a pertinent biological molecule causing the perturbation can be isolated, an agent can be designed to target this molecule and ultimately stop expression of the symptom. This is a fairly straightforward process in the development of cancer therapeutic drugs because tumor tissue is readily obtainable, whereas specific tissues associated with symptoms are rare. It is therefore crucial to find more of these pivotal targets in all types of cancer-related symptoms, so that agents can be tailored to inhibit them. For example, some circulating cytokines, such as tumor necrosis factor (TNF)-α and interleukin (IL)-6, are potential targets because antibodies against them have been created. Cytokine antibodies are under study for symptom reduction. Active malignancy or infection can produce a continuous endogenous supply of inflammatory proteins; therefore the resultant consequences of cytokines on a cellular level may represent additional specific targets to consider.

Biological pathways to treatment-related toxicity

Malignancy was once thought to be a surgical condition only; however, multimodal treatments often greatly affect survival. For example, survivors of early-stage breast cancer usually will undergo surgery, radiation therapy, combination chemotherapy, and sometimes monoclonal antibody administration before their approximately 1-year treatment program is completed; for patients with hormone-positive tumors, daily adjuvant hormonal therapy will continue for another 5 years or even longer. The exposure to multiple treatments increases the probability of toxicity both during therapy and years later. This toxicity is generated from any of the anticancer treatment modalities. The benefits of combined-modality therapy – increasing numbers of survivors – outweigh the risks. However, as more and more people are burdened with long-term and often-significant toxicities related to treatment, it becomes imperative that acute and chronic adverse events be precisely delineated.

In oncology, where toxicities of treatment have made it difficult to deliver the full complement of cancer therapies, attempts to address this issue have resulted in new agents to diminish the severity of toxicities (eg, antiemetics) or to prevent toxicities altogether (eg, hematopoietic growth factors). The development of these agents was based on significant basic science research that sought to better understand the pathophysiology of the underlying issue (eg, the neural signals for emesis or the growth factors for hematopoiesis). Further, the spectrum of toxicities from anticancer therapies is expanding with the development of novel therapies.

New cancer therapeutic agents are developed with a clarified mechanism of action, which allows for early prediction of toxicity. Preclinical drug testing in several species of animals uncovers adverse events and their severity; drugs often need to be redesigned or abandoned if animal toxicity is too great. Phase I studies of a new anticancer drug enumerate the type and intensity of toxicities in humans and are tested in diverse populations, such as healthy volunteers and cancer patients who are heavily pretreated. These early-phase studies can help discern a plan for toxicity management for drugs that appear to be destined for phase III trials. This plan may include evidence-based guidelines utilizing existing drugs for problems such as emesis, or might require a new compound to be developed as in the case of epidermal growth factor receptor (EGFR) inhibitor-induced rash, or chemotherapy-induced neuropathy.

Molecularly targeted agents are briskly being identified and have numerous treatment applications; some of the varying toxicities exert a "class effect," or common toxicity among similar agents. Knowing these patterns, pharmaceutical companies and researchers can tackle toxicity-control issues simultaneously with emergence of new agents in the same class. For example, the most prevalent toxicities of the class of EGFR inhibitors are rash and diarrhea.[11] EGFR-1, an EGFR subclass, is found not only in the tumor, but also in the skin and intestinal tract. These small molecules cause cellular dysfunction and cancer stabilization without a considerable change in measurable tumor parameters. Patients may derive benefit from EGFR-1 inhibitors for an extended period of time and resulting toxicity may appear as a chronic medical condition. Patients have reported intolerance of cutaneous manifestations of EGFR-1 inhibitors, such as the papulopustular rash; treatment discontinuation for this reason is well known. The pathophysiology of this cutaneous manifestation is blockade of EGFR-1 activity in the dermis, preventing normal keratinocyte function, with the resultant rash.[12] Researchers have drawn upon experience with other types of skin conditions, such as acne vulgaris, to explore available drugs to treat or prevent the rash systemically and topically, but with minimal success.[13] Although treatments could target EGFR-1 inhibition, re-establishment of EGFR activity may accelerate tumor growth. Therefore, cutaneous treatments would appear to be a feasible course of action for study as opposed to a systemic intervention.

The challenge in side effect management is to isolate the affected organ, such as the skin in the example above, to preserve treatment efficacy. The use of symptom-control agents must be proven not to prevent optimum cancer cell death or dysfunction. There is no patient gain if these agents impair survival, response rate, or any other vital parameter. Agents may need to be studied in combination with anticancer therapies for changes in pharmacokinetics (analogous to combination phase I trials) and decrements in therapeutic efficacy. Unfortunately, large randomized trials are required to obtain survival information, which occur late in the drug development process. For example, erythropoiesis-stimulating agents were developed to improve anemia, as anemia in malignancy was found to interfere with treatment efficacy and HRQOL, especially in regard to fatigue. Conflicting data has emerged from several large studies, with some studies noting a decrease in overall survival. A 2009 meta-analysis from the Cochran Collaboration assessed almost 14 000 patients from randomized trials and concluded that patients treated with erythropoiesis-stimulating agents had worse overall survival.[14] Even though toxicity was established in earlier trials, thousands of patients were necessary to uncover this survival effect. Late toxicity from today's novel targeted agents also may require years of observation to manifest. Post-marketing surveillance is vital for both anticancer therapies and symptom management agents.

Symptom management refers to the alleviation of the entire symptom burden without additional, cumbersome problems; thus, the ability of an agent for symptom or toxicity management to potentiate another adverse effect is of prime concern. An example is megesterol acetate, which is prescribed as an appetite stimulant. The increased risk of thromboembolic events makes megesterol acetate unsuitable for some hypercoaguable cancer patients, especially patients with pancreatic cancer who are anorexic but at high risk for thromboembolic disorders. In the development of medical drugs, especially symptom control agents, the risk-to-benefit ratio for the patient must be considered.

Developing novel therapies for symptom control

If a potential symptom mechanism of action is defined, preclinical studies can proceed in a manner analogous to the National Cancer Institute (NCI) Developmental Therapeutics Program[15] and the Translational Research Working Group (TRWG) plan for treatment development.[16] The TRWG was formed by NCI to advance the structuring of translational research, which produces targeted therapies and biologics, on a national level. This group documented the essentially universal course of drug development, referred to as the Agent Pathway, for anticancer and preventative therapy. The hope for implementation of this pathway is to speed the process of translational research, validate drug targets before proceeding with further development, coordinate drug development with government, academia, and pharmaceutical companies, and assimilate all components of drug development not only step wise but with appropriate concomitant testing before proceeding in the clinical trial arena.[16] Not all the steps are performed sequentially. However, if particular criteria are not achieved, one would have diminished confidence in the clinical appropriateness of a target or an agent.

This organized pathway, although developed for curative agents, can be applied to symptom drug development. A suitable example of translational research for symptoms is the testing of eicosopentaenoic acid for cancer-associated unintentional weight loss, as outlined in Table 27.3. Although these studies were performed and published some time ago, they outlined the development of a new agent formulation based on presumed biological pathways for cachexia.[17–19]

Ideally, symptom drug development trials would not proceed until they have "target validation" per the first step of the TRWG pathway.[16] Target validation for symptoms may not include tumor cell lines, but instead assessment of damaged cells, such as neuronal axons for chemotherapy-induced peripheral neuropathy. Some symptoms clearly are not easily generalized

Table 27.3. Potential development pathway for eicosapentaenoic acid in the treatment of cachexia

Phase of development process[a]	Example: eicosapentaenoic acid (EPA) in cancer cachexia
• **Credentialing** Identify target and assess relevance Does a target have clinical potential? Can agents be developed to affect target?	Cachexia/unintentional weight loss is an important clinical problem without effective treatments Putative inflammatory mechanism with potential targets: • Increased cytokines[b] • Increased eicosanoid formation • Increased nuclear factor-κB • Activated ubiquitin-proteasome system • Increased gluconeogenesis • Potential tumor release of PIF Malnutrition and neuroendocrine targets not as well delineated **SUMMARY:** Inhibiting inflammation is clinically relevant target; potential drug development
• **Supporting tools** Parallel development of agent and assays Pharmacodynamic assay to measure target inhibition Validate endpoints Which classes of patients may benefit?	Anti-inflammatories decrease cytokines and increase weight in mouse model MAC-16 with cachexia EPA n-3 essential fatty acid in diet for cell membrane, enzyme function; average human intake ~0.1 g/day Higher dose EPA reduces inflammatory markers, PIF with less weight/muscle loss in MAC-16 mouse Serum assays detect cytokines, EPA levels ; lean body mass, weight easily measured Pancreatic cancer patients with high incidence of cachexia **SUMMARY:** Agent identified with assays; effective in mouse model
• **Creation of modality** Develop lead agent for human use	EPA capsule or liquid form difficult to take in large quantity Formulated oral nutritional supplement with higher doses of EPA Patient input on taste/flavors Develop best vehicle in lowest physical volume; drug stable in vehicle **SUMMARY:** Agent formulated in improved delivery system
• **Preclinical development** Assess metabolism, bioavailability, toxicity Is manufacturing product consistent?	Dose-finding tests in animals; check bioavailability of EPA No dose-limiting toxicities found Standard manufacturing practices for 1.0g EPA per can of supplement **SUMMARY:** Agent without severe toxicity; solid manufacturing plan
• **Clinical trials** Test in humans Test in targeted patient population	**Phase I** noncancer population: EPA safe, tolerable, palatable **Phase I/II** patients with cancer: statistically significant increase in lean body mass, decrease in IL-1, IL-6, PIF **Phase III** patients with advanced pancreatic cancer: not statistically significant **SUMMARY:** Randomized trial without statistically significant conclusions

EPA indicates eicosapentaenoic acid; PIF, proteolysis-inducing factor; IL, interleukin.
[a]Categories based on drug development plan by the Translational Research Working Group.[16]
[b]Mainly IL-1 and IL-6.

into existing animal models, requiring discovery of appropriate models. For instance, there are nerve ligation models for diabetes mellitus and traumatic neuropathy; how closely these models correlate to human chemotherapy-induced peripheral neuropathy is unknown. Although extremely challenging scientifically, animal models for other cancer-related symptoms, such as fatigue and disease-related cognitive impairment, need to be developed.

Finding physiological biomarkers for symptom management will enhance drug development for symptoms. Most current or potential biomarkers are direct measurement of some tumor component (ie, PSA, CA-125, circulating tumor cells, beta-catenin). Prospective physiological biomarkers are being investigated in studies of functional brain MRI in cognitive dysfunction,[20] fat-free or lean body mass in unintentional weight loss,[21] and circulating cytokines in depression.[22] However, the correlation between any current biomarkers and symptom severity is far from perfect.

Translating the subjective into the measurable

When feasible, elucidating the genetic alterations and pathophysiology behind the "symptom phenotype" (that is, the patient's expression of his or her symptoms) can lead to development of rational interventions to offer patients. As seen in clusters of symptoms, the symptom phenotype is diverse and interrelated with a host of environmental and psychosocial factors. Appropriate assessment questionnaires can aid in categorizing some of these important issues into tangible components.

Symptoms by patient report

If the symptom under study has no observable component, then the measure of the symptom is completely the patient's report. Many oncology clinical trial endpoints are objective, measurable, and rated by health care professionals. The more subjective information is best supplied directly from patients, collected by patient-reported outcome (PRO) instruments. Validated PRO instruments are developed to measure specifics of subjective symptoms and are utilized as an objective or endpoint of symptom trials. The PROs become the "target" in the assessment and measurement of the symptom. The US Food and Drug Administration (FDA) report *Guidance for industry. Patient-reported outcome measures: use in medical product development to support labeling claims*[23] highlights the problems with quantifying subjective endpoints and suggests methods for developing effective PRO assessment tools.

Several well-validated PRO instruments for measuring cancer pain (eg, The Brief Pain Inventory[24]) have been tested in a manner analogous to the TRWG Supporting Tools concept. In some cases, specific agents such as gabapentin have been approved for medical use based upon subjective improvement of pain.[25] Finding the most appropriate measurement for a particular symptom involves refinement and re-evaluation of patient-reported "assays," as well as validation. Use of a PRO, as with any biomarker or tumor measurement, in a clinical trial requires objectives and endpoints to be relevant, succinct, and measurable.

Measurement of patient-reported outcomes

PRO measurements must encompass the essential aspects of a symptom, and symptoms can have several components. For example, chemotherapy-induced neuropathy usually consists of pain, diminished deep tendon reflexes, and neuropathic sensory and motor changes such as numbness, tingling, and burning. Alterations in motor function may include diminished hand–eye coordination and balance. These nonpainful components of neuropathy may be disabling for patients even in the absence of pain. In the case of such multicomponent symptoms, one instrument is insufficient and several measures are required to capture the patient experience in a study. If measures do not exist for a particular endpoint, they must be developed in an early phase of clinical trial planning.

All PRO measurements must be well defined during protocol development to ensure that the collected data will be statistically relevant. PROs can be used to define eligibility (ie, the symptom needs to be present and of a sufficient severity to respond to treatment) and should be measured at baseline and in response to the intervention. Assessing toxicity of therapies may require several assessments over the trial period. As subjective reports, PROs are subject to many biases; therefore these trials, unlike therapeutic studies, need to incorporate randomization of interventions with blinding. Even so, as of 2009 seven cancer therapeutic agents for managing symptoms or functional status have been approved by the FDA on the basis of PROs.[26]

Some standardization may aid in the reporting of PROs. The National Institutes of Health (NIH) Roadmap Initiative to advance the clinical trials process[27] has developed the Patient-Reported Outcomes Measurement Information System (PROMIS).[28] The PROMIS Network includes primary research sites and the NIH and aims to produce standardized and validated patient-report tools in many domains for various chronic conditions. To validate instruments for the cancer population, the NCI has joined the PROMIS effort to format the domains of physical functioning, fatigue, pain, and emotional distress for all cancer patients and survivors. With a concerted effort, PROMIS is assessing its Cancer Fatigue Short Form; the final version will be readily available to all cancer researchers and clinicians, even as ongoing study of minimal important differences for this form continues.[28] Given instruments that are valid, relevant, precise, consistent as to the results provided, and not excessively burdensome for patient or researcher, the research community will have a useful method of communicating trial results that will enhance the research process.

Further considerations in clinical trial design

Hypothesis testing

Sound trial design is the key to obtaining meaningful data for any type of clinical trial. The FDA has Guidelines for the Format and Content of the Clinical and Statistical Sections of an Application for testing new agents that are the cornerstone to experimental design.[29] A frequent design for cancer symptom trials has been randomized, placebo-controlled studies of agents, often at several dose levels, as in a parallel group design. In phase II studies of this nature, an overestimation of benefit often occurs, with a false-positive rate of 20% to 40%.[30]

Crossover designs are commonly used. In a crossover design, one group of patients receives the treatment and another group receives placebo for a specified time period, after which the subjects "crossover" to the opposite modality. Crossover designs have several advantages over randomized controlled trials: they are simpler to conduct and employ noncomplex statistical analyses, and acute or chronic conditions can easily be studied. In contrast, some of the patients in a parallel group design receive only placebo, which may not be appropriate. The crossover design can quickly test agents with short half-lives and determine efficacy and safety,[31] and all patients ultimately receive the study drug. For this design to be truly effective, the primary endpoint must be ascertained before the crossover. Crossover designs may be difficult to apply for some symptomatic agents, as the course of disease-related and treatment-related symptoms may change during the trial period, confounding the outcome.

To improve results from symptom management trials, other designs could be considered. One example is the randomized discontinuation trial (RDT) design, suited for studies with a nonhomogeneous cohort, as often seen in symptom control trials. The RDT can rapidly decrease the number of patients exposed to an ineffective drug and enrich the cohort with patients who can potentially benefit. All eligible patients receive the study drug and at a certain time point, patients not benefiting by *a priori* measures are discontinued from the trial. The remaining patients are then randomized to continue on therapy or on placebo. After a second assessment, patients on placebo may crossover to drug if symptoms recurred on placebo. The advantages of RDT can include quick accrual with early abandonment of an ineffective agent, less dosing of placebo, which is utilized more extensively in symptom control trials, and the continuation of patients on the study based on clinical response/benefit and not more arbitrary factors.[32] A similar set of advantages might be offered by the use of a Bayesian adaptive trial design for symptom research, as described in Chapter 24.

Criticism of the RDT design for anticancer therapeutic trials would also hold true for symptom management trials: (1) there are ethical concerns about proceeding to placebo-controlled phase III trials, especially in symptomatic patients; (2) there is the possibility of a positive crossover effect in a truly negative outcome; and (3) additional investigation into the biological make-up of the enriched group is required to select eligibility criteria for further studies.[33]

Establishing endpoints

Defining suitable self-report or biological endpoints to test a particular hypothesis for a symptom-management trial can be an arduous task. Unlike a relatively tangible improvement, such as overall survival from 12 months to 24 months in a cancer therapeutic trial, the degree of actual clinical benefit reflected by a specific change in patient report is often difficult to define before a trial, because symptom management trials lack the typical endpoints (overall survival, disease progression) that clinical trialists are more comfortable with. Investigators have to decide *a priori* what amount of change in reported symptoms will be hypothesized as significant. For example, is a reduction in patient-reported severe dyspnea from 10 to 8 on a numeric rating scale clinically different from a reduction from 10 to 7?

The minimally detectable difference, or minimally important difference (MID), is defined as the minimum benefit that could influence a patient's therapy. The MID is an integral concept for determining the change in an outcome before and after an intervention.[34] Some investigators are proponents of utilizing one-half of a standard deviation or standard error of measurement in the population symptom severity to characterize the MID,[35] although there is support for other methods.[36] The importance of the MID is central to the interpretation and generalization of trial results (see Chapter 23).

Finally, many symptom-control trials have been designed without much forethought regarding the changes that are expected, on the basis of biology, from the trial agent. For example, with cancer-related fatigue, does the biology of the agent potentially affect the mood, cognitive impairment, or diminished alertness that contribute to the patient's report of fatigue? This issue requires careful consideration of endpoint selection.

Future directions

One direction for expanding the development of symptom management drugs is to solicit increased involvement from basic science researchers. Many of the chapters in this book present overviews of what this basic science contribution might look like. Clinical and basic researchers recruited from other areas where symptoms are problematic, such as rheumatology, immunology, endocrinology, cardiology, and neurology, will help discern shared symptom mechanisms across diseases. Preclinical studies for biologically based symptoms will enhance drug development and lead to more meaningful clinical trials.

The National Cancer Institute has reevaluated their approach to symptom management clinical trial development. The Clinical Trials Working group,[37] with a goal of prioritizing correlative science and symptom management protocols, devised disease-specific steering committees for this task. One such committee is the Symptom Management and Health-related Quality of Life (SxQOL) Steering Committee. The SxQOL Steering Committee is charged with evaluation of clinical trials from the NCI Community Clinical Oncology Program research bases. Additionally, the committee will focus on the use of HRQOL endpoints in cooperative group phase III clinical trials.[38] This committee is composed of members from multiple backgrounds (such as government-funded investigators, outcomes researchers, NCI scientists, biostatisticians, patient advocates, and community research investigators) with diverse expertise. The SxQOL Steering Committee has identified the lack of specific agents for symptom control as a critical impediment to improving symptom management. It recently convened the Drug Development Task Force to strategically promote drug development research and to interface with stakeholders in symptom-drug development.

The SxQOL Steering Committee is taking inventory of the current state of the science. It sponsored a Clinical Trials Planning Meeting regarding chemotherapy-induced peripheral neuropathy in March 2009.[39] The meeting delineated the need for collecting basic science data, devising evidence-based therapies against key targets in the pathogenesis of the condition, and validating appropriate clinical measures of outcome. Workshop meetings of this kind may be helpful in stimulating the development of agents for other cancer-related symptoms.

Conclusion

Pertinent measurements for symptoms can unify the often diverse conceptual definitions of symptoms and may allow future correlations between physically measured components of symptoms and the patients' subjective reports. Thus, enrichment of both biologically based and subjective-report assessments is key to deriving succinct endpoints for drug development.

The goal of symptom amelioration can be further advanced by examination of available data to acknowledge what is known and to identify knowledge gaps. More research is warranted to better comprehend the wide array of symptoms, symptom clusters, and symptom pathophysiology to achieve rationally designed approaches for reducing the burden of cancer symptoms and treatment-related toxicity.

Acknowledgment

We acknowledge Ann O'Mara, PhD, Ms. Pamela Maxwell, and Kara Smigel-Croker, MS for their important contributions to this chapter.

References

1. National Cancer Institute, Division of Cancer Control and Population Sciences, Office of Cancer Survivorship Research. Estimated US cancer prevalence counts: who are our cancer survivors in the U.S.? Available from: URL: http://dccps.nci.nih.gov/ocs/prevalence/. Accessed Aug 31, 2009.
2. Ng AK, Bernardo MP, Weller E, et al. Long-term survival and competing causes of death in patients with early-stage Hodgkin's disease treated at age 50 or younger. *J Clin Oncol* **20**(8):2101–2108, 2002.
3. Ott MJ. Complementary and alternative therapies in cancer symptom management. *Cancer Pract* **10**(3):162–166, 2002.
4. Cleeland CS. Symptom burden: multiple symptoms and their impact as patient-reported outcomes. *J Natl Cancer Inst Monogr* **37**:16–21, 2007.
5. Miaskowski C, Dodd M, Lee K. Symptom clusters: the new frontier in symptom management research. *J Natl Cancer Inst Monogr*(32):17–21, 2004.
6. Dodd M, Janson S, Facione N, et al. Advancing the science of symptom management. *J Adv Nurs* **33**(5):668–676, 2001.
7. Morrow GR, Hickok JT, Roscoe JA, et al. Differential effects of paroxetine on fatigue and depression: a randomized, double-blind trial from the University of Rochester Cancer Center Community Clinical Oncology Program. *J Clin Oncol* **21**(24):4635–4641, 2003.
8. Konsman JP, Parnet P, Dantzer R. Cytokine-induced sickness behaviour: mechanisms and implications. *Trends Neurosci* **25**(3):154–159, 2002.
9. Cleeland CS, Bennett GJ, Dantzer R, et al. Are the symptoms of cancer and cancer treatment due to a shared biologic mechanism? *Cancer* **97**(11):2919–2925, 2003.
10. Miller AH, Ancoli-Israel S, Bower JE, Capuron L, Irwin MR. Neuroendocrine-immune mechanisms of behavioral comorbidities in patients with cancer. *J Clin Oncol* **26**(6):971–982, 2008.
11. Shepherd FA, Rodrigues Pereira J, Ciuleanu T, et al. Erlotinib in previously treated non-small-cell lung cancer. *N Engl J Med* **353**(2):123–132, 2005.
12. Lacouture ME. Mechanisms of cutaneous toxicities to EGFR inhibitors. *Nat Rev Cancer* **6**(10):803–812, 2006.
13. Jatoi A, Rowland K, Sloan JA, et al. Tetracycline to prevent epidermal growth factor receptor inhibitor-induced skin rashes: results of a placebo-controlled trial from the North Central Cancer Treatment Group (N03CB). *Cancer* **113**(4):847–853, 2008.
14. Bohlius J, Schmidlin K, Brillant C, et al. Erythropoietin or Darbepoetin for patients with cancer: meta-analysis based on individual patient data. *Cochrane Database Syst*Rev3:CD007303, 2009.
15. National Cancer Institute, Division of Cancer Treatment and Diagnosis. *Developmental therapeutics program (DTP)*. Available from: URL: http://dctd.cancer.gov/ProgramPages/dtp/default.htm. Accessed Aug 31, 2009.
16. Schilsky RL, Gordon G, Gilmer TM, et al. The Translational Research Working Group developmental pathway for anticancer agents (drugs or biologics). *Clin Cancer Res* **14**(18):5685–5691, 2008.
17. Wigmore SJ, Ross JA, Falconer JS, et al. The effect of polyunsaturated fatty acids on the progress of cachexia in patients with pancreatic cancer. *Nutrition* **12**(1 Suppl):S27–S30, 1996.
18. Babcock T, Helton WS, Espat NJ. Eicosapentaenoic acid (EPA): an antiinflammatory omega-3 fat with potential clinical applications. *Nutrition* **16**(11–12):1116–1118, 2000.
19. Fearon KC, von Meyenfeldt MF, Moses AG, et al. Effect of a protein and energy dense N-3 fatty acid enriched oral supplement on loss of weight and lean tissue in cancer cachexia: a randomised double blind trial. *Gut* **52**(10):1479–1486, 2003.
20. Vardy J, Wefel JS, Ahles T, Tannock IF, Schagen SB. Cancer and cancer-therapy related cognitive dysfunction: an international perspective from the Venice cognitive workshop. *Ann Oncol* **19**(4):623–629, 2008.
21. Simons JP, Schols AM, Westerterp KR, ten Velde GP, Wouters EF. The use of bioelectrical impedance analysis to predict total body water in patients with cancer cachexia. *Am J Clin Nutr* **61**(4):741–745, 1995.
22. Mikova O, Yakimova R, Bosmans E, Kenis G, Maes M. Increased serum tumor necrosis factor alpha concentrations in major depression and multiple sclerosis. *Eur Neuropsychopharmacol* **11**(3):203–208, 2001.
23. US Food and Drug Administration, Center for Drug Evaluation and Research, Center for Biologics Evaluation and Research, Center for Devices and Radiological Health. Guidance for industry. Patient-reported outcome measures: use in medical product development to support labeling claims. Available from: URL: http://www.fda.gov/downloads/Drugs/GuidanceComplianceRegulatoryInformation/Guidances/UCM071975.pdf. Accessed Dec 18, 2009.

24. Cleeland CS, Ryan KM. Pain assessment: global use of the Brief Pain Inventory. *Ann Acad Med Singapore* **23**(2):129–138, 1994.
25. US Food and Drug Administration, Center for Drug Evaluation and Research. Drugs@FDA: FDA Approved Drug Products. Available from: URL: http://www.accessdata.fda.gov/scripts/cder/drugsatfda/. Accessed Jun 8, 2009.
26. Rock EP, Kennedy DL, Furness MH, Pierce WF, Pazdur R, Burke LB. Patient-reported outcomes supporting anticancer product approvals. *J Clin Oncol* **25**(32):5094–5099, 2007.
27. National Institutes of Health, Division of Program Coordination, Planning, and Strategic Initiatives. *NIH roadmap for medical research*. Available from: URL: www.nihroadmap.nih.gov. Accessed Oct 2, 2009.
28. Garcia SF, Cella D, Clauser SB, et al. Standardizing patient-reported outcomes assessment in cancer clinical trials: a patient-reported outcomes measurement information system initiative. *J Clin Oncol* **25**(32):5106–5112, 2007.
29. US Food and Drug Administration. New drug application (NDA). Available from: URL: http://www.fda.gov/Drugs/DevelopmentApprovalProcess/HowDrugsareDevelopedandApproved/ApprovalApplications/NewDrugApplicationNDA/default.htm. Accessed Oct 19, 2009.
30. Chow S-C, Liu J-P. Designs for clinical trials. In: Chow S-C, Liu J-P, eds. *Design and Analysis of Clinical Trials: Concepts and Methodologies*. Hoboken NJ: Wiley-Interscience, 2004:167–214. Wiley Series in Probability and Statistics.
31. Chow S-C, Liu J-P. Designs for cancer clinical trials. In: Chow S-C, Liu J-P, eds. *Design and Analysis of Clinical Trials: Concepts and Methodologies*. Hoboken NJ: Wiley-Interscience, 2004:215–238. Wiley Series in Probability and Statistics.
32. Stadler WM, Rosner G, Small E, et al. Successful implementation of the randomized discontinuation trial design: an application to the study of the putative antiangiogenic agent carboxyaminoimidazole in renal cell carcinoma – CALGB 69901. *J Clin Oncol* **23**(16):3726–3732, 2005.
33. Freidlin B, Simon R. Evaluation of randomized discontinuation design. *J Clin Oncol* **23**(22):5094–5098, 2005.
34. Jaeschke R, Singer J, Guyatt GH. Measurement of health status: ascertaining the minimal clinically important difference. *Control Clin Trials* **10**(4):407–415, 1989.
35. Norman GR, Sloan JA, Wyrwich KW. Interpretation of changes in health-related quality of life: the remarkable universality of half a standard deviation. *Med Care* **41**(5):582–592, 2003.
36. Dworkin RH, Turk DC, Wyrwich KW, et al. Interpreting the clinical importance of treatment outcomes in chronic pain clinical trials: IMMPACT recommendations. *J Pain* **9**(2):105–121, 2008.
37. National Cancer Institute, Coordinating Center for Clinical Trials. Report of the Clinical Trials Working Group of the National Cancer Advisory Board: restructuring the national cancer clinical trials enterprise. Available from: URL: http://restructuringtrials.cancer.gov/files/ctwg-report.pdf. Accessed Oct 2, 2009.
38. Minasian LM, O'Mara AM, Reeve BB, et al. Health-related quality of life and symptom management research sponsored by the National Cancer Institute. *J Clin Oncol* **25**(32):5128–5132, 2007.
39. National Cancer Institute, Coordinating Center for Clinical Trials. Restructuring the clinical trials enterprise: symptom management and health-related quality of life steering committee. Available from: URL: http://restructuringtrials.cancer.gov/steering-committees/symptom-management. Accessed Oct 2, 2009.
40. Casciato DA. Cancer chemotherapeutic agents. In: Casciato DA, ed. *Manual of Clinical Oncology*. Philadelphia: Lippincott Williams & Wilkins, 2004:49–101. Spiral Manual.
41. Abeloff MD, Armitage JO, Niederhuber JE, Kastan MB, McKenna WG. *Abeloff's Clinical Oncology*, 4th ed. Philadelphia: Churchill Livingstone/Elsevier, 2008.

Section 5 Chapter 28

Government & Industry Perspectives

Cancer-related symptoms: issues for consideration in drug and therapeutic biological product label claims in the United States

Jane A. Scott

Previous chapters of this book have emphasized the importance of symptoms and symptom management in the clinical care of patients with cancer. Given the complexity of cancer and its treatment, as well as the many symptoms that could be the targets of treatment for cancer patients, it is surprising that relatively few treatments have been approved in the United States specifically for the treatment of cancer symptoms or for the treatment or prevention of symptom-producing toxicities of anticancer treatments. This is due in part to the fact that accurately documenting the effectiveness of treatments for symptoms is particularly challenging when the presence and severity of a symptom is often determined by both the cancer and the complex regimens used to treat it.[1]

The pharmaceutical, biotechnology, and medical technology industries that develop, produce, and market products to treat or prevent cancer-related symptoms in the United States must adhere to the laws enacted by the US Congress and to the regulations established and enforced by the US Food and Drug Administration (FDA). These laws and regulations specify the research required to demonstrate the safety and efficacy of a cancer treatment. Medical product development research necessary to secure the FDA's approval to market a product in the United States requires significant investment in studies that are costly to implement and that require years to complete.

This chapter provides an overview of the legal and regulatory requirements for symptom claims, with emphasis on the special challenges that must be overcome to meet regulatory requirements for the approval and marketing of products for treatment or prevention of cancer-related symptoms in the United States. An understanding of these requirements should be helpful for those wishing to design clinical trials where reduction or prevention of symptoms is a potential endpoint.

Product labeling and advertising claims

Legal and regulatory requirements

Companies that develop and sell medical products must secure FDA approval before marketing their products in the United States. As described in the Federal Food, Drug and Cosmetic Act (FD&C Act), the label – the written, printed, or graphic material on the product container or included with the product container[2] – describes the product and lists the claims regarding its use, as approved by the FDA. A "claim" in this context is any statement in the label or in advertisements (including print and broadcast advertisements) that describes an FDA-regulated product – how it should be used, who should use it, what it can do, and what problems patients may experience from using the product.[2] The product label serves as the primary source of information for health care professionals and the general public about evidence the FDA has reviewed and found adequate to include in the approved prescribing information for the product.

The FDA authorizes product claims on the basis of evidence that meets the regulatory requirements for rigorous research design and measurement. In a summary of the endpoints used by the FDA to approve new cancer drug applications, Johnson et al.[3] cite federal regulations requiring that marketing approval for all drugs and biological agents be based on substantial evidence of efficacy from adequate and well-controlled investigations. The attributes of such investigations needed to secure FDA approval are described in various FDA regulations and guidance publications. Statutes and regulations used by the FDA to evaluate product safety and efficacy ensure valid comparison to a control based on a quantitative assessment of the product's effect. The clinical benefit of the treatment must be demonstrated by prolongation of life, a better life, or an established surrogate for at least one of these.

Cancer Symptom Science: Measurement, Mechanisms, and Management, eds. Charles S. Cleeland, Michael J. Fisch, and Adrian J. Dunn. Published by Cambridge University Press.

The safety of the product for the intended use and population must be well characterized. Careful deliberation during product approval determines whether risks associated with the product's use are offset by the benefits the product is likely to provide to the patients targeted for the treatment.

Once the FDA approves a label claim, the company selling the product can include the claimed characteristics in its advertising and promotional marketing messages. All claims stated in the approved product label can be used in advertising. Statutes prohibit labeling claims that relate to benefits that are promotional in nature and do not reflect a clinical benefit to the patient.[4] However, a company may advertise benefits of its product that are important to patients but that are not listed in the approved product label if these have been adequately documented (ie, with substantial evidence from well-controlled studies using well-defined and reliable endpoints) in patients in the population referenced in the advertisement. The company that manufactures or markets the product can submit for FDA review a supplement to the original product application containing the new evidence of the additional benefit. If FDA review finds that the information meets evidence requirements, the approved product label may be revised to reflect these added product benefits.

Advertisements should describe the benefits observed in the trials using language appropriate for the target audience, as long as nothing stated or implied in the advertisement is false or misleading.[4] The FD&C Act makes illegal the "introduction or delivery for introduction into interstate commerce of any food, drug, device, or cosmetic that is adulterated or misbranded."[5] "Misbranding" refers to the inclusion of any information that is false or misleading in any particular in the approved product label or advertisements.[6] It includes overstated or exaggerated claims of benefits and promotion of unapproved ("off-label") use of the products, such as claims promising benefits that have not been documented or claims indicating benefits in patients other than those studied. An advertisement also misbrands the product if it fails to provide an adequate balance between the information promising benefits of the treatment and a fair presentation of the side effects or toxicities associated with the treatment.

For example, assume the FDA approves a product for treatment of a symptom on the basis of clinical trials in patients with a particular condition, such as migraine headache, but without other comorbid illnesses. Clinicians may prescribe the product for the management of migraine headache in patients with cancer, and may even explore its usefulness for the treatment of headaches other than migraine headache in their patients. However, the company that sells the product cannot advertise or promote the use of the product for any indication or population not specified in the approved product label. So, if the company distributes promotional materials stating appropriateness for treatment of migraines in patients with cancer, these promotional materials would misbrand the product by promoting an off-label use of the product (treatment of migraines in cancer patients) that had not been rigorously demonstrated. Companies that promote off-label uses of their products are subject to FDA censure, ranging from public warning letters or notices of violation of the FD&C Act, to requirements to provide "Dear Doctor" letters to inform doctors of the misinformation in prior advertisements, seizure of the product, criminal prosecution, or court-ordered injunction to stop marketing or distributing the product.[5,7]

Thus, describing clearly the value of the product as observed in clinical studies, without implying a benefit that was not demonstrated, is a critical consideration for descriptive information in the product label and advertising materials. Companies generally try to avoid making advertising claims that are not reflected in the approved product label; even so, describing the measured benefit of the treatment observed in clinical trials in a way that is appropriate for advertisements can be challenging. The rise of advertisements targeted for the general public – "direct-to-consumer," or DTC, advertisements – has increased the challenge for the FDA and for medical product manufacturers and advertisers to clearly word label claims to avoid misbranding. For example, product claims based on patient, clinician, or caregiver satisfaction or preferences for treatments, as well as evidence of the effects of the treatment on those other than the patient (eg, caregivers or family members of the patient), are not considered clinically important benefits to the patient and therefore are inappropriate for inclusion in approved product labeling. These benefits of a treatment may be suitable for marketing if adequately demonstrated with substantial evidence from adequate and well-controlled studies using well-defined and reliable endpoints.

Cancer-related symptom claims in product labeling

To promote a product as a treatment for symptoms caused by cancer or cancer treatments, the manufacturer must submit evidence based on well-designed and carefully conducted clinical studies demonstrating that, when used as directed, the product effectively treats symptoms in patients with cancer. Trials documenting the effect of the treatment also must show that benefits to the patient outweigh the risks of treatment-related toxicities or substance abuse.

Establishing clinical benefit: a history

Johnson and Temple[8] note that "Improvements in symptoms or physical signs thought to represent symptomatic improvements have been accepted as primary evidence of a benefit to patients sufficient to support oncology drug approval since the 1950s." However, until the early 1990s the FDA approved many products used to treat cancers based on tumor response rate, "the assessment of observable tumor burden based on laboratory tests or physical signs as a surrogate for clinically meaningful endpoints that measure directly how the patient feels, functions or survives."[9]

The appropriateness of tumor response rate as the sole basis for anticancer-product approval began to be challenged in the mid-1980s. Because many cancer therapies are highly toxic, identifying the response rate that would justify serious adverse events that patients must endure to secure some reduction in the size of the tumor becomes an ethical concern, particularly if reduction in tumor size may not translate directly to improvement in survival. In the early 1990s, the FDA Oncology Drugs Advisory Committee (ODAC) – a panel of experts enlisted by the FDA to provide advice on the review of clinical safety and efficacy evidence – recommended that tumor response rate was not a sufficient surrogate indicator of clinical benefit to the patient and should not be the sole basis for approval of anticancer treatments. To address these concerns, the FDA and the National Cancer Institute reviewed other endpoints that potentially demonstrate clinical benefit to the patient.[10] Improvement in overall survival or symptom palliation was confirmed as direct evidence of clinical benefit sufficient for approval for marketing. Two surrogate markers of tumor response were sufficiently linked to clinical benefit to be considered adequate for approval:

- If most recurrences were symptomatic, improvement in disease-free survival was sufficiently linked to clinical benefit to serve as an endpoint for approval of adjuvant therapies.
- Durable complete response also was interpreted as a validated surrogate endpoint on the basis of its strong association with increased survival and with other clinical outcomes.[3]

Both of these surrogates were considered to be adequately validated on the basis of the impact on symptoms.

In 1992, new FDA regulations introduced accelerated approval for marketing products to address the growing call for more rapid access to new anticancer therapies.[11] Evidence that a treatment improved outcomes on a surrogate marker that was reasonably likely to predict clinical benefit could be sufficient to secure accelerated approval when there was an unmet medical need (eg, the product promised benefits beyond those provided by available treatments for a serious or life-threatening condition). Companies were allowed to market a product prior to demonstrating its clinical benefit so long as additional research demonstrating the clinical benefit to patients was submitted for FDA review within a specified time. Evidence of improvement in symptoms of cancer continued to be sufficient for full approval.

Table 28.1 lists oncology product indications approved by the FDA from January 1995–June 2009 either partially or completely on the basis of symptom palliation.

The rise of patient-report in symptom assessment

A review of approved cancer-related symptom claims shows that until the mid-1990s symptoms were almost exclusively assessed in clinical trials by clinicians who queried the patient and then rated the symptoms based on their own clinical judgment. Advocates for patient self-assessment of symptoms challenged the appropriateness of using clinician judgment to evaluate symptoms that can be experienced only by the patient.[12] They argued that, unlike clinical signs of disease that could be rated by multiple, blinded clinicians, symptoms were best assessed by patients themselves using carefully developed and validated patient-reported outcome (PRO) assessment tools integrated as endpoints into clinical trials. Photofrin® (porfimer) became the first oncology treatment based on a PRO symptom assessment to secure FDA approval. FDA reviewers who have tracked the interest in and use of PRO measures as

Table 28.1. Treatments approved by the US Food and Drug Administration[27] based partially or completely on improvement in cancer-related symptoms

Drug	Year Approved	Indication	Symptom Endpoint	Other Endpoints	Study Design
Altretinoin gel (Panretin®)	1999	Kaposi's sarcoma	Clinician-assessed improvement in skin appearance	Tumor response rate	Double-blind, vehicle-controlled randomized trial
Amifostine (Ethyol®)	1999	Xerostomia from radiotherapy for head and neck cancer	PRO-assessed xerostomia	Saliva production	Open-label randomized controlled trial
Aprepitant (Emend®)	2003	Prevention of chemotherapy-induced nausea & vomiting (CINV)	Composite: clinician-assessed emesis episodes + PRO-assessed nausea episodes	PRO-assessment of impact of CINV on patient's daily life	Randomized, parallel, double-blind, controlled trial
Bexarotene capsules (Targretin® capsules)	1999	Cutaneous T cell lymphoma	Cutaneous manifestations (clinician-assessed composite index lesion severity)	Tumor response rate	Single-arm trial
Bexarotene gel (Targretin® gel)	2000	Cutaneous T cell lymphoma	Cutaneous manifestations (clinician-assessed composite index lesion severity)	Tumor response rate	Single-arm trial
Daunorubicine citrate (DaunoXome®)	1996	Kaposi's sarcoma	Clinician-assessed improvement in skin appearance	Tumor response rate	Open-label randomized controlled trial
Dolansetron mesylate (Anzemet®)	1997	Prevention of chemotherapy induced vomiting	PRO-assessed severity of nausea and vomiting episodes	PRO-assessed need for rescue medication	Randomized, double blind trial comparing multiple doses
Eculizumab (Soliris®)	2007	Paroxysmal nocturnal hemoglobinuria	PRO-assessed fatigue and health-related quality of life	Hemoglobin; number of transfusions	Double-blind randomized controlled trial
Fentanyl citrate (Fentora®)	2006	Management of breakthrough pain in patients with cancer who are already receiving and are tolerant to opioid therapy for underlying persistent cancer pain	PRO-assessed breakthrough pain		Double-blind randomized controlled trial
Fosaprepitant dimglumine (Emend®)	2008	Prevention of vomiting associated with highly emetogenic chemotherapies	PRO-assessed nausea; Clinician-assessed emetic episodes	PRO-assessed impact of CINV on patient's daily life; use of rescue medications	Double-blind randomized controlled trial
Gemcitabine (Gemzar®)	1996	Pancreatic cancer	PRO-assessed pain intensity; clinician-monitored weight gain	Survival; "clinical benefit response" as measured by a composite of pain, performance status, and weight gain	Single-blind trial

Table 28.1. (cont.)

Drug	Year Approved	Indication	Symptom Endpoint	Other Endpoints	Study Design
Gemcitabine (Gemzar®)	1998	Non-small cell lung cancer	PRO-assessed health-related quality of life, including symptoms and function measures	Survival	Single-blind randomized controlled trial
Imatinib mesylate (Gleevec®)	2003	Philadelphia-chromosome-positive chronic myeloid leukemia	PRO-assessed symptoms of interferon toxicity	Complement to safety data	Open-label randomized controlled trial
Leuprolide acetate (Eligard®)	2002	Prostatic neoplasms	PRO-assessed bone and urinary pain, urinary signs and symptoms	Testosterone levels; WHO performance status	Open-label, multiple dose comparison trial
Methoxsalen (Uvadex®)	1999	Cutaneous t-cell lymphoma	Clinician-assessed overall skin scores, improvement in edema, and scaling and fissure resolution		Single-arm trial
Mitoxantrone (Novantrone®)	1996	Pain from hormone-refractory advanced prostate cancer	PRO for pain	Use of rescue medicines	Open-label randomized controlled trial
Ondansetron (Zofran®)	1992	CINV	PRO for emetic episodes, composite emesis+nausea		
Ondansetron sodium chloride (Ondansetron®)	2006	Prevention of nausea and vomiting associated with cisplatin-based chemotherapies	PRO for severity of nausea; clinician-reported number of emesis episodes	PRO-assessed satisfaction with control of nausea and vomiting	Randomized, blinded active and placebo controlled trials
Paclitaxel (Taxol®)	1997	Kaposi's sarcoma	Clinician-assessment of clinical benefit based on improvements in ambulation, edema, and ulcer resolution	Tumor response	Single-arm trial
Paclitaxel (Taxol®)	2000	Non-small cell lung cancer	PRO-assessed FACT-L Lung cancer specific symptom scale	Tumor response Time to progression	Open-label randomized controlled trial
Palifermin (Kepivance®)	2004	Prevention of severe oral mucositis after bone marrow ablation	PRO-assessed mucositis (mouth and throat soreness)	Analgesic use	Randomized, double-blind, placebo-controlled trial

Table 28.1. (cont.)

Drug	Year Approved	Indication	Symptom Endpoint	Other Endpoints	Study Design
Palosetron hydrochloride (Aloxi®)	2003	Reduction of nausea and vomiting associated with moderately or high emetic chemotherapies	PRO-assessed metic episodes, severity of nausea	Use of rescue medications; global satisfaction with treatment; FLIE (health-related quality of life)	Randomized, double-blind, active controlled trail
Pilocarpine hydrochloride (Salagen® tablets)	1994	Xerostomia in Sjorgen's syndrome and head and neck cancer	PRO-assessed global evaluation of dryness of mouth; PRO for specific symptoms of xerostomia		Randomized, double-blind, placebo-controlled trial
Porfimer sodium (Photofrin®)	1995	Photodynamic therapy for completely obstructed esophageal cancer	PRO-assessed dysphagia	Esophageal luminal response	Single-arm trial
Porfimer sodium (Photofrin®)	1998	Photodynamic therapy for completely or partially obstructed endobronchial non-small cell lung cancer	Clinician-assessed severity of nine pulmonary symptoms	Luminal response	Open-label randomized controlled trial
Topotecan (Hycamtin®)	1998	Small-cell lung cancer	PRO-assessed pulmonary symptoms	Response rate; response duration	Open-label randomized controlled trial

PRO indicates patient-reported outcome and here refers to a PRO assessment measure; CINV, Chemotherapy-Induced Nausea and Vomiting; WHO, World Health Organication; FACT-L, Functional Assessment of Cancer Therapy–Lung questionnarie; FLIE, Functional Living Index–Emesis.

endpoints for documenting the impact of oncology treatments reported that between 1995 and 2006, seven products were approved for symptom palliation on the basis of PRO endpoints.[13]

Efficacy of more than half of the products with approved indications for use in oncology treatment shown in Table 28.1 involved evidence based on PRO symptom assessments or on composite endpoints that included PRO symptom data. Clinician-reported endpoints were used to provide evidence for evaluating clinically observable signs, such as skin lesions, and to substantiate the use of radiation therapy for managing localized pain.

Symptom palliation vs. tumor-reduction treatments

Effective treatment of the cancer may be the only way to adequately relieve symptoms induced by the disease. In this case, improvement in symptoms could be evidence of treatment of the cancer itself (eg, reduction in Kaposi's sarcoma lesions). However, a treatment that improves symptoms without affecting the underlying cancer could be indicated for managing or treating symptoms in the cancer population studied in a particular trial (eg, prevention of emesis in cancer patients undergoing chemotherapy). In fact, FDA regulations state that the "relief of symptoms associated with a disease or syndrome" can be the indication for a product.[14] In this case, the symptom claim equals the indication. Some examples from currently marketed therapies:

- Targretin® (bexarotene) gel 1% is indicated for "the topical treatment of cutaneous lesions in patients with cutaneous T cell lymphoma (Stage 1A and 1B) who have refractory or persistent disease after other therapies or who have not tolerated other therapies," (from approved product label for Targretin® accessed June 9, 2009).[15]
- Ethyol® (amifostine) is indicated to "reduce the cumulative renal toxicity associated with repeated administration of cisplatin in patients with advanced ovarian cancer" and to "reduce the incidence of moderate to severe xerostomia in

patients undergoing post-operative radiation treatment for head and neck cancer, where the radiation port includes a substantial portion of the parotid glands" (from approved product label for Ethyol® accessed June 9, 2009).[15]
- Photofrin® (porfimer sodium), a photosensitizing agent used to augment the effect of photodynamic therapy, is indicated for "palliation of patients with completely obstructing esophageal cancer, or of patients with partially obstructing esophageal cancer who, in the opinion of their physician, cannot be satisfactorily treated with Nd:YAG laser therapy"; for "reduction of obstruction and palliation of symptoms in patients with completely or partially obstructing endobronchial nonsmall cell lung cancer (NSCLC)"; for "treatment of microinvasive endobronchial NSCLC in patients for whom surgery and radiotherapy are not indicated"; and for "ablation of high-grade dysplasia in Barrett's esophagus patients who do not undergo esophagectomy" (from approved product label for Photofrin® accessed June 9, 2009).[15]

Symptom improvements also are considered to be evidence of clinical benefit associated with the reduction tumor size or other clinical signs of treatment effectiveness.

Examples:

- Hycamtin® (topotecan hydrochloride) for injection is indicated for the treatment of "metastatic carcinoma of the ovary after failure of initial or subsequent chemotherapy"; of "small cell lung cancer sensitive disease after failure of first-line chemotherapy"; and, in combination with cisplatin, for "stage IV-B, recurrent, or persistent carcinoma of the cervix which is not amenable to curative treatment with surgery and/or radiation therapy" (from approved product label for Hycamtin® accessed June 9, 2009).[15] Hycamtin® was approved based on tumor response and tumor response duration supported by improvement in nine pulmonary symptoms that provided evidence of a clinical benefit.
- Gemzar® (gemcitabine) is indicated for treatment of breast cancer, NSCLC, and pancreatic cancer. In addition to improvement in survival, Gemzar® also had better clinical benefit response, defined as improvement in a composite of pain, performance status, and weight gain, than 5-fluorouracil (as described in the approved product label for Gemzar® accessed June 9, 2009).[15]

Changes in symptoms also provide evidence about the toxicity of anticancer treatments (eg, xerostomia in patients with head and neck cancer treated with radiotherapy). If clinical trials demonstrate that a treatment significantly reduces symptomatic toxicities while providing comparable survival or tumor response, this would be evidence of a safety benefit that could justify product labeling and marketing claims. For example, Gleevec® (imatinib) is indicated for treatment of many different neoplasms. In open-label studies comparing Gleevec® to interferon-containing regimens, patients receiving Gleevec® reported fewer symptoms of interferon toxicity (as described in the Gleevec® product label approved as of May 27, 2009).[15]

The FDA approval process for securing symptom claims

A product secures FDA approval for marketing only after it has been painstakingly evaluated to ensure it can be used safely in the intended patient population, that there is adequate evidence that the product provides a clinical benefit to the patient, and that the appropriate dosing regimen balancing the effectiveness of the product against its side effects and toxicities (its safety) has been documented. In life-threatening illnesses like cancer, information about symptoms helps address a critical challenge in regulatory decision making: determining an acceptable balance between treatment-related toxicities and survival benefits of the treatment.

The reviewers

Medicines used to treat cancer or its symptoms are reviewed by the FDA's Office of Oncology Drug Products (OODP), which has primary responsibility for ensuring that drug and therapeutic biological treatments for cancer that are available to the US public are safe and effective. OODP oversees the development, approval, and regulation of drug and biological treatments for cancer, therapies for cancer prevention, drug and biological products used for medical imaging, and products for treatment of nonmalignant hematological conditions.[16] Within OODP, the Division of Oncology Drug Products and the Division of Biological Oncology Products review new pharmaceutical therapies and biological therapies, respectively, targeted for the prevention or treatment of cancer.

FDA review divisions work together to provide advice to research sponsors during development, to review evidence to determine eligibility to support market approval, to develop labeling language, and to review initial marketing materials prior to market launch of the product for the indication. Oncology treatments and studies conducted primarily in oncology patients are reviewed by one of the divisions in OODP. Other divisions at FDA have primary review responsibility for symptom management therapies that may include cancer patients but that are not targeted specifically for use in cancer. For example, a treatment for nausea and vomiting that is used for post-operative treatment as well as for management of chemotherapy-related toxicity may be reviewed by OODP with consultation from the Division of Gastroenterology Products. Similarly, a hormone replacement therapy that seeks an indication for reduction of symptoms due to bilateral oopherectomy used to treat or prevent ovarian cancer would likely be reviewed by OODP with consultation from the Division of Reproductive and Urology Products. Conversely, during other divisions' reviews, OODP provides consults about the oncology-specific implications of proposed indications and labeling.

Product development

When a research sponsor seeks to initiate studies of a new drug in human subjects, they begin by submitting an Investigational New Drug (IND) application to the OODP's Division of Oncology Drug Products to secure permission to begin studies.[17] All FDA correspondence and communication with the sponsor uses the IND number to ensure accurate record keeping of the drug development research. When the sponsor has completed all of the research required to assess the safety and efficacy of the drug, they submit a New Drug Application (NDA) containing all the evidence collected to substantiate the dosing, the pharmacology and pharmacodynamic studies, the manufacturing process, and clinical efficacy and safety data. If the FDA concurs that the application meets basic requirements for review, the NDA is accepted for filing. A similar process is used by the Division of Biological Oncology Products to track the development of and application for approval to market a new biological agent: the development research is conducted under a BB (blood and biologics)-IND and the full documentation of the development research is submitted as a Biologic Licensing Application (BLA) for review by the division.

Throughout the development phase, meetings between the sponsor and the FDA and the submission of key documents to the FDA serve as milestones for the product development. Figure 28.1 presents these milestone meetings and events as they occur throughout the clinical development phase.[18] The sponsor-FDA interactions occur along what the FDA has labeled the "critical path" for drug development,

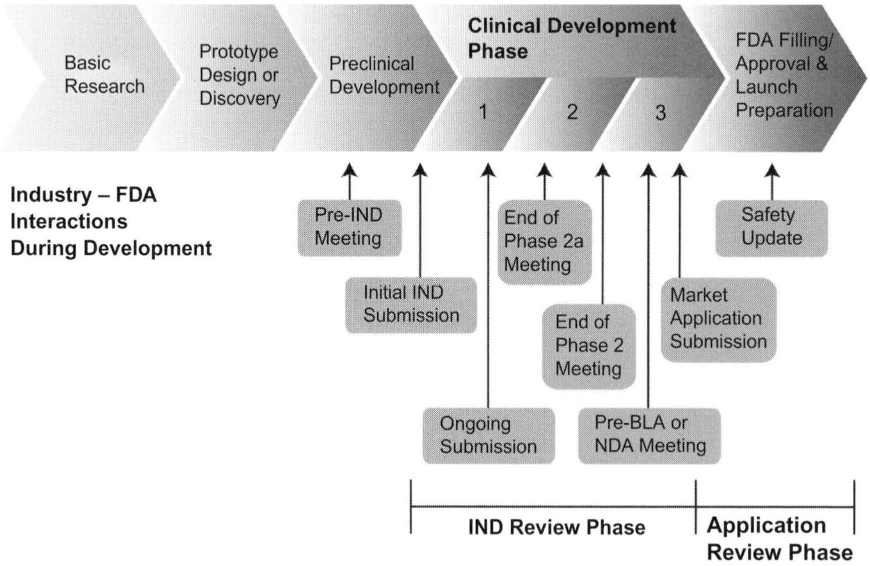

Figure 28.1. FDA review in medical product development.
Source: Adapted from Rock 2006.[18]

beginning with the pre-IND meeting where research sponsors present the rationale for human studies, the expected benefit, and the proposed research program to initiate preliminary safety data in relevant patient populations. The pre-IND meeting generally is followed by submission of the IND application. If the application is accepted by the FDA, the sponsor can initiate the proposed studies with proper FDA oversight of all safety issues and protocol designs throughout the clinical development phase.

Before initiating the phase 3 studies that will be the basis for approval of the product, sponsors submit information collected from phase 1 and phase 2 studies for FDA review to confirm appropriateness of initiating large-scale studies. Upon completion of phase 2 studies, the sponsor is expected to present evidence that they have identified the minimum effective dose for the drug, the maximum safe dose, a dosing regimen that is expected to produce the maximum evidence of efficacy with the least toxicities, and appropriate (well-defined and reliable) endpoints for assessing safety and efficacy outcomes in the phase 3 trials. A combined phase 2–3 trial can be conducted when the affected patient population is quite small because the condition is rare. Upon completion of the phase 3 studies, sponsors preparing to submit the NDA or BLA will often seek a meeting with the FDA to review the development research conducted, review preliminary evidence from the data analysis regarding the targeted claims, and discuss additional analyses required to clarify issues raised in study designs or interim reports. The FDA often uses this meeting to set expectations about the package required to support the desired claims and to provide advice to the sponsor about submission requirements for the marketing application. When the research, analysis, and documentation are complete, the sponsor submits these with the application for marketing (NDA, BLA, supplemental NDA, etc.) to the FDA for evaluation.

The FDA is expected to meet certain timelines for review and response as established in the Pharmaceutical Drug Users Fee Acts, which were enacted to help speed FDA review cycles by supporting FDA budgets with application fees paid by the research sponsors for the reviews. The Food and Drug Administration Amendments Act of 2007 (FDAAA) is the most recent legislation intended to improve both the funding of FDA and its ability to oversee the safety of the public health in the United States.[19] The FDAAA reauthorizes user fees and increases the resources available to the FDA Center for Drug Evaluation and Research for ensuring product safety in the drug review process, monitoring drug safety after product marketing, and reviewing consumer television ads that are voluntarily submitted to the FDA.[19] The FDAAA also reauthorizes key programs for ensuring safe use of drug products in children by encouraging more research into developing treatments for children, including pediatric oncology treatments.[19]

Guidance documents and guidance meetings

The FDA commonly relies on three tools for regulation of medical product development and marketing: (1) legislation passed by the US Congress that the FDA enforces; (2) regulations published by the FDA that explain how it will undertake its enforcement tasks; and (3) regulatory guidance documents published by the FDA that describe the agency's current thinking about how regulations and laws are interpreted. Guidance documents can serve as valuable tools for understanding current FDA thinking on how to interpret statutes and regulations in relation to particular disease areas or as part of continual efforts to improve the process and outcomes of FDA's regulatory decision making, including those related to medical product development and marketing.[20]

An FDA regulator's task of enforcing legislation can at times be difficult to reconcile with advancing medical innovation. Embracing new methods, new products, and new goals for therapy is essential to address threats to public health that the FDA was commissioned to protect. However, existing regulations or statutes do not always provide sufficient guidance to the pharmaceutical industry or to the FDA to address innovative new methods used in clinical research. When this occurs, the FDA and other regulatory agencies around the world use guidance documents to provide general advice on how to comply with legislative and regulatory requirements.[20] Often, these guidance documents are couched as advice that is "generally recommended, but not required." Their intent is to publicly convey information that applies to a wide audience. Guidance documents may serve as precursors to regulations, but this is not always the case. The guidance documents published by the FDA to provide significant new information about its current policies require extensive internal review to ensure all aspects of the recommendations in the guidance comply with existing laws and regulations. FDA regulations address the process and requirements for commenting on guidance documents when they are initially published.

The FDA's Center for Drug Evaluation and Research recently published guidance documents that are of particular value to researchers seeking to measure the impact of treatments on cancer-related symptoms:

- Guidance for Industry. Clinical trial endpoints for the approval of cancer drugs and biologics. Final published May 15, 2007.[21]
- Guidance for Industry. Clinical studies section of labeling for human prescription drug and biological products – content and format. Final published January 18, 2006.[22]
- Guidance for Industry. Patient-reported outcome measures: use in medical product development to support labeling claims. Final published December 2009.[12]

The 2007 guidance on clinical trial endpoints in cancer drugs and biologics includes a significant discussion on the use of symptom assessments as endpoints in cancer trials,[21] much of which focuses on the importance of being able to distinguish between the symptoms of cancer and the toxicities related to anticancer treatments. Endpoints that focus on time to symptom progression are considered acceptable endpoints to support an indication for an anticancer treatment. For example, a composite endpoint of skeletal metastases that included pathological fractures, radiation therapy to bone (for pain palliation), surgery to bone, and spinal cord compression provided evidence on skeletal-related events that were the basis for approval of Aredia® and Zometa®. The clinical endpoints guidance suggests various ways to document a symptom benefit in an oncology trial and emphasizes the importance of prespecifying methods to minimize symptom data and of prospectively defining the testing of endpoints to control for type II error due to multiple comparisons in trial analysis.

The clinical studies section of an FDA-approved drug or biological product label contains a summary of the information describing the effectiveness of the product as documented in clinical studies, which forms the basis for the FDA's approval of an indication for the product. In keeping with the FDA's mandate to ensure that product labeling does not include information that is false or misleading, the final guidance on content and format of the clinical studies section of FDA-approved product labels highlights the importance of unambiguous statements about the observed effects of the treatment for prescribing information:

> Words or phrases that lack a commonly understood meaning (eg, imprecise quantitative terms), are not easily defined, are vague, misleading, or promotional in tone should be avoided. Examples include *large* or *small* (instead, use actual size or amount), *well-designed* (instead, provide specifics about the study design), *extensively studied* (instead, provide specifics about the database), *rapid* (instead, specify change/unit time), *trend* (instead, provide specifics about the outcome), *potent* (instead, give the size of the effect), *pivotal study* (instead, describe as major effectiveness study), and *highly significant* (instead, provide the confidence interval).[22]

Effective methods for presenting various types of data, as well as the nature and extent of information appropriate for the clinical studies section, are addressed in this guidance.

The guidance on the use of PRO endpoints to support labeling claims[12] is particularly important for the measurement of symptoms in clinical trials, in that symptoms are best assessed by the patient. Therefore, well-defined and reliable symptom endpoints should be based on valid assessments that patients can complete. The PRO guidance provides the FDA's current thinking on the proper development and validation of PRO endpoints that would be recommended for symptom assessment in clinical trials, as well as on issues the FDA will review in evaluating PRO endpoints as they are implemented in clinical trials. These include questions about the adequacy of the implementation of the PRO in clinical trials to support the product claims the research sponsor seeks to include in the labeling.

To be useful for clinical trials, PRO assessments must be clearly worded and relevant to the patients who will complete the assessment in trials, and they must have demonstrated that they have adequate measurement properties (ie, validity, reliability, and ability to detect change) in studies in the target patient population for the indication, that changes in the endpoint can be interpreted as a true clinical benefit to patients, and that the PRO assessments have been implemented in adequate and well-controlled clinical studies. Unblinded and nonrandomized study designs (ie, open-label studies, single-arm trials) are not adequate to support claims for symptom endpoints because of the subjectivity inherent in evaluation of symptoms. Because modifications, translations, or adaptations of PRO assessments can undermine the reliability or validity of the assessment, sponsors are encouraged to provide information showing that a revised or translated instrument is valid and reliable. If data from multiple versions of a PRO are combined (eg, multiple translations, long and short forms, paper-and-pencil self-completion and electronic or interviewer administration), the FDA will need documentation confirming that the comparability of the versions is suitable for combined analysis from multiple versions.

Given the importance of each of these guidance documents for the evaluation of symptom claims in cancer products, topics addressed therein will be discussed in more detail in the following section of this chapter, to highlight specific concerns for measuring cancer-related symptoms intended to support product claims.

Measuring symptoms in oncology trials

The recent FDA guidance documents have encouraged the use of PRO assessment for monitoring symptoms in trials that aim to support claims about symptom improvement or prevention. Product claims for treatments that improve or prevent cancer-related symptoms will likely be based primarily on clinical trial endpoints assessed using PRO data that show how symptoms changed over time in the study. Identification of valid assessment tools that patients can use to systematically describe symptoms they are experiencing is fundamental to development of new treatments for symptoms.

Defining symptoms

Clinical terms used to refer to symptoms or symptomatic syndromes are not always clearly defined, which can lead to questions about what the symptom assessment must include (content validity) as well as which terms to use when asking patients to report their symptoms. A classic example is fatigue, often cited as a major symptom of cancer and its treatment. Researchers and published diagnostic systems disagree about the specific manifestations of fatigue and whether it is a unidimensional symptom with many alternative descriptors (eg, fatigue, tiredness, weariness, lack of energy) or a multidimensional symptom that is quantified primarily through its impact on a patient's physical functioning, cognitive functioning, and emotional state.[23] Evidence from interviews with cancer patients indicates that they experience cancer fatigue as qualitatively and quantitatively different from their experience of "normal" fatigue that arises from exertion or lack of sleep.[24] The FDA's guidance on PRO endpoints,[12] as well as the final guidances on clinical endpoints in oncology[21] and on content and format of the clinical studies section of the approved product label,[22] suggest that reference to "fatigue" in a product label could be misleading because the term is not consistently defined or measured.

The reviewer discussions noted in the medical review for Soliris® (eculizumab) for treatment of paroxysmal nocturnal hemoglobinuria highlight the challenges that the FDA faces in measuring complex symptoms like fatigue in cancer. The medical reviewer noted that the FDA's Study Endpoints and Label Development (SEALD) team review questioned the ability of quality-of-life assessment tools (in this case, the FACT-F and EORTC QLQ-C30) to measure the multidimensional attributes of fatigue. Despite this concern, the clinical studies section of the approved Soliris® label included the following language: "After 3 weeks of Soliris treatment, patients reported less fatigue and improved health-related quality of life." This decision was driven by the substantial treatment effects that were observed for all endpoints, including the fatigue assessment.

Measuring symptoms

Valid symptom assessment requires a clear objective. What is it about the symptom that is important to capture? This should align with the expected effects of the treatment in the target population. That said, it is often unclear what aspect of the symptom should be assessed to demonstrate a clinical benefit to patients. A review of the natural history of the disease, coupled with expert advice and qualitative research in patients, provides the best starting place for understanding which symptoms are likely to matter to patients and when these symptoms evolve in the natural history of the cancers targeted or treatment regimens of interest.

Both the oncology endpoints guidance[21] and the PRO endpoint guidance[12] state that the most appropriate person to report on symptoms is the patient. Although clinician assessment of observable signs can be useful for standardization across patients and sites, it does not reflect the patient's experience of the symptom, which is important for understanding effective management of the disease.[12] Interviews or focus groups with patients provide initial insight into what patients value, but the ultimate evidence of clinical benefit of observed individual changes in symptoms or differences between groups must be established through clinical studies using assessments that have a demonstrated ability to provide valid and reliable information in the population of interest.

Symptoms can be assessed in trials in a variety of ways, such as:

- A single-item PRO measure (eg, a daily diary or log of the symptom's severity; a current-status assessment at each clinic visit).
- A PRO symptom scale assessing current status of multiple symptoms or multiple characteristics of a single symptom (eg, frequency, severity, duration, timing, impact on functioning); these also can be included in a diary or log, but more often are used at key patient visits throughout the trial.
- A symptom assessment that is a domain or item within a larger PRO instrument intended to measure burden of disease, health-related quality of life, or other concepts related to symptoms; these assessments are typically only administered during clinic visits as their length can make them onerous to complete on a daily basis.

In the case of a symptom scale, the FDA's guidance on oncology endpoints cautions that a "*composite symptom endpoint* should have components of similar clinical importance and the results should not be exclusively attributed to one component."[21] If three questions in the PRO instrument assess dyspnea and only one question each is used to assess cough and chest pain, a summed score of all item responses will emphasize the impact of the treatment on dyspnea and be less linked to cough or chest pain. This inadvertent weighting can be overcome by averaging the items measuring a single symptom and then scoring the sum or average symptom scale score using the average (eg, lung cancer symptom score = three-item mean dyspnea score + cough score + chest pain score).

FDA PRO guidance recommends that PRO symptom assessments avoid recall bias by focusing on evaluation of the current status or recent experience of the symptom characteristic (eg, severity of the symptom right now, or the worst severity experienced in the last 24 hours).[12] Cognitive studies have shown that "worst" severity is easiest to recall accurately, so that an assessment of worst severity over the past 24–48 hours for a symptom assessment should provide reliable and valid measurement for clinical trials. The appropriate recall period for a PRO endpoint must be determined and agreed with the FDA to ensure adequate evidence to support a product claim.

Some symptoms are always evidence of pathology. Pain is the classic example. Other symptoms are the pathological extension of normal states, in intensity, duration, context, etc. For example, breathlessness is normal if a person just ran a 10-kilometer race, but if the person is breathless without exertion or takes a long time to recover normal breathing, the breathlessness is a symptom worthy of investigation. Diagnosis of a pathological level of symptoms that extend into the continuum of healthy states is essential for symptom trials.[21]

The process for identifying or developing a multi-item symptom scale or a single-item symptom assessment is essentially the same, although the tasks required expand for multi-item assessments.[12] Briefly, the FDA encourages sponsors to provide an indication of the proposed labeling claims, then to develop or identify a conceptual framework for how each endpoint will be measured. This framework guides the selection or identification of measures for inclusion in the trials. Evidence of the adequacy of the measurement properties for the symptom assessment and justification for what change or difference in scores would be evidence of a clinical benefit to patients must be demonstrated prior to initiating phase 3 trials.

Study design considerations

Previous chapters in this volume have addressed many of the issues related to study design and analysis that should be considered to support symptom claims in a submission to the FDA for market approval of a new product. Ultimately, how a symptom assessment is incorporated in the trial will determine what can be claimed from it in the product label or advertisements. It is therefore important that study designs anticipate how best to ensure that the statements they hope to make about the product can be demonstrated using the study design, patient population, instrumentation, and analysis prespecified for the phase 3 trials.[22]

Quantifying subjective or observed experiences inherent in symptom assessment can be difficult, as it is never possible to directly compare the subjective experience of one person with that of another. For this reason, symptom claims should be substantiated based on randomized, double-blinded, well-controlled clinical trials using standardized assessments that accurately (with minimum recall error) record the patient's experience of the symptom throughout the study. Open-label trial designs make the use of perceptual endpoints challenging because there is no way to blind the patient or clinician to minimize subjectivity bias.

Study designs that mix patient self-assessment with assessment by a proxy (anyone other than the patient who reports "for" the patient) are difficult to interpret because of well-established biases in proxy reports. Patient report of symptoms should thus be used, and wherever possible, patients should complete the same version of the assessment throughout the trial to avoid problems interpreting results due to known biases associated with mode of administration[25] or nuances in meaning from different wording or language versions.[12]

Just as symptoms can be manifestations of the cancer or its treatment, changes in symptom severity over time may reflect changes in an individual tumor (reduction or progression), metastases, a reaction to a toxic therapy, or a combination of disease progression and side effect of treatment. When symptoms are used as primary endpoints to evaluate anticancer treatments, the study design must provide ways to differentiate changes in the symptoms that are likely to be evidence of toxicity of the treatments studied from those likely to result from treatment failure.

Timing of symptom assessments during trials should be selected so as to enable the FDA to evaluate the effect of the treatment and, ideally, the durability of that effect.[21]

A critical component of clinical trial design is determining how much change in a symptom assessment could be considered a benefit that is clinically important to the patient. Various methods have been proposed for evaluating what is a meaningful change or significant difference between groups. To approve an indication for clinical benefit based on symptom scores, the FDA often requests that sponsors document what change in the score would be evidence of a clinical benefit to the patient, ie, how much improvement is required to classify a patient as a "responder." "Responder" criteria also require validation to be useful, but clinicians find them more intuitive to use in determining what the likely effect of the treatment will be in a specific patient than they find interpretation guides based on effect sizes associated with group mean differences. However, the FDA has indicated that for new measures lacking a long history of use in clinical research and clinical practice, it is helpful to provide evidence of what would be a benefit of treatment based on multiple approaches.[12]

Example: selection and use of a symptom scale

Assume that a sponsor seeks to demonstrate efficacy of a lung cancer treatment by targeting improvement in lung cancer symptoms. The sponsor will need to do the following:

- Identify the likely product effect that will serve as a "target claim" for planning endpoints and measurements in trials, along the lines of "product x improves lung cancer symptoms."
- Identify all the symptoms of lung cancer that are important to patients with lung cancer.
- Confirm that the symptoms the product is expected to improve are among those noted as important to patients.
- Identify or develop a lung cancer symptom assessment (either a set of individual symptom scores or a scale summarizing the important symptoms in one score) that assesses all the symptoms identified as important on the dimensions (eg, reduction of severity, frequency, number of symptoms experienced, duration of symptoms, etc.) required to document the target claim. Often researchers will propose that the symptoms of a particular cancer or cancer treatment toxicity can be best understood as a composite based on the sum or average of a list of individual symptoms. This approach is reasonable if each symptom is equally important to patients and if the list does not include various symptom terms that are simply alternative ways of asking about the same symptom.
- Confirm that the measurement properties of the lung cancer symptom assessment are adequate for the patient population targeted for the clinical trials:

- Demonstrate that all important symptoms are included (content validity). For scales, it is important to make certain that none of the symptoms are overrepresented (eg, measuring dyspnea with three items – breathlessness, shortness of breath, difficulty breathing – but measuring all other symptoms with only one item each).
- Confirm that the adequacy of the assessment's measurement properties – reliability, validity, ability to detect change – have been demonstrated in the target patient population for the clinical trials and for the ultimate indication sought.
- Confirm that patients with lung cancer comprehend the items in the assessment and are attuned to the symptoms so that they can assess them reliably. This generally involves a process known as cognitive debriefing, which is used to test comprehension of questionnaires and surveys.[26]
- Identify the amount of change in individual symptom scores or the symptom scale score that would be clinically meaningful as a clear benefit to patients.

- Implement the symptom assessment in a way that adequately captures expected improvement with treatment in well-controlled studies conducted in patients with lung cancer:
  - Fully integrate the assessment into the protocol and analysis plans for two randomized, blinded treatment trials.
  - Incorporate symptom assessment score(s) in the endpoint hierarchy and prespecify the method that will be used to control for multiple testing.
  - Ensure that procedures are in place to minimize missing PRO data and to document the reason PRO assessments were missing when this occurs.
- Conduct analyses of the PRO symptom data using a prospectively defined analysis plan with stated endpoint hierarchy that properly accounts for multiple endpoints.
- Report results from each study that provide evidence of the measurement properties for the PRO assessment and how this compares with prior studies using the same assessment.
- Develop a draft product label and sample advertisements that accurately describe the study designs, population, assessments, and results observed for efficacy and safety outcomes in the clinical trials.
- Submit these materials and documentation to the FDA for review at relevant advisory meetings or at standard application submission time points during the development of the product and application for its market approval.

As can be seen by this very simplified example, the process for securing symptom claims is very consistent with that recommended in the PRO guidance for documenting the adequacy of any PRO measure that will be used to support product claims.[12] The specific considerations for cancer trials and endpoints noted in the guidance on endpoints for oncology trials[21] are helpful in flagging the likely pitfalls for study design, instrumentation, and interpretation of symptom data for claims based on cancer trials.

Conclusions

Developers of new treatments that improve cancer-related symptoms must overcome a host of research design and analysis challenges that can undermine the integrity of the evidence of their products' safety and effectiveness:

- They must provide evidence that assessment of the symptoms the medication is intended to treat is valid.
- They must design clinical trials that will generate data that is useful for regulatory decision making.
- They must analyze the clinical trials using methods that enable regulators to evaluate the impact of the treatment on the targeted disease process without confounding the toxicities of treatment with efficacy assessments.
- They must provide clear and comprehensive documentation of the research conducted.

If these obstacles can be overcome, what remains is the difficult task of accurately describing the research evidence of the product's safety and efficacy in the labeling and advertising of the product when it is approved. Drug developers must work with the

FDA to generate a description of the development research that is accurate and informative and that provides sufficient information about the risks and likely benefits of the treatment.

Effective use of FDA guidance and advisory meetings can help streamline the clinical development of a treatment and ensure a clear understanding of the regulatory requirements that must be addressed to gain FDA approval of symptom claims.

Acknowledgments

Research for the development and writing of this project was supported by Mapi Values, LLC. The author appreciates the help of Jeanie Woodruff for helpful editorial suggestions, Barath Rao in assembling information about cancer product claims, and Nicola Moss and Daria Pelech for assistance with references cited.

References

1. Williams G, Pazdur R, Temple R. Assessing tumor-related signs and symptoms to support cancer drug approval. *J Biopharm Stat* **14**(1):5–21, 2004.
2. Federal Food, Drug and Cosmetic Act (FD&C Act), 21 USC §321 (2009).
3. Johnson JR, Williams G, Pazdur R. End points and United States Food and Drug Administration approval of oncology drugs. *J Clin Oncol* **21**(7):1404–1411, 2003.
4. Prescription Drug Advertising, 21 CFR §202.1e (2008).
5. Federal Food, Drug and Cosmetic Act (FD&C Act), 21 USC §331 (2009).
6. Federal Food, Drug and Cosmetic Act (FD&C Act), 21 USC §352 (2009).
7. Federal Food, Drug and Cosmetic Act (FD&C Act), 21 USC §355a (2009).
8. Johnson JR, Temple R. Food and Drug Administration requirements for approval of new anticancer drugs. *Cancer Treat Rep* **69**(10):1155–1159, 1985.
9. Temple R. A regulatory authority's opinion about surrogate endpoints. In: Nimmo WS, Tucker GT, eds. *Clinical Measurement in Drug Evaluation*. Chichester, West Sussex, England: J. Wiley, 1995:3–22.
10. O'Shaughnessy JA, Wittes RE, Burke G, et al. Commentary concerning demonstration of safety and efficacy of investigational anticancer agents in clinical trials. *J Clin Oncol* **9**(12):2225–2232, 1991.
11. US Food and Drug Administration. Fast Track, Accelerated Approval and Priority Review. Available from: URL: http://www.fda.gov/ForConsumers/ByAudience/ForPatientAdvocates/SpeedingAccesstoImportantNewTherapies/ucm128291.htm. Accessed Jun 9, 2009.
12. US Food and Drug Administration, Center for Drug Evaluation and Research, Center for Biologics Evaluation and Research, Center for Devices and Radiological Health. Guidance for industry. Patient-reported outcome measures: use in medical product development to support labeling claims. Available from: URL: http://www.fda.gov/downloads/Drugs/GuidanceComplianceRegulatoryInformation/Guidances/UCM071975.pdf. Accessed Dec 18, 2009.
13. Rock EP, Kennedy DL, Furness MH, Pierce WF, Pazdur R, Burke LB. Patient-reported outcomes supporting anticancer product approvals. *J Clin Oncol* **25**(32):5094–5099, 2007.
14. Specific Requirements on Content and Format of Labeling for Human Prescription Drugs, 21 CFR §201.57c (2008).
15. US Food and Drug Administration, Center for Drug Evaluation and Research. Drugs@FDA: FDA Approved Drug Products. Available from: URL: http://www.accessdata.fda.gov/scripts/cder/drugsatfda/. Accessed Jun 8, 2009.
16. US Food and Drug Administration, Center for Drug Evaluation and Research. Office of Oncology Drug Products (OODP). Available from: URL: http://www.fda.gov/AboutFDA/CentersOffices/CDER/ucm091745.htm. Accessed Jun 9, 2009.
17. US Food and Drug Administration. How drugs are developed and approved. Available from: URL: http://www.fda.gov/Drugs/DevelopmentApprovalProcess/HowDrugsareDevelopedandApproved/default.htm. Accessed Jun 9, 2009.
18. Rock E. FDA response to Paper 1: Patient-reported outcomes: conceptual issues [abstract]. Podium presentation at the FDA-Mayo Clinic co-sponsored conference "FDA Guidance on Patient Reported Outcomes: Discussion, Dissemination, and Operationalization," Chantilly VA, February 23, 2006.
19. Food and Drug Administration Amendments Act of 2007(FDAAA), 21 USC §105–115 (2007).
20. Good Guidance Practices, 21 CFR §10.115 (2000).
21. US Food and Drug Administration, Center for Drug Evaluation and Research, Center for Biologics Evaluation and Research. Guidance for industry. Clinical trial endpoints for the approval of cancer drugs and biologics. Available from: URL: http://www.fda.gov/downloads/Drugs/GuidanceComplianceRegul

atoryInformation/Guidances/UCM071590.pdf. Accessed Jun 9, 2009.

22. US Food and Drug Administration, Center for Drug Evaluation and Research, Center for Biologics Evaluation and Research. Guidance for industry. Clinical studies section of labeling for human prescription drug and biological products –content and format. Available from: URL: http://www.fda.gov/downloads/RegulatoryInformation/Guidances/ucm127534.pdf. Accessed Jun 9, 2009.

23. Wu H-S, McSweeney M. The assessment and measurement of fatigue in people with cancer. In: Armes J, Krishnasamy M, Higginson I, eds. *Fatigue in Cancer.* Oxford: Oxford University Press, 2004:193–222.

24. Richardson A, Ream E, Wilson-Barnett J. Fatigue in patients receiving chemotherapy: patterns of change. *Cancer Nurs* **21**(1):17–30, 1998.

25. Unruh M, Yan G, Radeva M, et al. Bias in assessment of health-related quality of life in a hemodialysis population: a comparison of self-administered and interviewer-administered surveys in te HEMO study. *J Am Soc Nephrol* **14**(8):2132–2141, 2003.

26. Willis G, Reeve BB, Barofsky I. Invited Paper C. The use of cognitive interviewing techniques in quality-of-life and patient-reported outcomes assessment. In: Lipscomb J, Gotay CC, Snyder C, eds. *Outcomes Assessment in Cancer: Measures, Methods and Applications.* Cambridge UK: Cambridge University Press, 2005:610–622.

27. US Food and Drug Administration, Center for Drug Evaluation and Research. Drugs@FDA: FDA Approved Drug Products. Available from: URL: http://www.accessdata.fda.gov/scripts/cder/drugsatfda/. Accessed Jun 8, 2009.

Section 6 Chapter

29

Conclusion

Symptom research: looking ahead

Charles S. Cleeland, Michael J. Fisch, and Adrian J. Dunn

Both cancer and cancer treatment produce multiple, disabling symptoms, the most prominent and distressing of which are addressed in this book. Our aim in assembling this volume has been to balance information from clinical research in cancer-related symptoms, including pain, fatigue, appetite and weight loss, sleep disturbance, cognitive impairment, and cancer-related affective changes, with basic laboratory research that explores, often in animal models, the potential mechanisms responsible for these symptoms.

Several chapters have considered new approaches to studying symptoms, including developing more-pertinent animal models and approaching symptoms from molecular, genetic, and neuroimaging perspectives. Other chapters have focused on issues of symptom assessment by self-report, longitudinal modeling of the relationship between symptom report and biology, and novel clinical trial designs. Finally, several chapters have addressed such real-world issues as obtaining funding for symptom research, establishing the cost-benefit of symptom management, integrating symptom research into collaborative cancer research groups, understanding regulatory guidelines for stating that symptom-relieving drugs really are effective, and exploring pathways for the development of new symptom-management agents. Together, these chapters lend support to the real possibility of a multidisciplinary collaboration that could become a science of symptoms – at least, of symptoms related to cancer.

Current challenges in symptom research

The subjective nature of symptoms

As reviewed in Chapter 23, the subjective basis upon which symptoms are known and graded has been a major barrier to the development of effective symptom research. A high degree of variability in the severity of symptom reports in the face of similar signs of objective disease is relatively commonplace in practice. This variability often leads to distrust in the only data – subjective report – that best represent most symptoms. The subjective basis of symptoms has curbed interest in innovative research that examines the mechanisms underlying these symptoms and in novel ways of treating or preventing symptoms. Particular difficulties include the subjective nature of many of the measurement and outcome variables, the poor fit of current disease models of research for doing this type of health-related investigation, and lack of statistical models that integrate "rough" self-report data with biological data. Nonetheless, substantial progress in symptom measurement has been made of late: self-reported symptoms have been recognized as legitimate primary outcome variables for clinical trials[1] and are becoming a standard for measuring the symptoms and toxicities of cancer therapies.[2]

The need for mechanism-focused research

In discussions preparing for this volume, we noted that many researchers working in areas relevant to symptom science understand that cancer produces multiple symptoms, yet they do not have the clinical experience to appreciate the level of distress that symptoms cause and do not recognize the ultimate effects that symptoms may have on survival. Other researchers have little knowledge of the potential biological mechanisms that may be responsible for symptoms.

Until relatively recently, the study of symptoms other than pain has consisted primarily of (1) cross-sectional descriptive studies of self-report from patients at specific stages of specific types of cancer; and (2) clinical trials that examine the reduction of a specific symptom. For example, a typical descriptive study might identify patients with stage IV breast cancer, measure the patient-reported severity of fatigue, look

Cancer Symptom Science: Measurement, Mechanisms, and Management, eds. Charles S. Cleeland, Michael J. Fisch, and Adrian J. Dunn.
Published by Cambridge University Press.

for the relationship of fatigue to measures of other symptoms and to function and mood (such as global or health-related quality of life), and determine whether other variables (age, sex, cancer type and stage, minority status) influence the pathway between fatigue and more complex dimensions, such as function and quality of life. Only very rarely – mostly in studies of pain or depression – have symptoms been addressed from the standpoint of their biological origins.

Clinicians sometimes lack information about the biological basis of symptoms and knowledge about specific symptoms that are legitimate targets for both prevention and treatment. As a result, clinical trials in symptom management may be formulated without enough appreciation of the mechanistic effects of the symptom-relieving agents that are to be tested. As illustrated in several of these chapters, the approaches to symptom reduction can be both biological (pharmaceutical) and behavioral. Given that the symptoms of cancer occur together in clusters in a predictable manner and might therefore share common underlying mechanisms, improved understanding of such mechanisms may well lead to an effective, systematic approach to controlling multiple symptoms. Animal preclinical studies can help determine the efficacy and appropriate dosage of symptom-focused drugs; however, few opportunities exist to conduct preclinical evaluation of the mechanistic effects of candidate agents for relieving symptoms other than pain (for which there are credible animal models of clinically painful conditions).

The lack of an interdisciplinary approach

The fundamental principle organizing this volume is that symptom research is, by necessity, an interdisciplinary science. The foregoing chapters have collectively provided evidence for this fact. However, in the editors' experience there has been insufficient consideration of the possibility that symptom prevention and symptom management might improve if subjected to the same aggressive multidisciplinary scientific effort that has been applied to understanding the biology of and developing treatments for cancer. As we considered various topics to include in this book, it was clear to us that interdisciplinary symptom research lacks a long-term, ongoing framework in which to apply and generalize the results of research into symptom mechanisms.

The field of symptom research has just begun to provide a biobehavioral understanding of the mechanisms underlying the symptoms experienced by patients with cancer, yet its momentum is challenged by its own set of barriers. Although progress has been made in some aspects of symptom research, research into the mechanisms of symptoms has been difficult to conceptualize, organize, and fund. Perhaps the most salient challenge we face is bringing together, and keeping together, the diverse disciplines needed to understand complex biological and behavioral phenomena leading to symptom expression. The study of symptoms requires interrelated studies involving, among others, behavioral scientists, molecular biologists, immunologists, behavioral geneticists, neurocognitive and comparative neuroscientists, statistical modelers, and cancer clinicians. Many disciplines that could make major contributions to understanding symptoms (eg, molecular imaging) have not yet been fully engaged in this enterprise.

Crosstalk among researchers is essential for improving cancer symptom control. Busy, highly productive scientists are already engaged in their own research programs and will naturally have commitment conflicts, especially in regards to maintaining an ongoing commitment to a new area of investigation. They may come from more than one institution, bringing with them different institutional cultures and perspectives. An interdisciplinary program will need to provide appropriate incentives and recognition to attract, retain, and pull together top-flight researchers.

Despite these challenges, a long-term interdisciplinary approach to symptom research will contribute synergistically to clarifying the nature of and mechanisms underlying symptom clusters in a way that cannot be achieved by single disciplines working separately. An important aspect of this approach will be providing avenues for cross-training investigators in a variety of disciplines. This will pave the way for researchers to deal with a significant health care problem for millions of people, a problem that has not yielded to current single-discipline efforts.

Future directions

Forward progress in symptom science can be accelerated using available research methods and developmental strategies to produce tangible benefits for cancer patients via symptom reduction within a realistic time frame. We endorse the development of a "translational pathway" for discovery and evaluation of better symptom-control agents that includes: (1) focusing on treatment-related symptoms; (2) exploiting what we have learned about inflammation and symptoms; (3) increasing efforts to produce animal models of cancer-related symptoms; (4) examining genetic determinants of risk for high symptom expression; (5) using neuroimaging to study the expression of symptoms in the central nervous system (CNS); and (6) investigating symptom interventions through clinical trials.

Studying symptom development during treatment as a model for understanding symptom mechanisms

Studying symptom expression during cancer treatment provides a unique window for understanding the mechanisms that promote symptoms and for testing agents that might prevent or control symptoms. Patients with cancer, even those who have more advanced disease, often come to the treatment setting feeling relatively healthy and asymptomatic. However, once treatment is started, many patients begin to experience multiple symptoms caused by the therapy (be it surgery, chemotherapy, radiotherapy, or a combination of these). Symptom severity is variable across patients with the same cancer and subject to the same treatment. It is this variability that provides us a research target in gaining a better understanding of what causes symptoms.

Figure 29.1 presents an illustration of how multiple symptoms can be tracked across the trajectory of treatment with the specific methodological contributions of several disciplines. At each step across the treatment where differences in symptom severity are present, from diagnosis through survivorship, we can use combined input from longitudinal patient report, cognitive and neurosensory testing, longitudinal biostatistical modeling, genetics (eg, polymorphisms in cytokine genes), protein analysis, and neuroimaging to identify patients at greater or lesser risk for high symptom levels and to yield markers and potential mechanisms of symptom burden. This information can inform the use of animal models of behaviors that reflect symptom expression in additional discovery studies of symptom mechanisms and in preclinical testing of agents that might modulate symptom expression. The ultimate goal of this integrated approach would be to develop a menu of candidates to move into phase 1–2 symptom-focused clinical trials.

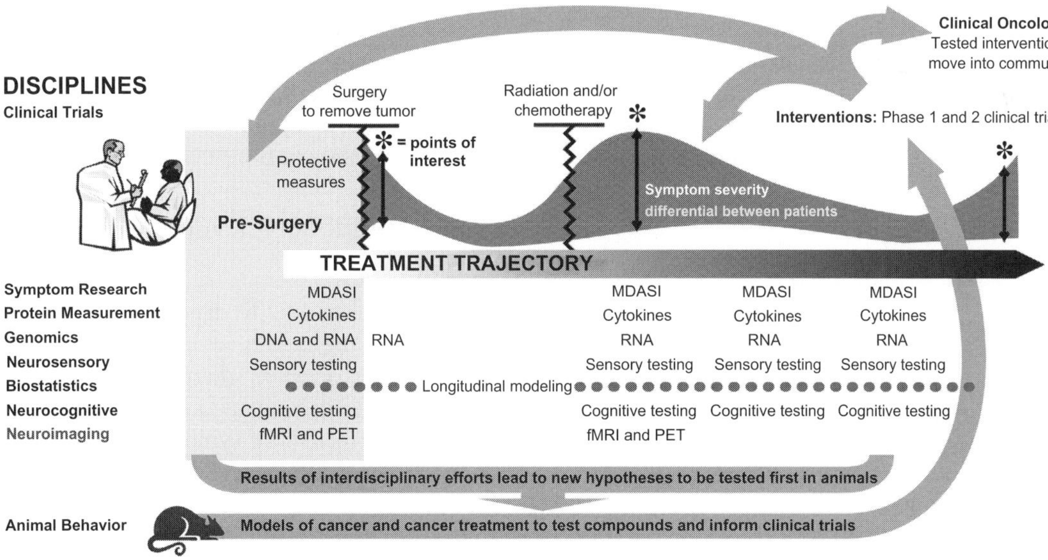

Figure 29.1. Trajectory of interactions among interdisciplinary groups in the study of treatment-related symptoms. Most patients with early disease have relatively low levels of symptoms before treatment. The points of interest (*) are the expected points of high symptom severity in response to the insults of cancer treatment (surgery, chemotherapy, radiation, and biological therapies), influenced by the variability among patients. In this conceptual approach, symptoms are monitored frequently, along with assays performed to track protein changes, and neurosensory testing conducted. DNA and RNA are collected before surgery, and RNA is collected several times after surgery. Cognitive and affective assessment are done at baseline and at peak symptom expression, coincident with imaging studies. Resulting hypotheses for symptom prevention and treatment move ultimately into clinical testing. Animal studies parallel the human studies, and inform and are informed by the human studies.

Investigating the effects of inflammation on symptom production

One direction that multidisciplinary research should take is to continue pursuing the role of inflammation in response to both disease and treatment as a mechanism underlying symptom production. A common thread throughout this book is the accumulating evidence that inflammatory mechanisms may be involved in the genesis of multiple cancer-related symptoms. It is well known that symptoms and increases in specific proinflammatory cytokines, primarily interleukin (IL)-1, IL-6, and tumor necrosis factor (TNF)-α, are produced by both disease and treatment. The exaggerated production of endogenous cytokines can lead to inflammatory reactions in which activation of transcription factors such as nuclear factor kappa B (NF-κB) promote still more inflammation. Recent studies of rheumatoid arthritis, inflammatory bowel disease, and depression have suggested that inflammation plays a central role in the production of multiple symptoms in diseases other than cancer, and that reduction of inflammation by targeted cytokine therapies can ameliorate pain and other symptoms.

The tight interaction between the pathways involved in inflammation and other pathways associated with symptoms, such as neuroendocrine and neuromodulatory pathways, has been illustrated in several chapters of this book. Although cytokines can be effective in cancer treatment, the symptoms they produce interfere with the patients' tolerance for therapy and thus diminish their therapeutic effects.[3] Among the most profound adverse symptoms related to cytokine treatment is fatigue, which involves physical (anemia, muscle weakness, cachexia, fever, and night sweats) and mental (anhedonia) manifestations that can lead to cognitive and affective impairments.[4,5] Cancer-related cachexia has been associated with TNF-α, IL-1, IL-2, and IL-6 therapies (Chapter 12). Cytokines, particularly IL-6 and IL-8, correlate strongly with symptom burden after transplantation and other aggressive therapies such as combined chemotherapy and radiation, with fatigue being the most common symptom.

As a result of our understanding of inflammatory mechanisms and sickness behavior, we have already postulated several approaches to ameliorate or block the development of sickness behaviors in animals. These might well be effective in reducing treatment-related symptoms. CNS proinflammatory cytokines are viable targets for the "treatment" of sickness behaviors. Blockade of proinflammatory cytokine receptors (most notably IL-1 receptors) and proinflammatory cytokine synthesis (by inhibiting the cleavage of proinflammatory cytokine prohormones to mature protein) within the brain, selective glial inhibition, and the administration of anti-inflammatory cytokines such as IL-10 (either as protein or via viral vectors) have all proven successful in reducing a variety of sickness behaviors.[6]

Gaining further understanding of the mechanisms underlying symptom production could be accomplished through well-designed clinical trials with symptoms as outcomes using agents already approved for clinical use for other indications. One motivation to pursue the inflammatory basis of symptoms is the existence of approved therapeutic agents that modulate specific cytokines, and other agents such as minocycline that induce broad-spectrum reduction of inflammation. Interventions might focus on reducing production of unwanted activities of proinflammatory cytokines with treatments directed at the immune system, such as the use of inhibitors of cytokine action (eg, TNF-α inhibitors), NF-κB inhibitors, or cytokine receptor antagonists (eg, IL-6 antibodies). This strategy of blocking critical biomarkers linked to the development of distressing symptoms associated with disease-induced or treatment-induced cytokine production could provide valuable information for confirming or refuting the impact of specific cytokines on specific symptoms or symptom clusters under certain clinical pathophysiological conditions.

Developing additional relevant animal models

Biomedical research is largely dependent on having animal models of the targets of interest. The same applies to symptom science, where exploratory and confirmatory studies in humans can be conducted in parallel in animal models of symptom translational research in a bedside-to-bench and bench-to-bedside collaboration. Fatigue research is an excellent example: as many have pointed out, we cannot ask animals if they are tired. But many of the components of fatigue that patients describe – lack of motivation, increased effort in problem solving, decreased motivation to be social – can be modeled in animals (Chapters 3 and 11) and many are typical components of what is studied in animals as sickness behavior. Animal models of disease-induced cancer pain and the pain produced by cancer therapies (Chapter 5) have suggested both potential mechanisms of pain development and novel ways of treating cancer pain.[7–9] Animal models of cachexia have also been helpful in understanding poor appetite and wasting (Chapter 13), leading to testable hypotheses about what might attenuate cachexia in patients (Chapter 12).

Animal models are necessary for discovery, but they also are requisite for preclinical testing of symptom agents. As has been shown in pain research, animal models provide an efficient approach for preclinical testing of novel immunological and pharmacological combination therapy strategies against symptom expression that will generate hypotheses for human clinical trials. Although animal models have been used in pharmaceutical development for psychiatric disease and dementia, the validity of these models is often based on response to agents already established as effective in humans or on morphological changes in animal CNS. In contrast, animal models that reflect symptomatic behaviors in a way that "makes sense" to both patients and clinicians need to be developed on the basis of patient self-report of symptom severity and behavioral assessment of patients, and linked to animal behavioral, CNS, and systemic changes that reflect these symptoms. Not surprisingly, there is a need for investment in intellectual resources and laboratory effort to produce such models.

Identifying genetic markers of risk for severe symptoms

As reviewed in Chapter 17, cancer-related symptoms are affected not only by disease and treatment, but also by individual genetic characteristics. Carcinogenesis, multiple self-reported symptoms, autoimmunity, and neurodegeneration may share common endogenous inflammatory pathways or similar treatment-related mechanisms in response to exogenous agents; such pathways or mechanisms can be studied using advanced molecular genetics technologies such as high-throughput genotyping and gene profiling (microarrays), which are being used in the discovery of genetic markers in humans. Analysis of genetic predictors for symptom occurrence and severity during treatment will help us to understand the biological basis of symptoms, identify susceptible individuals, develop tests with prognostic power, design novel drug targets, and predict therapeutic outcomes.

Polymorphism analysis can help describe the genetic background for each patient. Gene expression pattern determines function. Gene expression is a dynamic process which can be both transiently and permanently changed, reflecting both temporary and lasting changes in the biological state of cells, tissues, organs, and organisms. Thus, gene expression analysis may lead to more precise identification of patients at risk for severe symptoms and may aid in grouping patients into clusters with more predictable treatment responses.

Hypothesis-driven study of genetic polymorphisms affecting specific pathways may help achieve the goal of identifying genetic markers for cancer-related symptoms. Genome-wide association studies will provide novel candidate genetic markers by scanning the entire genome for millions of genetic polymorphisms, without hypothesizing specific biological pathways that might be associated with cancer-related symptoms.

Investigating brain networks involved in symptom expression

Processing the wealth of peripheral physiological information that underlies the expression of symptoms is ultimately a function of the brain. Symptoms may be conceptualized as functional disorders of the central nervous system.[10] However, our understanding of the mechanisms that take place inside the brain as a result of the development and impact of symptoms is in its elementary stages. A convergence of research suggests that the brain is organized to process many symptoms in similar ways.[11] Rapid advancement in techniques of imaging brain structure and function has allowed us to examine symptom-related events in the central nervous system (Chapter 18). Newer neuroimaging techniques have capitalized on progress made in visualizing the anatomical structures of the brain to show how these structures interact as networks in a functional context, and are beginning to open the door to understanding brain changes at the molecular level. Molecular imaging using positron emission tomography, widely used in understanding cancer biology and the action of anti-cancer agents, has only recently been employed in the examination of pain and depression, and has yet to be deployed in understanding fatigue, cognitive impairment, appetite changes and disorders of sleep.

Pursuing clinical investigation of symptom interventions

Finally, mechanistic symptom hypotheses and therapies that have a high probability of preventing or modulating symptoms need to be studied clinically. This will require academic, medical, radiation, and surgical oncology and hematology researchers who have interest and skill in symptom research. It will also require research staff and data managers who have been trained in symptom research, and biostatisticians who have an appreciation of the nuances of this realm of research where both biology and subjective report are the primary outcomes.

For example, if the inflammatory avenue for symptom production were confirmed, several novel methods of treatment could be explored. As a first step, interventions might be directed at reducing the production of unwanted activities of proinflammatory cytokines with treatments essentially directed at the immune system. An example of such treatments might be the use of immunosuppressants and inhibitors of cytokine action such as cyclo-oxygenase inhibitors or cytokine receptor antagonists. A second level of intervention might be directed at attempting to restore equilibrium to brain areas already affected by cytokine surges, such as through the use of antidepressants to restore central nervous system balance in biogenic amine metabolism, which is altered by the effects of cytokines on the brain. A third level of symptom-directed treatment would be the more typical use of analgesics, psychostimulants, and behavioral interventions. Finally, therapies might be designed to take advantage of the normal endogenous feedback circuits that limit sickness responses in more common settings, such as in response to a viral illness. In this regard, supplementation of the normal neuroendocrine response to illness may have benefit.

There are several potential pathways other than inflammation that are no doubt involved in symptom expression, and research into the mechanisms of symptoms needs to investigate these pathways as well. For example, neuromodulators and neuroprotectants may offer substantial benefits in symptom prevention and reduction.

A translational pathway to develop symptom-focused therapies

The steps outlined above are aimed at improving control of cancer-related symptoms through more effective therapy. Accomplishing this will require a translational pathway that incorporates (1) information from both animals and patients about genetic predisposition to risk for high symptom expression and to response to candidate agents; (2) neuroimaging of the CNS expression of symptoms and the modification of symptoms by candidate agents in animals and patients; and, especially, (3) translation of symptom behavior into animal models for high-throughput development of agents that reduce or even prevent cancer-related symptoms.

The difficulties inherent in translating laboratory findings to patient benefit are widely recognized in every disease area. In 2005, The National Cancer Institute created a Translational Research Working Group to speed the application of the findings of molecular oncology to patient care. In response, the working group developed a model for a translational research pathway. Although the model was developed for new curative therapy, a similar model might be used to conceptualize how to move the collective basic and clinical symptom research into the clinic. A schematic illustrating such a translational pathway for symptom research is presented in Figure 29.2.

Early components of the pathway include discovery research steps and decision points based on longitudinal observational studies of patients. Correlational studies showing the covariation of biomarkers and symptom expression, although an important step, do not provide sufficient information on the mechanistic basis of symptom production for the development of potential agents targeted at symptom control. Hypotheses about mechanisms underlying symptom expression are developed through examination of longitudinal symptom data, clinical correlates, biomarkers (genes, proteins), and imaging data obtained from patients. These hypothesized mechanisms are then tested in animal models. Candidate agents that may affect these mechanisms are developed in the laboratory, then applied in animal models of the specific disease. Agents that give some signal of effectiveness in preventing or reducing the specific cancer without excessive toxicity then move forward into patient research to determine appropriate dose, effectiveness, and toxicity in humans.

The chapters in this book suggest that the elements of a translational pathway for symptom-focused agents are available. For some symptoms, such as neuropathic or bone-related pain (Chapter 5), sufficient progress has been made in animal models to provide a basic

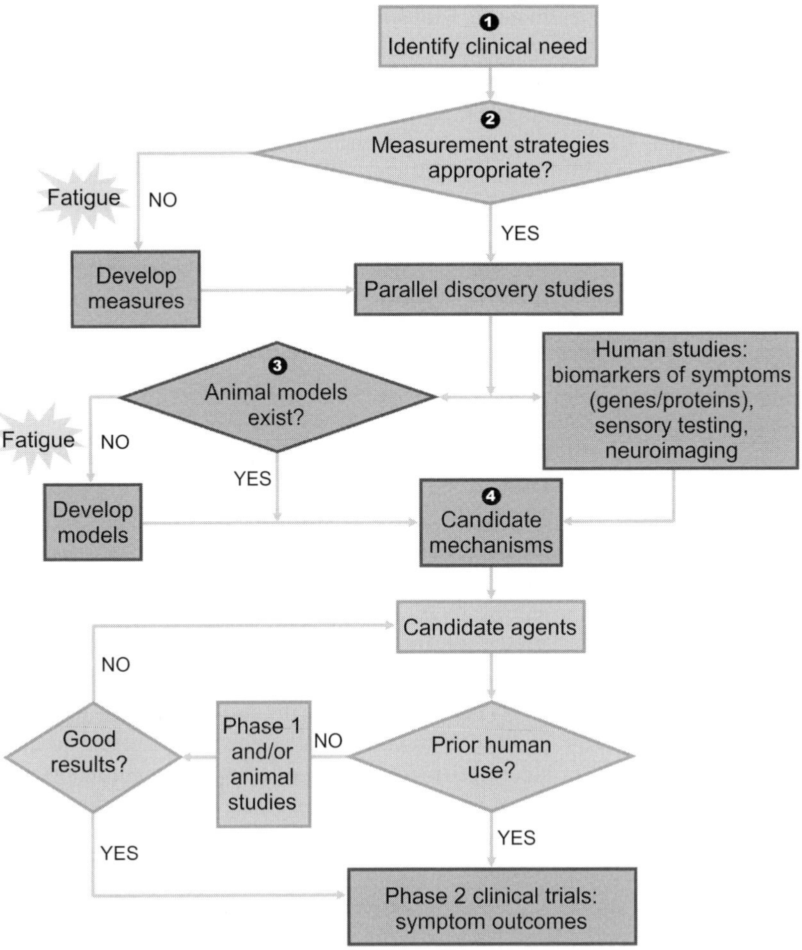

Figure 29.2. Discovery and translational pathway for symptom research.

Pathway Notes

❶ **Identify clinical need:** Sapported by symptom/toxicity prevalence studies

- Chemotherapy-induced peripheral neuropathy – significant
- Fatigue – significant
- Neurocognitive impairment – significant

❷ **Agreement on measurement strategies:** patient-reported outcomes (PROs), clinical findings

- Chemotheraphy-induced peripheral neuropathy – some consensus on neuropathic pain (patient-reported outcomes, clinical findings), less on painful neuropathy
- Fatigue – lack of conceptual and measurement consensus
- Neurocognitive impairment – established consensus on clinical criteria

❸ **Animal models**

- Chemotherpy-induced peripheral neuropathy – several models avaliable
- Fatique – little agreement on animal models
- Neurocognitive impairment – several models available

❹ **Mechanisms:** Suggested by patient and animal biomarker/symptom or toxicity studies. Symptom outcomes are generally self-report, but process mirrors mechanistic study for curative theraphyes understanding of the involved mechanisms and to test agents that might have a clinical benefit. In contrast, much less is known about the development of animal models of such symptoms as treatment-related cognitive impairment, fatigue, and treatment-related distress. Animal models of depression are available, but the effects on these models of having cancer and being treated for cancer have not been assessed (Chapter 9). Considerable effort will need to be expended on developing animal models that reflect the patient's experience of fatigue and cognitive impairment; suggestions of what these models might look like are presented in Chapters 6, 7, and 11. Neuroimaging and biomarker information from patients experiencing these symptoms should enhance the discovery process.

Better symptom clinical trial designs

It has been noted that a high percentage of trials dealing with chronic pain are trial failures, with negative results that add little information for decision making. An unacceptable number of trials focused on other symptoms end in this type of failure as well. Components of the translational pathway we have described may reduce the number of failed trials. Fortunately, the steps outlined above should yield more knowledge of symptom mechanisms and promote focused clinical investigations that allow for a better specification of behavioral and self-report outcomes. Moreover, preclinical models should help with providing a range of dosing for effectiveness. It is also important to examine issues in the design of clinical trials and consider design elements that can increase trial yield, such as adequate baseline assessment, trial duration, fixed versus flexible dosing, titration during the trail, "enriched" trials that only study those responsive to the treatments. For a comprehensive review of these issues, see Dworkin et al.[12]

A final word

Cancer-related symptom burden affects many thousands of patients with cancer, both during and after cancer therapy and into survivorship. We owe them the best research we can provide. As illustrated in this volume, symptom research will best be conducted within an interdisciplinary framework that encompasses the contribution of information from several sources. Many exciting new scientific technologies are available to address the problem. If this book has succeeded in encouraging new investigators to consider the mechanisms of symptom expression and modulation as a primary research focus, it has served its purpose.

References

1. US Food and Drug Administration, Center for Drug Evaluation and Research, Center for Biologics Evaluation and Research, Center for Devices and Radiological Health. Guidance for industry. Patient-reported outcome measures: use in medical product development to support labeling claims. Available from: URL: http://www.fda.gov/downloads/Drugs/GuidanceComplianceRegulatoryInformation/Guidances/UCM071975.pdf. Accessed Dec 18, 2009.
2. Basch E. The missing voice of patients in drug-safety reporting. *N Engl J Med* **362**(10):865–869, 2010.
3. Cleeland CS, Bennett GJ, Dantzer R, et al. Are the symptoms of cancer and cancer treatment due to a shared biologic mechanism? *Cancer* **97**(11):2919–2925, 2003.
4. Kurzrock R. The role of cytokines in cancer-related fatigue. *Cancer* **92**(6 Suppl):1684–1688, 2001.
5. Valentine AD, Meyers CA. Cognitive and mood disturbance as causes and symptoms of fatigue in cancer patients. *Cancer* **92**(6 Suppl):1694–1698, 2001.
6. Bilbo SD, Biedenkapp JC, Der-Avakian A, Watkins LR, Rudy JW, Maier SF. Neonatal infection-induced memory impairment after lipopolysaccharide in adulthood is prevented via caspase-1 inhibition. *J Neurosci* **25**(35):8000–8009, 2005.
7. Ledeboer A, Jekich BM, Sloane EM, et al. Intrathecal interleukin-10 gene therapy attenuates paclitaxel-induced mechanical allodynia and proinflammatory cytokine expression in dorsal root ganglia in rats. *Brain Behav Immun* **21**(5):686–698, 2007.
8. Cata JP, Weng HR, Dougherty PM. The effects of thalidomide and minocycline on taxol-induced hyperalgesia in rats. *Brain Res* **1229**:100–110, 2008.
9. Xiao WH, Bennett GJ. Chemotherapy-evoked neuropathic pain: abnormal spontaneous discharge in A-fiber and C-fiber primary afferent neurons and its suppression by acetyl-L-carnitine. *Pain* **135**(3):262–270, 2008.
10. Kroenke K, Harris L. Symptoms research: a fertile field. *Ann Intern Med* **134**(9 Pt 2):801–802, 2001.
11. Craig AD. How do you feel? Interoception: the sense of the physiological condition of the body. *Nat Rev Neurosci* **3**(8):655–666, 2002.
12. Dworkin RH, Turk DC, Peirce-Sandner S, et al. Research design considerations for confirmatory chronic pain clinical trials: IMMPACT recommendations. *Pain*:e-pub ahead of print, 2010.

Index